The SAGE Encyclopedia of
HUMAN COMMUNICATION SCIENCES AND DISORDERS

Editorial Board

Editors

Jack S. Damico
University of Louisiana at Lafayette

Martin J. Ball
Bangor University

Editorial Board

Elizabeth Armstrong
Edith Cowan University

Judith A. Gierut
Indiana University

Nicole Müller
University College Cork

Greg A. O'Beirne
University of Canterbury

Michael Perkins
University of Sheffield

Nelson Roy
The University of Utah

Sara Miller McCune founded SAGE Publishing in 1965 to support the dissemination of usable knowledge and educate a global community. SAGE publishes more than 1000 journals and over 800 new books each year, spanning a wide range of subject areas. Our growing selection of library products includes archives, data, case studies and video. SAGE remains majority owned by our founder and after her lifetime will become owned by a charitable trust that secures the company's continued independence.

Los Angeles | London | New Delhi | Singapore | Washington DC | Melbourne

The SAGE Encyclopedia of
HUMAN COMMUNICATION SCIENCES AND DISORDERS

Edited by

Jack S. Damico
University of Louisiana at Lafayette

Martin J. Ball
Bangor University

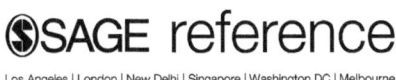

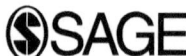

FOR INFORMATION:

SAGE Publications, Inc.
2455 Teller Road
Thousand Oaks, California 91320
E-mail: order@sagepub.com

SAGE Publications Ltd.
1 Oliver's Yard
55 City Road
London, EC1Y 1SP
United Kingdom

SAGE Publications India Pvt. Ltd.
B 1/I 1 Mohan Cooperative Industrial Area
Mathura Road, New Delhi 110 044
India

SAGE Publications Asia-Pacific Pte. Ltd.
18 Cross Street #10-10/11/12
China Square Central
Singapore 048423

Acquisitions Editor: Maureen Adams
Editorial Assistant: Jordan Enobakhare
Developmental Editor: Sanford Robinson
Production Editor: Kimaya Khashnobish
Reference Systems Manager: Leticia Gutierrez
Copy Editor: Hurix Digital
Typesetter: Hurix Digital
Proofreaders: Larry Baker, Theresa Kay, Ellen Brink, and Rae-Ann Goodwin
Indexer: Joan Shapiro
Cover Designer: Candice Harman
Marketing Manager: Jennifer Jelinski

Copyright © 2019 by SAGE Publications, Inc.

All rights reserved. No part of this book may be reproduced or utilized in any form or by any means, electronic or mechanical, including photocopying, recording, or by any information storage and retrieval system, without permission in writing from the publisher.

All trade names and trademarks recited, referenced, or reflected herein are the property of their respective owners who retain all rights thereto.

ISBN: 978-1-4833-8083-4

19 20 21 22 23 10 9 8 7 6 5 4 3 2 1

Contents

Volume 3

List of Entries *vii*

Entries

L *(Contd.)*	*1079*	P	*1309*
M	*1125*	Q	*1539*
N	*1213*	R	*1557*
O	*1273*		

List of Entries

Abstraction
Academic Impact of Communication Disorders
Accent Modification
Acclimatization to Hearing Aids
Accountability in Therapy for Communication Disorders
Acoustic Admittance
Acoustic Ecology
Acoustic Phonetics
Acoustic Reflex
Acoustics
Adaptation Theory
Adjectives and Adverbs
Adolescent Language Disorders
Adpositions and Conjunctions
Advocacy
Affect
African American English
Age and Aging
Age-Related Hearing Loss
Agnosia
Air and Bone Conduction
Airflow Measurement
Airstream Mechanism. *See* Phonetics
Alaryngeal Voice
Allocation of Resources
Allomorph. *See* Morphology
Allophone. *See* Phoneme
Altered Auditory Feedback and Stuttering
Alzheimer's Disease
Ambulatory Phonation Monitoring
American Sign Language
Amplitude Compression
Amplitude Envelope
Amusia
Amyotrophic Lateral Sclerosis
Anatomy of the Hearing Mechanism and Central Audiology Nervous System
Anatomy of the Human Articulators
Anatomy of the Human Larynx
Anatomy of the Human Neurological System
Anchored Assessment
Anomia
Aphasia
Aphasia Assessment
Aphasia Intervention
Applied Linguistics
Apraxia of Speech
Arthritis: Laryngeal Involvement
Articulation (Phonetic) Assessment
Articulation Disorders. *See* Speech Sound Disorders; Articulation (Phonetic) Assessment; Articulation Therapy (Phonetic Intervention)
Articulation Therapy (Phonetic Intervention)
Articulatory Phonetics
ASL. *See* American Sign Language
Aspiration: Swallowing
Assistive Listening Devices. *See* Hearing Assistive Technology
Attention
Attention Deficit Hyperactivity Disorder (ADHD)
Attitudes in Stuttering
Atypical Speech Sounds
Audiology
Audiometry. *See* Diagnostic Audiological Assessment; Hearing Screenin; Hearing Tests
Audiovisual Integration
Auditory Brainstem Implant
Auditory Brainstem Response
Auditory Development
Auditory Neuropathy Spectrum Disorder
Auditory Phonetics
Auditory Processing
Auditory Processing Disorder
Auditory Scene Analysis
Auditory Steady-State Response
Auditory Training
Augmentative and Alternative Communication (AAC)
Australian Aboriginal Languages

Australian Sign Language (Auslan)
Autism Spectrum Disorder

Babbling
Background Noise
Baselines
Behaviorism
Bernoulli Effect
Bias
Bibliotherapy
Bilingual Aphasia
Bilingual Children With Specific Language Impairment
Bilingual Education
Bilingualism
Binaural Hearing
Biofeedback
Blindness, Impact on Communication
Book Clubs, Communication-Adapted
Boyle's Law
Brain Imaging
Breathing Exercises
British Sign Language (BSL)
BSL. *See* British Sign Language (BSL)
Bullying and Teasing

Cancer of the Head and Neck
Captioning
Cascade Effect
Case Studies
Caseload
Categorical Perception
Causation
Ceiling Effect in Testing
Cepstral Analysis of Voice
Cerebral Palsy
Childhood Apraxia of Speech
Chronic Cough
Chronological Age. *See* Age and Aging
Circumlocution and Avoidance in Stuttering
Classification Systems
Classroom Acoustics
Clauses and Phrases
Cleft Lip and Palate: Speech Effects
Clinical Linguistics
Clinical Phonetics
Clinical Phonology
Clinician
Cluttering
Coaching

Coarticulation
Cochlear Hearing Loss
Cochlear Implant (Re)habilitation
Cochlear Implants
Code Switching and Mixing
Cognition
Cognitive Behavioral Therapy
Cognitive Development
Cognitive Impairment
Cognitive Linguistics
Cognitive Neuropsychological Approach to Intervention
Cognitive Processes and Operations
Cognitivism
Cohesion and Coherence
Collaboration in Speech–Language Therapy
Communication Disorders
Communication Partner Training
Communicative Competence
Compensatory Adaptation and Strategies
Compensatory Strategies: Swallowing
Competence and Performance
Comprehensibility
Comprehension
Computer-Aided Rehabilitation
Concussion
Concussive Injury
Conductive Hearing Loss and Its Treatment
Connected Speech
Connectionist Models
Consonant Clusters
Consonants
Constructivism
Context
Conversation
Conversation Analysis
Cooperative Learning
Cooperative Principle
Coping Hypothesis
Corpus Linguistics
Counseling in Speech–Language Pathology
Covert Contrast
Covert Stuttering
Craniofacial Anomalies
Critical Discourse Analysis
Critical Period for Language Acquisition
Crosslinguistic Manifestations of Disordered Speech and Language
Cued Speech and Language

Cultural and Linguistic Informants
Culture

Databases in Communication Disorders
Deaf Culture
Decibel
Deixis
Delayed Auditory Feedback. *See* Altered Auditory Feedback and Stuttering
Delayed Language Development
Delayed Phonological Development
Dementia
Depression
Descriptive Assessment
Descriptive Linguistics
Determiners
Developmental Apraxia of Speech. *See* Childhood Apraxia of Speech
Developmental Language Disorder (DLD). *See* Language Disorders in Children
Developmental Verbal Dyspraxia. *See* Childhood Apraxia of Speech
Diagnosis of Communication Disorders
Diagnostic and Statistical Manual of Mental Disorders (DSM)
Diagnostic Audiological Assessment
Diagnostic Reasoning
Dialects and Dialectology
Dichotic Listening
Digital Signal Processing
Diglossia
Discharge From Therapy
Discourse
Discourse Analysis
Discourse Impairments
Distortion
Distributed Cognition
Diversity
Down Syndrome
Dual Sensory Impairment (DSI)
Dynamic Assessment
Dysarthria
Dysphagia. *See* Swallowing Disorders; Swallowing Assessment; Swallowing Intervention
Dysphonia

Early Literacy Development
Earphones and Other Transducers
Echolalia
Educational Audiology

Efficacy and Effectiveness of Treatment Studies
Elderly: Communication Disorders of Aging
Electrocochleography (ECochG)
Electroencephalography (EEG)
Electroglottography (EGG) / Electrolaryngography (ELG)
Electrolarynx
Electronsytagmography (ENG) and Videonystagmograhy (VNG)
Electropalatography (EPG)
Emergence and Human Communication
Emergentism
Emotional Impact of Communication Disorders
Enculturation Into the Profession
Endoscopy
Epidemiology of Communication Disorders
Epilepsy
Esophageal and Tracheoesophageal Speech
Essential Vocal Tremor
Ethics in Communication Disorders Research
Ethics in Communication Disorders Service Delivery
Ethnographic Approaches in Research
Etiology
Evidence-Based Practice
Executive Function and Communication
Experimental Research
Expressive and Receptive Language
Eye-Tracking Technology

Feedback in Therapy
Felicity Conditions
Fetal Alcohol Spectrum Disorder
Fiberoptic Endoscopic Evaluation of Swallowing (FEES)
Fingerspelling
Fluency and Disfluency, Typical
Fluency and Fluency Disorders
Focus Groups
Foreign Accent Syndrome
Forensic Speech–Language Pathology
Formulaic Language
Fortition. *See* Lentition and Fortition
Foundations for Language Learning in the Neonatal and Early Infant Period
Frequency Compression and Transposition
Frequency Resolution
Frequency Response
Functional Assessment
Functional Communication Skills

Functional Hearing Loss
Functionalism

Gatekeeping
Gaze
Generative Linguistics
Genetics
Genetics and Stuttering
Genetics of Hearing Loss
Geriatric Audiology
Glossectomy
Grammar. *See* Syntax and Grammar; Universal Grammar
Grammatical Development
Grounded Theory
Group Therapy

Hard of Hearing
Hearing. *See* Audiology; Hard of Hearing; Hearing Disability and Disorders
Hearing Accessibility
Hearing Aid Earmold
Hearing Aid Fitting
Hearing Aids
Hearing Assistive Technology
Hearing Disability and Disorders
Hearing Screening
Hearing Tests
Hemiplegia
Hydrocephalus
Hyperacusis

Imitative Response
Implicature
Incidence of Communication Disorders
Inclusion Models in Special Education
Indigenous Languages
Indigenous Languages of Central and South America
Indigenous Languages of North America
Indigenous Languages of the Pacific
Individual Differences
Infectious Diseases and Communication Disorders
Information Structure
Instrumental Analysis of Speech
Instrumental Assessment of Voice Disorders
Intellectual Disability
Intelligence
Intelligibility
Intelligibility Enhancement

Intensive Stuttering Programs
Intentionality
Intercultural Communication
International Adoption: Impact on Speech and Language Abilities
International Classification of Functioning, Disability and Health
Internet Resources
Interviewing
Intonation
Irritable Larynx Syndrome

Jargon and Jargon Aphasia
Jitter and Shimmer
Joint Attention
Journaling

Key Word Signing Systems
Kinesics

Labeling of Communication Disorders
Language
Language Acquisition
Language Assessment
Language Delay
Language Difference
Language Disorders in Children
Language Disorders of People With Hearing Impairment
Language Families
Language Register
Language Sampling
Language Therapy and Intervention
Languages of Africa
Languages of Central, South, and West Asia: Urdu and Persian
Languages of East Asia
Languages of Europe
Languages of Mainland South East Asia
Languages of North Asia
Languages of South Asia
Languages of the Caucasus
Languages of the Middle East and North Africa
Languages of West and Central Asia: Turkic
Laryngeal Disorders: Benign Vocal Fold Pathologies
Laryngectomy
Laryngopharyngeal Reflux (LPR)
Late Auditory Evoked Potentials
Late Talkers
Learned Helplessness

Learning Disabilities
Lenition and Fortition
Lexicon
Linear Phonology
Linguistic Profiles
Linguistic Typology
Linguistics
Listening Effort
Locus of Control
Loudness

Magnetic Resonance Imaging (MRI). *See* Instrumental Analysis of Speech
Makaton Sign System. *See* Key Word Signing Systems
Manual Circumlaryngeal Techniques in Voice Disorders
Mapping Hypothesis
Markedness
Masking
Mean Length of Utterance (MLU)
Meaning
Mediation in Therapy
Medical Management of Voice Disorders
Memory
Memory Disorders
Memory Impairments in Aphasia
Ménière's Disease
Meta-Analysis
Metacognition
Metalinguistics
Metaphonology
Metaphor
Miscue Analysis
Modality
Modified Diet
Modularity
Morpheme. *See* Morphology; Mean Length of Utterance (MLU)
Morphology
Motherese
Motivation
Motor Speech Disorders
Multidimensional Scoring
Multilingualism
Multilingualism and Speech Sound Disorders
Multimodal Communication
Muscle Tension Dysphonia (MTD)
Myasthenia Gravis

Naming
Narratives
Nasalance and Nasometry
Nasality
Nativism
Neuroconstructivism
Neurogenic Communication Disorders
Neurogenic Stuttering
Neurolinguistics
Neurophonetics
Neuropragmatics
Noise-Induced Hearing Loss and Its Prevention
Nonlinear Phonology
Nonpulmonic Consonants
Nonverbal Communication
Normal Aging. *See* Age and Aging
Nouns and Pronouns

Observation
Occupation-Related Dysphonia
Operationalism
Optimality Theory
Oral Language
Origins of Language
Orofacial Myofunctional Disorders
Otitis Media
Otoacoustic Emissions (OAE)
Ototoxicity
Outcome Measurement

Paradoxical Vocal Cord Dysfunction (PVCD)
Paralinguistic and Prosodic Impact on Stuttering
Paraphasia
Parkinson's Disease
Pathophysiology of Stroke
Pathophysiology of Traumatic Brain Injury
Pediatric Audiological Assessment
Pediatric Audiological Rehabilitation
Perception
Person-Centered Care
Pharmacological Interventions in Hearing Disorders
Pharmacological Interventions in Speech and Language Disorders
Phenomenology
Phonation. *See* Phonetics; Voice Quality
Phoneme
Phonetic Transcription
Phonetics
Phonological and Phonemic Awareness

Phonological Development
Phonological Disorders
Phonological Processes
Phonological Treatment
Phonology
Physiological Basis of Hearing
Physiological Basis of Swallowing
Physiological Basis for Voice
Pidgin and Creole Languages
Pitch
Placebo Effect
Plasticity of the Brain
Play
Play Therapy
Positive Psychology and Wellness
Post-Polio Syndrome (PPS)
Posttreatment Relapse in Stuttering
Poverty and Language
Power Relations in Service Delivery
Pragmatic Development
Pragmatic Impairment
Pragmatics
Premorbid Level
Prenatal Drug Exposure. *See* Speech, Language, and Learning Difficulties Associated With Prenatal Drug Exposure
Preschool Language Intervention
Prescriptive and Descriptive Approaches
Prevalence of Communication Disorders
Prevention of Hearing Disorders
Prevention of Speech and Language Disorders
Primary Progressive Aphasia
Priming
Professional Associations
Prognosis
Prompts
Prosodic Disorders
Prosody
Prosthetics for Structural Deficits
Proxemics
Psychiatric Disorders With Communication Disorders
Psychoacoustics
Psychogenic Voice Disorders
Psycholinguistics
Psychological Stress and Speech Disorders
Psychosocial Impact of Aphasia
Psychosocial Issues Associated With Communication Disorders

Puberphonia
Pulmonic Ingressive Speech
Pure-Tone Audiometry

Qualitative Research
Quality of Life and Neurogenic Communication Disorders
Quality of Life and Stuttering
Quantitative Research

Radiation Therapy and Communication Disorders
Readability
Reading and Reading Disorders
Reading Fluency
Receptive Language. *See* Expressive and Receptive Language
Recovery From Aphasia
Recursion
Reference
Referral Issues
Regional Cerebral Blood Flow (rCBF)
Rehabilitation
Rehabilitative Audiology
Reinnervation of the Larynx
Relational Analyses
Relaxation Therapy
Relevance Theory
Reliability
Research
Residual Speech Sound Errors
Resilience
Resonance Disorders
Response to Intervention (RtI)
Retrocochlear Hearing Loss
Revaluing Reading
Right Hemisphere Cognitive–Communication Disorders
Room Acoustics
Rule-Governed Alternations

Sampling Rate
Saturation Sound Pressure Level (SSPL)
Schemata
Scientific Realism
Screening for Speech and Language Disorders
Scripts
Second-Language Acquisition
Segmentation of Speech
Seizure Disorders

Selective Mutism
Self-Advocacy
Self-Assessment, Audiology
Self-Assessment of Speech Disorders
Self-Correction
Self-Help Groups
Self-Management
Semantic Development
Semantic Disorders
Semantic Field
Semantics
Semi-occluded Vocal Tract Techniques
Semiotics
Sense
Service Delivery Models
Signal Detection Theory
Signed Languages
Significance
Singing and Performing Voice
Skills Versus Strategies
Sleep: Effects on Language Learning
Social Development
Social Stories
Socialization
Sociolinguistics
Sociolinguistics of Sign Languages
Sonority
Sound Localization and Auditory Spatial Perception
Sound Spectrography
Special Education
Specific Language Impairment (SLI). *See* Language Disorders in Children
Speech Act Theory
Speech Audiometry
Speech Intelligibility Index (SII)
Speech Mechanism Examination
Speech Naturalness
Speech Perception, Theories of
Speech Production, Theories of
Speech Recognition
Speech Sampling
Speech Sound Development and Disorders in Multilinguals
Speech Sound Disorders
Speech Synthesis
Speech Tracking
Speech, Language, and Learning Difficulties Associated With Prenatal Drug Exposure
Speech–Language Pathology

Speechreading
Spontaneous Recovery
Standardized Testing
Statistical Learning
Statistics: Descriptive
Statistics: Inferential
Stereotypy
Stigma
Stimulability
Stroke
Stuttering. *See* Fluency and Fluency Disorders; Stuttering, Causes of; Stuttering, Effects of
Stuttering, Causes of
Stuttering, Effects of
Stuttering, Motor Control in
Stuttering, Response to
Stuttering and Adolescence
Stuttering and Emotional Reactions
Stuttering and Language Complexity
Stuttering Treatment
Stylistics
Support Groups
Supported Conversation for Adults With Aphasia (SCA)
Suprasegmental Aspects of Speech
Swallowing Assessment
Swallowing Disorders
Swallowing Disorders: Prophylactic Therapy
Swallowing Rehabilitation in Adults
Syllable
Syntactic Disorders
Syntax. *See* Syntax and Grammar; Syntactic Disorders
Syntax and Grammar
Systemic Functional Linguistics

Tardive Dyskinesia
Technology and Communication Disorders
Telehealth
Telepractice
Temperament, Anxiety, and Stuttering
Temporal Fine Structure
Temporal Imperative
Temporal Processing
Teratogens
Test–Retest Approach
Texts
Theories of Language Acquisition
Theory of Mind
Thickened Liquids

Threshold
Timbre
Tinnitus
Tissue Engineering
Tone Languages and Communication Disorders
Tongue Thrust
Tourette Syndrome
Tracheostomy
Transcranial Stimulation
Transgender Voice and Communication
Translation
Trauma to Speech and Hearing Mechanisms
Traumatic Brain Injury
Treatment Research
Type Versus Token

Ultrasonography
Ultrasound. *See* Ultrasonography
Universal Grammar
Usage-Based Approach to Language Acquisition

Validity
Variable Speech Production
Varieties of English
Velocardiofacial Syndrome (VCFS)
Ventilator-Assisted Speech Production
Verbs
Vestibular Assessment
Vestibular Disorders
Vestibular Rehabilitation

Vestibular System
Videofluoroscopic Swallow Study
Virtual Reality
Vocabulary
Vocal Hygiene
Vocal Production System: Evolution
Vocal Quality: Perceptual Evaluation
Vocalization
Vocoding Techniques
Voice Acoustics
Voice Disorders
Voice Production: Physics
Voice Quality
Voice Therapy
Voice Therapy for the Professional Singer
Vowels

Williams Syndrome
Word Deafness
Word Frequency
Writing and Writing Disorders
Writing Systems

Xenophone
X-radiography. *See* Instrumental Analysis of Speech

Yawn-Sigh Technique

Zone of Proximal Development

Late Auditory Evoked Potentials

Since the mid-1990s, electrically measured late auditory evoked potentials, otherwise known as *cortical auditory evoked potentials* (CAEPs), have become widely used in clinical research and practice as measures of auditory perception and discrimination and as biomarkers of cortical plasticity across the life course and cortical dysfunction. More recently, there has been a broader focus on the role of oscillatory cortical potentials and their clinical utility as neural markers of cognitive effort during an auditory task or online speech tracking. This entry explores these different types of cortical potentials, with a focus on CAEPs that are more commonly used in clinical practice, particularly in infants or adults who are unable to provide a reliable behavioral response. Understanding how the cortical potentials are affected by stimulus and subject characteristics is important in determining the most appropriate stimuli to select, the importance of subject alertness, and how to interpret the response that is obtained.

Obligatory CAEPs are characterized by the electrically generated P1/N1/P2 complex (where P1 is the first positive peak, N1 is the first negative peak, and P2 is the second positive peak) or their magnetically recorded equivalent, namely P1m/N1m/P2m. In adults, these responses typically occur between 50 ms and 300 ms poststimulus onset. Based largely on information from intracranial recordings in animals as well as measurements taken from humans with known disruptions to the auditory pathway, these scalp-recorded peaks measured in awake humans are assumed to arise from the sum of temporally overlapping contributions from spatially separate generators in the thalamocortical portion of the cortex. The amplitude of the CAEP is graded in frequency, with larger responses measured for lower frequencies. This is consistent with the tonotopic organization of the primary auditory cortex where low frequencies are represented laterally, or closer to the surface of the scalp, and high frequencies more medially. The good signal-to-noise ratio (SNR) and longer temporal integration window of neural information, compared with the auditory brainstem response, makes it less vulnerable to physiological movement and to disorders of rapid temporal processing, such as auditory neuropathy. These responses can be measured at the onset and offset of a tone burst as well as during a change in spectral or temporal characteristics of an ongoing tone burst, where the latter is typically referred to as the acoustic change complex.

CAEP morphology, amplitude, and latency reflect the duration, intensity, and spectral and temporal characteristics of the sound stimulus as well as the history of stimulation. For example, the N1-P2 amplitude increases as stimulus duration (above hearing threshold) increases up to 30 ms and then plateaus so that stimulus durations greater than 30 ms have minimal impact on response amplitude. As this is not consistent with temporal integration times needed to perceive a suprathreshold stimulus, it suggests that it is not a measure of the psychoacoustic characteristic of loudness perception. Longer latencies have also been observed for slower tone burst rise times and for plateau durations less than 3 ms. Several studies suggest that N1 latency is sensitive to temporal characteristics of the sound stimulus, such as changes in voice-onset time, where N1 latency increases linearly with increases in voice-onset time for synthesized stimuli for adults. Similar changes in P1 and N2 latencies have been observed in young children (where the N1 peak is not yet fully developed) to changes in voice-onset time. However, it has also been suggested that such changes might not occur for nonsynthesized speech unless the consonant is preceded by another sound (e.g., vowel).

Other than stimulus characteristics, waveform morphology is also affected by the wakefulness and attentiveness of the person being assessed. During sleep or in a deeply anesthetized state, the CAEP cannot be reliably obtained. Light general anesthesia causes a prolongation of P1/N1 peaks, reduction in amplitude, and disruption to the waveform morphology. Different types of general anesthesia, such as halothane or enflurane, also may affect the CAEP waveform differently so that utilization of these potentials, or their earlier mid-latency potential counterpart, as a marker of depth of anesthesia is not yet possible. A more recent study has demonstrated that the level of alertness can influence the waveform morphology. Certainly, it has been known since the earliest studies of CAEPs that attention toward the eliciting stimulus increases the amplitude and reduces the duration of the P1/N1 peaks.

Electrode configuration is also an important factor that affects the morphology of the CAEP waveform. The cortical waveform is elicited from the primary and secondary auditory cortices, distant from the recording electrodes, and is typically measured using a configuration of three electrodes: active, reference, and ground electrodes. Its two-dimensional representation on the scalp is influenced by the location of the active (typically noninverting) and reference (inverting) recording electrodes selected to evaluate the potentials, and it is the comparative voltage measured between these electrodes that determines the waveform morphology. While configurations of 32, 64, or 128 channels are often used for source localization or to obtain the best morphology waveform in cases where there is electrical interference or artifact from another source (such as a cochlear implant where advanced statistical algorithms are used to identify and remove the electrical artifact produced by the implant from the averaged CAEP waveform), the waveforms from each active electrode are the comparative waveforms from this and the reference electrodes. The CAEP is the sum of multiple generators that partially overlap in time; therefore, the scalp location at which the response is measured can influence both the morphology of the waveform and the relative contribution from each of the different sources. Therefore, for waveform comparisons across individuals, it is important to ensure that the electrode configurations are the same.

While CAEPs measured within clinical practice are typically evoked by a transient tone or click, speech-evoked cortical potentials are now in clinical use as an objective method of verifying hearing aid fitting in babies or infants. With the introduction of universal newborn hearing screening in many countries, babies are often fitted within the first few months before they are able to provide a reliable behavioral response. Certainly, in Australia, considerable research has been undertaken to evaluate the feasibility of obtaining cortical responses to brief tokens of consonants from infants and the association of a select sample of these with varying spectral emphasis (30 ms token of /m/ and /t/ and 21 ms token of /g/) with behavioral responses in developmentally normal infants >8 months of age with hearing loss. In addition, the relationship between the presence or absence of these potentials with parent report has been assessed, suggesting that they may be a useful tool in supporting hearing aid fitting in infants.

However, the amplitude of the CAEP is more closely related to the SNR rather than to the absolute signal level. This is an important factor to consider if one is relying on this measure to evaluate hearing aid fitting. That is, amplitude and latency growth functions of N1 and P2 peaks predictably follow the changes in the SNR rather than the signal level per se. While P1 latency is affected by SNR, its amplitude appears to be insensitive to SNR. Curtis Billings and colleagues demonstrated that the latencies of P1 and N1 peaks are also sensitive to the type of noise presented, where the shortest latencies were observed for interrupted noise, then continuous noise, and the longest latencies measured for 4-speaker babble. Significant amplitude changes were only observed for the N1 peak, which was largest for interrupted noise, then continuous noise, and smallest for 4-speaker babble. Such effects are important when considering the use of CAEPs for estimating the neurophysiological effects of hearing aid gain that may not accurately demonstrate the level of the signal reaching the auditory cortex but the SNR of the amplified signal to the internal noise of the hearing aid. Therefore, care should be taken when using this as a clinical measure.

Changes in amplitude of the CAEP with changing stimulus onset intervals (SOIs), the interval between the start of first stimulus to the start of the second stimulus, have also been observed. The CAEP amplitude reaches a minimum at approximately 0.5 ms, increasing in amplitude for longer and shorter stimulus onset intervals. Based on the changes measured in the N100m magnetic response with increasing stimulus onset intervals, Norman Zacharias and colleagues developed a transient reduction of excitability model that qualitatively and quantitatively reflects their measured data. Using two exponential functions, they modeled the changes to the existing pool of neurons (or neurotransmitter), with one having a short delay and decaying rapidly and the other with a longer delay increasing more slowly.

As the CAEP matures over approximately the first 20 years of life, where only a large P1 peak of prolonged latency is measureable in infants, the P1 latency has been used as a biomarker of auditory pathway maturity. It is assumed that the changes in amplitude and latency of this peak result from the development and maturation of the N1 potential, which continues to develop through to adolescence. Studies in children born congenitally deaf have demonstrated good correlation between the age of cochlear implantation, or duration of auditory deprivation, and changes in the duration of the P1 latency. Specifically, Anu Sharma and colleagues have demonstrated that children implanted before the age of 3.5 years show prolonged P1 latencies at implantation; however, within 6–8 months, these reach normal latencies. On the other hand, children implanted over the age of 7 years show prolonged P1 latencies that do not reach normal latencies even years after implantation. Similar trends in the development of spoken language in children implanted early versus late have been observed, supporting the idea that a sensitive period before approximately 3.5 years of age exists for implantation and language development.

Using a life course perspective, aging can also cause changes in the CAEP morphology, where it is assumed that declines in neural synchrony can reduce the morphology and increase the latencies of the cortical waveform. That is, increased N1 latencies have been observed in cases of disruptions to temporal processing ability, such as that produced by physiological declines from aging and disorders of auditory neural synchrony, such as auditory neuropathy. Kelly Tremblay and colleagues showed that older adults with normal hearing and those with hearing loss showed greater difficulties discriminating 10 ms voice-onset time contrasts for the synthesized /ba/–/pa/ continuum. These perceptual differences compared with younger adults correlated with prolonged CAEP response latencies. The authors assumed that prolonged N1 latencies were the result of age-related declines in temporal processing ability.

Similar effects of CAEP amplitude and N1 latencies have been observed in disorders where temporal processing has been disrupted. One study that investigated adults diagnosed with auditory neuropathy showed that N1 latencies, measured using a 1-kHz tone at levels between 80 dB SPL and 100 dB SPL, were significantly delayed compared with normal hearing adults, although the slope of the input–output curves was not significantly different. Interestingly, when the 1-kHz tone was presented in broadband noise (fixed at 90 dB SPL), the N1 latencies of normal hearing adults were similar to the latencies of the auditory neuropathy group when the tone was presented in quiet. The authors suggest that the presence of noise may simulate the perceptual and psychophysical characteristics of auditory neuropathy.

Discriminatory potentials, including mismatch negativity (MMN), which peaks at 50–150 ms after stimulus onset, and P300, a positive peak appearing at 250–300 ms after stimulus onset, provide neurophysiological measures of auditory discrimination rather than detection. Both utilize an *oddball paradigm* where a deviant sound is presented randomly with low probability in a sequence of repetitive standard auditory stimuli. MMN, an automatic response that has been linked to auditory memory, can be observed as a negative displacement on the fronto-central and central electrodes by subtraction of the standard waveform from the deviant waveform. Whereas the MMN does not require attention to be elicited, the P3a (a component of the P300, as described below) can only be elicited when the individual is attending to the sound stimuli and can be seen in the averaged waveform to the deviant stimulus (i.e., it does not require subtraction of waveforms to be perceived). MMN has been used widely to better understand the effect of clinical disorders on auditory discrimination as well as the effects of speech sound training on perceiving speech contrasts and the perception of native and nonnative contrasts. While considerable attention has been focused on the MMN as a neurophysiological marker of auditory discrimination, Dorothy Bishop's (2007) review of the role of MMN in dyslexia and specific language impairment demonstrates the variability in the measurement and detection of the MMN. In some cases, even where behavioral measures of discrimination show a perceptual difference of a phonetic or tonal contrast, the MMN is not detectable.

The P300 potential can be reliably recorded across the auditory, somatosensory, and visual systems and is assumed to reflect attentional and working-memory processes in perceiving deviant stimuli. Its amplitude is affected by the probabilistic nature of the oddball response as well as the discriminable difference (context and contrast) between the standard and deviant stimuli (i.e., greater amplitudes with low probability and high discrimination differences). In addition, enhanced amplitudes are observed for emotional stimuli suggesting that motivational relevance may play a role. Therefore, it is considered to reflect working memory or, more specifically, a context-updating process. The P300 is characterized by a frontally located early involuntary orienting or attention-switching response (P3a) followed by a temporoparietal attention-based response to the deviant stimulus (P3b). Interestingly, P300 amplitude reductions are commonly linked with externalizing disorders associated with disinhibiting behavior, such as substance use disorders, and may provide an early indicator for problem behavior. Further, in a study of 1,196 adolescent male twins, it was demonstrated that this association between P300 amplitude reduction and externalizing disorders is effectively predicted by genetic influences. This suggests that P300 can be used as a genetic marker of such disorders.

While many auditory studies have focused on the role of the time-locked synchronous cortical waveforms, more recently, the role of synchronized slow cortical oscillations has been applied to better understand the neurophysiological mechanisms of subjective tinnitus and the perceptual *effortful* effects of listening to spectrally and temporally degrading a sound stimulus. For example, Nathan Weisz and colleagues showed that alpha power (8–12 Hz) measured in the magnetically recorded spontaneous cortical activity was significantly lower in tinnitus, compared with nontinnitus participants. Further, alpha power was associated with the amount of tinnitus-related distress reported by the participant (measured using the German adaptation of the Tinnitus Questionnaire). While Weisz and colleagues also report increases in gamma power (40–90 Hz) and delta power (1.5–4 Hz), effect sizes appear to be smaller than those observed with alpha power. In a separate series of studies looking at effortful listening, they evaluated changes in alpha power during and immediately after presenting spectrally and temporally degraded speech sounds (German mono-, bi-, and tri-syllabic nouns) in normal hearing young adults and correlated this with a four-point rating of comprehension, which shows high correlation with speech recognition scores. Within these studies, they demonstrated that alpha power was reduced with spectral degradation and that reductions in alpha power were also related to temporal envelope smoothing, although the effect was not as great as that observed with spectral degradation. This suggests that alpha power may be a biomarker of effortful listening, which could increase the sensitivity of current clinical tests. That is, assessing not only which speech sounds or sentences individuals with hearing loss can comprehend but also the effort that they needed to invest in understanding this may enable clinicians to develop more personalized rehabilitation programs. This could include the fine-tuning of hearing devices or the evaluation of auditory training programs. However, at this stage, the clinical utility of cortical oscillations remains unclear. That is, the trajectory of change in the oscillatory activity during changes in task difficulty is not consistent across studies, and high interindividual variability is observed within studies. Therefore, further research is needed prior to utilizing cortical oscillations as a clinical marker of cognitive load. Other studies have investigated the role of cortical entrainment to speech as a neural marker of online speech processing. Such studies demonstrate the influence of the spectral quality of the speech signal and attention on cortical entrainment, although, similarly, more work is needed prior to utilizing this as a clinical measure.

In summary, the CAEPs can be used as a marker of auditory perception, discrimination, and the maturation and decline of the auditory cortical pathway. More recent studies have focused on the potential use of cortical oscillations as an indicator of cognitive load, which could ultimately increase the sensitivity of existing clinical tests. These potentials have been well integrated into clinical diagnostic environments given their ease of measurement and robustness as a measure in awake individuals.

Catherine McMahon

See also Anatomy of the Hearing Mechanism and Central Auditory Nervous System; Audiology; Auditory Brainstem Response; Dual Sensory Impairment (DSI)

Further Readings

Bishop, D.V.M. (2007). Using mismatch Negativity to study central auditory processing in developmental language and literacy impairments: Where are we, and where should we be going? *Psychological Bulletin, 133,* 657–672.

Hall, J. W. (2007). *New handbook of auditory evoked responses* (Vol. 1). Boston, MA: Pearson.

Weisz, N., Hartmann, T., Müller, N., & Obleser, J. (2011). Alpha rhythms in audition: Cognitive and clinical perspectives. *Frontiers in Psychology, 2,* 73. Retrieved from https://doi.org/10.3389/fpsyg.2011.00073

LATE TALKERS

Late talkers is a term used to refer to 2-year-olds who have delayed expressive language. Interest in this group stems from research in the late 1980s and 1990s by Leslie Rescorla, Donna Thal, and Rhea Paul, which sought to determine the prognosis for 2-year-olds who were late in acquiring their first words. Since this time, numerous studies have examined the lexical, morphosyntactic, and phonological characteristics of late talkers; the risk factors associated with being a late talker; and the long-term outcomes of this group.

Definition

A late talker is commonly defined as a 2-year-old child who has a productive vocabulary of fewer than 50 words and no two-word combinations, or who falls below the 10th percentile on a parent-report inventory such as the MacArthur-Bates Communicative Development Inventories. Using these criteria, approximately 10–18% of 2-year-olds will be identified as late talkers. By definition, late talkers do not have neurological, cognitive, socioemotional, or sensory deficits; however, a proportion of them may have limited receptive vocabulary and deficits in social skills. Children who are delayed at age 2 years but catch up to developmental norms by age 3 are referred to as *late bloomers*.

Language Characteristics of Late Talkers

Lexical

Lexicon size is the central inclusionary feature for identifying late talkers. Apart from quantitative differences in vocabulary size, the qualitative aspects of lexical acquisition appear to be similar between late talkers and typically developing children. Late talkers acquire words from a wide range of semantic categories, and they acquire words that have similar word frequencies to those acquired by typically developing children. Detailed studies of the lexical growth patterns of late talkers show that some late talkers may exhibit a lexical explosion shortly after their second birthday, whereas other late talkers continue to have very low vocabularies at age 2 and a half showing little evidence of a lexical explosion.

Morphosyntax

In addition to reduced vocabulary size, the absence of two-word combinations at age 2 often serves as a criterion for identifying late talkers. Interestingly, late talkers may manifest more conspicuous delays in morphosyntax (morphology and syntax) than in vocabulary development. Several studies report smaller mean lengths of utterances, delayed use of morphemes, and less advanced syntactic structures in late talkers at ages 3–5 than in typically developing children.

Phonological

The phonological skills of children with low vocabularies (i.e., late talkers) are less well developed than those of children with medium or high vocabularies. Late talkers have smaller phonetic inventories, lower scores for percentage of consonants correct, and less complex syllable structure than age-matched children who are not late talkers. The close relation between phonological and lexical abilities of late talkers has led to discussion on the direction of causation of this relation. Late talkers may have reduced vocabularies because of their slow oral motor and phonological processing abilities. Alternatively, late talkers may have depressed phonological skills because they talk less. Most recent accounts emphasize the bidirectional nature of the relationship between phonology and the lexicon.

Risk Factors

A number of factors may increase children's risks of being late talkers (e.g., gender, socioeconomic status, family history, and presence of siblings). Boys are more likely than girls to be late talkers. Children from low socioeconomic status are more often associated with late talker status than children from middle socioeconomic status, an effect that may be related to other factors such as low birth weight, quality of parenting, and time spent in day care. Children with a family history of language, speech, or learning problems are more frequently classified as late talkers than children without a family history. The number of siblings is a risk factor for vocabulary delay at age 2. A late talker is significantly more likely to have one or more siblings than to be an only child.

Long-Term Outcomes

A substantial proportion (approximately 50%) of late talkers continues to display expressive language delay at 3 years. A smaller proportion of late talkers (25%) evidences delay at 5 years. Late talkers followed through primary and secondary school often score within the normal range on standardized language measures but still score significantly less than age-matched controls. Age and gender are factors predictive of developmental outcomes. Older (vs. younger) late talkers and boys (vs. girls) are less likely to overcome initial delays. Some studies find that the language outcomes of children with receptive and expressive language delay are different from those with expressive language delay only: Children with receptive language difficulties are more susceptible to having long-term difficulties. Late talkers who are faster and more accurate in lexical processing are also the ones to display accelerated vocabulary growth later on and to overcome their delay. The subset of children who continue to experience language difficulties through the school years is labeled as having specific language impairment.

Summary

Late talkers is a general descriptor for toddlers who exhibit delay in the onset of expressive language. It does not define a clinical disorder but the manifestation of a potential one. Most late talkers will score within the average range on language measures when tested at school age but will score significantly less than a comparison group, suggesting ongoing weaknesses in language skills. Findings concur that late talkers are not a homogeneous group, and future research should delineate subgroups of late talkers with the aim of establishing differentiated intervention programs for these children.

Margaret Kehoe

See also Language Disorders in Children; Lexicon; Morphology; Phonological Development; Vocabulary

Further Readings

Desmarais, C., Sylvestre, A., Meyer, F., Bairati, I., & Rouleau, N. (2008). Systematic review of the literature on characteristics of late-talking toddlers. *International Journal of Language & Communication Disorders*, 43(4), 361–389. Retrieved from https://doi.org/10.1080/13682820701546854

Hammer, C. S., Morgan, P., Farkas, G., Hillemeier, M., Bitetti, D., & Maczuga, S. (2017). Late talkers: A population-based study of risk factors and school readiness consequences. *Journal of Speech, Language, and Hearing Research*, 60(3), 607–626. Retrieved from https://doi.org/10.1044/2016_JSLHR-L-15-0417

Hawa, V. V., & Spanoudis, G. (2014). Toddlers with delayed expressive language: An overview of the characteristics, risk factors and language outcomes. *Research in Developmental Disabilities*, 35(2), 400–407. Retrieved from https://doi.org/10.1016/j.ridd.2013.10.027

Zubrick, S. R., Taylor, C. L., Rice, M. L., & Slegers, D. W. (2007). Late language emergence at 24 months: An epidemiological study of prevalence, predictors, and covariates. *Journal of Speech, Language, and Hearing Research*, 50(6), 1562–1592. Retrieved from https://doi.org/10.1044/1092-4388(2007/106)

Learned Helplessness

Learned helplessness is a psychological condition in which patients feel they are in an unescapable or uncontrollable situation after enduring unpleasant, adverse, or painful experiences. In communication sciences, learned helplessness may be observed in pediatric, adult, and geriatric patient populations with communication, cognitive, or swallowing disorders. The etiology of this behavior may be related to their deficits, or it may be rooted in previously unrelated negative experiences that manifest during rehabilitation, treatment, recovery, or generalization/maintenance. This entry discusses the theory of learned helplessness, how it relates to communication sciences and disorders, and relevant clinical application and impact.

The theory of learned helplessness was first developed, through animal models, by psychologist Martin Seligman in the early 1970s, and then reformulated for application to humans by Lyn Abramson, Martin Seligman, and John Teasdale later in the decade. The theory postulates three parameters of causal explanations for negative events: internality (internal vs. external), stability (stable vs. unstable), and globality (global vs. specific). The combination of each of the three causal explanations determines an individual's explanatory style. See Table 1 for examples of explanatory style and causal explanations.

The first parameter, internality, refers to whether the negative event is attributed to *internal* causes (distinctive to an individual) or *external* causes (inflicted upon an individual from outside forces). For example, a man reports debilitating tinnitus to his audiologist after working in a loud machine shop for many years. He may have an internal locus of causality if he believes the tinnitus is because he didn't wear ear protection in the shop. If he has an external locus of causality, he might blame his employer for not providing hearing protection.

The second parameter, stability, relates to the way in which the cause of the negative event persists over time. A *stable* cause would be attributed to some personal deficit that persists no matter the situation, while an *unstable* cause is attributable to a transient situation or insufficiency. An example of stability would be a young girl with a learning disability who does not do well on her first speech therapy task. If she has a stable causal explanation, she would believe she can never do well because she thinks she is not smart enough. If her causal explanation was unstable, she would believe she did not do well because she was tired that day. For the stable cause, all future performance will be stably impacted by their learned helplessness, while the

Table 1 Examples of Causal Explanations for the Event "I stuttered a lot during my conversation with my boss"

Internality	*Stability*	*Globality: Example Explanation*
Internal	Stable	Global: "I always stutter."
		Specific: "I'm disfluent on words beginning with B, P, or vowels."
	Unstable	Global: "I've worked long hours this week and I stutter more when I'm tired."
		Specific: "I stutter more when I talk to my boss."
External	Stable	Global: "All bosses make their employees uncomfortable."
		Specific: "My boss always cuts people off."
	Unstable	Global: "The negative environment the last two weeks has everyone on edge."
		Specific: "My boss was in a bad mood today."

Source: Table format based on Peterson and Seligman (1984, pp. 347–374).

unstable cause would not indicate future success or failure.

The third parameter, globality, determines if the causal explanation is *global* and will affect an individual over a variety of situations and outcomes, or *specific* and is exclusive to a particular situation or outcome. With global causes, although all the negative experiences that caused the behavior may have been related, the learned helplessness will carry over and affect many situations and outcomes unrelated to the causal events. If that carryover does not exist, the cause is considered specific because the learned helplessness is expressed only during particular situations or outcomes that relate directly to the causal events. A 70-year-old man, for example, with a global causal explanation for his expressive aphasia may believe that he will never be able to communicate again. That same patient with a specific causal explanation may feel his speech may not improve back to normal, but he can find other ways to communicate effectively.

There are two tests for determining a patients' explanatory style, the Attributional Style Questionnaire for adults and the Children's Attributional Style Questionnaire. As these tests are psychological in nature, their results do not correlate directly to communication sciences; however, inferences can be made. In general, a person who scores as internal, global, and stable would be considered to have a more pessimistic explanatory style and therefore may be at a higher risk of depression. People with communication, cognition, or swallowing disorders who score in this range may have a more pessimistic outlook on their deficits, which in turn, may negatively impact their participation in treatment and their prognosis for recovery. People who score as external, unstable, and specific may be more optimistic about their recovery and may engage in treatment more effectively.

The scope of practice for a speech-language pathologist or audiologist includes counseling patients on their psychological state only as it relates to their communication deficits. Therefore, understanding the etiology of patients' learned helplessness behavior is important. Counseling persons exhibiting learned helplessness during treatment can help to optimize their performance in the clinic. However, if the root cause for their behavior is extrinsic in nature and globally applied to their current state, the appropriate course of action is to refer the individual to the appropriate psychological professionals.

Learned helplessness can frequently be seen in clinical populations treated by both speech-language pathologists and audiologists. This type of behavior may have a negative impact on patients' prognosis, progress of treatment, and recovery and, therefore, should be addressed, when appropriate, by the clinician. Although explanatory style questionnaires may allow for a better understanding of how patients may view the cause for their deficits, each patient's personal experiences and history should be taken into account before making any inferences or assumptions based on these tests. With the appropriate care and counseling, patients with learned helplessness can be effectively treated.

Nicholas A. Barone

See also Cognitive Behavioral Therapy; Cognitive-Neuropsychological Approach to Intervention; Depression; Prognosis; Rehabilitation

Further Readings

Abramson, L. Y., Seligman, M. E., & Teasdale, J. D. (1978). Learned helplessness in humans: Critique and reformulation. *Journal of Abnormal Psychology*, 87(1), 49–74. Retrieved from http://dx.doi.org/10.1037/0021-843X.87.1.49

Ellis, D. W., & Christensen, A. L. (Eds.). (2012). *Neuropsychological treatment after brain injury* (Vol. 1). Norwell, MA: Springer Science & Business Media.

Lubusko, A. A., Moore, A. D., Stambrook, M., & Gill, D. D. (1994). Cognitive beliefs following severe traumatic brain injury: Association with post-injury employment status. *Brain Injury*, 8(1), 65–70. Retrieved from https://doi.org/10.3109/02699059409150959

Peterson, C., Maier, S. F., & Seligman, M. E. (1993). *Learned helplessness: A theory for the age of personal control*. New York, NY: Oxford University Press.

Peterson, C., & Seligman, M. E. (1984). Causal explanations as a risk factor for depression: Theory and evidence. *Psychological Review*, 91(3), 347–374. Retrieved from http://dx.doi.org/10.1037/0033-295X.91.3.347

Seligman, M. E. (2006). *Learned optimism: How to change your mind and your life*. New York, NY: Vintage.

Uomoto, J. M., & Fann, J. R. (2004). Explanatory style and perception of recovery in symptomatic mild traumatic brain injury. *Rehabilitation Psychology, 49*(4), 334–337. Retrieved from http://dx.doi.org/10.1037/0090-5550.49.4.334

LEARNING DISABILITIES

Learning disability (LD), *global LD*, *learning difficulty*, and *intellectual disability* are all labels currently used to describe children and adults who have difficulties in their learning of new skills and understanding of information combined with difficulties in their adaptive functioning. These difficulties are considered developmental as they start or are identified at birth or in childhood, and are pervasive, impacting on all aspects of the child's development continuing through the life span.

People with LDs have difficulties in their development of speech, language, and communication. Some syndromes of LD such as Down syndrome (DS) have specific developmental profiles of communication development. Identifying these profiles is helpful in understanding the nature and trajectory of communication development in these syndromes and how to support these individuals to be the most effective communicators they can be throughout their lives. Communication is a key life skill and fundamental to quality of life. Yet, people with LD have historically been marginalized and excluded from society in part due to their reduced communication abilities. Here, society needs to know how to communicate with people having LD to ensure that their views are represented. The study of communication in people with LD informs theories of communication development and the impact of communication difficulties on everyday life. Moreover, this knowledge is used to inform approaches to enable people with LD and those around them to be the best communicators they can be, thus optimizing their life chances.

This entry explains how perspectives of LD have changed over time; details the communication development identified in LD; describes two profiles of communication development, the first specific to a syndrome of LD and the second as an example of emerging communication ability in profound and multiple LDs; and finally, explains approaches that enable people with communication difficulties to be effective communicators. The terms *communication development* and *communication difficulties* will be used to encompass development of and difficulties in speech, language, and communication.

Historical Perspectives of LD

The medical perspective has dominated understanding of people with LD. Intelligence was used to identify people with LDs where severity of an LD was defined based on an individual's level of intelligence. Such an approach depended on assessing IQ often using standardized measures to derive an intelligence score for a person, and this determined levels of severity into categories such as mild, moderate, severe, and profound. Terminology used reflected this perspective where terms included *endogenous imbecile*, *feeble minded*, *mental subnormality*, *backward*, and *mental retardation*.

Historically, people with LD have been marginalized from society. In the 1800s, no distinction was made between mental health and learning difficulties reflected in early government legislation such as the 1890 Lunacy Act in the United Kingdom. Much stigma still surrounds people with LD. The social movement of the 1970s moved understanding on from the medical perspective to understand people with LD as equal members of society. Here, emphasis is placed on society to change our attitudes and behaviors toward people with LD. In the developed world, legislation has attempted to address this; however, it is generally acknowledged that people with LD are still vulnerable members of our society, often treated unequally, with significant health and well-being challenges leading to a reduced quality of life.

Today, medical, social, and psychological models are used to understand and support the needs of people with LD. Different terminology still exists although the terms *learning disability* and *intellectual disability* are preferred. *Mental handicap* and *retardation* continue as terms in the medical profession. An individual's adaptive functioning is equally if not more important than level of intelligence. Adaptive functioning refers to managing everyday life such as education, social relationships, and communicating, and being risk aware is also taken into account. The social movement embedded fundamental changes into how health, education, and social care services consider and meet the needs of people with LD reflected in key legislation. Nevertheless, inequity continues to exist in both the developed world and more so in developing countries.

The medical perspective has an essential role in meeting the complex health needs of people with LD. LD is often part of an individual's complex medical diagnoses or can be a syndrome of LD. Often there is no obvious medical cause of LD, particularly for people described with a mild LD. Complex medical diagnoses can include abnormalities of development while the infant is in utero or during birth. Prematurity is a known risk factor for LD where the incidence of people with multiple and profound LD is increasing due to more infants born prematurely now surviving. A syndrome of LD is where there is a known medical cause such as a chromosomal disorder and this cause is accompanied by a specific profile or phenotype of physical, cognitive, and behavioral development that can be differentiated from other syndromes.

Health, education, and social care services are required to coordinate their care to offer cohesive provision led by the individual's desires and wishes. However, the amount and quality of provision differ across the world with developed countries aiming at being more cohesive and person centered than developing countries where there is still much stigma surrounding people with LD.

Communication Development in LD

People with LD are a very heterogeneous population with respect to their level of learning, the extent of and range of associated medical needs such as epilepsy, impairments in hearing and vision, and physical health needs such as feeding and movement often requiring intensive medical intervention in hospital. All of these contribute to a very heterogeneous profile of communication development. Some people with LD never develop verbal communication, and others may develop verbal communication but this level of development plateaus or stops developing in the usual way much earlier than expected. Therefore, the range and severity of communication difficulties across the population are very wide.

In typical early child development, the emergence and development of speech, language, and communication (the term *communication* will be used to encompass these three aspects) usually occur with ease and in conjunction with other areas of development, that is, cognition, physical/motor, and socioemotional competence. Such typical development is marked by the emergence of significant milestones in the first year of life such as communicative intent or the desire to interact and communicate, pointing, and first words, followed by combining two words together in the second year. It is accepted that the dynamic interaction between development in cognition, physical ability, and socioemotional competence results in the child becoming a competent communicator ready for learning in school by 5 years of age.

In infants with LD, communication can be one of the first aspects of development observed not to develop as expected. Such observations can include early communicative behaviors such as communicative intent, joint attention, smiling, response to sound, pointing, vocalizations, and first words to be absent when expected to emerge and to then develop much more slowly. For some infants, these early communicative behaviors may never fully develop. Early communicative behaviors are the foundation for further development of communication abilities and so delays in or absent communicative behaviors have significant implications for further development in communication ability.

At 5 years of age, children are expected to be competent communicators who are ready to use their communication skills to learn. Children with LD may never achieve this and so continue to have difficulties for the rest of their lives. Such difficulties impact negatively on their learning, their psychosocial development, and life chances. People with LD are less likely to achieve in terms of education, to gain employment, and to live independently, and they experience higher levels of health needs including mental health. People with LD often present with challenging behaviors where limited communication ability leads to the individuals using these behaviors to express themselves.

Profiles of Communication Development in LD

Having acknowledged the heterogeneity of people with LD and general considerations about communication development, this entry now describes two profiles of communication development. The first profile is specific to a syndrome of LD, and the second profile is an example of emerging communication ability in profound and multiple LDs.

A Syndrome of LD: DS

DS was first identified by John Langdon Down in the 1860s and is one of the more common causes of LD. DS is a congenital chromosomal syndrome, which means the child is born with the syndrome and the syndrome is caused by a chromosomal abnormality. In DS, the infant is born with an extra copy of Chromosome 21, and this leads to the specific physical, cognitive, and behavioral phenotype found in DS.

The physical phenotype includes low muscle tone, referred to as hypotonia, a shortening of the front-to-back dimension of the head known as *brachycephaly*, *cardiac problems*, and *abnormalities* in the development of the ear and its mechanisms. Recent evidence confirms a higher risk of early dementias than in the general population.

In terms of learning, the cognitive phenotype encompasses a mild to moderate LD with intelligence scores declining over age. Research shows impairments in specific aspects of cognition, namely, working memory and executive functioning. Working memory refers to the process of how people store and manipulate complex information needed for learning. Executive functioning describes the process involved in how people plan, initiate, and execute behaviors. Visual abilities are considered superior to verbal abilities, and so people with DS have specific strengths in their visual abilities.

The physical and cognitive phenotypes have implications for how children with DS develop communication. For example, the brachycephaly means the ear canal is short and flat and so children with DS are more susceptible to ear infections leading to conductive hearing loss. This transitory but recurrent hearing loss can significantly reduce their language learning opportunities. Learning new words depends on children being able to store the sounds of a new word in their working memory while mapping or matching the word onto the object or concept it refers to. If a child has a reduced working memory, it is harder to learn new words at the same rate as other children.

The communication profile of DS is best considered as part of the behavioral phenotype, although reference should also be made to the interactions between and within physical and cognitive phenotypes. The profile is broadly characterized by delayed early communicative behaviors, and once these emerge subsequent milestones are also delayed. For example, first words are acquired at about 18 months of age. Communication development follows an expected pattern but is slower to develop plateauing at a level below that expected for the child's age. Development can be uneven so, for example, the language understanding of these children is often more advanced of their spoken language. Children with DS often learn to use simple sign language before being able to talk. This is thought to be due to their more advanced visual than verbal skills and so it is easier for them to sign early words than to say them. These examples of uneven development are unusual in terms of typical communication development and considered to be specific to the communication profile of DS.

Due to the brachycephaly and other differences in craniofacial structure such as a high-arched palate, speech difficulties are usually evident. It is harder for children with DS to use their speech muscles and articulators to learn and produce speech sounds clearly. For example, children with DS often have a relatively small mouth for the size of their tongue, which can protrude and so articulating speech sounds becomes more difficult. The hearing difficulties described above will also make it harder for children with DS to develop clear speech and will also impact on their phonological development (learning the sounds of the language they are learning). In terms of socioemotional competence, many people with DS have strengths in socialization but can be described as *overfriendly* and not discerning of their social relationships, thus increasing their vulnerability.

An Example of Emerging Communication Ability: Profound and Multiple LDs

The communication profile of people with profound and multiple LDs (PMLD) is different from the profile found in DS. Importantly, many people with PMLD may remain at a preverbal or preintentional stage of communication referred to here as emerging communication abilities and so never become verbal communicators. People with PMLD often have significant and complex medical needs. The individual may not be able to move independently, may need assistance with everyday functioning such as eating and drinking, and may not be able to engage in the everyday tasks that others take for granted such as interacting and communicating with others and making choices over their needs and desires.

The emerging communication stage is crucial to understanding people with PMLD. Infants usually move through this stage of development in the first 6–9 months of life. Here, important milestones are achieved that underpin subsequent communication development. The first is the shift from being a preintentional to an intentional communicator where the infant develops a conceptual understanding that engaging in a reflexive behavior such as crying, or looking or smiling at the primary carer, results in an action that the infant will usually seek to initiate again. For example, crying results in being fed or cuddled, and smiling initiates interaction. These behaviors are reflexive in the first months of life as they reflect the child's internal state and are not intentional. Over time, the infant learns that engaging in these behaviors results in a satisfactory outcome. The shift to intentionality then underpins the concept of intentional communication and so marks the transition to being an intentional communicator who then goes on to look, gesture, point, and vocalize to communicate. For infants with PMLD, this shift to intentionality may never or only partially be achieved, which significantly compromises subsequent development. Adults with PMLD can be at this stage of emerging communication ability for all of their life.

Therefore, communication often consists of nonverbal means such as head nods, grunts, other bodily movements, and vocalizations, behaviors that are not consistently communicative and so are difficult to identify and interpret to those not familiar with the individual. People with PMLD have to rely on others to understand their emerging and often inconsistent communication, and so they may never truly be able to express themselves and are dependent on others to make decisions about their lives, thus increasing their vulnerability. The *experts* at communicating with people with PMLD are often key family members who are attuned to how the individual communicates. This can place very high demand on parents and families.

Enabling Communication in People With LDs

As for all people, communication is a key life skill for people with LDs. Here, communication is verbal and nonverbal with all behaviors considered potentially communicative. Approaches aim to work directly with an individual to facilitate specific communicative abilities but more importantly to change the individual's everyday environment to ensure that individuals have opportunities to use their communication and that people in their environment know how to and are able to effectively understand the communicative behaviors of the individual. Furthermore, people in the individual's environment must learn to and competently be able to change their own communication to enable the most effective communication possible. Essential to this is ensuring that people with LDs understand and are actively involved in decisions about their lives and the services they receive.

Approaches to enable communication will differ in emphasis across education, health, and social care sectors. In education, communication must be enabled to ensure that individuals can learn to the best of their abilities. The language and communication demands of curricula need to be differentiated and individualized to meet the individual's learning needs. In health services, individuals need to be able to understand their medical needs and to be able to communicate their wishes about their treatment. In social care, people with LDs must be able to understand the provision they can receive and to express their needs and communicate their choices about their everyday life. The emphasis must always be on the services and not the individual, to ensure that this is achieved.

Summary

People with LDs are a very heterogeneous population who present with a wide range of communication difficulties. Evidence exists to support specific profiles of communication development in some types of LD. The communication difficulties of people with LD have significant implications for their well-being and life chances over their lifetime.

Judy Clegg

See also Down Syndrome; Intentionality; Language Acquisition; Language Delay; Language Disorders in Children

Further Readings

Atkinson, D., Jackson, M., & Walmsley, J. (Eds.). (1998). *Forgotten lives: Exploring the history of learning disability*. Kidderminster, UK: British Institute of Learning Disabilities.

Bunning, K., (2009). Making sense of communication. In J. Palwyn & S. Carrnaby (Eds.), *Profound intellectual multiple disabilities* (pp. 46–61). Oxford, UK: Wiley-Blackwell.

Fidler, D., & Daunhauer, L. (2011). Down syndrome: General overview. In P. Howlin, T. Charman, & M. Ghaziuddin (Eds.), *The SAGE handbook of developmental disorders*. London, UK: Sage.

Goldbart, J., & Caton, S. (2010). *Communication and people with the most complex needs: What works and why this is essential*. London, UK: Mencap.

Goldbart, J., Chadwick, D., & Buell, S. (2014). Speech and language therapists' approaches to communication intervention with children and adults with profound and multiple learning disabilities. *International Journal of Language and Communication Disorders, 49*(6), 687–701.

Goodley, D. (2010). *Disability studies: An interdisciplinary introduction*. London, UK: Sage.

Hostyn, I., & Maes, B. (2009). Interaction between persons with profound intellectual and multiple disabilities and their partners: A literature review. *Journal of Intellectual and Developmental Disability, 34*(4), 296–312. Retrieved from https://doi.org/10.3109/13668250903285648

Mansell, J. (2010). *Raising our sights: Services for adults with profound intellectual and multiple disabilities*. London, UK: Department of Health.

LENITION AND FORTITION

The sound changes known as *lenition and fortition* depend on a hierarchy of consonant strength. Such a strength hierarchy can be considered as the converse of the sonority hierarchy, that is, sounds that are high in sonority are low in strength and vice versa. Sonority is described elsewhere in this encyclopedia but may be thought of as the degree of sound clarity derived from the degree of opening of the vocal tract (the more open the more sonorous). The strength hierarchy, on the other hand, classifies the strongest consonants as those with the greatest degree of closure and those without vocal fold vibration. Thus, plosives are stronger than fricatives, and voiceless plosives are stronger than voiced. Sound changes that involve moving from a stronger to a weaker consonant are termed *lenitions* (weakening), while the opposite changes are termed *fortitions* (strengthening).

In most languages, rapid, casual, connected speech demonstrates examples of lenition, and thus, lenition is probably encountered in the literature on normal phonology more often than fortition. Commonly occurring lenition pathways are illustrated as follows:

Lenition
[t] → [ts] → [θ / s] → [h] → ∅   [or: [t] → [ʔ] → ∅]
↓   ↓
[d] →   [ð / z] → [ð̞ / ɹ] → ∅

The upper pathway can be called *opening*, and the lower pathway *sonorization*, but as can be seen, it is also possible to move from the upper to the lower through a process of voicing. The final step of lenition involves the deletion of the segment entirely, and this is termed *elision*. Fortition changes are the reverse of those shown above.

Synchronic Lenition and Fortition

Lenition and fortition have been responsible for sound changes diachronically, but this section will look only at synchronic examples. In English, one example of phonemic lenition is seen in certain plural forms of words ending in voiceless fricatives. Thus, the plural of *hoof* is usually *hooves* with a change from fortis /f/ to lenis /v/. Similarly, the verb equivalent of the noun *wreath* is *wreathe* with a change from fortis /θ/ to lenis /ð/. The flapping of medial /t/ in several varieties of English (e.g., *better* realized as [ˈbɛɾɚ]) is also lenition as a voiced flap is weaker than a voiceless plosive. However, in this case, as [ɾ] is not a phoneme of English, this would be classed as allophonic lenition. Spanish also demonstrates allophonic lenition, in that /b, d, g/ are realized as [β, ð, ɣ] when in noninitial position.

Examples of synchronic fortition in English are rare but can be seen in some varieties of English, where the phonemes /θ, ð/ may be realized as plosives (dental or alveolar) in certain word positions or in casual styles of speaking. Use of dental plosives would be considered allophonic, but the use of alveolar plosives would be a phonemic change, as English contains alveolar plosive phonemes in its system. Some English speakers have a fortition with the word *with*. This would usually be pronounced /wɪð/ but would be optionally realized as /wɪθ/ when followed by a word starting with a voiceless consonant.

In many Germanic languages, word-final consonants must be voiceless. Thus, German has a plural form *Räder* (meaning "wheels") pronounced /ˈʀɛːdɐ/; however, the singular, *Rad*, which lacks the "-er" ending, is pronounced /ʀaːt/, as the now word-final orthographic "d" is subject to fortition and realized as /t/. This fortition process affects all obstruents in the language and is deemed here as phonemic, as German has contrastive voiced and voiceless obstruents in other word positions.

Lenition in Rapid Speech

In rapid, casual speech, there may be a considerable amount of lenition of consonants as well as elision and omission of entire syllables. For example, the utterance "I'm going to be walking home tomorrow" might be reduced to [ˈaɪŋnə bɪ ˈwɔkŋ ˈəʊm tˈmɒɹə], where the initial /g/ of *going*, the initial /b/ of *be*, and the initial /h/ of *home* are all subject to varying degrees of lenition.

Grammaticalized Lenition and Fortition

In some languages, lenition and fortition may depend in some instances on the grammatical context rather than the phonological or stylistic context. Among such languages are the Celtic languages, and examples here are taken from Welsh, Breton, and Irish. In Welsh, a variety of syntactic contexts (such as direct object of an inflected verb, following certain personal possessives, prepositions, or conjunctions) will cause phonological changes to the initial consonant of the relevant word. Welsh has three types of initial consonant mutation, and two of them involve lenition. Soft mutation changes voiceless plosives to voiced (voicing lenition), voiced plosives to voiced fricatives (sonorization lenition), and voiceless fricative liquids to voiced nonfricative liquids (also sonorization). The aspirate mutation changes voiceless plosives to voiceless fricatives (opening lenition). Breton has a similar pattern but also has a hard mutation, which changes voiced plosives to voiceless (fortition). Irish mutations fall into only two groups: lenition (plosives change to fricatives) and eclipsis (voiceless plosives become voiced, and voiced stops become nasals—this also being lenition as nasals are weaker than plosives). Examples of these in use are, in Welsh: *cath* ("cat"), *eu cath*, *ei gath*, *ei chath* ("their cat," "his cat," "her cat"); in Irish: *cat* ("cat"), *a cat*, *mo chat*, *bhur gcat* ("his cat," "my cat," "your cat").

Lenition and Fortition in Disordered Speech

Lenition is often encountered in dysarthria, where many forms of this disorder exhibit weakening of consonants. This can result in target plosives being realized with very brief closure (e.g., [b̆]), or as fricatives (e.g., [β] or [v]), or fricatives with weak frication (e.g., [v̞]), or even lenited to an approximant ([ʋ]).

Fortition is seen in child speech disorders where, in delayed phonological development, patterns such as the realization of target fricatives and affricates as stops is commonly reported, as is stopping of liquids. Voicing may also be affected in child speech disorders with both voicing lenition in word-initial position and voicing fortition in word-final.

Martin J. Ball

See also Articulatory Phonetics; Consonants; Dysarthria; Sonority; Speech Sound Disorders

Further Readings

Ball, M. J., & Müller, N. (1992). *Mutation in Welsh.* London, UK: Routledge.

Ball, M. J., & Müller, N. (2005). *Phonetics for communication disorders.* Mahwah, NJ: Erlbaum.

Ball, M. J., Müller, N., & Rutter, B. (2010). *Phonology for communication disorders.* Hove, UK: Psychology Press.

Local, J., & Kelly, J. (1989). *Doing phonology.* Manchester, UK: Manchester University Press.

Lexicon

Lexicon refers to the inventory of words in a language and the set of structural rules that make up its grammar, that is, its semantics, phonology, morphology, syntax, and pragmatics. When the lexicon is assumed to relate to a core cognitive function in humans, it is called the mental lexicon. The mental lexicon is responsible for the activation, storage, processing, and retrieval of words and their use in utterances with language-specific word sequences. As a result, the mental lexicon is the primary catalyst for language use and acquisition, permitting meaningful communication between speakers of the same language. Several theoretical models in linguistics assess its function and organization differentiating between adult and child-developmental lexicon, as well as between monolingual and bilingual lexicon. The lexicon plays a crucial role in understanding the mechanisms of oral language as the most basic form of human communication. This entry elaborates on the lexicon in the following four sections: terms and definitions, how the mental lexicon works, bilingual mental lexicon, and mental lexicon in acquisition.

Terms and Definitions

The term *lexicon* originates from the Greek word λεξικόν [lɛ.ksi.kón], which generally means "relating to words" but also refers to "dictionary." Similarly to a dictionary, the lexicon of a given language comprises the sum of its words (lexemes, i.e., units of basic meaning). Individual words in the lexicon carry semantic, phonological, and morphological information and are categorized into lemmas, that is, headwords that comprise groups of semantically related though morphologically differentiated words; for example, the headword *talk* relates to *talk-s, talk-ing, talk-er, talk-ed, un-talked-of, un-talk-able, talk-ative, un-talk-ative, un-talk-ative-ness*, and so on. Studying the lexicon of a given language involves knowing its vocabulary and relevant pragmatic information associated with each specific word/concept pair. It also involves knowing what a *word* is and what the relationship of a word is to its meaning, pronunciation, structure, and syntactic role in utterances. On the other hand, studying the *mental lexicon*, that is, how the human brain stores and processes information, helps answer questions such as the following: are words accessed in spoken communication? Does the lexicon differ in bilingual speakers? What is the role of the lexicon in language acquisition? Despite being a central theme in linguistics, there is not unanimous agreement on the validity of the mental lexicon as a scientific concept.

How the Mental Lexicon Works

Human cognition is an advanced faculty typified by general interconnected logical structures. Information concerning lexical items (words, affixes, idioms, etc.) and their grammatical structure in a speaker's language is stored in the mental lexicon, which guides the comprehension and production of speech. Our brain functions much like a superior computer that processes information (auditory, visual, contextual, etc.), stores it, and is capable of retrieving it upon request. Mental representations for lexical items and their predictable grammatical properties (e.g., phonetic) in a particular language become dictionary entries for those words, while unpredictable properties are contextually specified by grammatical rules (e.g., phonological), rather than being entered ab initio as default information.

There are several linguistic models of lexical processing. To exemplify their theoretical scope, the monolingual speaker "blueprint" is briefly discussed here: the lexicon is the principal mediator between conceptualization (i.e., forming a concept) and grammatical encoding (a code-concept association permitting labeling, classification, and retrieval from memory). The lexicon identifies components that process *what* and *how* something is spoken, organizing lexical information into lexemes (morphophonology) and lemmas (semantics/grammar). Speech production begins in the *conceptualizer*, continues in the *formulator*, and ends in the *articulator*. This model differentiates adult and child lexicon by terminating the conceptualizer–formulator link at a known endpoint in linguistic development, the "critical period."

By and large, word meaning is learned and interpreted through competing cognitive mechanisms that compare the grammatical cues in utterances, and then compute and adjust them in real time, influenced by the speaker's evolving experience with language. Supporting this notion, psycholinguistic theory views language acquisition and use as a unified process across a speaker's lifespan, which includes acquisition of an additional language during infancy or adulthood.

Bilingual Mental Lexicon

Much interdisciplinary discussion focuses on how bilingual speakers process lexical items in their two languages, with an early assumption being that words and concepts are stored separately. Subsequent assumptions view bilingual lexicon organization to be *compound* (single concept/separate entries per language), *coordinate* (separate concept/entry pairs per language), or *subordinate* (single concept/no link for second language entry). Most theoretical stances range between *holistic* and *separated lexica* for bilingual speakers. Evidence of lexicon separation comes from separate language retrieval in bilingual patients who have brain damage. Although total lexicon integration is unsupported, completely independent lexica are also unlikely, as indicated by language interference phenomena and conversational code switching.

A bilingual adaptation of the "blueprint" assumes variable processing components and levels. While the conceptualizer is intermittently either language-specific or language-independent, there are different formulators per language, and the articulator employs non-language-specific motor strategies. The two languages are directly interconnected either via a shared concept depository, via lexical nodes, or both. Though this model was criticized for its static interpretation of bilingualism, subsequent postulations addressed dynamic properties in bilingual acquisition and use.

Mental Lexicon in Acquisition

Cognitive theory on child language acquisition discusses levels of grammar representation in the mind in terms of single/double lexica. In single-lexicon models, children have adultlike grammar representations but actual speech results from a two-level process: the *high* level differentiates *underlying* and *surface* grammar representations, and the *low* level differentiates *surface* representations and actual productions. Single-lexicon models fail to account for the variability in child developmental language, which is addressed by two-lexicon models in terms of *input* and *output* representations.

Accordingly, the three-level model differentiates between abstract grammar, storage of phonetic representations, and actual productions. A word is subject to selection rules before being stored in the *input lexicon*, while specific rules modify perceptual representations prior to entering the *output lexicon* for production. Thus, actual production is directed by the *output lexicon* rather than the original single lexicon, and processes are guided offline by memorized processing. The model was expanded to also account for psycholinguistic influences, like an individual child's "guesses" about the adult language, its varieties, and registers in the ambient environment. Other multilevel models discuss representations on different sets of parameters, like the fine-grained item-based level, the abstract level of sub-lexical grammatical patterns, and dynamic perspectives in which single words may have multiple representations.

With regard to bilingual lexicon development, an early hypothesis assumes three stages: a unified lexicon and syntax ensemble initially, lexicon separation with a single syntactic component midway, and complete lexicon/syntax differentiation finally. Vocabulary acquisition in both monolingual and bilingual speakers is grounded on the principle of mutual exclusivity, that is, new words refer to new referents. A bilingual person learns new words independently rather than through translating the earlier-acquired word into the subsequently acquired lexical item. Though early translation ability in bilingual children is supportive of lexicon/language separation, recent theoretical advancements assume distinct lexica that are variably interconnected on many levels. Similar arguments describe the multilingual lexicon, though the field is still embryonic.

In short, words in the brain carry the load of language. Despite our sketchy insights, lexicon theory helps pave the path of knowledge on human communication science and disorder.

Elena Babatsouli

See also Bilingualism; Code Switching and Mixing; Cognitive Linguistics; Critical Period for Language Acquisition; Language Acquisition; Linguistics; Multilingualism; Oral Language

Further Readings

Aitchison, J. (2012). *Words in the mind: An introduction to the mental lexicon*. Malden, MA: Blackwell.

Jarema, G., & Libben, G. (2007). *The mental lexicon: Core perspectives*. Oxford, UK: Elsevier.

Pavlenko, A. (Ed.). (2008). *The bilingual mental lexicon: Interdisciplinary approaches*. Clevedon, UK: Multilingual Matters.

Singleton, D. (1999). *Exploring the second language mental lexicon*. Cambridge, UK: Cambridge University Press.

Szubko-Sitarek, W. (2015). *Multilingual lexical recognition in the mental lexicon of third language users*. Berlin, Germany: Springer-Verlag.

LINEAR PHONOLOGY

Linear phonology is a method of studying the structure of the phonological components of language. Phonology is the branch of linguistics that explores how speech sounds are spoken and systematically organized within languages. Phonologists inventory the phonemes (i.e., the speech sounds) of a language and examine the features of these sounds and propose rules to describe how sounds are linked and patterned to form words. This entry discusses the differences between linear and nonlinear phonology; uses of linear phonology, for example, with children who have phonological delays; and the contributions of researchers, such as Noam Chomsky and Morris Halle.

Phonology entails several branches of study. Classical phonemics explores phonemes and phoneme combinations. Generative phonology is the study of the features of phonemes. Analysis within generative phonology focuses upon each segment of the linear sequence of sounds used to produce a stream of speech. Linear phonology provides the mechanism for this type of analysis of individual, discrete phonemes. In **nonlinear phonology**, a stream of speech is represented as multidimensional; it is an assembly that includes the overlapping features of phonemes along with linguistic units, such as syllables and morphemes, and suprasegmental features (such as sound, syllable, or word stress; changes in vocal pitch, loudness, and tone; and duration of sound production). Nonlinear models of phonology include the following:

1. autosegmental phonology, which explores speech sounds along with other independent features of speech, such as the tone and harmony that accompany speech sounds and that influence the production of groups or sequences of sounds;

2. metrical phonology, which describes how speech sounds are organized into syllables, how syllables become metrical feet, how feet become words, and how words are grouped in phrases and sentences; and

3. lexical phonology, which explores how sounds and morphemes are used to build words.

Speech–language pathologists are concerned with the diagnosis and treatment of speech sound production disturbances. Children who are acquiring speech and language may experience delayed or disordered development of the phonological system. These conditions characteristically have their onset in the preschool age range, result in systematic speech sound production errors, and are independent of physical or cognitive impairment, or of dialects, accentedness, cultural practices, or the influences of learning multiple languages. Children with phonological delays attain slower progress in acquiring the typical sequence of phonological development. Children with phonological disorders produce unusual speech sound errors and have a restricted phoneme repertoire. *Phonological impairment* and *speech sound disorder* are the umbrella diagnostic terms that describe phonological delay and phonological disorder. The term speech sound disorder globally encompasses the speech sound production difficulties that are due to motor origins (such as apraxia, dysarthria, and articulation delays or articulation disorders that are uncomplicated by language deficits), as well as speech production difficulties that are due to phonological impairment, that is, that have linguistic origins within the phonological system. In cases of phonological impairment, children appear to have difficulty producing speech sounds, but the cause of this difficulty is a language impairment within the phonological system. In this condition, children do not mentally represent speech sounds correctly; this difficulty perceiving, classifying, remembering, and activating speech sounds causes them to speak these sounds incorrectly.

Speech–language pathologists carefully analyze children's speech sound productions to determine the phonological patterns of error, known as *phonological processes*. Linear phonology and nonlinear phonology, as fields of linguistic study, historically informed the clinical research in the field of speech–language pathology. Linear phonology contributed to establishing the theoretical basis for how speech–language pathologists formally describe the linguistic features that underlie phonological impairments, and it influenced how speech–language pathologists diagnose the phonological behaviors of children who experience phonological delays or disorders.

A Historical Perspective on Linear Phonology

Linear phonology provided the theoretical basis for clinical study of speech sound production disorders throughout the middle decades of the 20th century. During the last two decades of the 20th century, nonlinear phonology supplanted linear phonology as the prevailing theory for the study of children's phonological development and as an explanation for the linguistic features that contribute to phonological processes and the phonological behaviors of children who experience phonological delays or disorders.

Although the study of the structure of language predates the 20th century by hundreds of years, a new scientific study of language emerged in Europe in the 1920s. Roman Jakobson, a philosopher of language, influenced the linguistic conceptualizations promoted by the scholars of the Prague school and drew attention to the emerging study of phonology as a system of language. Jakobson and other linguists advanced a theory of phonology and devised scientific methodologies to demonstrate the merits of this theory. The goal was to understand the function of the phonological system, but to make this discovery it was also necessary to explain the structural organization of the phonological system. Ensuing linguists explored paradigms for practical and complete analyses of the sound structure of language, with emphases on the functional or structural perspectives.

Chomsky and Halle: *The Sound Pattern of English*

Structuralism, as one theoretical framework and its empirical explanations came to be known, provided the preeminent approach to the study of linguistics through the 1970s. The accomplishments of the linguists in Europe and the United States who advanced the rigorous scientific study of language were situated within the structuralist approach. Generative phonology, which is the study of the features of phonemes, was devised by Noam Chomsky and Morris Halle, academicians at the Massachusetts Institute of Technology. Notable among their many publications was their 1968 book, *The Sound Pattern of English*. In the preface to the book, Chomsky and Halle stated that their intention was to provide a detailed investigation into English sound patterns and their underlying structure and to expose the rules of English phonology. Their methods established that a stream of speech is composed of sequences of discrete segments and that segments are composed of sets of phonetic features (speech sounds). The simultaneous and sequential combinations of these phonetic features and segments are subject to specific constraints that are predicated upon the multitude of ways that the sounds and segments can be spoken. They devised a "grammar" for phonology, that is, a linear sequence of rules for usage. The grammar represents the organization of the possible conditions under which the phonetic features of English could be used, one after the other, in a stream of speech.

Chomsky and Halle diagrammed phonetic representations within a two-dimensional matrix in which the rows lay out the sequences of phonetic features and the columns demarcate the consecutive segments of the utterance. The segments contextualize how the phonetic representations are being used and how they should be interpreted by a listener. A diagram might, for example, indicate the degree of intensity with which a given phonetic feature is present in a segment; for example, a "strident" feature might be indicated along a differentiated scale of degrees of stridency. The language context assigns to each phonetic representation a structural description that indicates how it is to be interpreted by a listener. This language context may govern the need for specific ways to produce a sound, for example, with intensity.

Chomsky and Halle acknowledged that the schematic of linear phonology is vast. The number of possible sequential phonetic representations is infinite, as is the number of possible sentences that can be constructed in each human language. However, the rules of a language must be finite, and the grammar must be attainable by the speakers of the language. Therefore, the system of grammar must be recursive, meaning that it must be constructed of rules that can be reapplied indefinitely and as needed, in new arrangements and combinations. As such, the grammar must be generative of the structural descriptions it needs. The rules must give rise to circumstances for applications of the rules. There is no limit to the number of applications of the processes, so the rules must be able to offer a structural explanation for any utterance.

In addition, Chomsky and Halle remarked on how every utterance is the externalized representation of the thoughts of a speaker. Each utterance is one possible manifestation of the ideas or concepts that the speaker is trying to convey. Chomsky and Halle described the spoken message, including its phonetic representations, as the surface structure of the message, and they labeled the speaker's thoughts or intentions as the deep structure. The surface structure is a transformation of the deep structure, meaning that the ideas are somehow transformed when they are put into language. The surface (i.e., overt) phonological properties of the utterance are determined by the mental representations of speech sounds that are inherent within the covert deep structure. The deep structure is transformed by the way that these properties are combined and exhibited as a surface structure. Chomsky and Halle described a "transformational cycle" that involves the rules that assign phonetic representations to each surface structure. Thus, the grammar of the phonological system must be transformational, in the sense that the rules allow for the transformation of thoughts into speech.

In sum, Chomsky and Halle accounted for certain "formal universals" that determine the structure of grammars and the form and organization of rules. They also accounted for "substantive universals" that define the sets of elements that figure into individual grammars, as within certain languages or dialects that have unique properties. They stated, "The theory of transformational generative grammar proposes certain formal universals regarding the kinds of rules that can appear in a grammar, the kinds of structures on which they may operate, and the ordering conditions under which these rules may apply" (Chomsky & Halle, 1968, p. 4). They proposed that there is a phonological component to generative grammar and observed it to occur in the linear patterning of the components of a fixed set of phonetic features. Their theory of universal phonetics specified the possible phonetic representations by determining the universal set of phonetic features and the conditions for their possible combinations within utterances. The phonetic form of each sentence in each language is drawn from this class of possible phonetic representations.

Linear phonology maintains that humans can innately and intuitively use patterns of sounds in rule-governed ways to generate words. The patterns and rules are the generative grammar of a given language, that is, the components that speakers use to generate language. There is a finite set of rules for stringing together phonological elements that allows for linguistic predictability. A speaker's phonological competence involves following the patterns and rules for effectively employing the elements of phonology to construct complex words.

The Utility and Applicability of Linear Phonology

Linear phonology provides an algorithmic description of the surface forms of the phonological properties of a language. It accounts for a multitude of phonological rules, and it allows for generating new forms by applying this set of phonological rules. The phonological representations within a language are explained as linear sequences and are diagrammed as matrices of features. As a structural system, linear phonology reveals the phonological contrasts that exist in a language and the conditions within a stream of speech under which these occur. However, linear phonology only marginally accounts for any other linguistic structures that occur outside of the linear structure of phonetic features and segments that are depicted in the matrices. For example, the morphology of syllables is not emphasized as a factor within the stream of speech that necessitates contrasts in pronunciation and inflection. This omission was addressed by the theory of lexical phonology, which emphasized the variations of sounds and structures that are operative within the inventory of the lexicon of a language, and which characterized how phonological rules could be governed by morphemic usage. Similar shortcomings of the linear model of phonological representations were identified by the theory of natural generative phonology, which adhered to the syllable as the unit of analysis and which saw the syllable as more suited to identifying the phonotactics of a language (i.e., the possible combinations of sounds within a language) as well as for distinguishing variations in how sounds are produced in words (e.g., as in the allophony and sonority of phoneme production).

Recent Perspectives: The Transition to Nonlinear Phonology

Nonlinear phonology accounts for spoken language as the assembly of phonemes, suprasegmentals, syllables, and morphemes. The phonetic features of language are one component within the multidimensional interactions of these linguistic constituents. A linear, left-to-right horizontal sequence of adjacent sounds has been supplanted by models that depict a speaker's dynamic coordination of many linguistic features, which may be adjacent or nonadjacent in an utterance. Nonlinear phonology provided the theoretical basis for the identification of the phonological processes produced by children with phonological impairments. Clinical assessment of children's phonological skills documents how children produce phonemes in the context of syllables, words, and phrases. Interventions for phonological impairments address developing children's mental representations of phonemic contrasts and the production of speech sound contrasts within these linguistic units.

Monica Gordon-Pershey

See also Linguistics; Nonlinear Phonology; Phonological Processes; Phonology; Speech Sound Disorders

Further Readings

Bauman-Waengler, J. (2016). *Articulation and phonology in speech sound disorders: A clinical focus* (5th ed.). New York, NY: Pearson.

Bernhardt, B. (1992). Developmental implications of nonlinear phonological theory. *Clinical Linguistics & Phonetics, 6*(4), 259–281. http://dx.doi.org/10.3109/02699209208985536

Bernhardt, B., & Stoel-Gammon, C. (1994). Nonlinear phonology: Clinical application. *Journal of Speech, Language, and Hearing Research, 37,* 123–143. http://doi.org/10.1044/jshr.3701.123

Chomsky, N., & Halle, M. (1968). *The sound pattern of English.* New York, NY: Harper & Row.

Goldsmith, J., & Laks, B. (2006). Generative phonology: Its origins, its principles, and its successors. In

L. Waugh, J. E. Joseph, & M. Monville-Burston (Eds.), *The Cambridge history of linguistics*. Retrieved May 17, 2017, from http://people.cs.uchicago.edu/~jagoldsm/Papers/GenerativePhonology.pdf

Iverson, G., & Wheeler, D. (1987). Hierarchical structures in child phonology. *Lingua, 73*(4), 243–257. https://doi.org/10.1016/0024-3841(87)90020-9

Language and linguistics—The structuralist era. (n.d.). Retrieved May 17, 2017, from http://science.jrank.org/pages/9907/Language-Linguistics-Structuralist-Era.html

McCarthy, J. J. (1982, February). Nonlinear phonology: An overview. *GLOW Newsletter 8*. Retrieved May 17, 2017, from http://www.meertens.knaw.nl/glow2002/mccarthy.pdf

Menn, L. (1983). Development of articulatory, phonetic, and phonological capabilities. In B. Butterworth (Ed.), *Language production* (Vol. 2, pp. 3–50). London, UK: Academic Press.

Linguistic Profiles

Today, a wide range of theoretically grounded and clinically useful assessments exists in a variety of languages that can be used to evaluate speech and language development and identify children with speech or language disorders. This entry focuses on the Language Assessment, Remediation and Screening Procedure (LARSP), conceived by David Crystal and his colleagues, and the non-English versions of LARSP that have been published. LARSP was developed with the explicit purpose of providing a platform for linguistically informed analyses of children's language skills that would be used by practicing clinicians working with children with speech and language disorders. The perennial challenge for any clinical assessment tool is that it be theoretically grounded and at the same time practical so that it would enjoy widespread clinical use rather than be treated as a linguistic curiosity by practicing speech–language pathologists. LARSP aims to address both of these issues by offering a practical, quick, informative, and linguistically sound language sampling and analysis procedure aimed at evaluating spontaneous samples collected from children.

Driven by the desire to provide language assessments with solid linguistic foundations that would also be used in clinical settings, the main tenets of LARSP are (a) to collect a representative sample of the child's speech and language, (b) to assign the collected utterances to well-defined developmental levels, and (c) to evaluate the interaction between the child and the clinician. Another, less prominent goal of LARSP is to offer much needed consistency across sampling sessions and different children so as to provide a uniform framework for language sampling and analysis.

For LARSP to be practical, the spontaneous language samples should contain a minimum of 50 utterances collected from the children during play sessions with the adult clinician or educator. Recommendations for these sessions range from naturalistic interactions between the child and the clinician to more topic-driven conversations between the interlocutors that could focus on the child's experiences. Even quasi-naturalistic productions are acceptable if obtaining 50 fully spontaneous utterances would prove challenging, especially when working with younger children or children with speech and language disorders. Whether completely spontaneous or quasi-naturalistic, conversational samples obtained via a uniform procedure offer a window onto the child's linguistic skills ranging from morphology to syntax that are relatively easy to administer in a variety of settings while providing information that would be useful for speech–language pathologists charged with assessing the child's language skills. Thus, over the years, LARSP has become a language sampling and analysis procedure that has enjoyed popularity among not only practicing speech–language pathologists but also researchers and other professionals.

David Crystal, Paul Fletcher, and Michael Garman's seminal publication of the English version of LARSP from over four decades ago has generated considerable interest among clinicians and researchers working with children with typical speech and language as well as their peers with various communication disorders. Since the publication of the original LARSP in the 1970s, a sizable number of analogous versions have been published in a variety of languages other than English, owing to the simplicity, practicality, ease of use, and linguistic grounding of LARSP. In 2016, a collection with 12 new languages was published, adding to the growing number of LARSP language varieties. Languages appearing in the 2016 volume vary both in terms of genetics (e.g., from Indo-European to Uralic) and geography (representing various continents). However, each new version shares the core principles and tenets of LARSP and also presents useful information about the linguistic structure of the language that it profiles as well as provides data about the acquisition of those structures with age-appropriate lexical and grammatical markers.

Versions of LARSP typically include a one- to two-page chart that is tailored to the language in which the assessment is being done. The typical LARSP chart is presented in sections where Section A usually includes items that cannot be easily interpreted (such as problematic or unanalyzed ones) so that clinicians can use their time more efficiently by not having to analyze responses that may not contain useful information from a grammatical standpoint. The following sections—usually B, C, and D—of LARSP charts contain information about the interaction between the clinician and the child. Subsequent to Sections A, B, C, and D, the majority of the LARSP chart is devoted to describing the stages of grammatical acquisition and to providing age-appropriate linguistic markers to which the child's production can be compared for the purposes of assessing her or his developmental stage relative to her or his peers. This section is language-specific and it varies both in age ranges and even the number of stages depending on the language being acquired by the child. For example, the English LARSP chart has seven stages ranging in age from 0;9 to 4;6+ compared to Hungarian with five stages and an age range of 1;0 to 3;6. Moreover, the linguistic markers themselves vary based on the target language and its grammar.

It is important to note that the various non-English versions of LARSP have been adapted and modified to meet the demands of the target language rather than the translated language, which enhances the validity of the measure. To illustrate the LARSP profile chart, the Hungarian version (HU-LARSP) and its English translation are displayed in Figure 1. These charts demonstrate that while HU-LARSP follows the general guidelines and adheres to the principles of LARSP previously noted, the adaptation makes the measure uniquely suited to assess and screen children acquiring Hungarian. The chapter on HU-LARSP by Ferenc Bunta, Judit Bóna, and Mária Gósy also provides a quick overview of the grammatical structures of Hungarian relevant to morphosyntactic development in children and also includes a brief review of how those structures are acquired by Hungarian-speaking children from the first words to 4 years of age. Thus, HU-LARSP and other non-English adaptations of LARSP are not only linguistically grounded, but the stages and markers of language development used by the assessment protocol are based on the literature and data from children acquiring the language for which the particular measure was developed.

While LARSP provides a linguistic profile of a child's language skills from a general perspective, linguistic profiles have also been developed to address more specific levels of analysis such as phonology (e.g., Pamela Grunwell's Phonological Assessment of Child Speech—PACS or Crystal's Profile of Phonology—PROPH), prosody (e.g., Crystal's Prosody Profile or PROP), or semantics (such as Crystal's Profile in Semantics—PRISM).

Grunwell's PACS was designed with the intent to provide a clinically viable comprehensive analysis of children's phonological systems that could be used to assess speech disorders using a standard procedure. PACS relies on spontaneous samples and emphasizes segmental analyses with a focus on consonants in the following positions: syllable initial word initial (SIWI), syllable initial within word (SIWW), syllable final within word (SFWW), and syllable final word final (SFWF). The analysis charts contain a phonetic inventory and distribution, systems of contrastive phones and contrastive assessments, phonological process analysis, and developmental assessments. Word-medial consonants, vowels, and other aspects of phonology (such as prosody or nonsegmental analyses) are not part of the PACS.

Another formalized assessment procedure of children's phonology is Crystal's PROPH, which shares similarities with PACS, but it is also different from it in nonnegligible ways. PROPH relies on analyzing 100 spontaneously produced words by the child, and it has segmental components as does PACS, but the analyses include both vowels and consonants unlike PACS, which focuses solely on the latter. The charts and the assessment goals are also different for the two

HU-LARSP Profile Chart in Hungarian

Név: _____ Életkor: _____ Adatgyűjtés napja: _____ Típusa: _____

A

Nem elemzett			Problémás	
1. Nem érthető	2. Egyéb reakciók (pl. nevetés, hangutánzó, stb.)	3. Nem tipikus	1. Befejezetlen	2. Félreérthető	3. Sztereotípiák

B Válaszok

			Tipikus válasz				Nem tipikus		
			Főbb (alanyt és állítmányt tartalmazó)						
		Ismételt	Kihagyásos			Hiányos	Teljes	Kevésbé fontos	Szerkezeti	Ø	Prob-lé-mák
Stimulus típusa	Össz		1	2	3+					
Kérdések										
Egyéb										

C Spontán

D Reakciók

	Általános	Szerkezeti	Ø	Egyéb	Problémák

I. szakasz (1;0 – 1;7)

Kevésbé fontos	Válaszok	Megszólító	Kijelentés	Egyéb	*Problémák*
Főbb (alany-állítm.)	Utasítás	Kérdés			
	'Ige'	'Kérdő'	Főnév:	Ige:	Egyéb	Problémák

Átlagos MLU-m: 1.1 (I szakasz)

(*Continued*)

(Continued)

Kapcs.	Megjelenő szófajok	Ragozás		Nyelvtani szerkezetek
II. szakasz (1;8 – 2;0)				*Kijelent mód:* *Felszólító mód:* *Tagadás "nem"-mel:* *Egyéb:* Átlagos MLU-m: 1.5 (II szakasz)
	Névmások: Személyes: Mutató: Birtokos:	*Főnév:* Tárgyragos: "-é" birtokjeles: Birtokos személyjellel: Helyraggal: Korai határozóragok (-ba, -be, -ban, -ben, -ra, -re):	*Ige:* Jelen idő: Általános: Határozott:	
és	*Névelő:* Határozott: Határozatlan: *Névmások:* Határozatlan: Kérdő: Melléknév:	*Főnév:* Többes szám (-k): Határozóragok (pl. -on, -en, -ön, -hoz, -hez, -nál, -nél):	*Ige:* Múlt idő: Általános: Határozott:	*Mondatok:* Mellérendelő összetett: *Tagadó szerkezet:* *Egyéb:* Átlagos MLU-m: 3.0 (III szakasz)
Egyéb				
III. szakasz (2;1 – 2;6)				
ha	*Határozószó:* *Névutó:* *Névmások:* Visszaható: Kölcsönös: *Segédige:* *Módosítószó:*	További határozóragok (pl. -val, -vel, -tól, -től, -ig):	*Ige:* Szám (valamennyi): Személy (valamennyi):	*Segédige:* *Módosítószó:* *Mondatok* Kérdő szerkezetek: Alárendelő összetett: Elváló igekötők: *Egyéb:* Átlagos MLU-m: 4.0 (IV szakasz)
Egyéb				
IV. szakasz (2;7 – 3;0)				
	Névmások: Vonatkozó:	További határozóragok:	*Ige:* Feltételes mód:	*Mondatok:* Feltételes szerkezetek: Többszörösen összetett: *Egyéb:* Átlagos MLU-m: 4.6 (V szakasz)
V. szakasz (3;0 – 3;6)				
Összes mondat száma:		Fordulónkénti mondatok száma:		MLU-m:

HU-LARSP Profile Chart in English

Name: _____ **Age:** _____ **Sample Date:** _____ **Type:** _____

A Unanalyzed

1. Unintelligible	2. Symbolic Noise	3. Atypical	Problematic		
			1. Incomplete	2. Ambiguous	3. Stereotypes

B Responses

			Totals	Repetitions	Elliptical			Major		Typical Response	Atypical		
					1	2	3+	Reduced	Full	Minor	Structural	Ø	Problems
Stimulus Type	Questions												
	Others												

C Spontaneous

D Reactions

	General	Structural	Ø	Other	Problems

Stage I (1;0 – 1;7)

Minor   *Vocatives*

Major   *Responses*

Comm.	Quest.	Statement	Other
'V'	'Q'	'N'	

Problems

Typical MLU-m: 1.1 (Stage I)
Other   Problems

Conn.   Emerging Parts of Speech   Inflection   Grammatical Structures

Stage II (1;8 – 2;0)

Pronouns:
Personal:
Demonstrative:
Possessive:

Noun:
Accusative:
Genitive "-é":
Possessive:
Positional:
Early adverb forming (-ba, -be, -ban, -ben, -ra, -re):

Verb:
Present:
Indefinite:
Definite:

Declarative:
Imperative:
Negation with "*nem*":
Other:
Typical MLU-m: 1.5 (Stage II)

(Continued)

1104 Linguistic Profiles

Stage III (2;1 – 2;6)	*és*	*Determiners:* Definite article: Indefinite article: *Pronouns:* Indefinite: Interrogative: *Adjectives:*	*Noun:* Plural (-k): Adverb forming (e.g., -on, -en, -ön, -hoz, -hez, -nál, -nél):	*Verb:* Past: General Past: Definite Past:	*Clauses & Phrases:* Coord. Complex Sent.: *Negation (various):* Other: Typical MLU-m: 3.0 (Stage III)
	Other			
Stage IV (2;7 – 3;0)	*ba*	*Adverbs:* Postpositions: *Pronouns:* Reflexive: Reciprocal:	Further adverb forming (pl. -val, -vel, -tól, -től, -ig):	*Verb:* All plurals: Persons:	*Aux:* *Modals:* *Clauses* Complex questions: Subordinate clauses: *Phrases* Detaching co-verbs: Other: Typical MLU-m: 4.0 (Stage IV)
	Other	*Aux:* *Modals:*		
Stage V (3;0 – 3;6)		*Pronouns:* Relative:	Further adverb forming:	*Verb:* Conditional Mood:	*Clauses:* Conditional structures: Complex subordinate: Other: Typical MLU-m: 4.6 (Stage V)
	Total Number of Sentences:		Mean Number of Sentences Per Turn		MLU-m:

Figure 1 HU-LARSP Charts

Source: Bunta, Bóna, and Gósy (2016, pp. 96, 97). Reproduced by permission.

measures. PROPH provides phonemic inventory analyses both from an accuracy and from an error pattern perspective. It also incorporates phonological feature analyses taking syllable structure into consideration, and phonological processes are also analyzed at the end of the chart. The phonological analyses of PROPH can be complemented by prosodic analyses (such as intonation patterns) that can be obtained via the PROP.

PRISM—also developed by Crystal—offers a range of analyses of a child's productions from a largely semantic point of view broken into two subtests: PRISM-L (Profile in Semantics, lexis) and PRISM-G (Profile in Semantics, grammatical). The former deals with the relationship between semantics and the lexicon, and the latter analyzes the relationship between semantics and grammar. PRISM necessitates the collection of language samples from a range of topics using various linguistic constructions so that the semantic aspects of the child's speech can be analyzed. The purpose of PRISM-L is to assess how vocabulary is organized into semantic fields by mapping the range of lexical items used by the child. PRISM-G, on the other hand, is used to analyze how meaning is conveyed by grammatical components of an utterance.

The legacy of the works discussed above is that today, no respected speech and language assessment could afford to be linguistically naive or ignore attested evidence-based patterns of speech and language development in children. In fact, a testament to the enduring nature of these classic linguistic profiles is that these measures not only continue to influence and inspire new assessments in the field of child speech and language and its disorders (such as new versions of LARSP in a growing number of languages), but they are still being used today as they were originally intended—a hallmark of seminal works that continue to have a significant impact on the field.

Ferenc Bunta, Judit Bóna, and Mária Gósy

See also Clinical Linguistics; Language Assessment; Language Sampling; Language Therapy and Intervention; Preschool Language Intervention; Syntax and Grammar

Further Readings

Bunta, F., Bóna, J., & Gósy, M. (2016). HU-LARSP: Assessing children's language skills in Hungarian. In P. Fletcher, M. J. Ball, & D. Crystal (Eds.), *Profiling grammar: More languages of LARSP* (pp. 80–98). Bristol, UK: Multilingual Matters.

Crystal, D. (2012). On the origin of LARSPecies. In M. J. Ball, D. Crystal, & P. Fletcher (Eds.), *Assessing grammar: The languages of LARSP* (pp. 4–11). Tonawanda, NY: Multilingual Matters.

Crystal, D., Fletcher, P., & Garman, M. (1976). The grammatical analysis of language disability: A procedure for assessment and remediation. London, UK: Edward Arnold.

Fletcher, P., Ball, M. J., & Crystal, D. (Eds.). (2016). *Profiling grammar: More languages of LARSP*. Bristol, UK: Multilingual Matters.

Grunwell, P. (1985). *Phonological assessment of child speech (PACS)*. San Diego, CA: College Hill Press.

Linguistic Typology

Linguistic typology is a discipline that studies linguistic diversity. Its main goal, as noted by Balthasar Bickel, is to explain "why linguistic diversity is the way it is." Linguistic typology is interested in both differences and similarities between the languages, because these are interrelated. Since languages can differ or be similar at various levels of language structure—phonology, syntax, morphology, semantics, and so on—linguistic typology is relevant for all these domains. This entry discusses language universals; the role of a language sample; synchronic, diachronic, and areal typology; and the issue of crosslinguistic comparison.

The history of linguistic typology as a discipline goes back at least 2.5 centuries. During this period it has been shaped by numerous scholars, with Friedrich von Schlegel, Georg von der Gabelentz, Nikolai Trubetzkoy, Edward Sapir, and Roman Jakobson among its founding figures. The discipline in its modern form took off in the 1960s influenced by Joseph Greenberg's study on word order universals.

Language Universals

What does linguistic typology encompass? A systematic comparison of language structures allows linguists to determine differences and similarities across languages. Every new difference that is observed between languages extends the limits of crosslinguistic variation, while every new similarity establishes new limits on structural variation within a human language. The two processes run hand in hand and form the core of linguistic typology. Similarities that constitute recurrent patterns across languages are used by linguists to formulate typological generalizations, or *language universals*. This term is used for linguistic phenomena that are found in most or, at least, in a significant number of human languages. Language universals fall into four following types. First, language universals can be *implicational* and *nonimplicational* (the latter is alternatively called *unrestricted*). The term *implicational* infers a correlation of two or more parameters, and this is what these universals are about. An implicational universal can be schematized as "If P, then Q." A nonimplicational universal, on the other hand, does not involve any correlation and focuses on just one linguistic parameter. Second, both implicational and nonimplicational universals can be *statistical* and *absolute*. Statistical universals hold for most, but not all, languages. They are alternatively called universal tendencies. Absolute universals, on the other hand, are assumed to hold for every single language. Absolute universals are few in number, and in principle, they have a highly hypothetical nature for the reason that that we do not (and never will) have information about all of the world's languages. All universals, in general, give us an idea about *preferences* of languages for certain structures. Implicational universals, in particular, provide additionally an insight on the structure and *dependencies* within a language system. Table 1 gives an example of each type of language universal.

In fact, all linguistic universals—either statistical or absolute, implicational or not— are hypotheses that are continuously being tested against data that emerge from previously unknown or under-described languages all over the globe. An example is the discovery of languages with object-before-subject basic word order. Greenberg's seminal study in the 1960s was the first to put forward a list of language universals, many of which hold until the current day. Greenberg was careful and cautious in his formulations, aware that most of them are tendencies rather than absolutes. However, the language sample that was used for the study did not contain any languages with object-before-subject word order, leading to a conclusion that such languages are nonoccurring at all or are excessively rare. It was generally assumed so, before Desmond Derbyshire demonstrated in the 1970s that the South American language Hixkaryana, spoken by about 350 people in northern Brazil, does have the object-before-subject as pragmatically unmarked (or regular) word order. Today, we know of more languages with this characteristic, leading to a rebuttal of an earlier suggested universal and, therefore, to an adjustment to our understanding of what is possible in a human language.

Explanations for language universals have been a matter of some debate among scholars. Explanations that have been proposed include cultural–historical, functional, and cognitive factors, or a combination of these. Some examples involve the notions of processing, economy, and iconicity. An explanation in terms of processing suggests that those linguistic structures that require less cognitive effort and are easier to process will be preferred by languages. The notion of economy refers to the tendency for frequently used elements to get reduced, as well as the tendency for highly predictable elements to get eliminated. The competing notion of iconicity proposes that the more complex the formal expression, the more complex is the semantic notion that is expressed, and vice

Table 1   Examples of Language Universals

	Absolute	*Statistical*
Implicational	In all languages, if there is /m/, there is also /n/.	If a language has object–verb word order, it is also likely to have postpositions.
Nonimplicational (unrestricted)	In all languages, there are stop consonants.	In most languages, the singular is the base form and the plural is the overtly marked form.

Source: Based on Moravcsik (2010, p. 70) and Velupillai (2012, pp. 31, 33).

versa. Historical factors relate to universal sources and constrains on language change, as well as long-term genealogical inheritance of language structures, or language contact in the past.

Language Sample

To search for similarities, differences, and dependencies among language structures, it is important to consider a large variety of languages. Not only is it undoable to include all documented languages in a comparison, it can be also problematic. Most linguistic characteristics show some kind of skewing in their distribution, whether it is a geographic skewing (clustering of unrelated languages with a certain characteristic in one area) or a genealogical one (retaining of a certain characteristic within a language family). It is therefore important to have a language sample that is representative and balanced from genealogical and geographic points of view. That is, a sample should contain languages from maximally different genealogical units and contain languages from diverse geographic areas (such as continents) but should also avoid clusters of languages spoken in a geographic proximity.

In general, the larger and the more diverse a sample is, the more robust the results are of a crosslinguistic comparison. However, the way a language sample is put together is determined by the exact purpose of a study.

Language typology depends considerably on the existence, quantity, and quality of data on the languages. It is often the case that a language sample has to be adjusted according to availability of sufficient data on a language. According to the overview by Harald Hammarström (the most systematic and thorough account of the current state of language documentation), about 30% of the world's languages have a full grammatical description and an additional 25% have a grammar sketch (which is, unfortunately, not always sufficient for typological research). Although there is lack of typological data for the other half of the world's languages, the overall picture now is more optimistic than 50 years before.

Synchronic, Diachronic, and Areal Typology

Language typology that has been considered so far is referred to as *synchronic* typology, that is, comparison of languages that are contemporaneous with each other. In synchronic typology, linguists are interested in language universals; however, for an explanation of exceptions to the universals, they may need to turn to diachronic typology or areal typology. *Diachronic* typology involves comparison of languages at various stages of their development. As argued by William Croft, in synchronic typology, language types are viewed as states that languages are in. In diachronic typology, on the other hand, language types are taken as stages that languages pass through. Since deep-time historical data are available only on a fraction of the world's languages, this is a handy solution in order to explore—at least hypothetically—a development of certain structures. Examining genealogically related languages can be particularly valuable here: Related languages can be the best approximations for different stages of development of one initial language type as found in their proto-language. But here, of course, typologists have to abstract from the fact that the rules of language can change too in the meantime. Finally, *areal* typology (a notion that combines areal linguistics and linguistic typology) is concerned with patterns in the geographic distribution of language structures. When speakers of two or more languages are in contact for a longer period of time, it is typical that characteristics of one language spread to another language. As a result, languages start to resemble each other. This leads to the emergence of *linguistic areas* or *Sprachbunds*, where unrelated or distantly related languages share linguistic characteristics that are not inherited from their respective proto-languages.

Issue of Crosslinguistic Comparison

One of the challenges in linguistic typology is the so-called problem of crosslinguistic identification. Since comparison of languages is central in the discipline, it is fundamental that linguistic phenomena that are being compared are indeed comparable. For example, a crosslinguistic study on word order of nouns and adjectives would likely run into a problem as to what can be taken as adjective in languages A, B, and C. In English, concepts such as "big," "old," and "red" are different from the concepts "eat," "grow," and "stand," denoting actions or states, for three major reasons. First, they show a different syntactic behavior (the role they play in a sentence or phrase). Second, they show different morphological behavior (use different sets of morphological markers). And third, the semantic notions they encode are, obviously, different. This gives us enough ground to identify adjectives in English. In the Sáliban language Mako, spoken in the Venezuelan Amazon, concepts such as big, old, and red differ neither syntactically nor morphologically from those such as eat, grow, and stand. Thus, using exclusively formal or structural criteria would not be helpful to identify a phenomenon crosslinguistically, particularly since structural variation among the world's languages is huge. A possible way out is to hinge the identification on semantic criteria or functional ones (taken broadly, with factors that are external to the language system). For a crosslinguistic comparison in phonology, one would likely use parameters based on articulatory–acoustic properties, and ultimately, speech organs.

Olga Krasnoukhova

See also Descriptive Linguistics; Diversity; Indigenous Languages; Language; Language Families; Language Sampling; Morphology; Phonology; Semantics; Syntax and Grammar

Further Readings

Allan, K. (Ed.). (2016). *The Routledge handbook of linguistics*. London, UK: Routledge.

Bickel, B. (2007). Typology in the 21st century: Major current developments. *Linguistic Typology, 11*(1), 239–251. https://doi.org/10.1515/LINGTY.2007.018

Comrie, B. (1989). *Language universals and linguistic typology* (2nd ed.). Oxford, UK: Basil Blackwell.

Croft, W. (2003). *Typology and universals*. Cambridge, UK: Cambridge University Press.

Derbyshire, D. (1977). Word order universals and the existence of OVS languages. *Linguistic Inquiry, 8*(3), 590–599.

Dryer, M. S. (1989). Large linguistic areas and language sampling. *Studies in Language, 13*(2), 257–292. http://doi.org/10.1075/sl.13.2.03dry

Dryer, M. S., & Haspelmath, M. (Eds.). (2013). *The world atlas of language structures online*. Leipzig, Germany: Max Planck Institute for Evolutionary Anthropology. Retrieved from http://wals.info

Greenberg, J. H. (1963). Some universals of grammar with particular reference to the order of meaningful elements. In J. H. Greenberg (Ed.), *Universals of language* (pp. 58–90). Cambridge, MA: MIT Press.

Greenberg, J. H. (1965). Synchronic and diachronic universals in phonology. *Language, 42*, 508–517.

Hammarström, H. (2014). *The status of description of the world's languages*. Nijmegen, The Netherlands: Radboud University.

Mithun, M. (2016). Typology, documentation, description, and typology. *Linguistic Typology, 20*(3), 467–472. https://doi.org/10.1515/lingty-2016-0019

Moravcsik, E. (2010). Explaining language universals. In J. J. Song (Ed.), *The Oxford handbook of linguistic typology* (pp. 69–89). Oxford, UK: Oxford University Press.

Muysken, P. (2016). Language contact: Trojan horse or new potential for cross-fertilization? *Linguistic Typology, 20*(3), 537–545. https://doi.org/10.1515/lingty-2016-0025

Plank, F. (Ed.). (2003). *The universals archive*. Electronic database. Retrieved from http://typo.uni-konstanz.de/archive/intro/

Song, J. J. (Ed.). (2010). *The Oxford handbook of linguistic typology*. Oxford, UK: Oxford University Press.

Stassen, L. (1985). *Comparison and universal grammar*. Oxford, UK: Basil Blackwell.

Velupillai, V. (2012). *An introduction to linguistic typology*. Amsterdam, The Netherlands/Philadelphia, PA: John Benjamins Publishing.

LINGUISTICS

Linguistics refers to the systematic study of human language: oral, written, and signed. It is an interdisciplinary scientific field whose aim is to construct a unified theory of human language by identifying the overt and covert mechanisms that make language an attribute unique to humans. Linguistics observes and describes human language aiming to find generalizable rules and representations of underlying structure, in order to draw conclusions about its general nature, and its development in individuals and in humankind.

The complexity involved in language as a genetic, cognitive, social, and cultural endowment in a single individual is amplified by the variability found in the languages of the world (over 7,000 living languages) across different groups of individuals, populations, and ages, on national scales, as well as worldwide. As such, linguistics is simultaneously related to the humanities and to the natural and behavioral sciences, hovering along an arts/sciences continuum. Linguistics combines both theoretically abstract and empirical approaches that influence each other in a two-way reciprocal regime, setting the study of the foundational principles of grammar within the more general framework of linguistic theory.

Limitations on actual evidence, in the form of linguistic data and scientific testimony, translate into limitations on the objectivity and universal applicability of linguistic theories. At the same time, such shortage catapults this fascinating field into a vibrant, continually evolving research industry, whose findings have fundamental significance and direct applications in fields such as human communication disorders, education, second-language pedagogy, bilingual education, translation, anthropology, and law, among others. This entry examines aspects in linguistics in the following five main sections: terms and definitions, linguistic subfields, linguistics as a relay race, advances in linguistic theory, and toward a unified theory of language.

Terms and Definitions

The term *linguistics* is a hybrid derived from Latin *lingua* meaning "language, tongue" and the English suffixes *-ist*, "the person practicing or concerned with," and *-ics*, "pertaining to." *Lingua* is argued to come from the Proto-Indo-European (PIE) putative root **dnghu-* "tongue" (4th millennium BCE); evidence of its existence are Old Latin *dingua* (before 75 BCE), Old English *tunge* (5th to 11th century), and Old Irish *tenge* (6th to 10th century). *Linguist* is first attested in the 1580s to mean "a master of languages" or "one who uses his tongue freely." By the 1640s, a linguist was a "student of language" and a linguister an early colonial interpreter between Europeans and American Indians. The adjective linguistic, meaning "of language" or "of linguistics," is first recorded in English between 1830 and 1840, possibly from German *linguistisch* (1807) or French *linguistique* (1833).

According to the *Oxford English Dictionary*, the use of *linguistics* to mean "pertaining to language(s)" (1847) is not supported by etymological considerations, having dominated over the earlier linguistry (1794) and the more appropriate lingual. Reversely, *linguistician* is attested from 1895 as a more accurate, though hardly used, synonym of *linguist*. *Linguist* has widely survived crosslinguistically to mean "expert or student of language science," for example, *linguiste* (French), *linguista* (Portuguese, Spanish), *linguïst* (Dutch), *lingvist* (Romanian, Swedish), *lingwist* (Polish), and *lingvista* (Czech).

Other synonyms of *linguistics*, meaning "the study or science of language(s)" (1847), are of Greek descent first attested in English as *philology* "love of speech/language" (1716) from *philos* "friend" and *logos* "speech, letters"; also comparative *philology* (1822); and *logonomy* from *logos* "speech" and *nomos* "law, rule" (1803). *Philologue* (1590s) and *philologer* (1650s) are disused terms for *linguist* these days. Similarly, *glossology* and *glottology* are less commonly used terms to mean *linguistics*, also derived from Ancient Greek *glossa* (Ionic dialect) or *glotta* (Attic dialect) "language, tongue" and *-logos*, loosely meaning "the study of." Interestingly, while the Latin-born *linguist* is singly adopted by several European languages, Italian (the direct descendant of Latin) also uses *glottologo*, much like the Modern Greek usage: *glossologos*.

Linguistic Subfields

Linguistics is concerned with the oral, written, and signed versions of human language. The fact that we speak before we learn to write is evidence of the primacy of spoken over written form. Contemporary linguists are primarily interested in investigating spoken language because it is, by default, closer to our original state as human beings and, thus, more revealing of what is involved in the language faculty per se. Written language data are secondary in the sense that they imitate or represent actual speech. Texts are customarily characteristic of better organization, well-formedness, and closer compliance to grammatical rules, because we have more time available to ruminate and write than when we speak.

Written language is also less liable to external influence and change over time. Sign language, that is, the language of manual (*cheremic*) rather than oral communication, displays, by and large, the same fundamental properties as spoken language.

There is a main distinction between *general*, *descriptive*, and *applied* linguistics that concerns concepts, description, and application of knowledge, respectively. Linguistics investigates language and its use both synchronically and diachronically. *Synchronic linguistics* observes, compares, and describes the current state of affairs in languages and individuals as snapshots in time. *Diachronic linguistics* investigates the origins and evolution of human language in the history of humankind, but also how language develops in individuals longitudinally in the course of months or years, focusing on both the process of transition and its end result.

Mirroring language itself, linguistics covers several areas, at higher and lower levels of structural complexity. To elucidate this, the *tree metaphor* is mentioned that is historically used to illustrate linguistic classifications since ca. 1800. Historical linguist August Schleicher first suggested striking similarities between biological and linguistic families. Though not all-encompassing, tree models help illustrate various concepts as branch points; sets of dependent features attached to each of these branch points distinguish among objects at other levels, above and below. Like a trunk that splits into two parts, linguistics separates into *theoretical* (abstract) and *applied* (functional). The theoretical part includes traditional grammar and theoretical stances originating in psychology, sociology, philosophy, logic, anthropology, mathematics, computer science, language pathology, and so on. The applied part separates into two sections: the *descriptive* (meaning "practiced/exercised") and the *applied* (meaning "relating or bearing to other domains").

In a bottom-up approach (A), linguistic theory derives from applied linguistics by means of descriptive linguistics (see Figure 1). It is an oxymoron (B) that "applied linguistics" is customarily suggestive of a priori theoretical elaborations that are actually applied to the understanding of language.

What actually holds is a loop action (Figure 2): Information gained from applied linguistics feeds specific theoretical postulations that come back in the form of a more generalizable theory to inform understanding of the language faculty, all via the medium of linguistic description that itself incorporates methodology (how), systemic theory (what linguistic concept), and evidence (what linguistic fact).

In short, the scope of each one of these subareas is hardly distinct and their sustained interaction is inevitable. Classifying and numbering distinct linguistic areas is admittedly an arbitrary process, because there is some divergence and overlap in what linguists recognize as areas in linguistics. The present entry aims to be comprehensive but not categorical or exhaustive.

Theoretical Linguistics

Theoretical linguistics encompasses the study of *grammar* (the framework describing the structural composition of languages and their *typology*, i.e., concepts, rules, and functional features) as well as *theoretical hypotheses* on core issues such as what language is, how it works, what its properties are, the role of universal characteristics and the brain, and the role of communicative contexts

A	B
LINGUISTIC THEORY	LINGUISTIC THEORY
↑	↓
DESCRIPTIVE LINGUISTICS	DESCRIPTIVE LINGUISTICS
↑	↓
APPLIED LINGUISTICS	APPLIED LINGUISTICS

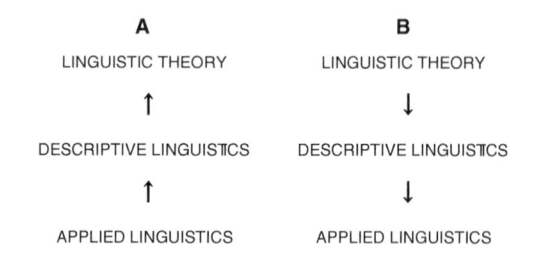

Figure 1 Bottom-Up and Top-Down Approaches in Linguistics

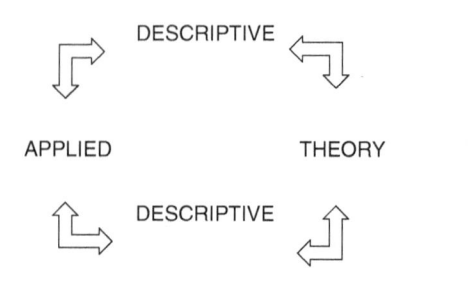

Figure 2 The Loop Approach in Linguistics

in language use, among others. Answers to such questions have taken millennia along a slow but continuous relay race that has led to the development of theoretical models about language. These are discussed in more detail in the section Linguistics as a Relay Race, below.

Systemic Theory

The four classical levels of grammatical representation are *phonology, morphology, syntax*, and *semantics*, dividing language into four main tiers on the systemic level; *lexicon* is also added to these because of the grammatical and representational significance of the inventory of words in a language; *pragmatics* and *discourse analysis* are also examined nowadays on the usage-based level.

- Phonology studies human speech sounds as the ultimately fundamental units of language and the contrastive relationships between them.
- Morphology studies the internal structure of words and their formation and modification in relationship to other words in the language.
- Syntax studies word order and word combinations in utterances.
- Semantics studies the meanings of words and fixed phrases and how these combine to form meaning in utterances.
- Lexicon studies both the inventory of words in a language and the set of structural rules that make up its grammar. The *mental lexicon*, as a primary cognitive function in humans, is responsible for several processes (e.g., activation, storage, processing, and retrieval of words) that are involved in the acquisition and use of language.

Usage-Based Theory

- Pragmatics studies how the meanings of words and of word combinations interact with contextual and other nonlinguistic information during language use. *Speech acts* (e.g., threats, requests, apologies, declarations) provide essential information on subtle features of language, such as communicative intent and hearer inferences.
- Discourse analysis studies language in natural settings (e.g., informal conversations, office documents, televised debates), mainly aiming to reveal the sociopsychological characteristics of the speakers, rather than the structure of the text itself.

Descriptive Linguistics

Descriptive linguistics has marked a significant change in the way that linguists approach the study of language, in that it is interested in language for its own sake; this is opposed to an earlier approach whereby linguists decided on a single standard (usually based on literary texts) and prescribed all language use based on that standard. Through observation and description, linguists nowadays discover the rules and principles that govern language use in different individuals and groups of people in all likely contexts. Major areas in descriptive linguistics include *comparative linguistics, historical linguistics, etymology, field linguistics,* and *experimental linguistics*.

- Comparative linguistics compares the similarities and differences of languages in terms of *linguistic typology*, that is, the structural and functional features of their grammatical representations (phonology, morphology, syntax, semantics, and their interfaces).

- Historical linguistics is interested in linguistic prehistory and recorded history studying known languages and their families in order to determine the origins of language and the properties of its evolution. Linguistic history is investigated both *externally* (social and migration influences on the speakers of a language) and *internally* (changes in the language itself).

- Etymology is a subarea in linguistics that is dependent on both historical and comparative linguistics. Etymology investigates the origins and historical evolution of words by utilizing the *comparative method* to analyze older and contemporary texts in related languages and make inferences regarding their common features and meaning.

- Field linguistics (or *fieldwork*) refers to a methodological stance that is indispensable for the development of the field of linguistics; primary linguistic data in unknown or little-studied languages (e.g., primitive/indigenous languages, dialects, non-Western languages) are collected in natural settings by personal contact, are analyzed in terms of linguistic phenomena, and are disseminated. Though "fieldwork" is a rudimentary aspect of linguistics, in general, in the sense of data collection in experimental and naturalistic settings, field linguistics is mostly concerned with prolonged and intensive investigations that amass extensive and detailed pools of data, commonly referred to as *corpus/corpora*.

Corpus/corpora. There are several corpora comprising collections of recorded utterances as linguistic evidence to be used for descriptive language analysis. Such data sets are *cross-sectional*, meaning that data are collected (without regard to differences in time) from many different speakers who share at least one common attribute, such as monolingualism, bilingualism, tongue slips, foreignness, or a communication disorder. Among these, the Max Planck Institute's IMDI-corpora of spoken and written crosslinguistic data are worth noting. Also, corpora on child language data—monolingual/bilingual, phonological—are represented by the *CHILDES* database, BilingBank, and PhonBank, respectively. Fromkin's Speech Error Database at the Max Planck Institute is a repository of crosslinguistic tongue slips in adults. The largest collection of crosslinguistic examples of second-language (L2) English speech can be found in the Speech Accent Archive, but the LeaP corpus is also concerned with nonnative German and English data. Digital archives of linguistic data characteristic of a communication disorder are the DisorderedSpeechBank and AphasiaBank. Online depositories of phonological resources, such as the UCLA Phonetics Laboratory Archive and VoxForge, also exist. Alongside publicized (and unpublicized) cross-sectional corpora, there also exist *single case study corpora* of longitudinal, uninterrupted, and dense records of child monolingual or bilingual speech over several consecutive months of linguistic development.

Among the largest and denser ones are those recorded by Werner F. Leopold and Neil Smith (in diary notes) and M. A. Macken and Elena Babatsouli (in audio recordings).

Annotation. The analysis of spoken linguistic data requires its transcription in *orthographic* (e.g., graphemes, pictographs, ideographs) and *notational* (graphics representing technical terms and standards) symbols that are decided upon by convention. Orthography, which may include spelling, hyphenation, capitalization, and punctuation, can be one of three types based on the primary grammatical unit represented: *alphabetical* (speech sound or phoneme), *syllabic* (syllable), and *logographic* (word or morpheme). All European languages have alphabetical writing systems, for example, Latin, Greek, and Cyrillic. Japanese and Cherokee are languages using a *syllabary*, while Chinese is a logographic language. In some cases, a language can be written in all three writing systems (e.g., Japanese). Linguistics also uses a *gloss* or *glossaries* as brief *marginal* (on the same line) or *interlinear* (on different lines) notations. These can either be the translation of a term in another language, usually signified by 'single quotes' (marginal), or capitalized-letter abbreviations of grammatical terms (interlinear). A well-established conventional system of interlinear gloss is the Leipzig Glossing Rules, of which an example is provided next with 1, PL, COM, PST, and ALL standing for 1st person, plural, comitative case, past tense, and allative, respectively:

Other types of notation include *phonetic transcriptions*, that is, visual representations of human speech sounds that may be either *phonemes* (abstract representations) or *phones* (actual sounds). The first phonetic transcription dates back to 500 BCE Sanskrit. The most widely used

Russian

My	s	Marko	poexa-l-i	avtobus-om	v	Peredelkino.
1PL	COM	Marko	go-PST-PL	bus-INS	ALL	Peredelkino
we	with	Marko	go-PST-PL	bus-by	to	Peredelkino

'Marko and I went to Perdelkino by bus.'

phonetic alphabets, comprising *graphemes* (smallest meaningful contrastive writing unit), *diacritics* (signs, accents, cedillas above or below a letter denoting pronunciation change), and *suprasegmentals* (contrastive elements beyond the segment, in the syllable or word) are the International Phonetic Association's International Phonetic Alphabet (IPA), which notates normal speech sounds across languages; the American Phonetic Alphabet (APA); utilizes a combination of standard graphemes (from Latin or Greek) and diacritics; the Extended IPA (ExtIPA), which accounts for disordered speech; and the Shriberg & Kent (SK) system for clinical phonetics, which informs both targeted speech and production. Nevertheless, phonetic transcription, even in its narrowest form, tends to be impressionistic and subjective. The IPA phonetic transcription of intended *linguistics* is /lɪŋˈɡwɪstɪks/; this may be pronounced as [lɪŋˈɡwɪstɪks] in native English speech, as *[lɪŋˈɡwɪstɪŋks] in a tongue slip, or as *[lɪɡuˈɪstɪks] and *[lɪŋˈɡvɪstɪks] in second-language English speech. The asterisk denotes *ungrammatical*.

Speech analysis software. Speech analysis software (SAS) is used these days to ease the management, organization, retrieval, and sharing of linguistic data in all representational notations, as well as to automate and enhance the reliability of analytic processes, such as frequency computations and interrater assessments. Such software include the Max Planck Institute's EUDICO Linguistic Annotator (ELAN), Computerized Language Analysis (CLAN), Phon (phonological analysis program), Systematic Analysis of Language Transcripts (SALT), Computerized Profiling (CP), Computerized Articulation and Phonology Evaluation System (CAPES), EXMARaLDA, ANVIL (for video annotation), and web-based archiving. Such software permit alignment of audio/video extracts to linguistic annotation and coding schemes for fast retrieval of specific information and allow researchers to include *metalinguistic* information, that is, how the researcher's own knowledge of language relates (or influences the interpretation of) pragmatic aspects of its use.

- Experimental linguistics investigates both the *production* and *perception* of speech during its acquisition and social use, utilizing a combination of comparative studies of data derived from text corpora, psycho/neurolinguistic laboratory experiments, quantitative methods (e.g., statistical techniques), and computational modeling. Experimental linguistics tests the legitimacy of hypotheses on real-time language representation in the mind/brain, utilizing inferential statistics. This approach complements formal and field methods in linguistics.

Applied Linguistics

Applied linguistics is a problem-driven domain, characteristic of both an *interdisciplinary* approach and a *practical* approach. The study of language overlaps with sociology, anthropology, psychology, mathematics/statistics, speech pathology, computer science, and acoustics, among other disciplines. This interdisciplinary perspective answers theoretical questions about the nature of language, which, in turn, provide applied solutions to language-related problems. Applications to concerns of professional practice are found in teaching, translation, lexicography, assessment and intervention for language/speech pathology, logopedics, and so forth. Major subfields in applied linguistics include the following:

- *Sociolinguistics* is concerned with the study of language as a social and cultural function. It examines how social identity (e.g., age, education, gender, class, race) affects language use in different contexts (*sociolects*). Sociolinguists observe and describe *vernacular* languages (the colloquial or informal versions of languages as opposed to their standard or literary varieties), *dialects* (language characteristics that are peculiar of certain social groups or geographic regions), and *idiolects* (i.e., the particular speech habits and language style of individuals).

- *Anthropological linguistics* (and *ethnolinguistics*), similarly, examines how the social life and cultural practices of individuals relate to language. Having its origins in the study of indigenous cultures and languages in the United States, this subfield of linguistics has spurred an interest in whether and how language and culture construct and/or preserve each other.

- *Quantitative linguistics* is an empirically based subfield that applies statistics and other mathematical methods to investigate laws operating behind language structure, diachronic change, and language acquisition and use.

- *Computational linguistics* is concerned with the development of computational models of language processing and learning in the brain that are neuroscientifically and cognitively probable. Such models formulate grammatical frameworks for the characterization and analysis of language and attempt to discover learning principles and processing techniques that represent the actual structural and statistical (distributional) properties of language. Ultimately, computational linguistics aims for the creation of computer systems that have human-like linguistic competence in language acquisition, machine translation, voice recognition, text analysis and summarization, and so on.

- *Phonetics* studies the physical properties of human speech sounds in production and perception.

- *Psycholinguistics* examines the psychological and cognitive influences involved in language perception, comprehension, production, acquisition, and use. It involves key fields such as biology, psychology, neuroscience, cognitive science, and information science; it also intersects with experimental and quantitative linguistics. Nevertheless, while psycholinguistics investigates executive functions (e.g., working memory) and general principles of brain processing, experimental linguistics primarily focuses on linguistic representations and the constraints that render representations variable. Subfields of psycholinguistics are the following:

  - *Neurolinguistics* studies the cognitive and physiological workings of human brain processes as they relate to the comprehension, production, and acquisition of language. Originating in *aphasiology* (i.e., brain damage), this subfield utilizes various experimental techniques such as electrophysiology, brain imaging, and computer modeling.
  - *Developmental linguistics* (or *language acquisition*) is concerned with how humans acquire language in various settings. These include children acquiring one language (*first-language acquisition* [FLA]), two languages/dialects (*bilinguals/bilectals*), or more languages/dialects (*multilinguals/multilectals*). This subfield also includes the study of how adults acquire a second (third, etc.) language in native or foreign language contexts, or how they acquire a second dialect, for example, Latin American Spanish rather than European Spanish (*second-language acquisition* [SLA]).
  - *Clinical linguistics* applies linguistic theories, methods, and findings to the understanding and intervention of language and speech pathology. *Language disorder* is a failure in the development and use of language, as in *aphasia*, *autism*, *developmental phonological disorder*, *dysarthria*, *dyspraxia*, and *specific language impairment* (SLI). *Speech disorder* involves a breakdown of the articulators (e.g., lips, tongue, palate), or of speech mechanisms, in general. Speech disorders are classified into disorders of *articulation* (relating to the movement of articulators, e.g., cleft lip/palate), *fluency* (relating to speech continuity, e.g., stuttering), and *voice* (relating to the failure of vocal mechanisms, e.g., resonance and phonation).

Linguistics as a Relay Race

The leitmotif of *similarity/difference* is undoubtedly pervasive in linguistics. It stems from a theoretical debate on anomaly and analogy, which exemplifies the continuity and steadfastness of fundamental notions in linguistics, such as universals and language-specific and individual-specific differences, since early times. Substantive evidence of linguistic prehistory is lost together with the original texts on logic, rhetoric, and religion that documented it. There is, overall, an agreement that recorded linguistic history in the Western world has evolved in an uninterrupted streak from the Sophists (3rd to 5th century BCE), to Hellenism (4th to 1st century BCE), to medieval Scholastics (12th to 16th century CE), to more modern times. Non-Western linguistic sources are found in China as early as the 13th century BCE, but non-Western formal grammatical tradition also dates back to the 4th century BCE in China and India. Panini's grammar for Sanskrit is monumental and has been very influential for modern Western linguistics. With its equal emphasis on literary and colloquial forms of language, it provides the earliest existing written grammar; it is also the most accurate code of language pronunciation than anything attempted until the late 19th century. Its core theoretical stances, however, do not diverge much from those of the Western tradition at the time. Grammars for Arabic, Armenian, and Hebrew developed subsequently, in the Dark Ages.

Traditional Grammarians

The Sophists. Linguistics as a *natural science* originates in traditional grammarians who started etymological reasoning: language has risen from *sound symbolism* such as *onomatopoeia*, that is, words imitating actual sounds such as *tweet*, *splash*, and *scratch*. Exceptions to this pattern led to a debate between the *analogists* and the *anomalists* (ca. 2nd century BCE) on the *regularity* of language. Dionysius Thrax (late 2nd century BCE) was the first linguist to write a comprehensive *grammar* in the Western world. Prior work carried out by the Sophists instituted the following distinctions: *gender* (Protagoras); *verbs/nouns* (Plato); *active/passive* verbs, *transitive/intransitive* verbs, *form/meaning*, and *case* (Stoics). Thrax expanded the systemic theory of grammar by adding distinctions for *adverb*, *pronoun*, and *preposition*.

Hellenistic grammarians. Hellenistic grammarians were the first to codify both *analogy* (similarity) and *anomaly* (difference) in the systematic grammar, also introducing principles of *syntax* (Apollonius Dyscolus). This era is responsible for the misconception of the *primacy of written language* as purer or more correct than spoken language, and for the *prescriptive approach* in linguistics. Hellenistic grammarians enforced a single *language standard* and prescribed how language ought to be spoken and written, largely ignoring linguistic variability in their systematic analyses. This stance dominated linguistic thought for more than two millennia.

The Romans. The Romans (2nd to 1st century BCE) espoused the earlier theoretical assumptions adapting Thrax's Greek grammar to Latin, mostly due to the similarities between the two languages. Donatus, Priscian, and Varro were the most notable grammarians during this period. Julius Caesar himself wrote a monograph, *On Analogy*, supporting the view of the existence of common patterns among languages.

The Scholastics. The Scholastics (or *Modistae*) (5th to 15th century BCE) introduced the notions of *science*, *metaphysics*, and *universal rules* in the study of language. Medieval scholars (such as William of Conches and Thomas of Erfurt) are also known as *speculative grammarians* in that they deduced grammatical categories from their causes. They suggested that language can be analyzed in terms of *modes* of *being*, *understanding*, and *signifying*, perhaps influenced by Aristotle's semantic hypothesis that things are represented by concepts that are themselves represented by words. Roger Bacon stood out as Doctor Mirabilis in advocating for a shared grammar among all languages, despite the presence of deviations. This is attributed to the high status Latin had at the time as *lingua franca* with many of the vernaculars actually deriving from it. This time also sees the beginning of grammars for vernacular languages such as Irish (7th century), Anglosaxon (10th century), Basque (10th century), Icelandic (12th century), and Provençal (13th century).

Humanists. Humanists (14th to 17th century), such as Petrarch and Erasmus, reintroduced the study of grammar as a means of comprehending ancient Greco-Roman classical literature (including Cicero's work), which continued to be considered more valuable and civilized than the existing vernaculars. With the advent of printing, the Renaissance revitalized and safeguarded ancient Greek and Roman texts, while also preserving Hebrew. At the same time, Dante's *De Vulgari Eloquentia* positively influenced grammarian endeavors to advance the study of vernaculars, leading to an abundance of new grammars.

Romanticists. Romanticists (18th century) further contributed to this trend publishing grammars for Old Germanic languages (Gothic, Norse, Old High German). They also advocated for a national character in language that affects its structure and its speakers' way of thinking, intricately relating race to language. Linguists of this era (e.g., Johann Gottfried Herder, Wilhelm von Humboldt) influenced 20th-century *relativity hypothesis* (language affects social and cognitive viewpoint), and *generative grammar* (language is rule governed), in visualizing language as "a system that makes infinite use of finite means" (Humboldt).

Main Schools of Thought

Despite the undoubtedly enormous effect of linguistic thought brewing since the dawn of human scholarship, pre-19th-century contributions are often considered theoretically meager. This section presents subsequent schools of thought.

Neogrammarianism

Comparative philologists (19th century) developed the *evolutional* point of view. August Schleicher assumed Proto-Indo-European as the common ancestor of all Indo-European (IE) languages, which led to the establishment of such concepts as *language family*, *language change*, and the *diachronic relationship* of languages. The discovery of *sound change laws* by neogrammarians (Jacob Grimm, Karl Verner) founded historical phonology and kindled an interest in dialects (*dialectology*). Languages are now assumed to diversify at different structural levels due to historical change.

Structuralism

Modern linguistics begins in the first half of the 20th century with Ferdinand de Saussure consolidating *structuralism* into a systematic linguistic theory: Linguistic units comprise a functional system of signs that are structurally interrelated (*langue*) and have a social and communicative function (*parole*). Key concepts introduced are *synchronic/diachronic relations* signifying a shift in grammatical correctness due to language change; *external/internal* distinctions based on the socially or crosslinguistic arbitrary and systemic nature of language; the *linearity* of linguistic units representing temporal reality; *syntagmatic/associative relations* of elements "inside" as opposed to "beyond" the utterance; and the dual physical (*signified*) and conceptual (*signifying*) nature of signs. Also, the primacy of spoken data over texts for linguistic theorizing is instituted.

Generative Theory

Noam Chomsky's generative theory advances the idea of language as a mental and abstract entity. According to *universal grammar*, languages share general characteristics that reflect fundamental properties of the mind. During language acquisition, there is an inherently human component (*language acquisition device*) that guides acquisition mechanisms crosslinguistically, as input triggers the *parameters* (switches) and sets the *principles* (grammatical rules) that determine language-specific particularities. Generative theory views language change as *rule change* in actual use across generations; mental processes and structures are influenced by external factors. Other principal concepts of generative theory include differentiations between *linguistic competence/performance*, *deep/surface* structures, and *conscious/unconscious* knowledge.

Advances in Linguistic Theory

These three schools of thought have had a paramount effect in modern linguistics introducing, by and large, the general scope of several other theoretical stances that have developed concurrently or subsequently, such as *constraint-based theory*, *functionalism*, *theory of mind*, and *cognitive* and *behavioral theories*. Subsequent advances in linguistics have been made by Martin Ball (*clinical linguistics*), Bickerton (*biolinguistics*), Roger Brown (*language teaching/learning*), Noam Chomsky (*psycho/cognitive theory*), David Crystal (*applied linguistics*), Wolfgang Dressler (*grammar and discourse*), Ralph Fasold (*sociolinguistics and variation theory*), James Emil Flege, David Ingram, and Brian MacWhinney (*language acquisition*), Malcolm Coulthard (*discourse analysis*), M. A. K. Halliday (*systemic linguistics*), Dell Hymes (*ethnographic linguistics*), Roger Keesing (*anthropological linguistics*), George Lakoff (*cognitive linguistics*), Peter Mühlhäusler (*field linguistics*), Michael Stubbs (*corpus-based studies*), and Yorick Wilks (*computational linguistics*), among others. Overall, contemporary linguistics aims at a multidisciplinary, crosslinguistic, and applied focus that enhances research on several plains (e.g., cognitive, neuro/psycholinguistic, social, pragmatic, quantitative, computational). Such advances will continue to impact understanding of the language faculty, as well as guide understanding of atypical use, which includes communication disorders.

Toward a Unified Theory of Language

A treatise of several volumes on linguistics might still fail to describe comprehensively the principles, directions of scope, and future paths of the field of linguistics. Thus, it is not surprising that leading linguists agree that we are still far from having developed a definite and unified theory of language. A contributing factor is the hordes of different languages, dialects, and contexts of language use, misuse, and disuse that still need to be considered in detail and integrated. The limited and compartmentalized knowledge of the physical mechanisms involved in the actual representation and cognitive processing of language is another such factor. What is certain, nevertheless, is that all progress relies on knowing what came before. Every single contributor to the field of linguistics has stood on the shoulders of giants.

Elena Babatsouli

See also Bilingual Education; Cognitive Linguistics; Descriptive Linguistics; Generative Linguistics; Language; Language Acquisition; Multilingualism; Psycholinguistics; Signed Languages; Sociolinguistics; Writing Systems

Further Readings

Aitchison, J. (2012). *Words in the mind: An introduction to the mental lexicon*. Malden, MA: Blackwell.
Aronoff, M., & Rees-Miller, J. (2017). *The handbook of linguistics*. Hoboken, NJ: Wiley/Blackwell.
Ball, M. J., Crystal, D., & Fletcher, P. (Eds.). (2012). *Assessing grammar: The languages of LARSP*. Bristol, UK: Multilingual Matters.
Ball, M. J., Perkins, M. R., Müller, N., & Howard, S. (Eds.). (2008). *The handbook of clinical linguistics*. Malden, MA: Blackwell.
Chelliah, S. L., & de Reuse, W. J. (2011). *Handbook of descriptive linguistic fieldwork*. Dordrecht, The Netherlands: Springer.
Dabrowska, E., & Divjak, D. (Eds.). (2015). *Handbook of cognitive linguistics*. Berlin, Germany: De Gruyter Mouton.
Davies, A., & Elder, C. (Eds.). (2008). *The handbook of applied linguistics*. Malden, MA: Blackwell.
Eddington, D. (Ed.). (2009). *Quantitative and experimental linguistics*. Munich, Germany: Lincom.
Fromkin, V., Rodman, R., & Hyams, N. (2014). *An introduction to language* (10th ed.). Malden, MA: Blackwell.
Geeraerts, D., & Cuyckens, H. (Eds.). (2010). The Oxford handbook of cognitive linguistics. Oxford, UK: Oxford University Press.
Hemforth, B. (2013). *Experimental linguistics*. Amsterdam, The Netherlands: John Benjamins.
Ingram, D. (1989). *First language acquisition: Method, description and explanation*. Cambridge, UK: Cambridge University Press.
Lidz, J., Snyder, W. & Pater, J. (Eds.). (2016). The Oxford handbook of developmental linguistics. Oxford, UK: Oxford University Press.
Lyons, J. (2012). *Introduction to theoretical linguistics*. Cambridge, UK: Cambridge University Press.
MacWhinney, B., & O'Grady, W. (Eds.). (2015). *The handbook of language emergence*. Malden, MA: Blackwell.
Pinker, S. (2007). *The language instinct: How the mind creates language*. New York, NY: HarperCollins.
Pütz, M. (Ed.). (1992). *Thirty years of linguistic evolution: Studies in honour of René Dirven on the occasion of his sixtieth birthday*. Amsterdam, The Netherlands: John Benjamins.
Rowe, B. M., & Levine, D. P. (2016). A concise introduction to linguistics. New York, NY: Routledge.
Whitaker, H. & Stemmer, H. (Eds.). (1997). *Handbook of neurolinguistics*. London, UK: Academic Press.

LISTENING EFFORT

The term *listening effort* has been defined as the deliberate allocation of mental resources to overcome obstacles in goal pursuit when carrying out a listening task. This definition of listening effort was proposed in a consensus paper based on the 2015 Eriksholm Workshop on Hearing Impairment and Cognitive Energy. It builds on the more general concept of mental effort that has been used widely in cognitive psychology. The general concept was described in Daniel Kahneman's seminal book *Attention and Effort* published almost a half century ago. In the last two decades, the term *listening effort* has been used increasingly in audiology. Its usage increased as the importance of cognition became recognized by both researchers investigating listening in complex realistic situations and clinicians providing rehabilitation to people who are hard of hearing. However, the rapid development of new behavioral, physiological, and self-report measures to assess listening effort created some confusion in the field. Defining listening effort was identified as a necessary step in resolving this confusion so that progress could be made in understanding the connections between auditory and cognitive processing during communication. Research on this topic continues to be very active, but no clinical tools have yet been standardized.

Pure-tone and speech audiometry are the core clinical measures used to assess hearing. However, individuals who perform similarly on audiometric measures obtained in a sound-attenuating booth can differ markedly in how they experience listening in complex everyday communication situations. Similarly, aided audiometric measures can be poor predictors of the degree of benefit hearing aid users experience from amplification in everyday life. Whether or not hearing is biologically impaired, how well people function as they participate in daily communication activities depends on cognition. Indeed, people who are hard of hearing often report that they find it effortful or tiring to listen, even when sounds are loud enough for them to hear or when they are able to understand speech. A key difference between hearing and listening is that listening involves cognition. Listening is the use of hearing for a purpose, and it entails attention and intention.

Cognitive hearing science unites research on hearing and cognition. This research includes studies to evaluate how difficulty hearing may deplete cognitive capacity or, conversely, how the deployment of cognitive resources may compensate for difficulty hearing. A key assumption is that individuals vary in their cognitive resource capacity and that it is limited. The quality of auditory input can be reduced by external factors such as environmental noise or internal factors such as hearing loss. As the quality of input decreases, auditory processing can become more demanding, such that listeners may need to expend increasing attentional effort to successfully achieve the goal of their intended task. As listening effort increases, individuals allocate more of their limited capacity of resources to listening. Consequently, fewer of the limited cognitive resources remain available for other processing tasks, such as remembering what was heard. Thus, by expending effort, listeners can achieve high performance on tasks such as repeating words in noise, but success comes at a cognitive cost.

Working memory is a cognitive system with a limited capacity that is responsible for temporarily storing and processing information. Behavioral tests of working-memory span are used to measure individual differences in cognitive capacity and to evaluate how much capacity individuals allocate to meet the processing demands associated with specific tasks. In a typical working-memory span test, an individual is required to both process and store information, for example, comprehending sentences and later recalling the sentence-final words. The tester infers that the working-memory span, or the number of words recalled, decreases if more capacity is diverted from storage and allocated to processing the information to be comprehended. Working-span tests have been introduced in audiology to measure individual differences in cognitive capacity. New tests of listening working-memory span have been developed to gauge how much listening effort an individual expends in processing information across varying conditions. Preliminary evidence based on measures of working-memory span demonstrates that people with larger cognitive capacities may benefit more than those with smaller capacities when using fast signal-processing hearing aids, especially in background noise such as speech. Other evidence suggests that improving the quality of the auditory input can reduce the effort a listener expends to meet the processing demands of listening. Importantly, differences in effort may be revealed even when performance on speech audiometry is near ceiling.

In addition to behavioral measures, physiological methods have been used to measure listening effort, including functional neuroimaging and event-related responses in the brain as well as measures of autonomic cardiac, skin, and pupil responses. Some studies have used self-report measures of listening effort. New measures of listening effort may offer insights into the everyday experiences of listeners that surpass those gained from traditional audiometry. Future research is needed to discover why and how these behavioral, physiological, and self-report measures are interrelated. Ultimately, measures of listening effort could be incorporated into rehabilitation and the design of technologies or communication environments. The relevance of such measures to everyday communication may drive innovations that improve the communication function and quality of life for people who are hard of hearing.

Margaret Kathleen Pichora-Fuller

See also Attention; Background Noise; Cognitive Processes and Operations; Memory

Further Readings

Arlinger, S., Lunner, T., Lyxell, B., & Pichora-Fuller, M. K. (2009). The emergence of cognitive hearing science. *Scandinavian Journal of Psychology, 50*(5), 371–384. Retrieved from https://doi.org/10.1111/j.1467-9450.2009.00753.x

Kahneman, D. (1973). *Attention and effort*. Englewood Cliffs, NJ: Prentice Hall.

Mattys, S. L., Davis, M. H., Bradlow, A. R., & Scott, S. K. (2012). Speech recognition in adverse conditions: A review. *Language and Cognitive Processes, 27*(7–8), 953–978. Retrieved from https://doi.org/10.1080/01690965.2012.705006

McGarrigle, R., Munro, K. J., Dawes, P., Stewart, A. J., Moore, D. R., Barry, J. G., & Amitay, S. (2014). Listening effort and fatigue: What exactly are we measuring? A British Society of Audiology Cognition in Hearing Special Interest Group "white paper." *International Journal of Audiology, 53*(7), 433–440. Retrieved from https://doi.org/10.3109/14992027.2014.890296

Pichora-Fuller, M. K., Kramer, S. E., Eckert, M. A., Edwards, B., Hornsby, B., Humes, L. E., . . . Wingfield, A. (2016). Hearing impairment and cognitive energy: The Framework for Understanding Effortful Listening (FUEL). *Ear and Hearing, 37*(Suppl.), S5–S27.

Locus of Control

Locus of control is defined as individuals' beliefs about the degree of influence they have over what happens to them. The term was coined by clinical psychologist Julian Rotter in 1954 and is a joint feature to his social learning theory. Locus of control is important to human communication because it has been tied to individuals' perceptions of how reinforcement in social situations may affect their behavior in the future. It is also a significant factor in the overall worldview and belief system of an individual. This entry details how locus of control is related to operant conditioning that may shape behavior, the types of locus of control that individuals may display, and how locus of control has been shown to affect different domains of individuals' lives.

The elucidation of locus of control came from Rotter's work in social learning theory. The term translates to location or source of influence; that is, it describes whether individuals think they themselves influence what happens to them, or if some external force or entity acts upon them and ultimately dictates outcomes related to their behavior. Social learning theory is based upon the principles of behavioral learning theories, namely, operant conditioning. In operant conditioning, popularized by well-known behaviorists such as Edward Thorndike and, later, B. F. Skinner, a specific behavior is more likely to recur in the future if it is followed with a positive outcome, whereas a behavior that is met with a negative outcome is less likely to recur in the future. Rotter applied these principles (reinforcement and punishment, respectively) to his social learning theory, specifically relating it to how individuals interact and communicate with others. The end result is essentially a theory of motivation within the context of social situations; individuals are more likely to engage in a behavior if they think it will be reinforcing, and they are less likely to engage in it if they think it will not be reinforcing. For example, if individuals normally experience a positive consequence after opening up and being vulnerable to their close friends, they will be more likely to continue to do that behavior. On the other hand, if they are normally met with ridicule or indifference after making themselves socially vulnerable, the theory dictates that the individual will not be likely to repeat that behavior in the future.

Locus of control refers to the extent to which individuals feel they influence the consequences they experience, either positive or negative. Rotter categorized locus of control on an internal–external (I–E) continuum. Individuals with an internal locus of control tend to believe that the things that happen to them are a result of something they themselves enabled to happen, such as through their own behavior, work, or way of being. Individuals with an external locus of control, on the other hand, credit luck, fate, other people, or another outside entity with what happens to them. Locus of control was thus included as an aspect of personality, mirroring Rotter's clinical interests. Although some personality theorists throughout history have postulated personality and encompassing traits as being somewhat concrete and unchangeable, Rotter's behavioral conceptualization of locus of control as a core foundational piece of personality suggests that it is, in fact, modifiable.

The reinforcement–punishment aspect of Rotter's social learning theory and locus of control are closely related because they can play a great role in an individual's social beliefs and behavior. Individuals with an internal locus of control feel that they have power over what consequences they experience; they choose whether they perform a behavior that may or may not be reinforcing. Conversely, individuals with an external locus of control believe that the behaviors they engage in have relatively little to do with the reinforcement they receive; they believe that they may or may not be reinforced, even if they perform a behavior that has been reinforced in the past. Individuals with the external type of locus of control, according to Rotter and other clinicians and researchers, are more prone to negative mood and affect during mental illness, as they feel that some "other" is controlling what happens to them, rather than feeling a sense of internal control. It is important to note, however, that locus of control is highly subjective and personal; that is, any irrational thoughts or connections individuals have made between their behavior and subsequent consequences may not be accurate to the outside world but may dictate their future behavior. Rotter also noted that some social situations are more salient than others; that is, individuals may weigh the behavior–consequence pattern more heavily for situations they deem more influential or important to their lives.

Because of these points of Rotter's theory, his application of locus of control to therapy was to focus on adjusting irrational thoughts about behaviors and their subsequent reinforcement, as well as to place more internal control with the individual. He hypothesized that if individuals feel they have more personal control over determining successes, negative outcomes, and other experiences, mental health may improve. More recent research has shown that an individual's locus of control may be situational; for example, in relationships, a person may characteristically display an external locus of control, while within the person's career that person displays an internal locus of control. These aspects of social learning theory and locus of control have been enveloped into contemporary therapies that seek to adjust both cognitions and behavior of individuals.

Rachel H. Messer

See also Behaviorism; Individual Differences; Learned Helplessness; Motivation; Positive Psychology and Wellness; Psychosocial Issues Associated With Communication Disorders

Further Readings

Monty, R. A., & Perlmuter, L. C. (1979). *Choice and perceived control.* Hoboken, NJ: John Wiley.
Phares, E. J. (1976). *Locus of control in personality.* Morristown, NJ: General Learning Press.
Rotter, J. B. (1954). *Social learning and clinical psychology.* Englewood Cliffs, NJ: Prentice Hall.
Rotter, J. B. (1972). *Applications of a social learning theory of personality.* New York, NY: Holt, Rinehart, and Winston.

LOUDNESS

Loudness is the level of a sound as perceived by a listener. Our lives are increasingly becoming more dominated by human-made sounds around us, and the loudness of such sounds becomes important when they interfere with the ability to comprehend speech, or to focus on listening to music or other wanted sounds, or to sleep or relax. Exposure to loud sounds can cause permanent hearing damage, which only manifests itself as an issue in future years when one needs a hearing aid earlier than the average population. Music is often listened to at high levels using electronic amplification via earphones or in music and dance venues when sound levels can easily be made sufficient to cause hearing damage. There is increased knowledge about the effects of high sound levels on human hearing, and sound engineers who control the volume of sound at public events should be monitoring the overall sound level to keep it within guidelines. This entry examines how the loudness of sounds is perceived and measured, including the monitoring of sound levels to guard against hearing loss.

Although the loudness of a sound is related to its acoustic energy, the relationship between perceived loudness and acoustic energy is not a simple one. It is affected not only by the acoustic energy level but also by the spectral content of the sound. The intensity or power of a sound can be measured directly as an absolute value, but loudness cannot, since it requires a judgment to be made by a listener of the loudness level of a sound. Thus, loudness is referred to as a subjective measure because it requires a human subject in its measurement. It should be noted that there is no right answer when making a subjective assessment such as rating the loudness of sounds since people's hearing and perceptual systems differ; it is an opinion that is being offered. Conversely, the measurement of sound intensity or power can be carried out with appropriate equipment and is referred to as an objective measure. Thus, any scale of loudness is based on an average of how a large group of listeners rate the loudness of the sounds being considered.

Loudness Variation With Frequency

Human perception of the loudness of pure tones reveals that tones of different frequencies and the same intensities do not sound equally loud. People are most sensitive in terms of perceived loudness for pure tone frequencies between around 2 and 4 kHz and progressively less sensitive for pure tones decreasing in frequency from around 300 Hz to 20 Hz. In addition, people are increasingly less sensitive for pure tones at frequencies above 5 kHz. These variations in the way in which the loudness of pure tones of different frequencies are perceived occur because of the acoustic resonances of the outer ear, the frequency response of the ossicles (the three small bones of the middle ear), and the manner in which the inner ear functions in converting the input sound into neural impulses.

Equal loudness, or Fletcher-Munson curves, can be measured and plotted for any listener, and these are typically used to quantify these effects. They provide the basis for a scale of loudness known as the phon scale. The phon scale has as its reference a pure tone at 1 kHz at a fixed level, and this fixed level is defined as its loudness in phons. Listeners are asked to judge when pure tones at other frequencies sound equally loud to the fixed-level 1 kHz pure tone when their levels are changed. When a pure tone is judged to be equally loud to the 1 kHz reference tone, both tones have the same number of phons. Thus, a pure tone with a loudness of 55 phons has the same perceived loudness as a 1 kHz pure tone at 55 dBSPL (sound pressure level).

The perceived loudness of complex tones depends on the frequencies of the components within the tone. If they fall within a critical band, their loudness is perceived as being lower than if they fall in multiple critical bands. The ear seems to add the loudness responses of all critical bands involved to provide a total loudness. For components that fall within one critical band, the overall loudness relates to the sum of the intensities of the components themselves. In practice, this means that it does not matter how many or how few components there are within one critical band; if their overall acoustic intensity is the same then so is their perceived loudness. The output from each critical band produces a peak in the basilar membrane motion response, so for components that lie within one critical band there is one peak, whereas for sounds that have components spanning a number of critical bands there are multiple peaks. These basilar membrane peaks are responsible for neural firings, which themselves contribute to the perception of loudness. Multiple peaks will trigger the perception of greater loudness.

Loudness Variation With Sound Level

Perceived loudness varies as a function of sound pressure level as might be expected (the higher/lower the sound intensity the higher/lower the loudness), but this variation is far from being linear. The equal loudness curves provide evidence that loudness does not have a simple relationship with sound level change and that it varies with frequency for pure tones.

Many facets of human perception are based on logarithmic change, and one might assume that a perceived doubling in loudness occurs when the level of a pure tone has its pressure doubled (raising it by 6 dB) or intensity doubled (raising it by 3 dB), but this is not the case. On average, a doubling in loudness for 1 kHz pure tones is perceived when the sound pressure level is increased by 10 dB. This is encapsulated in the sone scale, which is a subjective scale that is based on the definition of 1 sone as the loudness of a 1 kHz pure tone at 40 dBSPL. In deriving the sone scale, listeners are asked to indicate how much louder or softer test sounds are in comparison with a reference sound. The results indicate that, on average, listeners require a 10 dB increase/decrease in sound level to perceive a doubling/halving in loudness. A 10 dB increase indicates that a sound source 10 times as large is required for a doubling in loudness; hence, to double the loudness of one violin would require 9 more violinists to join in, and to double it again would require a further 90 violinists to join in.

Loudness Variation With Sound Duration

It turns out that the duration of a sound, whether a pure tone or a complex tone, affects its perceived loudness and that the effect is a logarithmic rise in perceived loudness for a tone of fixed amplitude over its first fifth of a second. Beyond that, the loudness remains essentially constant. This suggests that the loudness of any sound that is changing in level is not based on the instantaneous sound level but on an average of the sound level over about one fifth of a second.

This effect is employed musically by organists. Pipes in a pipe organ are either sounding or not sounding depending on whether their stop is selected and their note is depressed. There is no volume control (ignoring the swell box). An important aspect of performing music is to ensure that the main beat in a bar is clear to the listener, and normal musical practice is to accent (make louder) the first beat of each bar. This cannot be done on a pipe organ, but what can be done is to make the last beat of the bar quieter by shortening the note so that its perceived loudness is lower that the following first beat of the next bar. So the start of a bar is made clear to the listeners providing the note or chord of the last beat of each bar is shorter than one fifth of a second and the first beat of the next bar is longer.

Measuring Loudness and Hearing Function

There are many situations where is it necessary to be able to measure sound pressure level in practice in a manner that relates to perceived loudness, including confirming reported noise nuisance; monitoring sound levels where there are legal requirements to guard against hearing damage (e.g., in night clubs, rock concerts, theaters, rehearsal spaces, orchestral venues, factories); and testing appliances to specify their noise ratings and to perform periodic routine checks. To enable such a meter to be produced, its output needs to be weighted to compensate for the average equal loudness curves for which two weightings are commonly used. These are known as the "A" and "C" weightings, used for low-level and high-level sounds, respectively. The measured sound levels are given as dBA and dBC, respectively.

Where there is a requirement, usually based on legislation relating to noise exposure, to monitor sound levels that people are being exposed to, a measurement of sound level is made over time to establish that on average, the sound level will not cause noise-induced hearing loss. Such a measurement is known as the L_{eq} and the measured sound level is integrated over a specified time interval, usually 8 hours to enable comparison with stated legal limits.

Hearing tests to check whether there is a hearing loss make use of a pure tone audiometer. It presents pure tones at known calibrated sound pressure levels, and the person being tested indicates whether he or she can hear the tones, usually by pressing a button that informs the testing audiologist. The sound pressure level is reduced until the tone can no longer be heard, and this is confirmed typically three times in a formal hearing test. The audiometer itself is calibrated in dBHL (decibels hearing level) in which a fixed dBHL value against frequency indicates equal loudness. For example, zero dBHL equates to the threshold of hearing. To achieve this, the audiometer has to produce each pure tone at the correct level depending on its frequency. This is done so it is easy to read the results of a hearing test; a normally hearing subject should have results that are close to zero dBHL at all frequencies. A hearing loss would be indicated by positive dBHL values, which would indicate that the sound presented had to be higher than the average hearing threshold to be heard. Depending on how large this positive value is and over what frequency range enables an audiologist to decide if a hearing aid is appropriate.

Listening to loud sound over time can cause noise-induced hearing loss. A useful rule of thumb based on 2006 legislation in Europe indicates that listening to sounds that have an L_{eq} of 85 dBA for longer than 8 hours can potentially cause noise-induced hearing loss, and for every 3 dB added to the level, the time of exposure should be halved. Thus, listening to sounds with an L_{eq} of 88 dBA for longer than 4 hours, or sounds with an L_{eq} of 91 dBA for longer than 2 hours, or sounds with an L_{eq} of 94 dBA for longer than 1 hour, and so on, can potentially cause noise-induced hearing loss. Armed with this rule of thumb and a sound level meter app on a smartphone, one can make a judgment as to how long is appropriate to stay listening within that space. One way of mitigating the risk would be to cut out a proportion of the sound entering the ears; even a rolled up piece of tissue in each ear can cut 2–3 dB of sound energy and potentially offers a doubling of the exposure time.

David M. Howard

See also Background Noise; Decibel; Speech Perception, Theories of; Speech Production, Theories of; Voice Acoustics

Further Readings

Epstein, M., & Marozeau, J. (2010). Loudness and intensity coding. In C. J. Plack (Ed.), *Oxford handbook of auditory science: Hearing* (pp. 45–70). Oxford, UK: Oxford University Press.

Florentine, M., Popper, A. N., & Fay, R. R. (Eds.). (2011). Loudness. In R. R. Fay & A. N. Popper (Series Eds.), *Springer handbook of auditory research* (Vol. 37). New York, NY: Springer-Verlag.

Howard, D. M., & Angus, J. A. S. (2009). *Acoustics and psychoacoustics* (4th ed.). Oxford, UK: Focal Press.

M

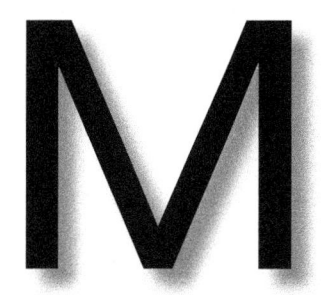

Magnetic Resonance Imaging (MRI)

See Instrumental Analysis of Speech

Makaton Sign System

See Key Word Signing Systems

Manual Circumlaryngeal Techniques in Voice Disorders

Poorly regulated paralaryngeal tension contributes to a host of voice problems and underlies a class of disorders referred to as hyperfunctional or musculoskeletal tension voice disorders. Although *paralaryngeal* tension typically implicates the extrinsic and intrinsic laryngeal muscles, this tension may extend to include the jaw, tongue, pharyngeal constrictors, and the muscles of the neck and upper back. The putative effect of such tightness is foreshortening and stiffening of muscles that restrict movements of structures related to voice production. Although the precise origin of abnormal paralaryngeal muscle activity is not well understood, most voice clinicians agree that (a) chronic tightness of the larynx can lead to cramping and stiffness of the hyolaryngeal musculature and voice mutation, (b) recognizing the adverse effects of such tension is an important part of assessment, and (c) restoring laryngeal muscular balance is essential to successful voice therapy. To this end, focal palpation and manual techniques, including circumlaryngeal massage, manual laryngeal reposturing, myofascial release, and laryngeal manual therapy, and osteopathic techniques, including laryngeal manipulation, mobilization, and postural manual therapy, have been offered as direct methods to assess and treat laryngeal hyperfunction syndromes. This entry provides an overview of common manifestations of excessive laryngeal muscle tension and then describes the use of manual circumlaryngeal techniques in the assessment and management of voice disorders.

Palpation of the Paralaryngeal Region

At rest, musculoskeletal tension can be appraised manually by palpation of the laryngeal area to assess the degree, nature, and location of focal tenderness, stiffness, muscle nodularity, and/or pain. Palpatory examination assesses laryngeal position, resting muscle tone, range of motion, ease of laryngeal mobility, and in some cases myofascial trigger points. It is important to acknowledge that palpation remains a qualitative assessment, and despite attempts to objectively quantify assessment findings, there are few data regarding the validity and reliability of various laryngeal palpatory methods. While considerable procedural variation exists surrounding this qualitative assessment, digital pressure is typically applied anteriorly (a) over the major horns of the hyoid bone, (b) over the superior cornu of the thyroid cartilage, (c) within the thyrohyoid and cricothyroid spaces, (d) along the anterior border of the sternocleidomastoid muscle, and (e) within the medial suprahyoid/submandibular regions. However, palpation may be extended beyond the anterior neck and laryngeal structures to include the craniocervical region such as the occiput and posterior muscles of the neck, upper back, and shoulder regions. The degree of compression applied during palpation is equal to the pressure required to cause the thumbnail tip to blanch when pressed against a firm surface. With this amount of pressure, focal sites of tension evoke discomfort or pain. Patients may wince, withdraw, or vocalize their discomfort when trigger points are identified. This exquisite tenderness in response to pressure within and outside the paralaryngeal region is considered a stereotypic feature of musculoskeletal tension voice disorders.

The extent of laryngeal elevation is also assayed by palpating within the thyrohyoid space from the posterior border of the hyoid bone to the thyroid notch. A narrowed or absent thyrohyoid space is suggestive of excess muscle tension whereby the larynx is suspended high in the neck. The mobility of the larynx is also tested by attempting to maneuver it side to side along the horizontal plane. Resistance to lateral movement is interpreted as generalized extralaryngeal hypertonicity. The clinician assesses not only resting muscle tone (i.e., static tension) but also contracted muscle tone and laryngeal position observed during specific voicing attempts (i.e., dynamic/phasic tension). Taut muscle bands, muscle stiffness, and disproportionate laryngeal elevation during voicing signal excessive muscle recruitment/activity. Excessive tone can also be detected in the suprahyoid and infrahyoid regions by palpating at rest, during voice produced at modal pitch, and then during upward and downward pitch glide maneuvers.

Manual Laryngeal Reposturing Maneuvers

Since 2000, a set of laryngeal reposturing maneuvers that can momentarily interfere with habituated patterns of muscle misuse has received attention. These laryngeal repositioning maneuvers are applied while the patient vocalizes and may inform the clinician regarding inappropriate extralaryngeal muscle activity, as well as provide insight regarding the potential for voice improvement. Thus, these manual reposturing maneuvers are considered voice stimulability testing techniques and an essential part of evaluation. The first maneuver involves compressing the larynx by exerting anterior-to-posterior pressure above, on, and below the hyoid bone. This is referred to as the *hyoid pushback* maneuver. The degree of the pressure applied is greater than what is applied during palpation, but this pressure will vary depending upon the degree of muscular resistance encountered. By virtue of its numerous muscular attachments below and above (i.e., jaw and tongue) and its connection to the larynx, the hyoid bone represents an important pivot point for the larynx. Because of shared attachments with the hyoid bone, which ostensibly serves as a biomechanical fulcrum for the suprahyoid structures above and the larynx below, excessive lingual and mandibular tension can affect voice function, and alternatively, laryngeal position and tension can potentially influence articulatory function. One goal of the pushback maneuver is to interfere with suprahyoid muscles exerting their influence on the hyoid, thereby manually releasing the hyoid and the larynx.

In addition to the hyoid pushback maneuver, other laryngeal reposturing techniques include physically impeding elevation of the larynx by applying downward traction over the superior border of the thyroid lamina (also known as the *pull-down* maneuver). Manually lowering the larynx during voicing can help to evaluate the adverse effects of laryngeal elevation on voice function. Finally, applying combined medial compression and downward traction over the superior cornu of the thyroid assesses the combined effects of laryngeal lowering and compression of the larynx, which can be particularly revealing in cases of nonadducted hyperfunction.

By manually repositioning or stabilizing the larynx during vowel productions, the clinician may stimulate improved voice and briefly interrupt patterns of muscle misuse. These moments can be further shaped using digital cueing or combined with tension reduction techniques. Digital cues are then faded, and the patient taught to rely on sensory feedback (i.e., auditory, kinesthetic, and vibrotactile) to maintain improved laryngeal posturing and muscle balance. According to some authorities, once the larynx is mobilized using these techniques, the recovery of normal voice can occur rapidly.

Circumlaryngeal Massage

Skillfully applied, kneading of the extralaryngeal region is thought to stretch muscle tissue and fascia, promote local circulation with the removal of metabolic wastes, relax tense muscles, and relieve pain and discomfort associated with muscle spasms. Once the larynx is *released*, and the range of motion/mobility is normalized, an improvement in vocal effort, quality, and dynamic range typically follows. By becoming aware of these laryngeal trouble spots, the patient can also begin to focus on relaxing them during self-massage, if necessary.

Once palpatory assessment has been completed, various manual laryngeal tension reduction techniques can be undertaken. Again, conceptual and procedural variation exists among these techniques, and opinions differ regarding the need for concurrent vocalization by the patient. Some authorities consider vocalizing to be an essential part of the procedure to (a) determine progress during therapy and (b) encourage the patient to continually self-monitor the quality and manner of voice produced so as to internalize and maintain improvements. These differences notwithstanding, kneading of the paralaryngeal region is a hallmark of most manual laryngeal therapies and is typically applied in a circular motion over the tips of the hyoid bone and suprahyoid region, as well as within the thyrohyoid space beginning from the thyroid notch and working posteriorly. The posterior borders of the thyroid cartilage medial to the sternocleidomastoid muscles are then located, and the procedure is repeated there. With the fingers over the superior border of the thyroid cartilage, the larynx is stretched downward and, at times, moved laterally. Sites of focal tenderness, nodularity, or tautness are given more attention. In general, manual procedures begin superficially, and the depth of massage and muscle/tissue stretching is increased according to the degree of tension encountered and the tolerance of the patient. It may be necessary to begin the technique peripheral to the sites of intense tenderness and then gradually direct attention proximal to these sites. When excess tension is encountered outside the paralaryngeal region, the clinician (depending upon his or her orientation and training) may extend the technique more peripherally to include the jaw, back of the neck, and shoulders. Some discomfort during the procedure is unavoidable; however, the goal is to achieve sufficient tension reduction without inducing reactive/reflexive muscle tension due to pain. Improvement in voice and reductions in pain (and laryngeal position) suggest a relief of tension and improved laryngeal mobility.

Research Evidence

There is growing evidence to support the clinical utility of manual circumlaryngeal techniques in the assessment and management of hyperfunctional voice disorders. In a series of early reports in the 1990s, the clinical effects of manual circumlaryngeal therapy (also known as circumlaryngeal massage) with a variety of hyperfunctional voice disorders were evaluated by Nelson Roy and colleagues. The results indicated a significant change in the direction of *normal* vocal function in the majority of patients with primary muscle tension dysphonia (pMTD) within one treatment session (with most patients considered by listeners as vocally normal following treatment). pMTD is defined as a voice disturbance in the absence of structural or neurological laryngeal pathology. Prior to treatment, almost all of the patients with pMTD reported pain and/or tenderness in the laryngeal region during palpation. During and immediately following the manual procedure, the majority of patients reported gradual reduction and then the resolution of laryngeal pain. These studies have been bolstered by those since 2010, which showed that manual circumlaryngeal therapy outperformed breathing exercises in the treatment of pMTD. Furthermore, several studies using acoustic analysis techniques have shed light on biomechanical correlates of voice improvement following successful manual circumlaryngeal therapy for pMTD. For instance, the acoustic analysis of vowel formants supported a decrease in laryngeal height and lengthening of the vocal tract, thereby providing evidence that improvement following manual circumlaryngeal therapy for muscle tension voice disorders is likely associated with lowered laryngeal position. In addition, the acoustic analysis of pre- and posttreatment speech samples from 111 women with pMTD who underwent manual circumlaryngeal therapy revealed that successful treatment benefitted both phonatory and articulatory subsystems, as evidenced by greater articulatory flexibility (i.e., expanded vowel space measures and steeper second formant trajectories) and increased speaking rate following treatment. The investigators explained that if mechanical coupling occurs via the hyoid between supralaryngeal articulatory structures (e.g., jaw and tongue) and the larynx, then mobilizing the larynx and hyoid via manual techniques likely produces desirable effects on articulation downstream. Collectively, these findings suggest that individuals with pMTD experience both articulatory and phonatory effects of abnormal muscle tension, and successful treatment using manual circumlaryngeal techniques overflows to the articulatory system.

Additional evidence to support the clinical utility of a variety of manual circumlaryngeal techniques has been reported since 2010. These reports (often based upon small samples) include laryngeal manual therapy, specific osteopathic-based laryngeal manipulations, as well as manual physical therapy approaches that include whole body/postural work. In some cases, manual therapies were combined with exercises to address general postural improvement (especially neck position), abdominal breathing, open-mouth approaches, and laryngeal manipulation (i.e., circumlaryngeal massage) of specific laryngeal muscles. While these combination approaches make identifying the active ingredient responsible for the reported success rates problematic, this research adds to a rapidly expanding literature that supports the clinical worth of manual techniques in voice disorder assessment and management.

Nelson Roy

See also Anatomy of the Human Larynx; Muscle Tension Dysphonia (MTD); Psychogenic Voice Disorders; Voice Disorders; Voice Therapy

Further Readings

Khoddami, S. M., Ansari, N. N., & Jalaie, S. (2015). Review of laryngeal palpation methods in muscle tension dysphonia: Validity and reliability issues. *Journal of Voice, 29*(4), 459–468.

Lieberman, J. (1998). *Principles and techniques of manual therapy: Application in the management of dysphonia* (pp. 91–138). In T. M. Harris, S. Harris, J. S. Rubin, & D. M. Howard (Eds.), *The voice clinical handbook*. London, UK: Whurr.

Mathieson, L. (2011). The evidence for laryngeal manual therapies in the treatment of muscle tension dysphonia. *Current Opinion in Otolaryngology & Head & Neck Surgery, 19*(3), 171–176.

Roy, N., Nissen, S. L., Dromey, C., & Sapir, S. (2009). Articulatory changes in muscle tension dysphonia: Evidence of vowel space expansion following manual circumlaryngeal therapy. *Journal of Communication Disorders, 42,* 124–135.

Roy, N. & Bless, D.M. (1998). Manual circumlaryngeal techniques in the assessment and treatment of voice disorders. *Current Opinion in Otolaryngology & Head and Neck Surgery, 6(3),* 151–155.

Roy, N., Bless, D.M., Heisey, D. & Ford, C.N. (1997). Manual circumlaryngeal therapy for functional dysphonia: An evaluation of short- and long-term treatment outcomes. *Journal of Voice*, 11, 321–331.

Roy, N & Leeper, H. A. (1993). Effects of the manual laryngeal musculoskeletal tension reduction technique as a treatment for functional voice disorders: Perceptual and acoustic measures. *Journal of Voice*, 7, 242–249.

Mapping Hypothesis

Mapping hypothesis is a model of word learning in early language development in which the child follows the adult's attention to identify the referent and create a mental map between the referent and the label that the adult provided. The model is increased to include a priori constraints on the possible hypotheses children test and to differentiate *fast* and *slow* mapping. Mapping hypothesis is an associative model of word learning, primarily used to describe the acquisition of object labels.

Some researchers have used the term *mapping hypothesis* to describe the interpretation of sentences with multiple subjects. This work led to a therapeutic approach to increasing sentence comprehension for individuals with nonfluent aphasia. Another separate use of the term *direct mapping hypothesis* is used by a faction of researchers in experimental research to refer to the process children undergo in the development of letter–sound correlations. This entry provides an overview of mapping hypothesis as it relates to the word learning process, as well as provides a critique of reducing the complexities of word learning down to mapping hypothesis.

Word Learning Process

Mapping hypothesis describes the acquisition of vocabulary using the associative metaphor of mapping between the referent and the label. The basic model includes a two-part process of word learning. First, the child is exposed to the ostensive definition, which means the adult and the child share attention on an unfamiliar object and the adult labels the object. The child creates multiple hypotheses about how the unfamiliar label may possibly map onto the real world. Then, the child tests these hypotheses to eliminate all but the correct referent. By eliminating all other possibilities, a process that has been explained with innate constraint principles, the child maps the word used to the real-world object.

At the completion of the mapping process, the child is assumed to have a similar mental concept mapped to the word as that of the adult partner. The metaphorical mapping of word to world achieves reference, and according to the theory of mapping hypothesis, this is assumed to mean that the child has achieved full conceptual knowledge of the meaning of the word.

Referent Constraints

In his 1960 book *Word and Object*, Willard Quine, using the adult linguist's attempt to learn an unknown language as a model for children's learning, argued that all possible hypotheses would be too much to eliminate. Experimental researchers have attempted to explain how mapping hypothesis could still explain word learning by adding to the model a priori principles that would constrain the child's attention and anchor him or her, preventing the child from being lost in a sea of all possible hypotheses.

In the 1980s, researchers concluded that these abstract constraints cause children's attention to shift to taxonomic relations to create hypothesis of the mapping relation of unfamiliar words. Later, this view was expanded to specify that children are more likely to assume labels refer to whole objects rather than parts or characteristics of objects.

Fast and Slow Mapping

In the 1980s, the mapping hypothesis model has been further expanded to contrast *fast mapping* and *slow mapping*. Fast mapping, also called *incidental learning*, is an initial stage of processing in which the child achieves the use of the word after only a minimum exposure. Slow mapping, also called *extended mapping*, is the clarifying process in which the child's understanding of the word continues to be refined with increased usage and exposure to the word.

Fast mapping is assumed to result in the child having a sense of the referential meaning of a label, but not a complete, adultlike conceptual understanding. Slow mapping follows the same theoretical process as fast mapping, but it specifically refers to word learning that requires multiple exposures for the child to create an adultlike map of the word-to-world relationship. The slow mapping process is idiosyncratic depending on the complex learning context in which the child is engaged.

Criticisms of Mapping Hypothesis

Mapping hypothesis as a model of word learning has been critiqued for limiting word learning to only object names and for its associationist focus. The ostensive associative mechanism, in which the adult points at an object and verbally labels the object while the child mentally creates a concept for the word-to-world map, only describes a limited number of interactions. Mapping hypothesis is limited in theoretical explanation of conceptual development because it assumes the ability to refer equals full conceptual knowledge of the meaning of words. Slow mapping seeks to remedy these limitations, but the reliance on a mapping metaphor assumes reference and conceptual knowledge are similar levels of meaning. Mapping hypothesis research relies on highly controlled experimental research, limiting its focus to in vitro learning instead of authentic in vivo learning. Notably,

Katherine Nelson's and Michael Tomasello's works present arguments against using the metaphor of mapping to describe early word learning in children, as well as presenting usage-based approaches to language acquisition which have more explanatory power than mapping hypothesis.

Kelly Koch

See also Language Acquisition; Lexicon; Naming; Usage-Based Approach to Language Acquisition; Vocabulary

Further Readings

Carey, S., & Bartlett, E. (1978). Acquiring a single new word. *Papers and Reports on Child Language Development, 15,* 17–29.

Nelson, K. (1985). *Making sense: The acquisition of shared meaning.* Orlando, FL: Academic Press.

Nelson, K. (2007). *Young minds in social worlds: Experience, meaning, and memory.* Cambridge, MA: Harvard University Press.

Tomasello, M. (2001). Perceiving intentions and learning words in the second year of life. In M. Tomasello & E. Bates (Eds.), *Language development: The essential readings* (pp. 111–128). Malden, MA: Blackwell.

Tomasello, M. (2003). *Constructing a language: A usage-based theory of language acquisition.* Cambridge, MA: Harvard University Press.

Markedness

The terms *marked* and *unmarked* are used to contrast linguistic oppositions in which one form, the *unmarked*, is more neutral, and usually more frequent, than the other. Consider, for example, the words *able* and *unable* or *polite* and *impolite*. In each case, the first form is more neutral, that is *unmarked*, whereas the second forms, which include the prefixes "un-" and "im-," are *marked*. The notion of markedness is a useful construct in studies of language acquisition and language disorders as it is often linked to developmental patterns and to types of errors. This entry provides an overview of marked and unmarked forms as seen in the three basic areas of language: morphology, semantics, and phonology. While all languages have the basic construct of markedness (although the surface representations may differ), the descriptions in this entry are based on English.

Morphology

Examples of markedness in the area of morphology include many word pairs that differ in the presence or absence of grammatical suffixes with the unmarked category lacking the suffix. Thus, singular nouns and present tense verbs are unmarked, while their counterparts are marked (e.g., *cat* vs. *cats*; *bush* vs. *bushes*; *talk* vs. *talked*; *go* vs. *going*). Some word pairs do not include an overt affix, but they are characterized by the same marked–unmarked (e.g., *mouse* vs. *mice*; *run* vs. *ran*; *he* vs. *him*). Word pairs with derivational suffixes can also be characterized as unmarked versus marked (e.g., *run* vs. *runner*; *red* vs. *reddish*; *coherent* vs. *incoherent*). In *syntax*, sentences in the active voice are unmarked in comparison to sentences in the passive voice (e.g., *The barking dog scared Joey* vs. *Joey was scared by the barking dog*).

Studies of early word use and sentence structure in young children acquiring English show that unmarked forms tend to be learned earlier than marked forms (e.g., singular vs. plural nouns; present vs. past tense; active vs. passive voice). Moreover, when errors occur, the unmarked form often occurs in place of the marked form (e.g., *Mary walk to school yesterday* or *I see two dog*).

Semantics

In the area of semantics, marked and unmarked word pairs in English are present, particularly in relationship to gender marking. Thus, the "male" term *mankind* includes both men and women and the pronoun *he* often stands for both males and females (e.g., *When attacked, a person should defend his rights*). English has a set of words for which the male terms represent the unmarked category, while their female counterparts are marked by a special suffix (e.g., *actor* vs. *actress* and *waiter* vs. *waitress*). In some cases, the female form is unmarked, for example, *nurse* is unmarked, and its counterpart, *male nurse*, is marked; *widow* is unmarked and *widower* is marked. In the past few decades, gender-neutral forms for some professions have been introduced (e.g., *police officer* and *firefighter* rather than *policeman* and *fireman*).

Other semantically related word pairs also show an effect of markedness, with the unmarked form used in a neutral context. Consider, for example, the pair *old* and *young*: old is unmarked and occurs in phrases like *How old are you?* The same relationship occurs with the pair *tall* and *short* (e.g., *How tall are you?*) and *big* and *small* (e.g., *How big is your dog?*).

Phonology

In the 1930s and 1940s, linguists and phonologists associated with the Prague School of Linguistics introduced the notion of markedness in the area of phonology, and discussions of phonetic and phonological markedness continue to be of interest. The defining features of the theory of markedness were based in part on frequency of occurrence in languages of the world and on order of acquisition of segments and features in young children learning to talk. In general, unmarked elements are characterized by simpler articulatory configurations and higher frequency of occurrence in the languages of the world.

A basic tenet of markedness for segments and features is that if a language includes a marked segment as part of its phonological system, it also includes the corresponding unmarked segment; however, the presence of the unmarked segment in the language does not imply presence of marked counterpart. Given this view, the following implicational relationships are expected: If a language has nasal vowels (marked), it also has oral vowels; if a language has fricatives (marked), it also has stops; if a language has palatal or interdental consonants, it also has alveolar/coronal consonants. Applying the concept of markedness to the category of consonantal voicing reveals interactions between sound class features: for obstruents (i.e., stops, fricatives, affricates), the unmarked category is voiceless; for sonorants, in contrast, the unmarked category is voiced. Thus, /s/ is unmarked compared with /z/ and voiceless unaspirated /k/ is unmarked compared with voiced /g/, but /m/ (which is voiced) is unmarked compared with voiceless /m̥/, and /l/ is unmarked compared with voiceless /l̥/.

The relationships posited for adult languages are also evident in phonological acquisition with unmarked categories present before their marked counterparts, as in the other areas of language. Thus, stops are acquired before fricatives (and the presence of fricatives in a child's phonological system implies the presence of stops); the presence of palatal consonants implies the presence of alveolar consonants; the presence of nasal vowels implies the presence of oral vowels, and so on. At the syllable level, unmarked consonant–vowel syllables appear in the child's repertoire before their marked counterpart: consonant–vowel–consonant syllables.

Substitution errors in child speech also conform to markedness patterns: when marked consonants are in error, the unmarked counterpart appears, as in target /v/ produced as [b], or target /s/ produced as [t]. Errors affecting syllable structure often reduce consonant–vowel–consonant syllables to consonant–vowel.

Carol Stoel-Gammon

See also Language Acquisition; Morphology; Phonetics; Phonological Development; Phonology; Semantics

Further Readings

Battistella, E. L. (1990). *Markedness: The evaluative superstructure of language.* Albany, NY: State University of New York Press.

Calabrese, A. (2005). *Markedness and economy in a derivational model of phonology.* Berlin, Germany: Mouton de Gruyter.

Jakobson, R. (1968). *Child language, aphasia, and phonological universals.* The Hague, The Netherlands: Mouton. (Original work *Kindersprache, Aphasie, und allgemeine Lautgesetze.* Uppsala, Sweden: Almqvist & Wiksell, published 1941)

MASKING

Masking is the process where one sound affects a person's ability to hear another sound. The masking effect can be total where the masked sound is unheard or partial where only part of the sound signal is heard. The masking can be simultaneous where the sound to be heard and the masking sound are provided at the same ear at the same time, and it can also be nonsimultaneous where the masker either precedes or follows the sound to be heard. The general effect of masking is a raised hearing threshold of the masked signal. This entry provides an overview of spectral, temporal, and informational masking as well as data from related clinical trials.

Spectral Masking

In its simplest form, masking of a pure tone is done by another pure tone in the same ear. If the masking tone is fixed in frequency and the test tone (i.e., the tone to be detected) is varied in frequency, the threshold level of the test tone is significantly lower than the masking tone level, when the frequency of the test tone is well below the masking tone frequency. When the frequency of the test tone increases and becomes closer to the masker tone, the test tone threshold increases monotonically with frequency. The curve formed by the masked thresholds at the different frequencies when the masker tone is held constant is known as the *masking pattern*. At frequencies very close to the masker frequency, the threshold of the test tone decreases forming a notch at the masker frequency. This notch originates in beats caused by the two tones at close frequencies resulting in an easier detection of the test tone. At test tone frequencies above the masker frequency, there is a reduction of the detection levels but not as sharp as at the lower frequencies, and the detection levels do not reach levels as low as those for the test tone at lower frequencies. This asymmetric behavior is most prominent when the masker has high levels and at low to mid frequencies and is less visible with low-level maskers or high-frequency maskers.

This asymmetry, which is also known as *upper spread of masking*, is caused by the mechanical vibrations in the cochlea. In the cochlea, the vibrations travel on the basilar membrane from the basal end where high frequencies are coded by the neurons and toward the apical end where the low frequencies are coded. The wave on the basilar membrane grows in amplitude with distance until it reaches the place where the frequency of the sound equals the mechanical parameters of the basilar membrane (resonance) and thereafter the wave amplitude rapidly decreases. This is seen in the masking where a masker wave with higher frequencies than the test tone does not reach the place on the basilar membrane where the test tone is coded (more apically than the masker). On the contrary, when a masker has lower frequency than the test tone, the masker wave on the basilar membrane travels over the place of coding for the test tone, and the masking affects the coding to a greater extent.

The same paradigm can be used, but the masking and test tones are switched so the test tone has a fixed frequency and the masker frequency is varied. In this way, the masker level needs to be high at frequencies lower or higher than the test tone in order to mask it but less high at frequencies close to the test tone frequency. This forms a notch-like behavior opposite to the configuration when the test tone frequency was varied. This type of testing is known as *psychoacoustic tuning curves*, but it is more common to use a narrow band noise as a masker than a tone as the detection is easier, especially when the test tone and masker tone are close in frequency since it can be difficult to distinguish two tones close in frequency, but a tone and a noise are easier to differentiate. Another benefit of using a narrowband noise as masker is that there are no beats between test tone and masker tone when the two are close in frequency and the curves are smoother at the fixed frequency, irrespective of whether the masker or the test tone frequency is varied. The asymmetry in masking between frequencies below and above the test tone frequency is also apparent when the test tone frequency is fixed, but in this scenario, the masking curve is steeper at the high frequencies than at the low frequencies.

The threshold measurement with a narrowband noise masker centered at a fixed frequency and varying the test tone frequency result in a function resembling a band-pass filter function. This measure is used as an estimate of the auditory filters. From a masking perspective, the auditory filter determines the ability to perceive sounds based on the presence of another sound (i.e., with the presence of the masker, sounds that fall below the threshold curve are inaudible). The caveat with varying the test tone frequency is that the masking pattern does not reflect a single auditory filter but an auditory filter for each test tone frequency. To resemble an auditory filter, the test tone frequency should be fixed and the masker frequency varied, resulting in a masking pattern that is the inverse of an auditory filter.

These filters are level dependent. Not only does an increase of the masker level increase the threshold with the same amount, but it also alters the threshold curve morphology. With a low-level masker at a fixed frequency, the threshold curve shows a steep slope on the low-frequency side and a slightly less steep slope on the high-frequency side. When the masker level increases, the steepness of the slopes decreases, resulting in a broader function. The broadening with level is especially prominent at the high-frequency side. This means that, at frequencies above the masker, an increase of the masker level by 10 dB requires an increase of the test tone of more than 10 dB to be detected. There is no single auditory filter that can be used for all frequencies and levels.

The masking of tones also depends on the spectrum of the masker. If the masker is a narrowband noise centered on the test tone, the masking level can be investigated as a function of the bandwidth of the masker. If the power density of the spectrum is constant, then the total masking power increases with the bandwidth of the masker. The masked threshold increases with bandwidth increase for small bandwidths, but at a certain bandwidth, the masked threshold becomes constant and is no longer a function of the masker bandwidth. This is another interpretation of the auditory filter. Only the noise spectrum of the masker inside the auditory filter affects the threshold of the test tone, and the sound power outside this filter does not affect the ability to hear the tone. Consequently, the detection ability is based on a constant signal-to-noise ratio between the masker and test tone inside the auditory filter determined by the frequency of the test tone. This hypothesis is called the *power spectrum model of masking*. When the noise bandwidth is less than the bandwidth of the auditory filter, an increase in bandwidth of the noise increases the masking effect, but once the noise bandwidth exceeds that of the auditory filter, there is no increase of the noise passing the auditory filter and hence no masking influence. The limit where no further increase of the noise bandwidth influences the masking effect is called the *critical bandwidth*.

Temporal Masking

In the previous examples, the masking sound and the test tone are applied simultaneously. Masking can also occur when the masking sound appears either before or after the test tone. This is often tested with a short sound, a probe, that either precedes the masker (i.e., backward masking) or comes shortly after the masker (i.e., forward masking). The masking effect only appears shortly before or after the masker, and around 100–200 ms before or after the masker, there is no temporal masking effect.

The reason for backward masking is still unclear, and it seems to be more pronounced in untrained than in trained listeners. This may suggest that the masking is a manifestation of confusion between the auditory signals, the probe, and the masker.

Forward masking is a result of several processes in the auditory system. Some of the threshold elevation of the probe can be attributed to fatigue and adaptation, which lead to a decrease of the sensitivity of the auditory system. But some of the masking is due to mechanical effects at the basilar membrane. A traveling wave on the basilar membrane does not die out immediately after the wave has passed but continues to vibrate a short time after its passing. This is known as *ringing* in a mechanical system. Consequently, if the probe excites the same place on the basilar membrane as the ringing occurs, the probe can be masked by the ringing. The ringing is most pronounced at low frequencies due to the smaller bandwidth of the resonance at those frequencies. Other explanations for the forward masking include persisting neural activity in the auditory system from the masker that can mask the probe or short-term adaptation and fatigue in the auditory system caused by the masker.

The smaller the time delay between masker and probe signal, the greater the masking effect for forward masking, and there is approximately a linear relation between the masking effect in dB and the logarithm of the delay (i.e., a doubling of the delay leads to a constant reduction of the masking in dB). The masking effect increases with the duration of the masker to somewhere between 50 and 200 ms, and no additional masking effect is found above this time limit. There is also an effect of masker level. However, for simultaneous masking, an increase of the masker by 10 dB results in a masked threshold increase by 10 dB (i.e., the signal to masker level is constant). For forward masking, a 10-dB increase of the masker level leads to an increase of the masked threshold by less than 10 dB.

Informational Masking

There is no clear distinction between what is meant by informational and energetic masking. One distinction between the two is that energetic masking is caused by the temporal and spectral overlap between the target sound and the masker; any additional masking effect is attributed to informational masking. Another way to separate the two is by assigning energetic masking to the processes in the peripheral auditory system and the informational masking to processes in the central auditory and cognitive systems.

Informational masking can be present in all types of sound stimuli together with a masker, but here, masked speech is the focus. The informational masking effect is greatest when the masker is as similar to the speech signal as possible. The greatest informational masking effect is obtained when the masker is the same voice as the target with meaningful linguistic sentences. A single talker as masker results generally in greater informational masking than multiple talkers. However, a single-talker masker results in silent intervals in the masking sound, which can be used effectively to comprehend the target speech by listening in the gaps. So multiple talkers as maskers result in greater energetic masking than a single talker because they give a smoother spectral content and less temporal modulation, while a single talker as masker results in more informational masking because the masker speech is more intelligible.

There have been several attempts to provide speechlike maskers without linguistic content. One such masker is time-reversed speech, that is, the speech from a talker is reversed in time to have the same long-term spectrum and modulation as normal speech but being unintelligible. However, such a masker is different from forward speech since the time reversal affects the way it spectrally masks the phonemes in time. Other maskers that have been used for this purpose include nonsense words and speech in another language. These types of maskers do not mimic the temporal variations and spectrum of the target and are therefore less efficient as energetic maskers. One attempt to provide a speech signal that temporally and spectrally resembles ordinary speech but is unintelligible is the International Speech Test Signal. This signal is derived from concatenating small segments of speech (i.e., 100–600 ms) from female speakers in six different languages. This makes the signal speechlike but unintelligible. Although the primary aim for the development of this speech material was for testing hearing aids, it has become popular as an unintelligible speech masker.

Masking in Clinical Tests

In clinical audiology, masking is used to ensure that a specific ear is tested. For pure-tone audiometry, the test ear receives the test tone, while the other ear is masked by a narrowband noise centered on the test tone frequency. It is important that the level of the noise is appropriate: It needs to be strong enough to totally mask the test tone in the non-test ear but not so strong that it causes detrimental effects such as central masking. When the masking is too strong, it is termed *overmasking*. One way to estimate the amount of masking required is to successively increase the masking level from a low level and measure the threshold at the test ear. If the sound is heard in the non-test ear, increasing the masking level increases the threshold. Once the masking is high enough, the threshold is constant with increasing masking level since it is now detected in the test ear and the masking is at a sufficient level. With further increase of the masking level, the threshold will increase once again, and the limit for overmasking has been reached.

Masking of one ear is usually done at situations in which the non-test ear may contribute to the perception. One such scenario is when the non-test ear has significantly better (i.e., 40 dB or more) sensitivity than the test ear when the hearing thresholds are obtained with earphones. The sound from the test-ear earphone can leak over to the non-test (i.e., better) ear and be perceived there. Another scenario is when the sound is provided in a sound field or the stimulation is by bone conduction, in which the sound reaches both ears with similar magnitudes. The masking ensures that only one ear responds to the stimulation.

If the masking level is too high, effects of central masking appear. Central masking manifests itself as a threshold raise at one ear when the other ear is simultaneously exposed to sound. The central masking is approximately 1 dB for every 10-dB increase above the threshold for the ear that is exposed to the masking.

Masking is also an integral part of speech in noise tests. In those tests, the speech signal is mixed with a noise signal, and the task is to find a speech-to-noise, SNR ratio level where the person has a preset speech recognition ability, often set to 50% correct recognition of the words. One of the most common test is the Hearing in Noise Test. In this test, an ordinary sentence is presented in noise. If the listener can repeat the sentence correctly, the SNR for the next sentence is reduced; otherwise, it is increased. Using this adaptive algorithm means that a speech-to-noise ratio can be computed for the test. The noise in these tests can be of any type, but a common type of noise is a speech-weighted noise with low or no modulation. The noise has the same long-term spectrum as the speech material to provide effective masking, but the masking can be speech-modulated noises or speech.

Stefan Stenfelt

See also Air and Bone Conduction; Audiology; Cognitive Processes and Operations; Frequency Resolution; Psychoacoustics; Speech Perception, Theories of

Further Readings

Holube, I., Fredelake, S., Vlaming, M., & Kollmeier, B. (2010). Development and analysis of an International Speech Test Signal (ISTS). *International Journal of Audiology, 49*, 891–903.

Katz, J. (2014). *Handbook of clinical audiology* (7th ed.). Philadelphia, PA: Lippincott Williams and Wilkins.

Kidd, G., & Colburn, H. S. (2017). Informational masking in speech recognition. In J. Middlebrooks, J. Simon, A. Popper, & R. Fay (Eds.), *Springer handbook of auditory research: Vol. 60. The auditory system at the cocktail party* (pp 75–109). Cham, Switzerland: Springer.

Kidd G., Jr., Mason, C. R., Richards, V. M., Gallun, F. J., & Durlach, N. I. (2007). Informational masking. In W. A. Yost, A. N. Popper, & R. R. Fay (Eds.), *Springer handbook of auditory research: Vol. 29. Auditory perception of sound sources* (pp. 143–189). New York, NY: Springer.

Moore, B. C. J. (2012). *An introduction to the psychology of hearing* (6th ed.). Bingley, UK: Emerald.

Nilsson, M., Soli, S. D., & Sullivan, J. A. (1994). Development of the Hearing in Noise Test for the measurement of speech reception thresholds in quiet and in noise. *Journal of Acoustical Society of America, 95*, 1085–1099.

Oxenham, A. J., & Dau, T. (2001). Reconciling frequency selectivity and phase effects in masking. *Journal of Acoustical Society of America, 110*, 1525–1538.

Stenfelt, S., & Goode, R. L. (2005). Bone conducted sound: Physiological and clinical aspects. *Otology & Neurotology, 26*, 1245–1261.

Mean Length of Utterance (MLU)

Mean length of utterance (MLU) is a measure that describes language production in terms of utterance length, initially as the average number of words and later as the average number of morphemes spoken per utterance. It is a language sample analysis tool that is used both clinically and in research. This entry provides an overview of MLU, including its history, calculation procedures, score interpretation, use with clinical populations, and application to other languages.

History

Early child language researchers noted a rise in the number of words spoken in a single utterance along with increases in chronological age, where younger children spoke fewer words per utterance than older children. This resulted in the use of utterance length as a measure of a child's language development. Given this general pattern of acquisition, the measure could be used to determine whether an individual's MLU is in line with what is expected of his or her chronological age. MLU counts shifted from words to morphemes (i.e., the basic unit of language), with the assertion that counting morphemes accounts for a child's knowledge of grammatical morphology in instances where the word count might overlook such richness in a child's production. In other words, an early two-word utterance contributes the same value to the count as a two-word utterance in which the child has inflected the verb. For example, a word count of the production *He walking* does not account for the syntactic complexity of that utterance.

In 1973, Roger Brown's stages of grammatical development created a framework to track the gains in grammatical structure that accompany increases in utterance length (in morphemes) and the age at which these coincide. The stages were thought to capture gains in linguistic knowledge as a result of increased utterance length, but a closer examination revealed the possibility of utterances with equal numbers of morphemes, but vastly differing in their grammatical complexity. Klee, for example, found that MLU was too variable when measures like utterance length and acquired structural complexity was analyzed for children of the same age. Despite this, however, Rice and others have appeared to confirm that MLU has good reliability and validity as an index of normal language.

Some conventions for counting morphemes are well established and widely accepted, such as counting past tense inflected verbs as two morphemes but irregular past tense verbs as a single morpheme. The *-ed* suffix is clearly added to a root verb (e.g., *jumped* and *laughed*), but there is no evidence of knowledge of either past tense morphology or the verb form's relation to its present tense form in irregular verbs such as *fell* and *saw*. Other scoring practices may be implemented by clinicians or researchers in accordance with their particular purposes. These decisions are customarily outlined in procedural descriptions and/or maintained with and across clients for consistency. For example, the first few minutes of every language sample may be disregarded to focus on the portion of the language sample collected after the child had settled into the new situation.

Calculating

MLU is calculated based on children's spontaneous language productions elicited via tasks ranging from free play to storytelling. A language sample of a minimum of 100 utterances is recommended to obtain a representative sample. MLU is computed as the total sum of words or morphemes divided by the total number of utterances. Below is a sample set to demonstrate the calculation of MLU (MLU = total words/total utterances).

Utterance	MLU *Morphemes*
I like the puppy.	4
He's my favorite.	4
I think he's hungrier.	6
It's big.	3
MLU TOTAL	17/4 = 4.25

A remaining challenge in preparing a transcription for MLU calculation is deciding what constitutes an utterance, particularly in the spontaneous language of a child. One may employ an utterance rule determined by linguistic boundaries (i.e., clauses) or a rule guided by paralinguistic cues such as intonation and pause. Other important considerations include the type of language sample elicited (e.g., free play vs. storytelling) as well as the choice of conversational partner (e.g., mother vs. experimenter). Great variability in children's performance as a function of these variables has been well documented. It is customary to specify the protocol implemented in research or practice consistency in clinical use. Once computed, it is then determined at what age a typically developing child produces a comparable MLU.

Language Impairment

Although MLU has shown to be a better indicator of the level of language development than age, the MLU score should not be the only measure used to diagnose language impairment. Rather, the score should be considered in combination with performance on other language assessments in order to determine the stage of language acquisition and make an informed diagnostic decision. As a result, an MLU calculation yielding a score that is below that which is expected of the child's chronological age signals the need for further evaluation, serving in a capacity similar to a language screener.

In addition to its use in assessment, the MLU is a useful tool in developing experimental control groups for research. In these studies, children with language impairment are compared with those of similar chronological age as well as children with comparable MLU levels. The MLU-matched group serves as a comparison group made up of children with language systems that are immature, yet typically developing. Similarities in errors between groups represent typical processes in development, whereas differences indicate a deviation in acquisition for the language-impaired group.

Crosslinguistic MLU

MLU was introduced as an index of grammatical development for monolingual English speakers. Due to its widespread utility, the application of the measure to other languages quickly followed. MLU was first calculated in other languages to test whether similar MLUs denote similar developmental stages in children who speak languages other than English. Extensive similarities in early syntactic development are noted across languages, namely children's early word combinations being composed of content words and largely void of function words. This speech is described as *telegraphic*. The precise procedure for identifying morpheme boundaries for the calculation of MLU must be adapted, or sometimes reformulated, for each language as a result of the structural differences across languages.

Sofia M. Souto

See also Language Acquisition; Language Delay; Lexicon; Morphology; Vocabulary

Further Readings

Bishop, D., & Adams, C. (1990). A prospective study of the relationship between specific language impairment, phonological disorders and reading retardation. *Journal of Child Psychology and Psychiatry, 31*, 1027–1050.

Brown, R. (1973). *A first language: The early stages.* Cambridge, MA: Harvard University Press.

Klee, T. (1985). Clinical language sampling: analysing the analyses. Child Language Teaching and Therapy, 1(2), 182–198.

Miller, J. F., & Chapman, R. S. (1981). The relation between age and mean length of utterance in morphemes. *Journal of Speech and Hearing Research, 24*(2), 154–161.

Rice, M. (2010). Mean length of utterance levels in 6-month intervals for children 3 to 9 years with and without language impairments. *Journal of Speech Language and Hearing Research, 53*, 333–349.

Meaning

Meaning of words, which is the subject of study in semantics, is one of the more controversial topics in linguistics. At a very simple level, considering the word as the unit of the language system and as a label or name for external world entities, there are two aspects to consider: the outer aspect, or sound form, and the meaning as the inner aspect of the word. A referential approach to word *meaning* makes this description clearer and distinguishes among three components: (1) *sound form* (symbol or linguistic sign); (2) *referent*, that is, the entity or aspect of reality to which the symbol refers; and (3) *concept*, that is, the notion or thought about the entity, singling out its characteristic properties, closest to meaning. Connection between sound form and referent is conventional and arbitrary; for instance, the concept of DOG (NB: in this entry concepts will be in all caps) is referred to in English as *dog*, in French as *chien*, in Spanish as *perro*, and in Italian as *cane*. Therefore, it seems that understanding the meaning and the process of meaning access requires a closer look at the underlying concepts and semantic memory where concepts are stored. This perspective is likely capable of explaining access to abstract meanings as well.

Role of Semantic Memory and Concepts

Semantic memory is a subset of long-term memory in which knowledge that individuals have acquired about the world including concepts (as well as facts, skills, ideas, and beliefs) is stored. Unlike *episodic memory*, which is a person's unique memory of events and experiences, semantic memory consists of memories shared by members of a culture. For example, whereas remembering the name and breed of one's first dog is dependent on episodic memory, knowing the meaning of the word *dog* and what a dog is relies on semantic memory. Presumably studying semantic memory and conceptual processing is a path that leads to an understanding of the way in which word meanings are accessed. When an individual has a concept for something, it means that he or she knows its meaning.

The Symbolic Versus the Embodied Approach to Semantic Memory and Concepts

Cognitive literature introduces two main constructs regarding the nature of concepts and how a concept is stored in semantic memory: *disembodied* or *symbolic* (amodal) and *embodied* (modal). The symbolic approach assumes that there is no similarity between components of experience (e.g., *objects, settings, people, actions, events,* and *mental states*) and relations and concepts stored in the mind. That is, perceptual information, including sensory, motor, introspective (e.g., *mental states* and emotional), about components of experience is transduced (reorganized) into arbitrary (language-like) symbols such that the final concept contains no reference to the actual experience per se. Thus, symbolic codes constitute concepts, and perceptual experiences do not play a role in knowledge representation. On the other hand, the embodied approach assumes that perceptual information about external world experiences is depicted in the brain's modality-specific systems. For example, when one sees a car, a group of neurons fires for color, others for shape, a third group for size, and so forth, to represent CAR in one's mind. Regarding the auditory and tactile sensory modalities, analogous patterns of activation can occur to represent how a car might sound or feel. Likewise, the activation of neurons in the motor system represents actions on the car, and activations that occur in emotion-related areas represent emotional reactions toward the car. Therefore, in the embodied milieu, concepts have the same structure as perceptual experiences.

A Third Approach: Integrative

Nevertheless, research provides support for a middle approach to concept representation, proposing that meaning is grounded in both words and in perceptual experiences, namely meaning access is accomplished through the involvement of two systems: a language-like system (i.e., linguistic system) and a perceptual or image-based system (i.e., simulation system). A detailed investigation into the role of these two systems is found in the work of Lawrence Barsalou's linguistic and situated simulation theory. According to the linguistic and situated simulation theory, the linguistic system helps individuals communicate the concepts stored in their mind and create a network containing semantically associated words. This network encompasses categories of words and relations among concepts. Simulation is the process by which concepts reevoke or produce perceptual states present when individuals are perceiving and acting in the real world. Hence, for example, being able to name different colors of APPLE is possible due to simulation. In fact, the linguistic and situated simulation theory holds that when a word is presented (heard or seen), both the linguistic and simulation systems become active immediately to access its meaning; nevertheless, the activation of the linguistic system peaks before that of the simulation system. The reason is probably that the linguistic forms of representation are more analogous to the perceived words than the simulation of related experiences.

Yet, the activation of the linguistic system is rather superficial because meaning is principally represented in the simulation system. For example, *car* first activates *vehicle* and *automobile*, and then, these associated linguistic forms act like pointers to related conceptual information. This process causes image-based simulation to occur, and meaning access is described as progressing deep and deeper.

Evidence for Contribution of Linguistic and Simulation Systems in Meaning Access

Two tasks that have provided evidence for the involvement of the linguistic and simulation systems in meaning access are the property verification task and the property generation task. In a property verification task, which is a passive and recognition-oriented task, the participant reads a word (e.g., *chair*) presented on a computer screen and verifies whether the next presented word represents a true or false property of its concept (e.g., *facet* vs. *seat*). Typically, the simulation system is expected to be involved because conceptual information must be retrieved that identifies whether the property is a part of the concept.

Nevertheless, task condition may cause participants to mostly rely on the linguistic system. That is, when information in the linguistic system is sufficient, participants do not utilize the simulation system. On true trials, the given property is always a part of the concept (e.g., ELEPHANT—*tusk*, SAILBOAT—*mast*). Consequently, the type of false properties presented is the factor that determines whether the processing is superficial or deep. On false trials, if the given property is unrelated to the concept (e.g., AIRPLANE—*cake*, BUS—*fruit*), the involvement of the linguistic system is sufficient for adequate performance. That is because correct responses in this condition are highly correlated with linguistic associativeness; that is, object and property being associated are equal to a *true* response, and being not associated is equal to a *false* response. Thus, participants consult only the linguistic system, and processing is superficial. In contrast, when true trials (e.g., ELEPHANT—*tusk*, SAILBOAT—*mast*) are mixed with false trials in which the property is associated with the concept but is not a part of its concept (e.g., TABLE—*furniture*, BANANA—*monkey*), consulting the linguistic system is not sufficient. Consequently, participants must simulate perceptual information for adequate performance.

In the property generation task, which is an active and production-oriented task, a word (e.g., *table*) is presented to the participant who is asked to verbally generate characteristic properties of its concept (e.g., *legs*, *surface*, and *eating on it*). In such a task, when words produced, for instance, in a 5-second period (usually one to three words) are analyzed, the properties that participants produce reveal the involvement of the linguistic system in meaning access. Typically, the linguistic origins of the produced words are shown when *compounds* (e.g., the response *hive* to *bee* comes from *beehive*), *synonyms* (e.g., *automobile* in response to *car*), *antonyms* (e.g., *bad* in response to *good*), *root similarity* (e.g., *selfish* in response to *self*), and *sound similarity* (e.g., *dumpy* in response to *lumpy*) are produced. In contrast, when words produced, for instance, in a 15-second period are analyzed, most produced words originate from the simulation system. In fact, the first responses are still linguistic-based, but they are followed by responses originating in the simulation system. Thus, later responses describe aspects of situations such as *physical properties* (e.g., *wings* in response to *bee*), *setting information* (e.g., *flowers* in response to *bee*), and *mental states* (e.g., *boring* in response to *golf*). Overall, the results of these two tasks suggest that both a faster-acting linguistic system and a slower acting simulation system are involved in conceptual processing and meaning access.

Access to the Meaning of Abstract Words

One main challenge in this area is related to access to the meaning of abstract words. Some experts claim that abstract concepts are represented only through associations with other concepts (i.e., language system). Barsalou casts doubt on this notion and believes that abstract words cannot be learned without the contribution of a simulation system. In effect, abstract concepts are represented in a wide variety of situations featuring predominantly introspective (emotional) and social information, whereas concrete concepts are represented in a restricted range of situations featuring chiefly sensory and motor information. This difference causes the situation to play a critical role in deep processing of abstract words. Therefore, when participants are asked to generate properties of concrete (e.g., BIRD, CAR, and SOFA) and abstract (e.g., TRUTH, FREEDOM, and INVENTION) concepts, in both cases, they produce relevant information about agents, objects, settings, events, and mental states. However, the emphasis placed on these types of information is different. For concrete concepts, the major focus is on information about *objects* and *settings*. In contrast, for abstract concepts, more information about *mental states* and *events* is produced. For instance, for an abstract word like *convince*, a variety of situations (e.g., political, sports, and school) may come to mind to represent events in which one person (agent) is speaking to another in order to change his or her mind. It seems to be difficult for people to process an abstract word without bringing personally relevant situations into their mind. For a concrete word like *rolling*, in contrast, the processing is simpler and more focused; hence, a ball rolling on the ground is imagined.

Therefore, linguistic and simulation systems contribute to meaning access not only for concrete words but also for abstract words. When the linguistic system is involved, meaning access is superficial, whereas meaning access via simulation system is deep.

Ensie Abbassi and Bess Sirmon-Taylor

See also Comprehension; Lexicon; Semantic Development; Semantics; Sense; Vocabulary

Further Readings

Abbassi, E., Blanchette, I., Ansaldo, A. I., Ghassemzadeh, H., & Joanette, Y. (2015). Emotional words can be embodied or disembodied: The role of superficial vs. deep types of processing. *Frontiers in Psychology*, 6, 975.

Barsalou, L. W. (1999). Perceptual symbol systems. *Behavioral and Brain Sciences*, 22, 577–609, 610–560.

Barsalou, L. W., Santos, A., Simmons, W. K., & Wilson, C. D. (2008). Language and simulation in conceptual processing. In M. De Vega, A. M. Glenberg, & A. Graesser (Eds.), *Symbols, embodiment, and meaning* (pp. 245–283). Oxford, UK: Oxford University Press.

Barsalou, L. W., & Wiemer-Hastings, K. (2005). Situating abstract concepts. In D. Pecher & R. Zwann (Eds.), *Grounding cognition: the role of perception and action in memory, language, and thought* (pp. 129–163). New York, NY: Cambridge University Press.

Solomon, K. O., & Barsalou, L. W. (2004). Perceptual simulation in property verification. *Memory & Cognition*, 32, 244–259.

Vigliocco, G., Meteyard, L., Andrews, M., & Kousta, S. (2009). Toward a theory of semantic representation. *Language and Cognition*, 1, 219–247.

Wilson-Mendenhall, C. D., Simmons, W. K., Martin, A., & Barsalou, L. W. (2013). Contextual processing of abstract concepts reveals neural representations of nonlinguistic semantic content. *Journal of Cognitive Neuroscience*, 25, 920–935.

Wu, L. L., & Barsalou, L. W. (2009). Perceptual simulation in conceptual combination: Evidence from property generation. *Acta Psychologica*, 132, 173–189.

MEDIATION IN THERAPY

Mediation in therapy is an application of constructivist thought to teaching and intervention for typically developing and impaired learners of all ages. It operates on the assumption that human learning takes place in the mind of the individual as he or she transacts with social partners and the environment for the purposes of both making sense of the world and functionally acting upon it. In this entry, *mediation in therapy* represents a conceptualization of the practitioner as a clinical arbiter between the person with a communicative disorder and the environment. It is through this mediation that the therapeutic effect is achieved. This entry provides an overview of the foundation of mediation in therapy and then explores the processes involved in accomplishing and implementing it.

Foundation of Mediation in Therapy

The Russian psychologist Lev Vygotsky recognized that the learning process was not a solitary phenomenon in which the individual constructed cognitive and interactional structures through the exploration of the environment. Rather, development and mental functioning are social affairs through which less expert learners transact with more expert learners via a process that leads to the construction of increased capacity and competence. Intellectuals such as Lev Vygotsky, Jerome Bruner, and many others realized that, in reality, most of the human learning occurs through mediated exposure to the world. Inherent in this belief is the recognition that the mental functioning in a human's development first appears socially before appearing at an individual level. That is, human psychological and cognitive development is constructed through transactions with others before it is internalized. In fact, it is through the transaction that the internal mental structures are created. The zone of proximal development was proposed by Vygotsky as a metaphor explaining the process learners go through as they experience the mediated effects of transacting with more competent meaning makers. The zone of proximal development is that area just beyond the individuals' level of independent functioning in which they can negotiate with the help of more capable and willing partners. It is within this zone that mediation occurs. It is through consistent functioning in this zone that the individual capacity of functioning expands as a result of the social negotiations of meanings and experiences.

The foundational belief that negotiated mediation is the key to the development of mental and interactional functioning is unique to constructivist approaches to therapy. In traditional behaviorist approaches to therapy, the client and clinician are often placed in adversarial relationship roles with specifically defined functions. Knowledge is viewed as a static product held by those who are competent. In clinical circumstances, the clinician holds the knowledge and repeatedly exposes the client to fragmented elements of it with an expectation of accurate and rapid mastery of increasingly complex skills. The eventual aim of traditionally behaviorist methods is the generalizability of skills to increasingly complex contexts until success in functional settings can be achieved by the client.

In contrast, mediation places an emphasis on establishing collaborative and integrative relationships with learners as they negotiate authentic contexts together. Mediators recognize that learners are resilient and bring a host of strengths and experience to every learning experience. They recognize that knowledge is ever changing and negotiated within social transactions. Efforts are made to facilitate the learners' ability to draw upon individual strengths as they construct strategies necessary to take increasingly more competent roles in the communicative context. Rather than fixing problems, mediators recognize that the clinician's role is to shape the context in a way that enhances opportunities for the learner's communicative success. Clinicians then do not teach; rather, they facilitate the construction of meaning. Learners, for their part, acquire and construct competency. Mediators facilitate therapeutic effects by making the environment and the client's contributions comprehensible.

Accomplishing Mediation in Therapy

Mediation in therapy is accomplished when the clinicians act as the meaning maker in an interaction by positioning their abilities between the learner and the environment and ensuring that both parties are comprehensible to each other. As the learner encounters the environment or context, the mediators take the incoming stimuli and modify them so that learners experience them within their zone of proximal development. The mediator is then responsive to the learner's efforts to act upon the environmental input. As the learner acts upon his or her context or environment, a mediator transforms, where necessary, the learner's output so that it is comprehensible. This negotiated dance of the mediator between the learner and the world ensures that interactions are effective, efficient, and appropriate. In order to do this, mediators must recognize the value of each party. The psychologist Kenneth Gergens suggests that mediated learning contrasts from behaviorist thought as a kinder and gentler understanding of human learning. Furthermore, he recognizes that it more accurately reflects the reality that humans experience as they develop mental, social, and cognitive functioning throughout their life.

The mediator assumes that an individual's behavior at any given time is driven by an internal logic system and makes sense, at least in some way, to him or her. Because of this underlying assumption of strengths, a mediator is primarily interested in understanding the process that leads to a learner's behaviors. By understanding a client's thoughts and interactional processes, the mediator can strategically facilitate the establishment of comprehensibility through modifying the context or the learner's response to the context. This is accomplished by focusing on the process of the interaction and guiding the client through questions, summarizations, and the use of predictions to promote the integration of previously addressed information in order to make logical expectations as to what might come. The mediator then assists the client in verifying or disproving these predictions after further transaction with the context occurs.

Implementing Mediation in Therapy

In order to implement mediation in therapy, clinicians should strive to operate within the individual's zone of proximal development to enhance the construction of meaning making. Mediated therapy strategies focus primarily on comprehensibility and secondarily on the structural elements of the interaction. That is, whether or not the social or intellectual transactions make sense is more important than the structural acceptability of an interaction. Importantly, issues of whether or not the transaction makes sense must be determined from the perspective of learner. For example, when a client is reading, the clinician looks for behaviors reflecting that connections are being constructed between what is being read and the background experience the client brings to the reading process. Any instruction provided by the clinician is tailored to helping the client connect the reading material with his or her background.

A number of programs and specific approaches have been proposed and carried out since the 1970s describing many ways in which mediation has been implemented in therapeutic and educational settings. Reuven Feuerstein developed mediated learning experiences as a programized approach to determine how a struggling learner can benefit from instruction and then through instrumental enrichment programs make strides toward improvement. Feuerstein's and similar formal approaches to mediation in therapy have shown significant success and have been well received in some settings. However, mediation in therapy does not always need to be as formally programized as these approaches in order to be successful. Most clinicians who embrace constructivist models of human learning are able to provide mediation in therapy by attending to the underlying principles of constructivism.

Ultimately, clinicians are responsible for creating contexts in which learning can occur and then mediating the learner's negotiation with those contexts. Jack S. Damico advocates that mediation in therapy is most readily and naturally accomplished as educators and clinicians strategically implement five guiding principles of constructivism in action. These principles represent mental reminders educators and clinicians can use as they create and reflect upon their efforts to provide learners with mediation in therapy.

- Meaningful—When aiming to provide mediation in therapy, all clinical activities and the materials and texts used to accomplish these activities should be intrinsically meaningful and functionally relevant to the learner and to the overall aim of the activity. This translates to the use of authentic experiences with various modes of meaning making (e.g., reading, writing, speaking, listening, and thinking). For example, when dealing with reading, whole, well-written texts are utilized. If oral language development is the therapeutic focus, then clients should experience authentic activities where oral language is used for real purposes to accomplish functionally relevant objectives. When the activities and supports of therapy are not meaningful, clients must spend time trying to figure out the functional relevance of an activity rather than experiencing the growth that comes from successfully participating in the activity. The mediator's role is to facilitate the learner's efforts to make sense of these authentic experiences.
- Contextually Embedded—When meaningful activities and materials are employed, the therapeutic value is found and constructed as the learner encounters the authentic context. Mediation embedded within functionally authentic contexts positions the learner as a successful and capable social agent. The learner is not left needing to generalize abstract skills to the real-world scenarios because the instruction is already embedded within contexts. An advantage of embedding instruction within authentic and meaningful contexts is that the contexts themselves end up functioning as a mediating therapeutic agent for the learner. Thus, the learner benefits from both the mediator and the context in which the activity occurs.
- Contrastive—Within therapeutic contexts, mediators ensure that the learner either is successful in his or her efforts or experiences reactions that facilitate success through the use of responsive strategies. The mediator's role is to help the learner recognize the difference between the unsuccessful interaction with the context and the mediated success. Mediators know that the learners will use these contrastive experiences to construct strategies that can be employed to achieve more effective, efficient, and/or appropriate future interactions. It is the recognition of contrastiveness in meaning making that allows learners to go beyond the information given and expand their zone of independent functioning.
- Active Engagement—Because learning is an active process of making sense of and through experiences, mediators ensure that therapeutic activities actively engage the learner in the meaning-making process. Again the use of meaningful and functional activities and materials is key in providing the social and cognitive motivation for the learner. Mediation in therapy is centered on the learner's process of actively engaging with materials and social partners presented in authentic contexts. Mediators facilitate this engagement by bridging gaps between the learner's transactional processes and the effects and responses of the environment, and those within it, to the learner's efforts.
- Recurrence—Mediators recognize that a functional recursiveness must exist in order for learners to develop the meaning-making strategies and mental operations necessary to function independently. Mediation in therapy

ensures that learners have many authentic opportunities to construct competence. Temporal and spatial saturation of meaning-making opportunities is provided to the learner by the efforts mediators make in ensuring that the first four principles are met. A specific criterion response rate is not the aim of recurrent opportunities; rather, a communicative and interactive competency with the concepts and contexts is the objective of mediation in therapy.

Ryan Nelson

See also Competence and Performance; Constructivism; Meaning; Positive Psychology and Wellness

Further Readings

Damico, H. L., Damico, J. S., Nelson, R. L., Weill, C., & Maxwell, J. (2016). Infusing meaning and joy back into books: Reclaiming literacy in the treatment of young children with autism spectrum disorder. In R. J. Meyer & K. F. Whitmore (Eds.), *Reclaiming early childhood literacies: Narratives of hope, power, and vision* (pp. 109–119). New York, NY: Routledge.

Feuerstein, R., & Lewin-Benham, A. (2012). *What learning looks like: Mediated learning in theory and practice, K–6*. New York, NY: Teacher College Press.

Vygotsky, L. S. (1978). *Mind in society: The development of higher psychological processes* (M. Cole, V. John-Steiner, S. Scribner, & E. Souberman, Eds. & Trans.). Cambridge, MA: Harvard University Press. (Original work published 1930–1933)

Medical Management of Voice Disorders

In caring for patients with voice disorders, medical management by an otolaryngologist or a laryngologist (i.e., an otolaryngologist with specialized training in care of voice, swallowing, and airway disorders) often serves to accompany behavioral management. Behavioral management involves voice therapy intervention performed by a certified speech–language pathologist with specialization in assessing and treating voice disorders. Medical management includes specific pharmacologic and surgical interventions for the voice-disordered population. This entry discusses the following laryngeal diagnoses and their medical management: laryngitis/upper respiratory infection (URI), vocal fold hemorrhage, phonotraumatic vocal fold lesion, vocal process granuloma, laryngopharyngeal reflux disease (LPRD), vocal fold paresis/paralysis, presbylarynx, spasmodic dysphonia (SD), and essential voice tremor (EVT).

Laryngitis/URI

Often, URI will manifest as symptoms of cold with associated dysphonia (laryngitis). The voice will drop in pitch because of vocal fold edema or swelling. As the vocal fold inflammation progresses, sometimes patients *lose their voice*, a result of the vocal folds losing their ability to vibrate normally. If coughing persists, eventual vocal fold thickening can develop along the vibratory surfaces. In this setting, vocal improvement can take several weeks beyond the resolution of the remaining URI symptoms. Frequently, URIs are viral and are, therefore, not responsive to antibiotic therapy. In the setting of voice changes that accompany a URI, it is most often recommended to rest the voice as much as possible, as continued voicing in this setting can lead to injury such as the development of a phonotraumatic vocal fold lesion. In severe cases, steroids can be prescribed to help decrease the vocal fold inflammation present; this intervention should be guided by laryngeal exam and may be coupled with a brief period of strict voice rest (e.g., 5–7 days) for optimal results. (Strict voice rest implies no voice use whatsoever, including no whispering.) Antitussive medications to help reduce coughing frequency and severity can be utilized as an adjunct. Room humidification, steaming, and adequate hydration efforts help contribute to a successful vocal recovery.

Vocal Fold Hemorrhage

Vocal fold hemorrhage is a phonotraumatic injury resulting from the rupture of a blood vessel and associated extravasation of blood into the superficial lamina propria of the vocal fold. As a result, the affected vocal fold does not vibrate normally, and dysphonia results. Historically, vocal fold hemorrhage has been regarded as a vocally emergent situation, requiring strict voice rest until recovery (confirmed by laryngeal exam). The urgency of this scenario centers on the risk of potential vocal fold scarring if the blood is not completely resorbed in a timely fashion; although this sequela is not strictly evidence based, laryngologists continue to treat vocal fold hemorrhage very seriously. Along with strict voice rest (typically 5–7 days), avoidance of medications (e.g., nonsteroidal anti-inflammatory drugs, full-strength aspirin) or supplements (e.g., ginger, ginkgo biloba, garlic) that have an effect of thinning the blood is important. The presence of varices, or dilated blood vessels, on the vocal folds increases the risk of vessel rupture with resultant hemorrhage. Laser ablation or surgical excision of the offending varix may be recommended for patients with a history of previous hemorrhage.

Phonotraumatic Vocal Fold Lesion

The development of a phonotraumatic vocal fold lesion is considered an injury related to mechanical trauma to the vocal folds. Many refer to vocal *overuse, misuse, and abuse* as the three varieties of phonotrauma. Care must be taken in communicating with the voice community about phonotrauma, however, as these labels can sometimes unnecessarily shame the patient. Typically, phonotraumatic lesions are located at the region of the *striking zone* or the middle portion of the vibratory surface, where the greatest shearing stress occurs during phonation. These lesions interfere with vocal fold closure and vibration patterns, often creating a raspy voice quality. Examples of phonotraumatic lesions include nodules, polyps, and cysts.

Nodules come in pairs and exist opposite to each other; they can be asymmetric in size and are associated with a variable amount of epithelial thickening. Stroboscopically, a typical hourglass closure pattern is seen. There is a nodular spectrum of severity including a diagnostic category of *prenodular formations*, when there is minimal thickening or fibrosis present. Nodules are analogous to a callus that can develop on a person's heel over time. Nodules are generally classed as nonoperative or inoperable lesions, meaning surgical removal is not recommended. Nodules are often chronic and respond well to efforts at decreasing the vocal dose, such as through vocal pacing efforts. Typically, as the nodules shrink and soften, they have less of an effect on voice quality.

Polyps are typically single lesions that can be hemorrhagic or translucent. Translucent polyps are also referred to as *pseudocysts*. Polyps involve the superficial lamina propria and vary in shape and size. Unlike nodules, polyps may require surgical intervention in the form of a microflap excision or laser ablation if they do not resolve through behavioral intervention.

Vocal fold cysts develop within a lining and exist in either fluid (mucus retention) or semisolid (epithelial inclusion) state. They are the least common of the benign vocal fold lesions. They can develop more superficially in the vocal fold or deeper and close to the vocal ligament. Stroboscopically, they are known to impair the mucosal wave. Like polyps, vocal fold cysts may also require a microflap excision, pending their response to behavioral intervention. Surgically, vocal fold cysts can sometimes be more challenging than polyps, especially if they develop deeper within the superficial lamina propria and require more extensive dissection for removal. Additionally, vocal fold cysts can recur, especially if the cyst lining is not removed in its entirety.

Microflap surgery is performed endoscopically through the mouth, using cold steel instrumentation and microscopy to delicately excise the polyp while preserving all surrounding normal tissue and minimizing scar formation. Strict voice rest in the postoperative period is typically employed to facilitate healing.

Vocal Process Granuloma

Vocal process granulomas are sequelae of perichondritis of the arytenoid cartilage. Granulomas can exist as unilateral or bilateral masses of granulation tissue and are centered on the vocal process of the arytenoid. They are a result of mechanical irritation to the posterior glottis. Patients often present with focal odynophagia, or pain with swallowing, that is on the same side as the granuloma. If the granuloma is large enough, it can also impair vocal function or, in some cases, obstruct the airway. One of the most common causes of vocal process granulomas is endotracheal intubation, as the endotracheal tube sits in the posterior glottis and can injure the vocal processes as a result. Other mechanical causes of granuloma formation include chronic coughing or throat clearing as well as a pressed voicing pattern with associated forceful adduction patterns. Chemical irritation at the posterior glottis may result from laryngopharyngeal reflux. Typically, nonoperative management of vocal process granulomas is recommended, as surgical manipulation can lead to recurrence and progression of disease severity. Simple observation in the case of intubation granulomas (that are not associated with new-onset coughing or throat clearing) may be sufficient, as these will often resolve spontaneously over time. Behavioral management in the form of cough and throat clear reduction therapy is often very effective. Additionally, antireflux measures such as dietary and behavioral changes, in combination with medications such as proton pump inhibitors and histamine blockers, are frequently prescribed for an 8- to 12-week period. Additionally, oral steroid inhalers can help to decrease the inflammation topically. In the office, intralesional steroid injections are sometimes effective. Laryngeal botulinum toxin injections can help to temporarily decrease the forceful adduction patterns. If necessary, especially if the granulomas are obstructive, laser ablation or even surgical excision may be required.

Laryngopharyngeal Reflux Disease

Laryngopharyngeal reflux exists when stomach contents travel in a retrograde fashion to the level of the larynx and pharynx. Especially if this happens repeatedly, this can cause irritation to these structures. The mucosal lining of the larynx and pharynx is more sensitive to acid exposure than the lining of the esophagus. Symptoms of LPRD can include a globus sensation, or the feeling of a lump in the throat, difficulty swallowing, chronic coughing or throat clearing, and a sour taste in the mouth. Typical chest burning symptoms of gastroesophageal reflux disease are not necessarily present with LPRD, which is why it is often referred to as *silent reflux*. Laryngoscopic findings of erythema and edema at the posterior larynx are nonspecific. There is not a perfect diagnostic study for LPRD; however, often pH/impedance testing can be performed using a probe placed in the oropharynx or hypopharyngeal region. Additionally, positive salivary pepsin testing may help confirm the presence of LPR.

Dietary and behavioral management, especially weight loss, is the most effective management strategy for those with LPRD. Proton pump inhibitors, sometimes in combination with histamine blockers, can also be prescribed for a 2- to 3-month period to allow for mucosal repair. In certain cases, surgical intervention may be required to help tighten the valve between the stomach and the esophagus.

Vocal Fold Paresis/Paralysis

Vocal fold weakness causes glottic incompetence, or underclosure, and an inability for the glottis to function normally. As a result, patients struggle with a breathy voice, a weak cough, and windedness with exertion and phonation due to constant air escape through the glottis. Similarly, thin liquid dysphagia results, as patients with vocal fold weakness have a *leaky valve* at the entrance to their tracheas. Vocal fold paralysis and paresis are both neurogenic in origin and are secondary to vagal or recurrent laryngeal nerve injury. Vocal fold paralysis is diagnosed when there is no movement of the affected vocal fold. Vocal fold paresis is associated with some, albeit reduced, movement of the affected vocal fold. Causes of both vocal fold paresis and paralysis include inadvertent nerve injury from surgical procedures of the neck or chest, tumors, trauma, pressure injuries from endotracheal tube cuffs, and even viral illnesses. Idiopathic vocal fold paresis/paralysis means there is no obvious root cause or etiology. Evaluation of vocal fold paralysis often includes neck and chest imaging to rule out the presence of a tumor. Treatment involves procedures to restore glottic competence. Within the first 9 months after injury, vocal fold injection augmentation procedures serve as a temporizing measure. By bulking up the immobile vocal fold, this in effect shifts it closer to the midline, which allows for easier approximation of the vocal folds. These procedures can be performed in the office setting or in the operating room, if patients do not tolerate the in-office approach. After 9 months, permanent interventions can be considered, including framework surgery such as a thyroplasty with a possible arytenoid adduction as an adjunct. The thyroplasty procedure involves the placement of an implant in the paraglottic space through a window created in the thyroid cartilage; this serves to shift the immobile vocal fold to a more medial position. The arytenoid adduction helps to tether the arytenoid joint in a more optimal position for voicing. Also, reinnervation procedures can help to restore tone in the setting of vocal fold paralysis. In the setting of vocal fold weakness, often maladaptive compensatory voicing habits result. These bad voicing habits should be addressed through voice therapy intervention. If they persist even after glottic competence has been restored, they can hinder vocal improvement.

Presbylarynx

Presbylarynx or *aging larynx* results from atrophy of the laryngeal soft tissues. Additionally, decreased tone and elasticity of the vocal folds leads to a thinner or weaker voice quality, decreased vocal range, and less stamina vocally. In men, especially, the speaking voice pitch will often increase. Stroboscopically, presbylarynx is notable for vocal fold bowing and prominent vocal processes. Behavioral intervention is often recommended initially to optimize the coordination of the vocal subsystems. Similar procedures to restore glottic competence in vocal fold weakness can be performed bilaterally in the setting of vocal fold atrophy. In-office vocal fold injection augmentations as a trial procedure can be useful, as these are temporary and do not require a general anesthetic, which is ideal for the elderly population. In cases where a permanent augmentation is desired, bilateral thyroplasty procedures can be performed under local anesthesia with sedation.

Spasmodic Dysphonia

SD is a neurologic voice disorder and more specifically, a focal dystonia of the larynx. SD affects connected speech and manifests as unpredictable spasms of the glottis. Adductor SD is characterized by voicing arrests caused by involuntary contractions of laryngeal adductors (i.e., the muscles that bring the vocal folds together); these voicing arrests are typically noted more with vowels. Abductor SD is characterized by breathy arrests caused by involuntary contractions of laryngeal abductors (i.e., the muscles that bring the vocal folds apart); these are typically noted more with consonants. Mixed SD presents with both adductor and abductor voice arrests. Adductor SD is the most common subtype of SD and the most easily treatable. The co-prevalence of clinically significant vocal tremor in patients with SD has been reported to be approximately 25–30%. It is not clear whether SD has a genetic basis; many report environmental triggers (such as significant stressors) at the time of onset. Treatment for SD involves the administration of laryngeal botulinum toxin injections. These are performed in the office setting with electromyographic guidance. Botulinum toxin targets in adductor SD are the thyroarytenoid/lateral cricoarytenoid complexes. In abductor SD, the targets are the posterior cricoarytenoid muscles. Botulinum toxin causes muscle weakening by reversibly blocking the release of acetylcholine (a neurotransmitter) at the nerve synapse. The larynx makes a well-suited target for botulinum toxin administration. Not only are the muscles accessible transcervically but also there exists a clear anatomic division between the adductors and abductors. A breathy period and thin liquid dysphagia often result for 1–3 weeks following injections for adductor SD, with therapeutic improvement lasting for 2–3 months thereafter. Surgical options are available for selected patients with SD; one example is the Selective Laryngeal Adductor Denervation-Reinnervation procedure. Voice therapy intervention can help to clarify the diagnosis and unload the supraglottic hyperfunction often seen with neurologic voice disorders. When combined with botulinum toxin, voice therapy may assist in further improving voice quality and prolonging the benefit of pharmacological effects.

Essential Voice Tremor

EVT, like SD, is a neurologic voice disorder. EVT has regular contractile activity (8–10 Hz) that is ongoing during active (e.g., phonation) and passive (e.g., respiration) laryngeal tasks. EVT can be produced by tremor involving different parts of the phonatory mechanism and can contain horizontal and/or vertical components. It is referred to as essential *voice tremor* instead of *laryngeal tremor* because other muscles of the phonatory apparatus are often variably involved, such as pharyngeal and palatal muscles. Botulinum toxin treatment to the vocal folds is generally considered first-line in the absence of tremor elsewhere in the body. Like adductor SD, the laryngeal targets for the horizontal component in EVT are the thyroarytenoid/lateral cricoarytenoid complexes. The strap muscles can be injected to address the vertical component. Adding oral therapy (such as propranolol or primidone) can be considered an adjunct in cases where botulinum toxin is not producing the desired result. As mentioned previously, tremor is present in approximately 25–30% of patients with SD. Therapeutic expectations for botulinum toxin treatment for tremor are different from those for SD. With adductor SD, specifically, botulinum toxin therapy can nearly eliminate the voicing arrests, whereas with EVT, botulinum toxin therapy serves to decrease the severity of the tremor and cannot eliminate it. This is because often multiple phonatory structures are affected by the tremor, yet typically, only the glottis is specifically targeted with botulinum toxin. Many patients with EVT report decreased effort with phonation after laryngeal botulinum toxin administration. Voice therapy for EVT can help the patient to both increase vocal awareness and adapt to the tremor through optimization of voice production.

Final Thoughts

The physical, emotional, and social burden of having a voice disorder is immense. A multidisciplinary approach serves the voice-disordered community well given that these disorders are multidimensional. Thus, medical management of voice disorders is best served in combination with behavioral management. This integrated approach is accomplished through the partnership of an otolaryngologist or laryngologist and voice therapist.

Lesley F. Childs

See also Anatomy of the Human Larynx; Laryngeal Disorders: Benign Vocal Fold Pathologies; Vocal Hygiene; Voice Disorders; Voice Therapy

Further Readings

Belafsky, P. C., & Rees, C. J. (2007). Identifying and managing laryngopharyngeal reflux. *Hospital Physician, 27*, 15–20.

Blitzer, A. (2010). Spasmodic dysphonia and botulinum toxin: Experience from the largest treatment series. *European Journal of Neurology, 17* (Suppl. 1), 28–30.

Kerwin, L. J., Estes, C., Oromendia, C., Christos, P., & Sulica, L. (2017). Long-term consequences of vocal fold hemorrhage. *Laryngoscope, 127*(4), 900–906.

Rosen, C. A., & Simpson, B. (2008). *Operative techniques in laryngology*. Springer. New York, NY

Memory

Memory is the process of encoding, storing, and retrieving information. Historically, psychologists have partitioned memory into two systems: short-term memory (STM) and long-term memory (LTM). STM memory refers to a temporary store for information that is held in mind for just a few seconds. STM has a very limited capacity of just 4–6 items. LTM holds information for much longer periods of time and has a much larger capacity. The term *working memory* (WM) is used to refer to multiple STM and LTM processes that are involved in holding information in an accessible state and then manipulating it for use in completing a task or solving a problem. The primary difference between WM and STM is that WM refers to moment-by-moment storage and manipulation, while STM refers to only the temporary storage of information. WM plays an important role in language acquisition, production, and comprehension because language development and use involves encoding, storing, and retrieving information related to sequences of sounds in words, sequences of words in sentences, and sequences of sentences in discourse (e.g., conversations, stories, and expository texts) that children are exposed to in their environment. This entry explores models of WM and how it is assessed, then provides an overview of LTM, the neuroscience of memory, and the relationship between memory deficits and speech disorders.

Models of WM

There are two main types of WM models: those that focus on the way information is stored and those that focus on the processes involved in storing information. A very popular storage model is the multicomponent model of WM by Alan Baddeley and his colleagues, in 2010. This model has four critical components: a phonological loop, a visuospatial sketchpad, an episodic buffer that interacts with information stored in LTM, and a central executive.

The phonological loop specializes in storing the serial order of verbal information. An example of a measure of the phonological loop is the nonword repetition test in which examinees must repeat multisyllable nonwords (e.g., *megilobon*) after hearing them. According to Baddeley's multicomponent model, verbal information in the phonological loop will fade rapidly unless it is rehearsed. Rehearsal, or subvocally thinking about the sequential order of items over and over, helps recall because it keeps the memory traces in an active conscious state. Because of the phonological loop, people can remember words that sound different better than they can remember words that sound the same, and they can remember shorter words better than longer words. The storage capacity of the phonological loop has been shown to be important for vocabulary development in young children and for second language learning in adults.

The visuospatial sketchpad holds information about the sequential order of visual, spatial, and kinesthetic information. An example of a visuospatial memory task involves showing participants 5 × 5 grids of empty squares. A series of Xs appear in certain squares in the grid in a sequential order. Upon command, examinees are shown and empty grid. Then, they must point to the squares where the Xs appeared in the correct sequential order. For some memory tasks, these memory representations may be organized spatially; for other tasks, they may be organized visually or even motorically. The visuospatial sketchpad plays an important role in learning how to read and write.

The episodic buffer is a processing system that holds chunks of multiple representations together, allowing people to bind together information from the phonological loop, the visuospatial sketchpad, and LTM. People who can only remember sequences of five or six unrelated words (representing phonological loop functions) can easily remember sentences that are more than 10 words long. This happens because the episodic buffer binds ideas and words into chunks (connections between words in the Noun Phrase and the Verb Phrase in LTM) that are used to remember sentences. Therefore, sentence imitation and story repetition tasks can be used to assess the episodic buffer, which plays an important role in communication. The episodic buffer is especially important for discourse because it is the component of memory that enables people to integrate contextual information with language knowledge in LTM.

Finally, the central executive controls attention and supervises the integration of information among the phonological loop, the visuospatial sketchpad, and the episodic buffer. Recall that WM tasks require people to simultaneously store and manipulate information. The central executive controls decisions to maintain attention on a stimulus or shift attention between multiple stimuli. It also regulates cognitive strategies because it decides between alternative plans of action for solving problems.

An example of a WM model that focuses on the processes involved in encoding, storing, and manipulating information is the embedded process model by Nelson Cowan. This model of WM has three principal components: LTM, a subset of information from LTM that has been activated, and the subset of activated information that is in the focus of attention. Cowan's embedded processes model revolves around LTM, which is composed of encoded and organized information about experiences, thoughts, and behaviors called *schemas*. Schemas help facilitate the regrouping and recoding of knowledge into *chunks* of information that become partially activated (available for storage and manipulation) when they are related to the task at hand. Those chunks of information that are the most relevant to the task become part of the focus of attention. From Cowan's prospective, memory capacity varies depending upon the nature of the information to be remembered, the characteristics of the task, the individual's familiarity with the information being stored and manipulated, and the individual's basic storage capabilities. Thus, limitations in WM could result from a combination of attention processes, storage processes, and the way knowledge is organized in LTM. For example, poorly organized knowledge in LTM would be less likely to be activated or would be activated more slowly than well-organized information, resulting in a capacity limitation.

Assessing WM

Researchers primarily assess WM using three types of memory span tasks: simple span, complex span, and running span. *Span* refers to the amount of information that can be stored and recalled within a particular time frame. A simple span task contains a list of sounds, words, or sentences that are presented auditorily or visually. Participants attempt to recall as many items as possible immediately after the last item in the list.

In a complex span task, participants complete a processing task between the time they store information and the time they retrieve it. For example, in a reading span task, individuals read lists of sentences aloud. After reading each sentence, the individual judges whether it is truthful or not. After reading and making truth judgments about a set of sentences, the individual is asked to recall the last word from each sentence in the set.

In the running span task, participants recall items from the end of long lists of words or numbers that vary in lengths. The key difference in the running span is that participants do not know when the list will end. The *n-back* task is an example of a variation of the traditional running span. In the n-back task, individuals listen to and/or see streams of letters or numbers and must decide quickly whether each item that is presented matches one that occurred a certain number of items before it. For example, in a one-back task, the individual indicates when a letter is the same as another letter that is 1 item back. In the following string, the underlined letters are the same as the letter that is immediately before it (1 item back), "B T M L L P K K S D." In a two-back task, the individual indicates when a letter in the string is the same as the letter that is 2 items back (B T M T D L P L S).

Long Term Memory

LTM is often divided into two systems: *declarative memory*, which contains explicit knowledge of facts and events, and *procedural memory*, which contains implicit (largely unconscious) knowledge of the sequences involved in sensorimotor activities (like playing basketball) and grammar. Knowledge in declarative memory can be readily expressed verbally and is often learned as a result of direct instruction. Knowledge in procedural memory is unconsciously acquired by repetition and practice, is difficult to explain verbally, and often lies outside conscious awareness. Declarative knowledge can be tested by a vocabulary test or having someone explain what he or she knows about a topic. Procedural knowledge is often tested with grammatical judgment tasks. Since the early 2000s, implicit learning tasks have been used to assess the ease with which information enters procedural memory. In an implicit learning task, individuals are exposed to a string of letters or numbers in a training phase. After listening to multiple patterns of letters and numbers that are consistent with a rule, participants engage in test phase in which they are asked if a particular string of letters or numbers violates the rule or not. Individuals with strong procedural memory abilities are good at recognizing which strings of sounds or syllables are consistent with the underlying (unstated) rule and which strings of sounds or syllables are not consistent with the rule.

Declarative and procedural memory play different roles in language learning. Declarative memory is hypothesized to play an important role in learning and using words. Procedural memory is hypothesized to play an important role in learning syntax and morphology.

Neuroscience of Memory

Memory ability probably depends on neural activation within complex circuits that vary according to the demands of the modalities (visual–spatial vs. phonological) and tasks (simple recall tasks, complex storage plus processing tasks, or running span tasks). Thus, it should not be surprising that there is a great deal of variability across neural imaging studies of memory. However, there are some consistent findings. In right-handed individuals, left hemisphere structures tend to be more active in verbal memory tasks, while right hemisphere structures tend to be more active in visual–spatial tasks. For verbal tasks, the left hemisphere supplementary motor cortex, the inferior frontal cortex (Broca's area), and the cerebellum are often activated while storing and rehearsing phonological information. The parietal cortex, especially the inferior parietal lobule, is involved in focusing attention on phonological information and storing it. The dorsolateral prefrontal cortex is commonly associated with central executive functions related to controlled attention, and the hippocampus plays an important role in the episodic buffer and LTM. A fertile area of research concerns the neural connections that play a role in different memory systems.

Memory Deficits and Language Disorders

WM limitations have been observed in adults with aphasia and children with specific language impairment (SLI) whether they are performing simple recall, complex recall, or running memory tasks. It appears that individuals with aphasia have restricted storage capacity as well as limitations in controlled attention, which vary in degree as a function of the severity of the aphasia. It is likely that binding functions between word and sentence knowledge in the episodic buffer play a large role in the WM deficits of adults with aphasia.

According to Ullman's Procedural Deficit Hypothesis, SLI in children results from a procedural memory deficit that is related to dysfunctions in underlying brain structures. However, it does not appear that procedural memory deficits are the only aspect of memory that are affected in children with SLI. Some researchers have hypothesized that a specific WM deficit related to remembering and storing phonological information may cause the WM deficit in SLI. Other researchers have hypothesized that WM deficits related to storing and manipulating information play an important role in SLI sentence comprehension. There is evidence suggesting that most children with SLI exhibit lower levels of declarative and procedural memory, WM storage, and attentional control than their same-age peers.

Final Thoughts

Memory is often divided into an STM, an LTM, and a storage and processing system known as WM. Models of these systems are represented by bottom-up models such as Baddeley's Multicomponent Model of memory and in top-down models such as Cowen's Embedded Processes Model of memory.

WM stores and processes are typically measured by three kinds of tasks: simple immediate recall tasks, complex storage and processing tasks, and running span tasks. WM has proven to be a key factor in language acquisition during childhood and in language production and comprehension across the life span.

Ronald B. Gillam and Allison Hancock

See also Aphasia; Brain Imaging; Cognitive Processes and Operations; Language Disorders in Children

Further Readings

Baddeley, A. D. (2003). Working memory and language: An overview. *Journal of Communication Disorders*, 36, 289–208. doi:10.1016/S0021-9924(03)00019-4

Baddeley, A. D. (2012). Working memory: Theories, models, and controversies. *Annual Review of Psychology*, 63(1), 1–29. doi:10.1146/annurev-psych-120710-100422

Cowan, N. (1999). An embedded-processes model of working memory. In A. Miyake & P. Shah (Eds.), *Models of working memory: Mechanisms of active maintenance and executive control* (pp. 62–101). New York, NY: Cambridge University Press.

Henderson, A., Kim, H., Kintz, S., Frisco, N., & Writher, H. H. (2017). Working memory in aphasia: Considering discourse processing and treatment implications. *Seminars in Speech & Language*, 38(1), 40–51.

Montgomery, J., & Evans, J. (2009). Complex sentence comprehension and working memory in children with specific language impairment. *Journal of Speech, Language, and Hearing Research*, 52, 269–288.

Ullman, M. T. (2004). Contributions of memory circuits to language: The declarative/procedural model. *Cognition*, 92, 231–270.

MEMORY DISORDERS

Memory is a cognitive ability particularly sensitive to any type of brain pathology. Focal brain damage can significantly impair memory, especially if mesial structures of the temporal lobes are involved, as well as extended global processes, such as traumatic head injury, dementia, and similar conditions. Memory defects are known as *amnesias*. There exists a basic distinction in amnesia: *specific* and *nonspecific* amnesia. Specific amnesia is a memory defect limited to a particular type of information, for instance, verbal amnesia, amnesia for faces, or amnesia for movements. Nonspecific amnesia refers to amnesia for every type of information. Patients with nonspecific amnesia can present an inability to store new information, that is so-called *anterograde amnesia*, and to recall previously learned information, that is *retrograde amnesia*.

Specific amnesias can be found in cortical lesions; in such cases amnesia for words, for places, and for movements can be observed, depending on the particular location of the damage. Nonspecific amnesias are more frequently found in cases where the mesial structures of the temporal lobe, such as the hippocampus, are damaged. They are also found in cases of diencephalic pathology. Nonspecific amnesias, associated with mammillary bodies and thalamic damage, are also known as *diencephalic* or *axial* amnesias. Diencephalic amnesias can be associated with *confabulation*, or false memories, as it is found in the Korsakoff syndrome.

There is a diversity of conditions associated with memory disturbances. This entry provides an overview of the principal conditions, including Korsakoff syndrome, hippocampal amnesia, amnesia associated with dementia, transient global amnesia, amnesia in traumatic brain injury, and frontal lobe amnesia.

Korsakoff Syndrome

The Korsakoff syndrome is characterized by remote memory impairments associated with severe anterograde memory disturbances. The most prominent memory disturbance is the anterograde amnesia involving both verbal and nonverbal information. In these cases, patients fail to memorize new information; even with multiple repetitions, they are unable to learn new words, names, faces, movements, or facts, and they rapidly forget what happened shortly before. Retrograde amnesia is also observed, commonly extending back for years and even decades. Regardless of the nature of the information, memories from childhood and early adulthood are remembered much better than memories from the recent past.

In addition, confabulations (production of distorted memories) may occur, particularly in the acute stage of the disorder. Two types of confabulation have been distinguished: provoked and spontaneous. The former is more frequently observed in Korsakoff syndrome. Spontaneous confabulation involves an unprovoked outpouring of unrealistic episodic autobiographical claims. These may represent a tendency for patients to fill in gaps in memory when faced with questions they cannot answer. However, confabulations are not specific to Korsakoff syndrome but are commonly seen in a variety of patients with lesions in the frontal lobes, basal forebrain, or both.

It is usually accepted that *declarative memory* (i.e., factual and semantic knowledge) is significantly impaired, whereas *procedural memory* (i.e., how to do something, that is, motor learning) is preserved. Visuoperceptual learning (e.g., the recognition of incomplete pictures) may be preserved in Korsakoff syndrome patients.

In addition, general intellectual abilities can be impaired, but there is a significant variability in the level of cognitive functioning and many patients perform in the average range on standard intelligence tests. Changes in personality traits are also observed in Korsakoff syndrome. Patients usually lack insight, are unconcerned about current events, and are uninterested in their personal appearance.

It has been established that Korsakoff syndrome is directly linked to a deficiency of thiamine (vitamin B1). It is most often related with chronic alcohol abuse, frequently associated with malnutrition. However, Korsakoff syndrome has also been described in the context of diverse disorders that cause malnutrition or malabsorption, including severe dysphagia, anorexia nervosa, persistent vomiting, and AIDS. Thanks to the generally improved standards of nutrition, Korsakoff syndrome of nonalcoholic origin is becoming more infrequent. Traumatic head injuries associated with bilateral lesions of the diencephalic structures may result in a memory disorder quite similar to the Korsakoff disease but frequently referred as *Korsakowian syndrome* or *mental syndrome of Korsakoff*.

Vulnerability to Korsakoff syndrome is highly variable. Among alcoholics with extensive drinking histories and malnutrition, only a minority develop the syndrome. Moreover, a genetic predisposition to impaired thiamine metabolism has been postulated. Treatment with thiamine is critical; this treatment usually results in a marked improvement in the neurologic symptoms but only modest recovery of the memory defects.

Some brain abnormalities can be found in these patients. Bilateral, symmetrically placed, punctate lesions in the area of the third ventricle, fourth ventricle, and aqueduct are characteristics of Korsakoff syndrome. Atrophy of the mammillary bodies, the mammillothalamic tract, and the anterior thalamus are considered responsible for the amnesia.

Hippocampal Amnesia

Bilateral lesions at the level of the hippocampus and the amygdala produce severe anterograde and a retrograde amnesia that could include the information acquired about 2–3 years before the lesion. Older memories, however, remain intact. Memory impairments are found in declarative memory for both episodic (experiential) and semantic (language mediated) information. Immediate memory (e.g., repeating digits or words) is normal and patients can generally keep information in working memory; however, if their attention is directed to another topic, that information disappears. Nonetheless, intelligence test results are typically normal. No attention disturbances are found, and these patients are aware of the memory defect and attempt to develop strategies to compensate for the deficit.

Unilateral injuries in the left hippocampus produce anterograde amnesia particularly in semantic memory, while lesions in the right hippocampus usually cause selectively impaired episodic memory. This type of amnesia could appear in patients with hypoxia (deficiency in the amount of oxygen reaching the tissues) or patients with epilepsy in the temporal lobe who have undergone surgery. It is also found in cases of herpes simplex encephalitis, which selectively affects the hippocampus.

One of the most studied cases of hippocampal amnesia was one of a patient referred to as HM who had epilepsy since the age of 16. At the age of 27, HM underwent a bitemporal lobectomy. After the surgery, HM was incapable of registering new experiences (anterograde amnesia), even though he was able to recall experiences before the surgery. Moreover, Brenda Miller, a researcher who studied his case very closely, had to reintroduce herself to him every session or else he would not recognize her. However, regardless of HM's memory defects, HM had a completely normal intellectual capacity and was very conscious of his memory deficits and often apologized. Ultimately, this patient managed to accomplish many motor tasks, such as learning to follow a maze using feedback. The way he executed these tasks and the time it took for him to accomplish them improved tremendously from session to session. Nonetheless, he was incapable of recognizing that task from the previous session, meaning each session felt like the first time he had accomplished the task. Therefore, HM had a preserved procedural (implicit) memory but an impaired declarative (explicit) memory.

The hippocampus' function is seen to be significantly related to structures of the limbic system, particularly the amygdala. Furthermore, the hippocampus and the amygdala are interconnected; the amygdala is directly linked to the dorsomedial nucleus of the thalamus, which plays an essential role in Korsakoff syndrome. Moreover, memory disturbances can be observed with bilateral injuries in the amygdala and the hippocampus. Injuries in the left hippocampus–amygdala cause the patient to be unable to remember simple sentences or stories or learn simple verbal tasks. On the other hand, right-sided lesions in the hippocampus/amygdala lead to visual learning defects, causing difficulty in identifying geometric figures, faces, and, in general, nonverbal information.

Traumatic Amnesia

Traumatic head injuries are associated to some degree with amnesia. Furthermore, posttraumatic amnesia is regarded as the best source of information for monitoring the impact and course of traumatic brain injury. In moderate traumatic brain injuries, there is a loss of consciousness for more than 5 minutes but less than 6 hours, while in severe traumatic brain injury the loss of consciousness lasts for 6 hours or more. In both types of brain trauma, there can exist a posttraumatic amnesia for more than 24 hours.

Traumatic brain injuries usually result from frontotemporal contusions and coup–contrecoup contusions. Memory deficits are the consequence of bilateral injuries to the basolateral and median frontal cortex as well as the temporal lobes. A significant diffuse traumatic brain injury is generally associated with evident frontotemporal contusions that impair both frontal functions (e.g., executive functions) and temporal functions (e.g., learning and memory). Frontal injury may cause disinhibition, inappropriate behavior, irritability, and personality changes.

Most traumatic brain injuries are closed (nonpenetrating) and result from motor vehicle accidents, falls, or fights. Nonpenetrating traumatic brain injuries are due to the linear or rotational acceleration of the head. Further brain injuries result from edema, hematomas, obstructive hydrocephalus, traumatic vascular injuries, subarachnoid hemorrhage, and systemic fat emboli. In general, the more severe the traumatic brain injury is, the greater the structural brain damage.

Traumatic head injuries may result in diverse cognitive disturbances, sometimes conforming to dementia. Older adults who present a significant cognitive decline and early-onset dementia quite often have traumatic head injury history. Dementia is also observed after repeated blows to the head; as a result, a significant percentage of professional boxers develop a so-called dementia pugilistica.

Evolution is variable. After the posttraumatic amnesia, there is a 6- to 12-month period of rapid recovery, after which improvement is slower. A healthy recovery depends on a diverse range of factors, including shorter duration of posttraumatic amnesia. Some degree of amnesia, both anterograde and retrograde, represents one of the major long-term sequelae of traumatic head injury.

Transient Global Amnesia

The fundaments characteristic of transient global amnesia is an episode of acute onset of transient global anterograde amnesia, with variable degree retrograde memory impairment; this memory disturbance is not associated with any other significant neurologic signs or symptoms. The onset usually is abrupt, and anterograde memory is severely impaired. Information is rapidly forgotten, and the patient can keep repeating the very same question over and over again. Global anterograde amnesia affects verbal and nonverbal memory in a similar way. The duration of retrograde amnesia varies from hours to years. Nonetheless, immediate memory (e.g., repeating digits) and procedural memory (e.g., driving) are preserved. Moreover, the patient's attention remains normal but can sometimes preset with anxiety. Nonetheless, general information and the ability to perform complex tasks, such as reading, writing, and solving arithmetical problems, are usually unaffected. Even personality traits and executive functions, such as abstract thinking and problem solving, are preserved; language also remains unimpaired. Resolution is gradual, usually occurring within 2–12 hours. During recovery, distant memories appear before more recent ones.

There are some potentially precipitating identifiable factors in about 50% of the events, such as intense emotion, sexual intercourse, pain, Valsalva-like activities, and extreme temperatures such as taking a hot bath or swimming in very cold water.

In an extensive study in France at the Caen University Hospital, Quinette and colleagues analyzed 1,495 cases, including those reported in the literature and their own cases, and concluded: (1) differences in gender ratio are observed when comparing different reports; risk factors may be different in men and women; (2) the vast majority of attacks occur between the ages of 50 and 80 years; (3) although recurrences have been reported, in most patients, transient global amnesia occurs only once; (4) the only factor significantly associated with an increased risk of transient global amnesia, particularly in younger patients, is migraine; (5) psychological and emotional instability history is frequently found in transient global amnesia patients; these patients may be particularly sensitive to psychological stress; (6) in addition, precipitating events (observed in more than 50% of the cases) include emotional stress, physical effort, water contact (temperature change), and sexual intercourse; (7) associated symptoms (more than 70% of the cases) include headache, nausea, and dizziness; (8) more frequently (more than 50% of the cases) the episode begins in the morning; duration is usually 1–9 hours; and (9) a hierarchical cluster analysis revealed different subgroups of patients; in women, episodes are mainly associated with an emotional precipitating event and certain personality traits, whereas in men, they are usually more frequently associated with physical precipitating events. In younger patients, a history of migraine represents an important risk factor.

Ultimately, the etiology of transient global amnesia is controversial. Different potential causes have been suggested including a transient ischemic attack, migraine, epilepsy, vein thrombosis, and some toxic and metabolic disturbances.

Amnesia in Dementia

The diagnosis of dementia requires a significant memory defect, plus other defects in cognition. Hence, amnesia is the cardinal element in dementia diagnosis. Alzheimer's disease, the most frequent type of dementia, usually begins with a progressive loss of memory, particularly episodic memory (i.e., memory for events). When advancing, the disease becomes an extended amnesia, so anterograde as retrograde. Here, the patient only recalls events that have occurred several years prior. In addition, language defects can be observed due to verbal memory defects.

In cases of general cognitive deterioration, most of the patient's memory capability is altered, including a decrease in immediate memory, as well as short-term and long-term memory defects. Patients with Alzheimer's disease are less capable of memory storage when compared to the average-aged adult.

In the second most frequent type of dementia, vascular dementia, the memory pattern varies correlating to the specific areas of brain infarcts. Frequently, there occur specific forms of amnesia that affect only one type of information. For instance, left temporal infarcts are associated with verbal memory defects, whereas right temporal infarcts are associated with spatial amnesia and amnesia for faces, where patients are incapable of recognizing places and faces, but no impairments in verbal abilities are observed.

In other dementia cases, in which the cerebral impairment is more prominent in subcortical structures (so-called frontal–subcortical dementias or simply subcortical dementias), the memory defect is observed particularly in retrieving or recovering information rather than storing it. Patients tend to store new information adequately, but they present with obvious difficulties when retrieving it; the normal access to memory traces already stored seems to be impaired. This defect has been described in patients with Parkinson's disease, Huntington's disease, and Wilson's disease.

Frontal Amnesia

Frontal lobe damage may result in memory disturbances associated with other cognitive defects, such as attention impairments. A pure amnesic syndrome is not frequent in cases of frontal lobe lesions. In addition to the amnesic syndrome, the patient usually presents attentional defects that do not allow adequate information storage. However, an overt amnesia is usually found in cases of bilateral frontal lesions; rupture of aneurysms of the anterior communicating artery is associated with nonspecific amnesia and frequently confabulation; in the acute phase, these patients are confused, experiencing a complete anosognosia (i.e., refusal to acknowledge) regarding the amnesic deficit. In addition to amnesia, behavioral changes characterized by disinhibition and behavioral inadequacy are observed.

Patients with frontal tumors also have difficulty storing recent memories. Some patients with frontal injuries could present amnesias similar to those found in Korsakoff syndrome. This could be the result of an interrupted connection between the frontal lobes and the structures of the limbic temporal lobe.

Some authors claim that these defects in memory in frontal lesion cases should not be considered *true* amnesia (primary amnesia) but instead would be considered secondary defects resulting from impairments in planning and regulating mental activity. As a result of their lack of programming and controlling a mnesic activity, that is, defects of metamemory, patients are unable to retain new information adequately; nonetheless, they are able to retain a general idea of a sentence or story. In this sense, a true amnesia does not exist but rather defects in memory strategies or metamemory.

It has been suggested that the main defect in patients with frontal injuries is the incapacity to adequately use previously acquired information. There exists a defect in storing memories, which would frequently be associated with confabulation. Patients are incapable of creating strategies to retrieve or recover the information. This lack of ability results from the inability to create a stable intention to remember or recall information. Usually, memory difficulties observed in frontal injured patients are primarily found in complex and lengthy memory tests.

In addition, these patients have difficulties in mentally manipulating information, often characterized as working-memory defect. Due to their difficulties in planning, they become forgetful of their intentions (prospective memory). By the same token, due to the loss of behavioral temporality, there is a defect in the ability to recall the correct sequence of events, as well as the temporal context of events; these difficulties ultimately result in the so-called sequential or temporal amnesia. Normally, memory traces contain a specific temporal and spatial location. We usually know when, how, and where we acquire a memory trace; in other words, we know its source. Patients with frontal lobe pathology can present an overt source amnesia.

Final Thoughts

Patients with frontal lesions have a complex memory defect that could include a nonspecific amnesia, frequently observed with frontal basal lesions. Metamemory disorders, which refer to the inability to develop strategies and control of memory, are frequently found. In addition, there exist impairments in working memory due to difficulties in internally manipulating the information. Moreover, intentions are often forgotten, resulting in a prospective memory defect. Finally, there is a loss in the ability to locate the temporal and spatial traces of memory, resulting in temporal and source amnesia.

Alfredo Ardila

See also Cognitive Impairment; Cognitive Processes and Operations; Memory; Neurogenic Communication Disorders

Further Readings

Baddeley, A. D., Kopelman, M. D., & Wilson, B. A. (Eds.). (2003). *The handbook of memory disorders.* New York, NY: John Wiley.

Borghesani, P. R., DeMers, S. M., Manchanda, V., Pruthi, S., Lewis, D. H., & Borson, S. (2010). Neuroimaging in the clinical diagnosis of dementia: Observations from a memory disorders clinic. *Journal of the American Geriatrics Society, 58*(8), 1453–1458.

Quinette, P., Guillery-Girard, B., Dayan, J., de la Sayette, V., Marquis, S., Viader, F., . . . Eustache, F. (2006). What does transient global amnesia really mean? Review of the literature and thorough study of 142 cases. *Brain, 129*(7), 1640–1658.

Scoville, W. B., & Milner, B. (2000). Loss of recent memory after bilateral hippocampal lesions. *The Journal of Neuropsychiatry and Clinical Neurosciences, 12*(1), 103–113.

Squire, L. R., van der Horst, A. S., McDuff, S. G., Frascino, J. C., Hopkins, R. O., & Mauldin, K. N. (2010). Role of the hippocampus in remembering the past and imagining the future. *Proceedings of the National Academy of Sciences, 107*(44), 19044–19048.

Tulving, E., & Markowitsch, H. J. (1997). Memory beyond the hippocampus. *Current Opinion in Neurobiology, 7*(2), 209–216.

Victor, M., Adams, R. D., & Collins, G. H. (1989). *The Wernicke-Korsakoff syndrome and related neurologic disorders due to alcoholism and malnutrition.* Philadelphia, PA: F. A. Davis.

Memory Impairments in Aphasia

Aphasia is a linguistic disorder that affects the understanding and productive use of verbal symbols in the spoken and/or written modalities. Historically, aphasia was viewed as a memory disorder. For example, Paul Broca's classification of aphasia included *verbal amnesia* where patients had forgotten the meaning of words. Modern studies on aphasia have also revealed strong connections between language and verbal short-term memory (STM) as well as working-memory (WM) functioning.

In this entry, two related impairments of memory that affect temporary (as opposed to long-term) encoding, processing, and storage of verbal information are discussed: STM and working memory. The focus is on verbal as opposed to nonverbal STM and WM, as these two constructs are defined in order to clarify similarities and differences. Then, STM and WM impairments that are seen in aphasia are discussed, as are the different experimental tasks of STM and WM that contribute to the identification of such impairments. (Aspects of clinical assessment and treatment of STM and WM deficits in aphasia are not covered.)

Defining STM and WM

STM and WM are temporary memory systems and both have limited capacity. STM governs the ability to encode, store, and recall information within a short time after its presentation in a relatively unprocessed state (i.e., without mental manipulation). WM is also a temporary memory system used for the mental manipulation of information. STM is usually tested with digits or words presented in a list format in ascending list lengths, in either serial (i.e., the order of the stimuli needs to be retained and recalled in the order of presentation) or free (i.e., the order of the stimuli does not need to be retained) recall conditions. For example, one of the most frequently used tasks to assess STM and WM is digit span. If the spoken digits need to be recalled serially (i.e., from the beginning to the end of the list), this involves STM. However, if the digits need to be recalled in reverse serial order (known as *backward recall*), from the end of the list to the beginning, thus involving manipulation, then WM is used. Clearly, in order to carry out backward recall well, one needs to have the ability to retain the order of the words for the period it takes to manipulate them from the end to the beginning of the list.

It should be pointed out that the terminology used in the aphasia literature can be confusing. Some authors talk about phonological WM and phonological STM and rightly assume that phonological WM is dependent upon phonological STM. Similarly, phonological STM can refer to either performance in STM tasks involving nonwords, or both words and nonwords.

Impairments of STM in Aphasia

An impairment of STM in aphasia can be defined and also identified by below age- and education-related performance in STM tests, provided the person with aphasia has understood the demands of the test and can cope with the speech or other test demands. This section focuses on two specific patterns of STM impairments: phonological and semantic. A ramification of STM in terms of input and output verbal processes, which can also be differentially impaired in aphasia, is also discussed.

Phonological and semantic STM impairments refer to impairments that relate to poor performance in phonological and semantic STM tasks and the way underlying linguistic representations influence phonological and semantic aspects of STM, respectively. There are two complementary approaches.

The first approach comes from Randi Martin's group. Table 1 shows the diagnostic features of phonological and semantic STM impairments. In

Table 1 Diagnostic Features of Phonological and Semantic STM Impairments

	Phonological STM impairment	*Semantic STM impairment*
1	Better performance in semantic probe than rhyme probe tasks	Better performance in rhyme probe than semantic probe tasks
2	Better performance in span tasks with short than long words (i.e., number of syllables)	Similar performance in span tasks with short and long words (i.e., number of syllables)
3	Better performance in span tasks with words than non-words	Similar performance between word and non-word span tasks
4	Better performance when information is presented in written than spoken modality	Better performance when information is presented in spoken than written modality

Source: Salis et al. (2015, p. 726). Copyright John Wiley & Sons. Reprinted with permission.

Table 2 Phonological and Semantic Probe Tasks

	Word lists	Probes
Phonological	chair, box, shoe	Does the word "hair" rhyme with any of the words you have heard?
Semantic	pen, train, bird	Is the word "car" in the same category as any of the words you have heard?

Source: Salis et al. (2015, p. 726). Copyright John Wiley & Sons. Reprinted with permission.

both types of impairment, the person has to demonstrate good single word processing ability and needs to have reduced STM in the range of 1–3 items.

One of the key diagnostic features is Criterion 1, based on differentiable performance in phonological and semantic probe tasks (Table 2). In these tasks, the person listens to lists of words. At the end of each list, there is an additional probe word. In the phonological task, the person decides if the probe word rhymes with any of the words in the list. In the semantic probe task, the person decides if the probe word belongs to the same semantic category with any of the words in the list.

The second approach comes from Nadine Martin's group and utilizes what is known in the STM literature as *recall curves*. In typical speakers, recall at the beginning of a word list is better for initial items (known as the *primacy effect*) than items in the middle of the list. Similarly, recall at the end of a word list is better than items in the middle of the list. These patterns are evident in both serial and free recall, in younger and older typical adults and give the curved U-shaped pattern when recall accuracy of word positions in lists is plotted.

Nadine Martin's group showed that phonological and semantic skills for lexical processing impact in a different way upon STM. In one study, aphasic speakers were divided into two subgroups, based on differential performance in lexical processing tasks: phonological (e.g., phoneme discrimination) and semantic (e.g., synonym judgments). Speakers' STM abilities were then tested. Two patterns of performance emerged: First, some participants were unable to recall items at the beginning of lists (i.e., absence of primacy effect). Second, some participants were unable to recall items at the end of the list (i.e., absence of recency effect). Lack of primacy effect was associated with lexical-semantic processing impairment (i.e., access to word meaning) and/or reduced semantic STM. Lack of recency effect suggested that access to phonology (i.e., access to word sound form as opposed to meaning) or phonological STM is impaired.

Another distinction that has been discussed in the context of phonological STM impairments in aphasia is that of input versus output processes. For example, patient GC reported by Cristina Romani presented with mild aphasia and showed strikingly different patterns in repetition and STM tasks that did not involve repetition. In repetition tasks of lists of words and nonwords, his performance was impaired compared to controls. He was able to repeat word lists of 2 items serially, with 90% accuracy and 80% accuracy for words and nonwords, respectively. However, performance deteriorated with lists of 3 items, with accuracy at 50% correct for words and 0% for nonwords. GC was also unable to repeat lists of 4 items irrespective of lexicality (i.e., no difference between words and nonwords). In tasks not needing speech output, GC had to indicate whether a probe word was featured in lists of words and nonwords he had previously heard. Performance was slightly below that of typical controls for words and within typical limits for nonwords. These patterns of performance were due to two different STM mechanisms: an input store, which was intact in GC, and an output store, which was impaired.

Impairments of WM in Aphasia

While different capacities for phonological and semantic abilities have been proposed for STM impairments and differences between input and output processes, this is not the case in WM impairments. The mental manipulation of verbal material that distinguishes STM from WM makes WM tasks more complex. Two such tasks are described subsequently: the listening span and n-back tasks. Both tasks have been used in aphasia to identify WM impairments.

The listening span task draws on the ability to process spoken information and, at the same time, store this information for a brief period before recall. Participants hear semantically congruous and incongruous sentences, for example, "you sit on a chair" and "trains can fly." The sentences are arranged in sets of two, three, four, and five sentences, incrementally. To ensure each sentence is processed as it is heard, the person has to respond true or false. Participants are instructed at the beginning of the task that they also have to remember the last word of each sentence (storage demand). Once each sentence set finishes, they are asked to recall the final word of each sentence in any order. This test provided a metric of WM capacity, which differentiated performance between a left hemisphere damaged group (76% of which presented with aphasia) and age- and education-matched typical controls.

In the n-back task, the person hears or sees words one by one, presented as a continuous list. He or she needs to keep track of the presented stimuli and identify the stimuli that he or she heard (or saw) at a prespecified interval. For example, in a 1-back task, the person has to remember an item that preceded another item before, that is, back. Table 3 shows an idealized example of a 1-back task with digits. The response modality is flexible depending on the version of the task. This means that in the example shown in Table 3, the person could either say the number that he or she heard before digits 4, 2, and 4 where heard or point to digits written on a card. In other versions of the task, there could be words, sounds, or other material, verbal or nonverbal. With regard to n-back, authors have commented that the flexibility, in terms of stimuli (verbal, nonverbal), response type, and interstimulus intervals, is also one of the greatest weaknesses. This is because it is difficult to assume that the feasibility and reliability estimates for one version of the n-back will be consistent across other versions of the task. In some studies, the n-back task indicated good clinical feasibility and high estimated test–retest reliability for the n-back task as utilized for adults with aphasia, consistent with reliability data of the n-back for typical speakers. However, other researchers found the n-back task to have poor psychometric properties.

Final Thoughts

Both STM and WM are temporary memory systems, and STM and WM impairments are prevalent in aphasia. Strong links between STM and WM and core language measures have been reported in aphasia. General STM and WM impairments are identified by below typical performance in STM and WM tasks. STM impairments can affect phonological or semantic aspects of STM. It has been argued that these aspects reflect underlying phonological or semantic aspects of word processing. In some patients, input and output aspects of STM can be differentially impaired.

Christos Salis, Helen Kelly, and Chris Code

See also Aphasia; Aphasia Assessment; Attention; Memory; Memory Disorders

Further Readings

Baddeley, A. (2012). Working memory: Theories, models, and controversies. *Annual Review of Psychology*, 63, 1–29.

Cowan, N. (2008). What are the differences between long-term, short-term, and working memory? *Progress in Brain Research*, 169, 323–338.

Table 3 Example of a 1-Back Task

Person hears	3	1	4	7	2	9	4
Correct response	None	None	3	None	4	None	2

Source: Salis et al. (2015, p. 729). Copyright John Wiley & Sons. Adapted with permission.

Dede, G., Ricca, M., Knilans, J., & Trubl, B. (2014). Construct validity and reliability of working memory tasks for people with aphasia. *Aphasiology, 28*, 692–712.

Lehman, M. T., & Tompkins, C. A. (1998). Reliability and validity of an auditory working memory measure: Data from elderly and right-hemisphere damaged adults. *Aphasiology, 12*, 771–785.

Martin, N., & Ayala, J. (2004). Measurements of auditory-verbal STM span in aphasia: Effects of item, task, and lexical impairment. *Brain and Language, 89*, 464–483.

Martin, R. C., & Allen, C. M. (2008). A disorder of executive function and its role in language processing. *Seminars in Speech and Language, 29*, 201–210.

Mayer, J. F., & Murray, L. L. (2012). Measuring working memory deficits in aphasia. *Journal of Communication Disorders, 45*, 325–339.

Romani, C. (1992). Are there distinct input and output buffers? Evidence from an aphasic patient with an impaired output buffer. *Language and Cognitive Processes, 7*, 131–162.

Salis, C., Kelly, H., & Code, C. (2015). Assessment and treatment of short-term and working memory impairments in stroke aphasia: A practical tutorial. *International Journal of Language and Communication Disorders, 50*, 721–736.

Tesak, J., & Code, C. (2008). *Milestones in the history of aphasia: Theories and protagonists*. Hove, UK: Psychology Press.

MÉNIÈRE'S DISEASE

Ménière's syndrome is a debilitating hearing and balance disorder with no known cause. It is commonly referred to as Ménière's disease. Despite several treatment options, those with Ménière's disease experience a reduced quality of life, and there is no cure for the gradual decline of hearing and balance in their affected ear(s). The incidence is reported to be 0.1–0.5% of the population, although this is biased by ethnic factors as it predominantly occurs in Caucasians. The average age of onset is 40–50 years, but the distribution is broad and children younger than 15 years are frequently diagnosed. Ménière's disease accounts for approximately ¼ of peripheral vestibular disorders observed clinically or close to 10% of all patients experiencing some form of dizziness. This entry provides an overview of Ménière's disease diagnosis, symptoms, potential causes, tests, treatments, and lifestyle changes.

The disorder was first recognized in 1861 when French physician, Prosper Ménière, described a number of patients experiencing sudden attacks of vertigo affiliated with a gradual hearing loss. Ménière also presented evidence in the form of postmortem temporal bone histology and drew upon earlier experimental research on pigeons by French researcher Marie Jean Pierre Flourens to propose that the syndrome was related to an inner ear pathology. Despite the span of years since Prosper Ménière first described the disorder, which now bears his name, the 21st-century understanding of this disorder remains limited.

Symptoms

Ménière's disease is clinically diagnosed on the basis of symptoms and only after the exclusion of other vestibular disorders. Because the symptomology varies and overlaps with other disorders, it can be difficult to establish a clear diagnosis of Ménière's disease in the early stages. Therefore, clinicians are directed to diagnose Ménière's disease as either *Probable* or *Definite*. A diagnosis of Probable Ménière's disease may be given if a patient has had at least two spontaneous vertigo episodes lasting between 20 minutes and 24 hours and has experienced fluctuating hearing dysfunction either in the form of hearing loss, tinnitus, or a feeling of pressure in the affected ear. A diagnosis of Definite Ménière's disease is given when there have been at least two vertigo attacks lasting 20 minutes to 12 hours, fluctuating hearing dysfunction, and a clinically documented hearing loss in the low- to mid-frequency (<2 kHz) range associated with at least one of the vertigo attacks.

While these specific criteria are used to clinically diagnose Ménière's disease, there are many other symptoms, phenomenon, and clinical observations associated with the disease. The vertigo attacks can vary in severity, duration, and form. Some attacks develop slowly over hours and last a full day, whereas others, such as *drop attacks*, occur instantaneously, causing the individual to fall violently. Furthermore, the attacks tend to cluster during the *acute* phase of the disease, with several occurring in a month, before long periods of respite. The vertigo experience also varies:

Individuals may either feel a strong rotational/spinning percept, or other times, they may experience a swaying perception. Due to this variability, the reported frequency of the attacks ranges between several per day and one or two per year. Moreover, this frequency will vary over time, and vertigo attacks are frequent during the first 4 years, becoming less frequent but more severe and long-lasting from years 10 to 20. Thereafter, the attacks will eventually abate in the *burn-out* phase of the disease, which is associated with a significant decrease in the overall function the affected ear.

The gradual, fluctuating hearing loss is relatively consistent among those with Ménière's, and it typically starts with a low-frequency loss, progressing to an overall severe broad loss, where hearing aids or cochlear implants may be required. Previously, it was believed that hearing fluctuation coincided with the vertigo attacks, but there is little evidence for this correlation. Various types of tinnitus are reported by individuals with Ménière's disease, ranging from a pulsatile gushing noise to a continuous ringing. The feeling of pressure in the ear and head, called *aural fullness*, also varies between individuals and usually coincides with the vertigo attacks. Individuals with Ménière's disease report difficulty with cognition during the acute phase of the disease, often referring to this mental state as *brain fog*, a phenomenon reported in many other disorders.

Approximately one third of individuals with Ménière's disease will eventually develop symptoms in their other ear. This can be particularly disabling because they can no longer rely on the balance or hearing of their *good ear*. There is also a weak familial inheritance of Ménière's disease, where approximately 7% of those diagnosed will have at least one immediate family member with the disorder. For many individuals, there are specific triggers for their vertigo attacks. Mental stress; a high dietary intake of salt, caffeine, chocolate, alcohol, tobacco; and changes in barometric pressure are often suggested as triggers for vertigo attacks and auditory dysfunction.

Causes

Although there is no clear cause of Ménière's disease, it is associated with a phenomenon called *endolymphatic hydrops*, which is an enlargement of the membranous fluid-filled compartment within the cochlea and vestibular system. The membranous compartment (called the *membranous labyrinth*) is filled with a unique fluid called *endolymph*, which has a relatively high concentration of potassium chloride. Via postmortem histology or magnetic resonance imaging (MRI), endolymphatic hydrops can be observed in almost all individuals with Ménière's disease. Endolymphatic hydrops can also occur in other hearing and balance disorders, either occurring without a clear cause (i.e., idiopathic, as is the case in Ménière's) or secondary to some other pathology or event. Moreover, damage to a small intracranial structure connected to the endolymph, called the *endolymphatic sac*, is often suggested as a cause of endolymphatic hydrops.

It is thought that any pathology that disrupts endolymph volume regulation may result in endolymphatic hydrops, which may then cause the symptoms of Ménière's disease. However, some studies have reported that endolymphatic hydrops can be observed in the ears of people who do not exhibit all the symptoms of Ménière's disease. This suggests that hydrops should perhaps be viewed merely as a histologic marker of the disorder, rather than directly forming part of the etiological pathway. With animal experiments demonstrating that endolymphatic hydrops can induce hearing fluctuation and a sudden loss of vestibular function, and an increasing number of MRI studies demonstrating a clear correlation between endolymphatic hydrops and the symptoms of Ménière's, it seems increasingly more likely that endolymphatic hydrops underlies many of the symptoms of Ménière's disease.

Regardless of the relationship between endolymphatic hydrops and Ménière's, scientists still lack a clear understanding of the root cause of the disorder. Evidence has supported the implication of several pathologies as the underlying cause, including viral infections, autonomic imbalance, autoimmune disorders, allergies, vascular abnormalities, genetic abnormalities, and structural disorders. There is also a strong association between Ménière's disease and migraine associated vertigo (i.e., a disorder in which individuals get Ménière's-like vertigo attacks but have no significant hearing loss, nor do they have endolymphatic hydrops), suggesting that the two disorders may share a common etiological pathway. To this end, many experts view Ménière's disease as a *multifactorial disorder*, that is, the root cause may differ among those with Ménière's, with endolymphatic hydrops possibly forming part of a common etiological pathway.

One reason why it has proven difficult to establish the pathology underlying Ménière's is that the inner ear is inaccessible, being housed in hard temporal bone. This prevents a simple scientific assay of the affected ear's tissues or fluids, which should ideally be performed during the acute phase of the disease when the underlying pathology is most evident. Blood tests, functional tests, postmortem analysis, noninvasive imaging, and assays performed during the remission phase only provide indirect markers of the pathology and can be difficult to interpret. Other methods for establishing the cause involve the response to treatments such as antivirals or antidiuretics. However, due to the cyclic nature of Ménière's disease symptoms, which can go into long periods of remission, along with the low prevalence, the high potential for misdiagnosis, a strong placebo effect, and the possibility that the syndrome may be multifactorial, performing clinical trials of treatments for Ménière's disease is an unreliable means for determining the cause. As of 2018, few studies if any have reliably demonstrated a statistically significant beneficial effect of any treatment.

Treatments

All treatments are aimed at reducing the severity or frequency of vertigo attacks rather than addressing the hearing symptoms. Treatments for vertigo attacks involve taking sedatives and anti-nausea or motion sickness drugs, such as diazepam, meclizine, lorazepam, betahistine, or promethazine. Other pharmacological treatments that theoretically reduce endolymphatic hydrops involve taking antidiuretics like furosemide, acetazolamide, or urea, along with a reduced salt diet. Still more treatments involve taking drugs, such as flunarizine and verapamil, used to treat vascular disorders. Increasingly, the injection of steroids, such as dexamethasone or prednisone, through the eardrum into the middle ear is being used to provide months of vertigo relief, theoretically reducing inflammatory mechanisms believed to underlie Meniere's. Some individuals claim relief of vertigo through the use of antiviral drugs (e.g., acyclovir) or homeopathic therapies thought to suppress an overactive immune system. There are also a few nonpharmacological therapies, such as a reduction of dietary salt intake, devices that manipulate middle ear pressure, and even chiropractic adjustments. However, none of these therapies have clearly demonstrated efficacy through rigorous clinical trials, and there is much debate as to whether any perceived benefit is due to the treatment or a placebo effect, which is known to be strong in individuals with Meniere's disease.

The only treatments that have clearly demonstrated a permanent relief from vertigo are aimed at completely or partially damaging the vestibular end organ. Injections of the antibiotic gentamicin into the middle ear or surgical destruction of the vestibular nerve or end organ (called a *vestibular neurectomy* or *labyrinthectomy*) can provide permanent relief from the vertigo attacks, but patients must adjust to a permanent loss of some vestibular function. However, due to the risk that patients may develop Meniere's symptoms in their other ear, caution is employed during the clinical decision to use these ablative therapies.

Testing

To improve the development of effective treatments, there is a need for objective measures that are specific for the presence of Ménière's disease. There has been an increasing use of MRIs as a means to visually demonstrate the presence of endolymphatic hydrops. Moreover, often the diagnosis of Ménière's disease is supplemented by the presence of an abnormal electrocochleography response. Electrocochleography responses are gross electrical responses to sound, measured by a clinical specialist who places an electrode on or through the patient's eardrum. However, because MRIs and electrocochleography testing require specialized equipment and expertise, they are not ideal for studying treatment efficacy. Since the year 2000, several noninvasive clinical tests of inner ear function have been developed and provide a promising approach to improve Ménière's diagnosis and track treatment efficacy. Many of these involve measuring vestibular reflexes, with a few providing objective measures of cochlear responses. Specific patterns of abnormal vestibular and cochlear function can be repeatedly demonstrated in individuals with Ménière's disease. Moreover, there is an increasing focus on measuring the immunological profile of individuals with Ménière's disease, which can be obtained from blood or saliva samples. However, there is still no test that accurately identifies Meniere's disease specifically.

Similar to most chronic disorders, there is a high correlation between symptom severity and the reduction in the quality of life for an individual with Ménière's disease. However, those who can manage the steep life adjustment and have a good support network typically cope better than those who have negative coping behaviors. The unpredictable and disabling nature of the vertigo attacks requires the largest adjustment. Lying down or sitting still for several hours in a quiet room, resting for a few days after a severe attack, managing personal stress, undertaking vestibular retraining therapies, and avoiding situations that may result in further injury during an attack (e.g., driving) can be helpful. Hearing aids may help some individuals with Ménière's disease, but the fluctuating hearing loss can complicate their use. Most individuals benefit from joining one of the numerous Ménière's disease support networks and community support groups, which can more broadly provide additional coping mechanisms and information on Ménière's disease.

Daniel J. Brown

See also Cochlear Hearing Loss; Cochlear Implants; Electrocochleography (ECochG); Experimental Research; Pharmacological Interventions in Hearing Disorders; Quality of Life and Neurogenic Communication Disorders; Spontaneous Recovery; Tinnitus; Treatment Research; Vestibular Assessment; Vestibular Disorders; Vestibular System

Further Readings

Espinosa-Sanchez, J. M., & Lopez-Escamez, J. A. (2016). Ménière's disease. *Handbook of Clinical Neurology, 137*, 257–277. doi:10.1016/B978-0-444-63437-5.00019-4

Gürkov, R., Pyykö, I., Zou, J., & Kentala, E. (2016). What is Ménière's disease? A contemporary re-evaluation of endolymphatic hydrops. *Journal of Neurology and Neurological Disorders, 263*(Suppl. 1), S71-S81.

Harris, J. P., & Salt, A. N. (2008). Meniere's disease. In T. D. Albright, T. D. Albright, R. H. Masland, P. Dallos, D. Oertel, S. Firestein, G. K. Beauchamp, . . . E. P. Gardner (Eds.), *The senses: A comprehensive reference* (pp. 157–163). New York, NY: Academic Press.

Haybach, P. J. (1998). In J. L. Underwood (Ed.), *Meniere's disease: What you need to know.* Portland, OR: Vestibular Disorders Association.

META-ANALYSIS

Meta-analysis is a method for systematically combining data from multiple studies to make statistical conclusions about a specific research question. As it involves an increased number and a greater diversity of subjects, the conclusions reached through meta-analysis are statistically stronger than the results of a single study. There are many strengths associated with conducting meta-analyses, including increased statistical power, increased accuracy, and reduced uncertainty regarding the conclusions from various individual studies. In addition, the process of conducting a meta-analysis can reveal additional context for understanding the results of individual studies as well as suggest potential questions for future research. For these reasons, a meta-analysis of well-conducted, rigorous studies is considered one of the highest levels of evidence in the literature. Although mathematicians and scientists have explored various methods for summarizing the results of different studies since the 17th century, in 1976 Gene Glass developed the formalized technique known today as *meta-analysis*. Since that time, researchers in many fields such as education, psychology, communication, and the biomedical sciences have employed the use of meta-analysis to combine data and make inferences from multiple studies.

This entry provides an overview of the steps involved with conducting a meta-analysis: (a) formulating the research problem, (b) searching the literature, (c) analyzing the data, and (d) disseminating the results as well as the strengths and weaknesses of this method. Formulating the research problem involves carefully defining the key constructs for the research question being studied. A detailed literature search requires outlining a set of inclusion and exclusion criteria that are used to retrieve and screen primary studies for analysis. The statistical analysis consists of extracting and coding the data, calculating the effect sizes for each primary study, examining the heterogeneity, and computing summary statistics. The methodology, results, and a detailed discussion of the meta-analysis are then compiled in a structured report for dissemination.

Steps in Conducting a Meta-Analysis

Formulating the Problem

The first step in conducting a meta-analysis is to formulate the research problem. Much like any other research methodology, meta-analysis begins with a research question or hypothesis. When formulating the problem, it is important to define key constructs that outline the boundaries for the question being studied. A clear formulation of the problem helps the researcher to decide which studies should be included in the meta-analysis as well as what data are relevant to answering the research question. Research questions for a meta-analysis are typically narrow and focused on a particular type of intervention. This is primarily because questions that are too broadly defined can limit the number of studies that can be effectively integrated through meta-analysis.

Sampling is another important consideration in the formulation of the research problem. In case of a meta-analysis, the study sample consists of the group of primary studies that address the research question. In formulating the problem, a researcher makes many decisions about the sample design, which are outlined in terms of inclusion and exclusion criteria. The criteria may explicitly identify specific variables of interest. Another concern is the study population. For example, in some instances, only studies containing certain age-groups of participants are included. The inclusion or exclusion criteria might also specify that only studies written in English, published after a certain date, or using specific experimental designs are considered.

Searching the Literature

There are a few important factors to consider before beginning a literature search. One is whether the meta-analysis will include both published and unpublished studies (such as dissertations and unpublished reports). In some instances, researchers may choose to include only studies that are published in peer-reviewed journals, because the peer-review system is regarded as a well-respected screening for relevant evidence. However, there are limitations associated with excluding unpublished studies in a meta-analysis. The main concern with excluding unpublished studies is publication bias. Publication bias refers to the tendency for published studies to overrepresent statistically significant findings. This occurs for many reasons: Researchers may be hesitant to publish studies with statistically insignificant findings, reviewers and editors may be reluctant to accept such articles, and readers may tend to ignore statistically insignificant findings that are published. Therefore, excluding unpublished studies in a meta-analysis can lead to publication bias that results in overestimating the statistical effects.

When conducting a literature search, it is important to obtain as many relevant studies as possible. Some effective search strategies include (a) conducting a manual search of relevant journals; (b) searching electronic databases such as PubMed, Medline, PsycINFO, ProQuest Digital Dissertation Database, Cochrane Reviews, Web of Science, and others; (c) reviewing abstracts from conference proceedings; and (d) searching foundations, corporations, and government agencies for published/unpublished reports. Once relevant studies are identified and obtained, they should be carefully reviewed and screened to determine whether they meet the inclusion criteria. This process occurs by first reviewing titles and abstracts, followed by reviewing the full text to eliminate nonrelevant studies from the sample.

Analyzing the Data

Once the literature search has been completed, the next step in conducting a meta-analysis is analyzing the data. This process begins by extracting and coding the data for analysis, which can be done conveniently through the use of a data extraction table. A data extraction table often contains column headings such as author(s) and year of publication, journal title and its impact factor, outcome measures, study design, sample size and population, data collection method, and a summary of findings. Additional details can also be included, such as the demographic characteristics of study participants and the type of intervention that was studied (if applicable). It is important that the data be extracted and coded by at least two people. This enables an assessment of intercoder agreement, which ensures that the recorded information is accurate.

Once the data are extracted and coded, the next step in analyzing the data is calculating the effect size for each study. In a meta-analysis, the data across various studies are compared through the calculation of a measure that quantifies the relationship between the independent and dependent variables in each study. Three common situations include (1) the comparison of two groups based on a continuous variable, (2) the comparison of two groups based on a dichotomous (i.e., Yes/No) variable, and (3) correlations between two continuous variables. When a study compares two groups based on a continuous variable, the effect size is typically calculated as the standardized mean difference. When comparing two groups based on a dichotomous variable, the effect size is often defined by the relative risk index, the odds ratio, or the absolute risk reduction. In other cases, when the primary studies report findings in the form of a correlation coefficient, this statistic serves as a measure of effect size. In many instances, statistical software can be used to conduct these analyses, and there is no need to manually calculate the effect sizes.

Once an effect size is calculated for each study, the next step is to synthesize the data. This involves calculating a weighted average of the effects for the primary studies. To compute the weighted average, each effect size is multiplied by a weight that corresponds to the amount of information that a given study provides. Therefore, studies with larger sample sizes are given greater weight than studies with smaller sample sizes. The sum of the weighted effect sizes is then divided by the sum of the weights to obtain the weighted average of the effects.

An important consideration in meta-analysis is the concept of heterogeneity. Heterogeneity refers to the extent to which the results of the primary studies are consistent. One approach to identifying heterogeneity is through the visual inspection of a forest plot. A forest plot graphs the estimated effect size for each study, along with the 95% confidence interval around each estimate. A situation in which there is low heterogeneity is indicated by overlapping confidence intervals, and high heterogeneity is indicated by confidence intervals that do not overlap. In addition to the visual inspection of a forest plot, heterogeneity can also be formally evaluated using a statistical procedure known as the *chi-squared* test. The chi-squared test yielding a low p value provides evidence of heterogeneity.

Understanding the heterogeneity across primary studies can help researchers determine which statistical analysis is appropriate. Two commonly used approaches to meta-analysis include a fixed-effects model and a random-effects model. In a fixed-effects model, the researcher assumes that there is a single true effect size underlying all primary study results. On the other hand, a random-effects model assumes that the estimates from the primary studies are different. When there is little heterogeneity, both the fixed-effects model and the random-effects model give nearly identical results. However, a random-effects model is typically recommended when the test for heterogeneity is statistically significant.

Disseminating the Results

The final step in conducting a meta-analysis is reporting the results and disseminating the findings. In many instances, the material contained in a meta-analysis follows the same format as a primary study, with sections outlining the introduction, method, results, and discussion. In particular, the method section contains detailed information about the literature search and data analysis, including the rationale for methodological and statistical decisions. In addition, the inclusion and/or exclusion criteria are outlined in the method section, along with the data extraction table. In some cases, a flowchart is included to illustrate the identification, screening, and inclusion of primary studies in the sample. The results section often contains tables and figures that summarize the statistical findings, including forest plots illustrating effect sizes and 95% confidence intervals. The discussion section includes an overall summary of findings as well as an assessment of the quality of the evidence and the consistency across studies. At the end of the meta-analysis, full citations for the entire sample of primary studies are included in the reference list. These references are often distinguished from other citations (i.e., with the use of asterisks).

Strengths and Weaknesses of Meta-Analysis

There are many strengths of conducting meta-analyses. First, meta-analysis provides a method for systematically combing data from many studies, which often results in large combined samples. This can lead to increased statistical power, increased accuracy, and reduced uncertainty regarding the conclusions from various individual studies. Therefore, the results derived in a meta-analysis can often be generalized to a larger population. In addition, meta-analysis can reveal flaws and sources of bias in research methods used in primary studies as well as suggest potential questions for future research.

Although there are many strengths associated with conducting meta-analyses for synthesizing data, there are some potential weaknesses. Because a meta-analysis does not involve an examination of the primary data obtained from the individual studies, the quality and validity of the results depend on the quality and validity of the individual studies. Another potential weakness occurs when researchers are not thorough in the selection of studies to include in the meta-analysis. The poor selection of studies (such as excluding unpublished results) may introduce publication bias and lead to results that are difficult to interpret. A potential solution for avoiding publication bias is to search for unpublished studies such as dissertations, conference proceedings, and governmental reports. Despite the potential weaknesses, the process of meta-analysis is an important mathematical tool for gaining a broader perspective on the cumulative results of studies on a specific research topic.

Taniecea Mallery

See also Outcome Measurement; Quantitative Research

Further Readings

Cooper, H. (2017). *Research synthesis and meta-analysis: A step-by-step approach*. Thousand Oaks, CA: Sage.

Cooper, H., Hedges, L. V., & Valentine, J. C. (2009). *The handbook of research synthesis and meta-analysis*. New York, NY: Russell Sage Foundation.

Ellis, P. D. (2010). *The essential guide to effect sizes: Statistical power, meta-analysis, and the interpretation of research results*. Cambridge, UK: Cambridge University Press.

Glass, G. V. (1976). Primary, secondary, and meta-analysis of research. *Educational Researcher, 5*(10), 3–8.

Hedges, L. V. (1992). Meta-analysis. *Journal of Educational Statistics, 17*(4), 279–296.

Hunter, J. E., & Schmidt, F. L. (2015). *Methods of meta-analysis: Correcting error and bias in research findings*. Thousand Oaks, CA: Sage.

Lipsey, M. W., & Wilson, D. B. (2001). *Practical meta-analysis*. Thousand Oaks, CA: Sage.

Polit, D. F., & Beck, C. T. (2012). *Nursing research: Generating and assessing evidence for nursing practice* (9th ed.). Philadelphia, PA: Lippincott Williams & Wilkins.

METACOGNITION

The ability to monitor and evaluate one's own thinking, often referred to as *metacognition*, is the hallmark of effective cognitive processing and an essential facet of learning across the life span. As a result, educational and psychological research studies are replete with explorations of the key components underlying individuals' capacity to engage in metacognitive processing. *Metacognition* is often succinctly defined as "thinking about one's own thinking," where the "meta" prefix represents the self-referential aspect of cognition. This entry provides a brief overview of the historical roots of metacognition; two perspectives on the primary components of metacognition; and principles gleaned from contemporary, empirical investigations.

Historical Development

Early philosophers and psychologists were aware of the importance of examining one's own thought processes long before the use of the term *metacognition*. Aspects of metacognition are evident in varied sources from the ancient Greek teachings of Socrates to 20th-century American philosophers like William James and John Dewey as well as influential educational scholars such as Jean Piaget and Lev Vygotsky. Yet John Flavell and colleagues only formally coined the term *metacognition* in the 1970s; they employed the term to describe the outcomes from a series of interviews evaluating children's thoughts and intuitions about memory, learning, and study strategies. The findings from this seminal study revealed prominent developmental differences such that older children had a greater ability to plan and were more self-aware than younger children.

Taxonomies of Metacognition

John Flavell also proposed a prominent taxonomy of metacognition comprising three types of knowledge (i.e., knowledge of the task, the person, and the strategy) that may be elicited through metacognitive experiences. *Task knowledge* includes information about the resources at hand, including the specific task demands and goals. For example, when an individual navigates public transportation in a foreign country, there are inherent differences as compared to the task of navigating in one's hometown (e.g., language, symbol convention, familiarity). *Person knowledge* includes the understandings that one has about one's abilities (e.g., "I am really bad with directions"); knowledge of other individuals (e.g., "My partner is really good at understanding maps"); and knowledge of human cognition in general (e.g., "Rehearsing the name of a train station may only help one recall the name for a short period of time"). *Strategy knowledge* includes the repertoire of techniques (e.g., mnemonic devices, rehearsal strategies, thinking aloud) that an individual can use while working toward a task.

Metacognitive experiences are instances where individuals reflect on their cognitive processes and engage in metacognitive thought. For example, an individual tasked with the goal of navigating public transportation back to his or her hotel may have a metacognitive experience when deciding to exit the train. The individual may be cognizant that he or she is uncertain of his or her exact location, causing the individual to consequently take action by asking another passenger about their location or by counting the number of stops traveled on the map.

An alternative framework of metacognition divides metacognition into two interrelated, but distinct, components: *knowledge of cognition* (i.e., self-appraisal of cognition) and *regulation of cognition* (i.e., self-management of thinking). Knowledge of cognition includes an individual's declarative, procedural, and conditional knowledge about cognition. Declarative knowledge includes the facts one knows about oneself as well as the knowledge of factors that influence learning. Procedural knowledge includes the strategies and processes one possesses for how to learn or complete a task. Conditional knowledge includes the ability for optimizing when to match varying environmental conditions to specific known strategies for success. Alternatively, regulation of cognition includes an individual's ability to plan, monitor or regulate, and evaluate one's processing. Planning includes the ability to select an appropriate strategy for a given task. Monitoring or regulating includes the in situ awareness of one's task performance, including one's awareness of the necessity to revise or modify the previously established plan, and evaluation includes gauging the success or failure of the learning.

Contemporary Findings

Contemporary researchers are also employing a variety of biobehavioral tools like brain imaging to gain a better understanding regarding the psychophysiological underpinnings of metacognition. Several early investigations in this area, around the 1980s, were conducted with participants diagnosed with some form of frontal lobe dysfunction or lesion. In one study, participants exhibiting amnesia due to Korsakoff's syndrome (i.e., a memory disorder caused by thiamine deficiency), participants prescribed electroconvulsive therapy, other amnesia participants, and control participants were asked to answer a question; if they were unsuccessful, they were asked to estimate their feeling-of-knowing (i.e., their perception of their ability to recognize the correct answer if it were presented to them along with distractor options). Only individuals with Korsakoff's syndrome evidenced stark impairments in their feeling-of-knowing, even when compared to other amnesia patients, which was a noteworthy finding that provided evidence differentiating memory from metamemory or metacognition.

Since the 1990s, rapid technological advances in neuroimaging through functional magnetic resonance imaging have led to an even greater proliferation of biobehavioral research on metacognition, which now allows researchers to inspect the brain activation patterns of individuals as they complete cognitive and metacognitive tasks. By investigating differences in the activation patterns of individuals completing diverse tasks, researchers can understand more about the variables that influence activation patterns in typically functioning adults. Emerging research has shown that individuals engaging in metacognitive processes (e.g., planning, evaluating) tend to exhibit activations in the prefrontal cortex. The anterior cingulate cortex is also activated when individuals are monitoring or processing feedback.

In the 21st century, a burgeoning area of research focuses on identifying ways to facilitate individuals' metacognitive capabilities. It is now understood that metacognition can be enhanced by (a) explicitly training individuals in a variety of effective task-relevant strategies, (b) ensuring individuals know the conditions under which to employ specific strategies, and (c) providing individuals with constructive, timely feedback about their performance.

Carla M. Firetto and P. Karen Murphy

See also Cognition; Cognitive Processes and Operations; Comprehension; Individual Differences; Theory of Mind

Further Readings

Alexander, P. A. (Ed.). (2008). Metacognition, self-regulation, and self-regulated learning: Historical roots and contemporary manifestations [Special issue]. *Educational Psychology Review.* 20 (4), 369–491.

Braver, T. S., & Ruge, H. (2006). Functional neuroimaging of executive functions. In R. Cabeza & A. Kingstone (Eds.), *Handbook of functional neuroimaging of cognition* (6th ed., pp. 307–348). Cambridge, MA: MIT Press.

Flavell, J. H. (1979). Metacognition and cognitive monitoring: A new area of cognitive-developmental inquiry. *American Psychologist, 10*(34), 906–911.

Metcalfe, J., & Shimamura, A. P. (1996). *Metacognition: Knowing about knowing.* Cambridge, MA: The MIT Press.

Shimamura, A. P., & Squire, L. R. (1986). Memory and metamemory: A study of the feeling-of-knowing phenomenon in amnesic patients. *Journal of Experimental Psychology: Learning, Memory, and Cognition, 12*(3), 452–460.

Weinert, F. E., & Kluwe, R. H. (1987). *Metacognition, motivation, and understanding.* Hillsdale, NJ: Erlbaum.

METALINGUISTICS

Metalinguistics or metalinguistic awareness involves *attention, awareness, reflection,* and, sometimes, *manipulation* of aspects of language form. This can be contrasted with everyday language use, where the content or meaning of a message typically is in focus. Metalinguistic awareness is an important feature of later language development, including literacy (reading and writing) development. Furthermore, metalinguistic awareness is a central concept in instructed second-language acquisition research, one reason being that most curricula involve metalinguistic strategies for teaching and learning, such as drawing explicit attention to linguistic rules. This entry provides an overview of metalinguistics, including its subtypes, the analysis and control model, the typical development of metalinguistic awareness in children, and its relationship to literacy and standardized testing.

Subtypes and Categories

Some subtypes of metalinguistic awareness are *morphological* and *syntactic awareness,* which is used, for example, when explaining grammatical rules or making grammaticality judgments, and *phonological awareness,* which involves awareness of the sounds that make up a language, including rhyme recognition and production, counting syllables, and segmenting words into phonemes. These types all belong to a metalinguistic awareness category that is related to the *systematic* nature of language (i.e., language as described by categories and rules). Another category relates to the fact that language is *arbitrary*, which enables metalinguistic skills such as differentiating a word from its referent, understanding that a word can have multiple meanings as well as synonyms, and understanding figurative language.

The Analysis and Control Model

One influential model of metalinguistic awareness was proposed by Ellen Bialystok and Ellen Ryan in the 1980s and has support from empirical data from many studies. They suggested that metalinguistic awareness is a combination of two interacting abilities: *language analysis* and *cognitive control*. Language analysis involves knowledge of language on both the implicit level (e.g., the use of grammar or phonology in communication) and the explicit level (e.g., using literacy-specific rules while reading or writing). Cognitive control involves attention and monitoring processes including executive functioning and working memory, and it is responsible for selection and integration of information. The model emphasizes that linguistic and metalinguistic tasks exist on a continuum and that the demands vary as a function of the communicative context and type of task. In general, metalinguistic tasks demand higher levels of both analysis and control compared to, for example, everyday communication. Metalinguistic tasks also vary in their demands. One example is the higher demands on cognitive control needed to perform a spoonerism task (i.e., exchanging the first sounds in two words such as *good morning* and *mood gorning*) compared to simply identifying the first sound in a word.

Using the analysis and control framework, research has shown that bilingual children have a metalinguistic (primarily syntactic) awareness advantage in tasks that are thought to involve high levels of cognitive control (e.g., judging the grammaticality of semantically implausible sentences such as "the pen *eat/eats a carrot"). This advantage has not been shown in tasks that are thought to load mainly on language analysis (e.g., judging the grammaticality of semantically plausible sentences such as "the child *eat/eats a carrot"). Other researchers, however, have challenged the bilingual metalinguistic awareness advantage, and whether this advantage exists is still an ongoing debate.

Development of Metalinguistic Awareness

Because metalinguistic awareness builds on linguistic skills, the development of metalinguistic awareness may start as soon as a child starts developing language. For example, early self-corrections in communicative breakdowns are signs of early metalinguistic awareness according to some researchers. Self-corrections can be performed by applying linguistic knowledge more or less automatically, however, and the act itself serves a pragmatic function. Therefore, other researchers want to reserve the term *metalinguistic awareness* for tasks and situations where *explicit* awareness and *conscious* reflection on language form have taken place.

Children with typical development start playing with and thinking about language from around 2 or 3 years of age, when they can, for example, learn to recognize and appreciate rhymes and word games that build on the arbitrariness of words/labels. Awareness on the whole-word level and syllable level generally precede awareness on the phoneme level. Importantly, the development of explicit metalinguistic awareness is highly dependent on the language environment of the child. One consequence is that children start school with varying degrees of metalinguistic awareness.

Relationship to Literacy Development and Standardized Testing

Metalinguistic awareness is a crucial part of literacy development. In alphabetic languages, *phonemic awareness*, the awareness that words can be divided into individual phonemes, is especially important. Examples of phonemic awareness tasks include segmenting and synthesizing words into phonemes, deletion of single phonemes, and spoonerisms. Phonemic awareness is a prerequisite for acquiring the *alphabetic insight* (sometimes called *grapho-phonological awareness*), which is the realization that letters can represent sounds, and is necessary for learning how to read and write in alphabetic languages. Phonemic awareness has been shown to be highly correlated with early decoding abilities, and phonological processing difficulties/weak phonemic awareness are put forth as one cause of specific reading impairment, *dyslexia*, which is characterized by lasting and significant decoding difficulties.

Later, oral and written language development is characterized by a refinement and expansion of various metalinguistic skills, which in turn are one driving force in language growth (e.g., expanding vocabulary and mastering production and comprehension of a range of oral and written genres). The academic context typically demands a high degree of metalinguistic awareness. Some examples are the use of *morphological awareness* to derive the meaning of unfamiliar words, *syntactic awareness* to revise a text, and *semantic awareness* to understand and create metaphors. For older children with developmental language disorders, failing to meet the metalinguistic demands may be one of the biggest obstacles to academic success.

Some researchers have pointed out that many standardized tests of language and language processing entail metalinguistic demands in addition to the linguistic demands. Thus, a poor result on a standardized language test can be a consequence of deficits in implicit linguistic knowledge as well as poor metalinguistic skills. This also includes tests of "auditory processing" with tasks such as auditory discrimination of minimal pairs (e.g., *pea–tea*). This involves making an explicit decision about language form—in other words, it is a metalinguistic task.

Even though metalinguistic awareness is a frequent concept in the language literature, definitions, tasks, and applications vary widely. It is therefore essential to always consider each researcher's definition of metalinguistic awareness.

Anna Eva Hallin

See also Language Disorders in Children; Phoneme; Phonological and Phonemic Awareness; Reading and Reading Disorders; Second-Language Acquisition

Further Readings

Bialystok, E., & Ryan, E. B. (1985). Toward a definition of metalinguistic skill. *Merrill-Palmer Quarterly, 31*(3), 229–251.

Gombert, J. E. (1992). *Metalinguistic development*. Chicago, IL: University of Chicago Press.

Kuo, L., & Anderson, R. C. (2008). Conceptual and methodological issues in comparing metalinguistic awareness across languages. In K. Koda & M. Z. Annette (Eds.), *Learning to read across languages. Cross-linguistic relationships in first- and second-language literacy development*. New York, NY: Routledge.

van Kleeck, A. (1994). Metalinguistic development. In G. P. Wallach & K. G. Butler (Eds.), *Language learning disabilities in school-age children* (pp. 53–98). Needham Heights, MA: Allyn and Bacon.

METAPHONOLOGY

In epistemology, the prefix *meta-* before a category (e.g., *meta-* before *phonology*) means "about" (or "with," "across," "after," "above," or "beyond") the rest of the word. *Meta-* also implies "the self." So, *metacognition* is the act of using cognitive skills to consider and speak about mental processes (cognition about cognition); *metalanguage* involves using language to reflect on and discuss language (language about language); and *metaphonology* refers to individuals applying *phonological knowledge*, *phonological awareness* (PA), and *phonological skills* to reflect on, talk about, and explain phonology, thereby revealing their understanding. This entry provides an overview of metaphonology.

Phonological Knowledge

In speech, there are four types of phonological knowledge: *perceptual knowledge* of the acoustic and perceptual characteristics of speech sounds; *articulatory knowledge* of the places, voicing, and manners of production of them; *metaphonological knowledge* of the system they comprise; and *social-indexical knowledge* of pronunciation variants conveying social identity. These knowledge types are addressed particularly in speech–language pathology/speech and language therapy intervention for children's speech sound disorders; in acquired speech disorders and accent modification in adults; and in working on pragmatics, voice, and speech with transgender and/or transsexual clients.

Phonological Awareness

In education, PA has a key role in literacy acquisition in typical and atypical school-aged learners, as well as speech–language pathology/speech and language therapy applications with children with speech sound disorders, where metalinguistic training and metaphonological therapy are often used. PA is the ability to attend to, recognize, label, and manipulate speech sounds, requiring conscious knowledge of the sound structure of the spoken words. *Phonemic awareness* is a part of PA, related to consciousness of the smallest speech units.

Phonological Skills and "Phon-Words"

Phonological skills incorporate the abilities to detect rhymes, alliteration, and other sound patterns; recognize that spoken words are reducible to smaller chunks such as syllables and phonemes; manipulate phonemes; and understand the relationship between speech and writing. Overt understanding of these things can be exhibited once individuals develop *metaphonological awareness*, as it allows them to talk about, discuss, and explain their use or knowledge of any aspect of PA that is under consideration. PA and phonological skills form an essential foundation for literacy acquisition, and as children become more experienced with text, they can increasingly use *metaphonology* to reveal their knowledge of phonology.

Phonology is among the jumble of important but inconsistently defined phon-words and expressions used in the fields of education, linguistics, psychology, and speech–language pathology/speech and language therapy. They include *phones*: spoken consonants and vowels; *phonetics*: the study of the production of speech sounds, within and across languages; *phonology*: the study of sound patterns, in terms of underlying representations of *phonemes* in the mind, their surface forms (phones), and the rules that "map" or communicate between the two; *phonemic awareness*: the ability to attend to, identify, and manipulate a variety of sounds within the speech stream; and *phonics*: a robustly evidence-based method of teaching children to read and spell, in which they learn, via explicit instruction, sound–letter links, or the relationships among phones and between graphemes.

Graphemes

Graphemes are the smallest meaningful units in a writing system and are represented by one letter or more. For example, the three graphemes in *couch* are "c," "ou," and "ch" (utilizing five letters), and the three in *through* are "th," "r," and "ough" (utilizing seven). In *phonetics*, which relates to *speech*, the word *through* has a consonant cluster, /θɹ/, and a vowel, /u/. In education circles, there is a tendency to call consonant clusters "blends." In *phonics*, which relates to early *reading and spelling* tuition in education contexts, *through* is conceptualized as a consonant digraph (the grapheme "th"), followed by another consonant (the grapheme "r"), then a vowel digraph (the grapheme "ough"), with "thr" referred to by teachers as "a blend."

Relationships Among Phonemes, Phones, Graphemes, and Letters

In Figure 1, the phonemes in /tʃaɪnə/ appear in Box 1, with an image of the human brain signifying that the *underlying* phonemic level is in the mind. In Box 2, the phones or *surface forms*, [tʃ] [a] [ɪ] [n] and [ə], are associated with pictures of a

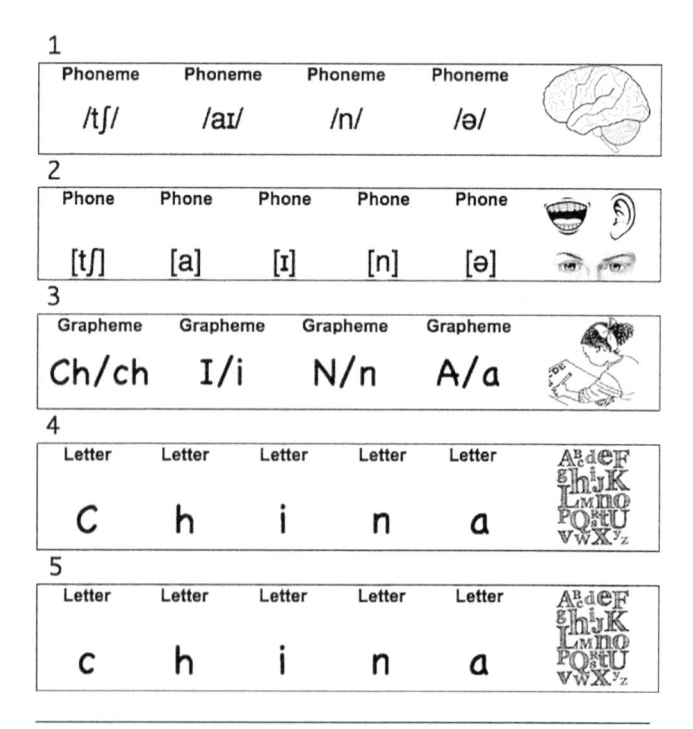

1	Phoneme	Phoneme	Phoneme	Phoneme	
	/tʃ/	/aɪ/	/n/	/ə/	

2	Phone	Phone	Phone	Phone	Phone	
	[tʃ]	[a]	[ɪ]	[n]	[ə]	

3	Grapheme	Grapheme	Grapheme	Grapheme	
	Ch/ch	I/i	N/n	A/a	

4	Letter	Letter	Letter	Letter	Letter	
	C	h	i	n	a	

5	Letter	Letter	Letter	Letter	Letter	
	c	h	i	n	a	

Figure 1 Phoneme–grapheme correspondences
Phonemes, phones, graphemes, and letters

mouth, ear, and eyes to show that typical speakers and listeners say them, hear them, and may look at the speaker, not simply to be courteous but also to aid comprehension, especially in background noise. Philip, who is 40 years of age, has impaired hearing and lip-reads to determine what a word is, depending more on vision than on hearing to detect tricky contrasts between auditorily and visually similar words like *Tom* and *Dom*, while Grace, a visually impaired preschooler, relies on her hearing alone.

Using Metalinguistic Skills in General and Metaphonological Skills in Particular

Elizabeth, who is 18 years of age, is an articulate speaker and an efficient reader, who processes the phonemic transcription, /tʃ/ /aɪ/ /n/ /ə/, and the broad phonetic transcription, [tʃ] [a] [ɪ] [n] [ə], with ease, by applying her metalinguistic skills. She understands that the addition of Box 3 represents the relationship between sounds and letters (i.e., phoneme–grapheme correspondences) and the existence of uppercase and lowercase letters. Still using metalanguage, Elizabeth *explains* in conversation that writers use orthographic knowledge, applying one of two spelling rules: starting /tʃaɪnə/ with capital C when it is the first word in a sentence and for China the nation (see Box 4) or small *c* for china the ceramic (see Box 5).

Elizabeth and her friend enjoy their metaphonology, finding humor in it. In wordplay, they combine rhyme, assonance, and cockney argot (i.e., rhyming slang: *me old china plate* for *mate*) in a silly fantasy scenario, with quotes around the word *china* denoting slang, in "My old 'china' buys fine designer china from guys with a myna in China."

Caroline Bowen

See also Phonological and Phonemic Awareness; Reading and Reading Disorders; Speech Sound Disorders

Further Readings

Hesketh, A. (2010). Metaphonological intervention: Phonological awareness therapy. In A. L. Williams, S. McLeod, & R. J. McCauley (Eds.), *Interventions for speech sound disorders in children* (pp. 247–274). Baltimore, MA: Paul H. Brookes.

Hesketh, A. (2015). Phoneme awareness intervention for children with speech disorder: Who, when and how? In C. Bowen (Ed.), *Children's speech sound disorders* (2nd ed., pp. 210–214). Oxford, UK: Wiley-Blackwell.

Metaphor

Up until the 1970s and 1980s, metaphor was generally regarded as a literary device and a tool for rhetorical flourish. From this perspective, metaphor definitions were in line with the work of Aristotle, who in the *Poetics* described metaphor as "the application of a word that belongs to another thing." Metaphor was, thus, traditionally considered an ornamental feature of language that was crafted by writers and speakers for creative and emotional effects. However, with the advancement of psycholinguistic research and cognitive linguistic theory since the 1970s, definitions of metaphor have shifted away from this idea of metaphor as exceptional language use. In fact, psycholinguistic and cognitive linguistic approaches concur that metaphor is used for mundane everyday talk, and it is generally this ubiquity of metaphor that is the reason for studies of metaphor comprehension, processing, and production in neurotypical individuals and in those with a neurodevelopmental disorder. However, it is important to note that psycholinguistic approaches tend to focus on metaphor as a form of linguistic expression, whereas cognitive approaches view metaphor as thought-based and conceptual in nature. This entry provides an overview of psycholinguistic and cognitive approaches to metaphor as well as metaphor comprehension, processing, and production.

Psycholinguistic Approaches

Earlier pragmatic models argued that metaphorical statements require more cognitive effort than literal statements to be understood and that they are only processed as metaphorical after initial attempts to process a literal meaning have failed. In contrast, current models of metaphor processing tend to agree that metaphors are understood when mappings between the target domain (the topic) and the source domain (the vehicle) give rise to new, emergent similarities. Explanations of how these features emerge fall into two major approaches: the comparison approach and the categorization approach.

In comparison approaches, such as the structure-mapping model, it is argued that metaphors are processed through a number of steps. First, the structures of the target domain and the source domain are aligned through a set of correspondences between the objects and their properties and relations in each domain. Alignment of structures is then followed by a projection of inferences from the source to the target. Within the target domain, novel inferences then occur that are formed primarily from the relational elements of the metaphorical mapping. In the metaphor *My job is a jail*, the metaphor is understood through inferences that the person's job is confining or constraining (relational properties) rather than inferences that the person's office is small and uncomfortable (physical properties). Studies utilizing the so-called perceptual metaphors and relational metaphors typically subscribe to the structure-mapping model.

In categorization approaches, such as the class-inclusion model, the topic is interpreted as a member of the superordinate category to which the vehicle belongs in the given context. Taking again the metaphor *My job is a jail*, the topic (*my job*) is interpreted as belonging to the category best represented by the vehicle (*a jail*). In the context of jobs, the vehicle category would be something along the lines of "places that restrict freedom" rather than any other category to which a jail could belong (such as "cramped accommodation with few luxuries"). Thus, the topic and the vehicle work together to attribute superordinate vehicle features to a contextually delineated topic. Relevance theory and its application to metaphor is an example of a class-induction model.

Cognitive Linguistic Approaches

In the cognitive paradigm, metaphor is not a surface-level linguistic feature but rather a mental mapping in the mind from one domain of experience to another. George Lakoff and Mark Johnson describe metaphor as "understanding and experiencing one kind of thing in terms of another." Known as *conceptual metaphors*, these metaphors in the mind typically structure an abstract domain of experience (the target domain) through a more concrete and often physical domain of experience (the source domain). People live through these metaphors; the mappings organize human perceptions, experience, and knowledge and make abstract concepts more familiar and understandable. Human language use is thus a reflection of these conceptual metaphors in the mind.

An oft-cited example is the conceptual metaphor ARGUMENT IS WAR, in which the metaphor organizes the entire lived experience of an ARGUMENT (the target domain) in terms of a WAR (the source domain). Metaphorical expressions such as *winning an argument*, *defending a position*, and *shooting down their claims* are not individual metaphors; instead, they are the linguistic realizations of the underlying conceptual metaphor. People experience these metaphorical expressions as literal as opposed to creative instances of metaphor; individuals often physically feel and experience that they have *won* or *lost an argument* rather than merely describing it using those words. Metaphorical expressions such as these are widespread in conventional, everyday language rather than being the reserve of creative and novel language use.

In addition to its role in organizing human experience, conceptual metaphor theory accounts for the origins of conceptual metaphors from early, embodied experiences; these very early metaphors are often referred to as primary metaphors. Emotions are often conceptualized via mappings from corresponding physical behaviors. As happiness is typically accompanied by an upright posture and sadness by a drooping posture, these embodied experiences generate the conceptual metaphors HAPPY IS UP (e.g., *I'm on top of the world*) and SAD IS DOWN (e.g., *I'm depressed*). In fact, many conceptual metaphors have been found to take these embodied, spatially oriented experiences as the source domain.

Most of the metaphors included as test materials in psycholinguistic studies are not conceptual metaphors, and this may explain some of the study outcomes.

Metaphor Comprehension

Several experimental paradigms have been used to study metaphor comprehension (e.g., forced-choice design in which the participant indicates understanding by selecting one option in the form of a word, definition, or picture, or the participant is required to explain his or her understanding or reword the metaphor). Of interest is how people with a language disorder understand metaphor quantitatively and qualitatively in comparison with typically developing individuals (e.g., onset of understanding, rate of development of understanding, and degree of understanding). There is a distinction between delayed comprehension (i.e., lower degree of understanding due to later onset and/or slower rate of development) and impaired comprehension (i.e., comprehension in the atypical group does not improve with time). It is also important to note whether the test materials contain lexicalized metaphors (i.e., metaphors used in everyday language that are stored in the mental lexicon) or novel metaphors, which due to their novelty are most likely harder to comprehend as the participant has to create a meaning for the metaphor, as opposed to searching for an existing one in the mental lexicon.

Metaphor comprehension in children with specific language impairment has been found to be intact when tested on the so-called dead metaphors (i.e., extremely lexicalized expressions) and lexicalized perceptual metaphors. In contrast, individuals with Williams syndrome (WS) do not start to understand lexicalized metaphor until around 6 years of age, compared to 3–4 years of age for neurotypical children, and their comprehension level remains low throughout life. Similarly, comprehension of novel metaphors begins to emerge around the age of 8 years, but comprehension levels neither improve with age nor with increasing verbal ability.

Studies of children and adolescents with autism spectrum disorder (ASD) have found that metaphor comprehension is impaired when tested on nonconceptual metaphors. However, a study published in 2014 tested children and adolescents with ASD on novel and lexicalized primary conceptual metaphors. Quantitatively speaking, the ASD participants did not perform as well as the neurotypical controls, but more importantly, the study found that they understood novel and lexicalized primary metaphors equally well and that verbal age contributed marginally to comprehension levels. This means that conceptual metaphor understanding in ASD differs from nonconceptual metaphor understanding; in short, it is not completely impaired.

Due to the later onset of schizophrenia, studies of metaphor comprehension have been carried out on adults. Studies have been limited to nonconceptual metaphors and show clearly impaired understanding.

Thus, most neurodevelopmental disorders display impaired metaphor comprehension, for novel and lexicalized metaphors alike.

Metaphor Processing

The main distinction between processing and comprehension studies is how the participants respond; in processing studies, participants are asked to simply indicate whether the test material is meaningful or not, while in comprehension studies they need to show what they believe the test materials mean. Processing tasks are online tasks and typically involve error rates, reaction time, or eye-tracking measures, often in combination with imaging techniques such as functional magnetic resonance imaging or event-related potentials.

Event-related potential studies with lexicalized metaphors have shown greater processing costs in adults with schizophrenia and longer reaction times. However, it is possible that this slower, yet costlier processing is typical in general for schizophrenia, which would mean that metaphor processing is not impaired but that semantic processing is deficient. Brain imaging studies of novel metaphor comprehension have found that processing is predominantly limited to the left hemisphere in adults with schizophrenia, while neurotypical controls also utilized the right hemisphere, which is a pattern specific to novel metaphor processing.

Adults with ASD have also displayed left hemisphere superiority for novel metaphors, and they also display a general semantic processing deficit for novel (and to some extent also lexicalized) metaphors when tested using event-related potentials.

Unfortunately, processing studies have been limited to ASD and schizophrenia, and conceptual metaphor comprehension is yet to be tested.

Metaphor Production

Production studies are very challenging for individuals with neurodevelopmental disorders, because many of these affect the person's speech and fluency. Consequently, there are few studies to date. The experimental designs used include sentence completion tasks and (re)telling of stories.

Production of lexicalized perceptual metaphors in children and adolescents with ASD, specific language impairment, and pragmatic language impairment has been found to be impaired when tested on a sentence completion task. However, some ASD studies have yielded contradictory results; another sentence completion task that encouraged participants to be creative found better production of novel metaphors in the ASD group compared to the typically developing controls. Interestingly, the novelty of the ASD metaphors differed qualitatively from the control group.

Adults with schizophrenia have been found to use surprisingly few conceptual metaphors; however, their production was similar to that of the neurotypical control group. Similar results have been found for WS, but for nonconceptual metaphors. In the WS study, neither the WS group nor the control group improved in performance with increasing age.

Unlike processing and comprehension studies, in which the experimenter controls whether novel and/or lexicalized metaphors are tested, production studies have little control over what is produced. Unfortunately, most production studies do not analyze and classify the types of metaphors created, nor do they list criteria for what counts as a novel metaphor as opposed to just being linguistically creative.

Final Thoughts

Most neurodevelopmental disorders show impaired metaphor comprehension and distinctly different processing of novel metaphors. In contrast, metaphor production may or may not be intact, as results depend largely on experimental design. Importantly for comprehension, processing, and production alike, atypical performance is most likely linked to the choice to utilize nonconceptual metaphors rather than conceptual metaphors in the tests.

Gabriella Rundblad and Olivia Knapton

See also Autism Spectrum Disorder; Psycholinguistics; Williams Syndrome

Further Readings

Gentner, D. (1983). Structure-mapping: A theoretical framework for analogy. *Cognitive Science*, 7(2), 155–170.

Glucksberg, S., & Matthew S. M. (2001). *Understanding figurative language: From metaphor to idioms.* Oxford University Press Oxford, UK.

Grice, H. P. (1991). *Studies in the way of words.* Harvard University Press Cambridge, MA.

Kircher, T. T. J., Leube, D. T., Erb, M., Grodd, W., & Rapp, A. M. (2007). Neural correlates of metaphor processing in schizophrenia. *Neuroimage*, 34(1), 281–289.

Lakoff, G., & Johnson, M. (2008). *Metaphors we live by.* University of Chicago Press Chicago, IL.

Rundblad, G., & Annaz, D. (2010). The atypical development of metaphor and metonymy comprehension in children with autism. *Autism*, 14(1), 29–46.

Van Herwegen, J., Dimitriou, D., & Rundblad, G. (2013). Development of novel metaphor and metonymy comprehension in typically developing children and Williams syndrome. *Research in Developmental Disabilities*, 34(4), 1300–1311.

Vance, M., & Wells, B. (1994). The wrong end of the stick: Language-impaired children's understanding of non-literal language. *Child Language Teaching and Therapy*, 10(1), 23–46.

MISCUE ANALYSIS

In 1963, educator and reading researcher Ken Goodman walked into a primary classroom and asked individual children to read a whole story aloud. In response to a sentence in the text: *A little monkey had it*, one child read: "The little monkey had it." Goodman was struck by the young reader's knowledge of English determiners to make such an error. With this and accumulated evidence from thousands of readers, Goodman discovered miscues and developed miscue analysis (MA) as a research tool. By the term *miscue*, he rejected the concept of error as a negative aspect of reading; rather, he defined it as a process of a reader making sense of a written text. Oral reading is not an accurate rendition of text, all readers make miscues, and linguistic understandings appropriately describe reading behavior. *Miscue* is now a common term in reading research, and MA is a research tool that builds knowledge about reading from in-depth analyses of reading miscues, while the process of teachers and readers engaging in conversations about reading is known as *retrospective miscue analysis* (RMA). This entry provides an overview of how MA works and then explores the knowledge that MA and RMA bring to the process of teaching and learning reading.

Research and scholarship on miscue theory and instruction include citations from 1965 to the present of thousands of English readings as well as readings in varied languages and dialects. Miscue is defined as points in oral reading where what the reader says (the observed or unexpected response) is not what is expected by the listener (the expected response). Unexpected responses are miscues categorized as substitutions, omissions, or insertions of words or phrases or intonation shifts that shift syntactic structures influenced by punctuation and reader's predictions. Miscues are not random and reflect readers' language (see second sample transcription line) and background knowledge.

How MA Works

MA illuminates the integral role of miscues in reading. MA analyses and discussions are a window into the reading process, providing understanding and knowledge for teachers, researchers, and readers.

MA involves selecting authentic reading material: well written with a beginning, middle, and end; interesting to the reader; and long enough to generate miscues and establish readers' patterns of miscues and strategies. The reader reads from the written text (e.g., book, article, digital), while the teacher marks miscues (i.e., unexpected responses) and other responses on a typescript preserving the text's format. The reading is recorded for research and instructional purposes.

The reader is informed of the following before he or she begins reading: He or she will receive no help during the oral reading and the student simply needs to do his or her best; the teacher marks miscues and takes notes on the typescript; after reading, the reader retells the story or article; the session is recorded. After reading, the reader provides an uninterrupted retelling followed by the teacher's open-ended questions to extend the retelling. The recording and typescript are analyzed to verify miscues and other markings and to determine the quality of miscues to enable discussion between the reader and the teacher.

Miscues are coded analyzing the degree to which they affect linguistic acceptability in sentences in which they occur and to establish a reader's patterns. Each sentence is analyzed including reader's miscues and self-corrections: Is the sentence syntactically and semantically acceptable in the reader's dialect within the entire selection? If acceptable, to what degree does the sentence change the meaning? How much do substitution miscues look or sound like the expected response? The analysis provides a reader's proficiency profile focusing on comprehension. Publications show how to mark miscues (e.g., omissions, insertions, substitutions, reversals) and reading strategies (e.g., self-corrections repetitions) to determine patterns of miscues and strategy use.

MA understandings expand reading knowledge and support the development of Goodman's model of the reading process. They help teachers develop knowledge about reading to evaluate and diagnose readers and to use MA with readers to develop their insights into reading—through RMA.

Building Knowledge About Reading

Goodman's model developed from MA research is informed by linguistics, psycholinguistics, sociolinguistics, and neurology as well as constructivist and sociocultural literacy practices of learning and teaching. Its latest iteration is in *Reading: The Grand Illusion* with coauthors Peter Fries, a linguist, and Stephen Strauss, a neurologist.

Without an understanding of language that includes literacy practices, it is easy to reduce reading instruction to the simplistic teaching of isolated skills. As a result, especially for learners convinced they cannot read, reading becomes sounding out and rereading, as they attempt to accurately recognize each word. As a result, such readers often do not see reading as a process of getting things done, answering their own questions, and engaging in reading as enjoyable.

Since the late 1800s, reading errors have been treated as evidence of serious reading difficulty. This led to the development of the concept of reading disabilities in which "good" reading is considered to consist of exact responses to words in a text or test rather than the construction of meaning or comprehension.

Goodman's insights from examining miscues as integral to language processing rejected the notion that unexpected responses were equally problematic. Brian Street calls narrow, word-oriented views of reading *autonomous literacy* where research, instructional practices and talk about reading are reduced to activities with little relation to authentic literacy use. MA clarifies varying beliefs about reading and provides alternative responses to errors or miscues in teaching and learning to read. MA illuminates individual patterns of readers' miscues, providing evidence that readers make sense as they read or that they pay most attention to surface cues that divert their attention from comprehension.

Gary, a 13-year-old sixth grader, considered the poorest reader in his school, had been in remedial reading since second grade based on a standardized reading test with a 2.2 grade level. For his MA, he read "The Stonecutter" taken from an unfamiliar fourth-grade basal reader.

The second sentence in the first paragraph of the story is:

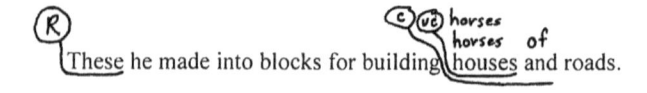

These he made into blocks for building houses and roads.

The markings show: Gary substituted *horses of* for *houses and*, repeated *horses*, then self-corrected to *houses and roads*.

Gary read the beginning of the eighth sentence without miscues (*He was sitting in a fine carriage and servants held a sunshade*) and came to the phrases at the end of the sentence. (Dollar sign [$] indicates an invented spelling for a reader's nonword.)

of turquoise silk with golden tassels over him.

Gary read *of turquoise silk with golden*, substituted $tisl- then $tessels, for *tassels*, repeated *over*, and completed the sentence with appropriate intonation. His miscues reveal linguistic knowledge (e.g., substitution of a noun, retaining plurality and orthographic and sound similarity to *tassels*). He provided a complete retelling with appropriate sequencing of events, a moral, and information revealing his background knowledge. After retelling, the teacher asked him whether he had trouble as he read. Gary responded, "*about little gold fringes on the sunshade.*" He also reported that his class was studying Troy and stone carvings people made at that time.

Gary's miscues, his strategy use, and his retelling reveal that he predicted appropriate language structures as he read, but when confronted with language that did not fit his predication, he regressed to select additional cues from the text and to continue to make sense. His miscues and retelling revealed his ability to construct concepts and comprehend as he read.

Courses in teacher education and professional development allow teachers to develop their own beliefs about literacy, reading, and how students read. They then capably plan for simultaneously embedding reading instruction that supports students' reading development and engages them in rich curricular experiences. Teachers engage readers in reflecting on their own reading processes using MA and encourage them to talk and think about how reading supports their development as literacy users.

Retrospective Miscue Analysis

The process of teachers and readers engaging in conversations about reading is called *retrospective miscue analysis*. Readers revalue themselves as they explore their miscues as a result of their knowledge about language and the world, not as a result of a disease or disability. MA with proficient readers reveals the high-quality nature of miscues. MA with younger and less proficient readers illuminates the power of MA and the universal nature of miscues. Teachers can discuss reading with their students and involve them in understanding their miscues.

When RMA became an instructional strategy, the analysis of the process resulted in research. RMA research shows that engaging readers in discussing their own reading, examining their own miscues, and reflecting on their literacy practices build understanding about the nature of their miscues and how miscues influence their reading. A major result is that they develop as confident readers.

When readers are able to revalue their own knowledge and literacy practices and processes in their discussions with their teacher, it lifts from the shoulders of vulnerable readers' negative views about themselves that interfere with a sense of control over their own learning. Once readers come to believe that they are not making miscues because they are lazy or incompetent, responses to their own high-quality miscues often include "I think the way I read it sounds better. It makes more sense that way." Debra Goodman developed the concept of a Reading Detective Club that results in readers becoming comfortable with making sense of texts from the perspective of reading detectives.

MA and RMA research show that as readers develop conscious awareness of their reading strengths, their reading problems diminish. They revalue themselves as readers and learners recognizing their strengths as language users with background knowledge and realizing the necessity to be actively engaged in their own learning and selecting interesting and personal reading opportunities. Such reading development is best supported by knowledgeable and experienced reading professionals who understand the nature of the reading process.

Yetta M. Goodman

See also Comprehension; Early Literacy Development; Language Assessment; Meaning; Revaluing

Further Readings

Crowell, C. (2015). Miscue analysis v. DIBELS: A tale of resistance. *Talking Points, 26*(2), 2–9.

Goodman, D. (1999). *The reading detective club.* Portsmouth, NH: Heinemann.

Goodman, K. (1976). Miscues: Windows on the reading process. In K. Goodman (Ed.), *Miscue analysis: Applications to reading instruction* (pp. 3–14). Urbana, IL: ERIC Clearing House on Reading and Communication Skills.

Goodman, K. (2003). Revaluing readers and reading. In A. Flurkey & J. Xu (Eds.), *On the revolution of reading: The selected writings of Kenneth S. Goodman* (pp. 421–429). Portsmouth, NH: Heinemann.

Goodman, K., Fries, P., & Strauss, S. (2016). *Reading: The grand illusion.* New York, NY: Routledge.

Goodman, K., & Goodman, Y. (2011). Learning to read: A comprehensive model. In R. Meyer & K. Whitmore (Eds.), *Reclaiming reading: Teachers, students and researchers regaining spaces for thinking and action* (pp. 19–41). New York, NY: Taylor & Francis.

Goodman, K., Wang, S., Iventosch, M., & Goodman, Y. (Eds.). (2012). *Reading in Asian languages: Making sense of written texts in Chinese, Japanese and Korean.* New York, NY: Routledge.

Goodman, Y., & Goodman, W. (2011). Eager young readers: A well constructed text and an insightful teacher. *New England Reading Association Journal, 46*(2), 9–16.

Goodman, Y., & Marek, A. (Eds.). (1996). *Retrospective miscue analysis. Revaluing readers and reading.* Katonah, NY: Richard C. Owen.

Goodman, Y., Martens, P., & Flurkey, A. (2014). *The essential RMA: A window into reader's thinking.* Katonah, NY: Richard C. Owen.

Goodman, Y., Watson, D., & Burke, C. (2005). *Reading miscue inventory: From evaluation to instruction.* Katonah, NY: Richard C. Owen.

Street, B. V. (1984). *Literacy in theory and practice.* Cambridge, UK: Cambridge University Press.

MODALITY

Modality is a notion that is understood in different ways within different approaches to human communication. Modality may be understood as a human sensory and/or motor channel, for example, vision, hearing, touch, voice, or speech. Often, however, modality is investigated in terms of ways of communicating or, alternatively, ways of *encoding information*. In the latter conceptualization, modalities are subdivided into bodily and material modalities. Whereas the former includes speech, gesture, facial expression, gaze, and body posture, the latter comprises graphic and electronic means. This entry provides a brief overview of the two principal forms of modality and the roles they play in communication disorders and their treatment.

In accordance with the two different notions of modality, communication disorders may be due to damage to the sensory-motor modalities or be the result of brain injuries that occasion so-called *impaired cognitive functioning*, a term that includes amnesia and difficulties with attention and abstract reasoning. Also, communication disorders or communicative disabilities may result from the coordination of modalities of communication that occasion a communicative action that cannot be typified as a specific one (e.g., a question), or though apt for typification, its details may not suffice to make sense of it. For example, if participants in face-to-face encounters do not combine speech in terms of "That's a gift?" with rising intonation, the communicative action may not be recognizable as a question. Furthermore, if it is not combined with a gesture or gaze that points to a material object, the recipient may not recognize what the question concerns *and* respond to it with a *yes*, as expected, rather than "What gift?" "Okay," or "Whose birthday is it?" which the recipient combines with different modalities (e.g., nodding, facial expressions, gaze). The combination of modalities in this case does not result in structures that make the action understandable. Neither does it constitute a context, which a responding action can be fitted to, so that the responding action makes sense too. From this perspective, ordered structured action and interaction, whether they include participants with diagnosed impairments or not, are the result of coordinated modalities within and, actually, across communicative actions produced by different participants. From this perspective, communicative disabilities result from social interactional structures and cannot simply be explained by reference to physical sensorimotor modalities in the individual.

Bodily behavior and written or electronic systems for communicative purposes are resources (e.g., for face-to-face communication) that are very different in nature. Individuals engage directly and bodily with the material world and with each other. Although the details of bodily behavior (e.g., body movements, speech, gaze, and gesture, including manual sign language) are not all the same every time, together the individuals manage to order elements of them and turn them into specific, recognizable, structured communicative actions. Actions of this kind may best be categorized as *embodied actions*. As research in social interaction has shown, embodied actions are ordinarily not treated as scripted and preplanned ideas that are being *encoded* in bodily *channels* of communication, and there is little evidence, if any, that a preplanned ideational complex prestructures what kind of bodily means are employed and how. Rather, individuals engage in interactional work that is incrementally developing and situated in the here and now of each and every situation.

Of course, this may also hold for communicative actions that are accomplished by spontaneously using graphic modalities, for example, making drawings or writing messages. By comparison, systems such as communication boards, picture exchange systems or Talking Mats, Bliss-Symbols, and Voice Output Communication Aid, however, are means that are prestructured and thus have embedded *encoded* communicative meanings and meaning potentials that to some extent prescript how the modalities can be used, for what purpose, and largely speaking, to what end. Modalities of this kind thus put constraints on the production, the structure, and thus the meaning of the spontaneous to-be-produced action, although of course they simultaneously provide possibilities for communication. This double-sided coin may occasion principles of use, according to which, communication aids are employed as much as needed but as little as possible.

Of course, embodied interaction may occasionally be pre-planned too. One may assume that in the moment of being hindered in spontaneous production of a communicative embodied multimodal action, one initiates a different kind of communicative process, which involves reflections and considerations of how to produce the action through different means and modalities. Hindrances may in effect also occasion consideration of the meaning that the obstructed action would otherwise have conveyed. Repair initiations of this kind have been shown to lead to sequences of embodied and multimodal action in which the participant with a diagnosed impairment tries to hint at what he or she *wants to say* and the coparticipant tries to guess *what he or she wants to say*. This indicates that in such cases, coparticipants may orient intersubjectively toward *pre-plans*. Still, the category *modality* seems inadequate to cover important constitutive features of embodied actions and material modalities respectively, and the conflation of the two categories in one may result in unfortunate approaches to the treatment of communicative challenges and the development of modalities in terms of communication aids that are not suitable for natural spontaneous communication.

Language plays a central role in human communication and may be considered a product of the human ability to create fine-grained, coordinated ordering and systematization of means for communication. Maybe for that reason, *linguistic* research traditionally concerns language structures in their own right that figure together in an independent autonomous system. Rather than being viewed as a component that combines together with other embodied and modal components, language is exclusively seen as being influenced by modalities of a physical and cognitive nature; they are treated as being highly conditioned by the individual's previously mentioned (brain-related) sensory-motor modalities that are involved in language perception and production, that is, so-called language modalities such as auditory comprehension, verbal (oral) expression, visual (reading) comprehension, and written (graphic) expression.

From the perspective of *communication* research, the development and the training of any modality for communication, in whatever way the notion is understood, must, however, take the complex interplay between different components of spontaneous communication processes into account.

Gitte Rasmussen

See also Augmentative and Alternative Communication (AAC); Communication Disorders; Emergence and Human Communication; Multimodal Communication

Further Readings

Kress, G., & van Leeuwen, T. (2001). *Multimodal discourse: The modes and media of contemporary communication*. Oxford, UK: Oxford University Press.

Rasmussen, G., Hazel, S., & Mortensen, K. (Eds.). (2014). A body of resources-CA studies in social conduct. *Special Issue for Journal of Pragmatics, 65,* 1–156.

von Tetzchner, S., & Martinsen, H. (2006). *Introduction to augmentative and alternative communication*. UK: John Wiley London, UK.

Modified Diet

There have been several attempts to standardize the definitions of a modified diet, ranging from no restrictions, to severe restrictions, and everything in between. One of the most frequent complaints about any modification to a patient's diet is that each individual speech–language pathologist (SLP) may have his or her own definition of what any specific adjustment is (i.e., *honey-thick* liquid may mean one thing to one SLP and a different thing to another). Nursing homes and others who care for patients with a modified diet have sometimes been at a loss to understand exactly how to prepare any specific modification. This entry provides an overview of the history of the treatment of dysphagia, including modified diet, then explores the National Dysphagia Diet standard and International Dysphagia Diet Standardisation Initiative (IDDSI).

History

In the early 1970s, SLPs began to work with individuals who had swallowing disorders in response to interest from dysphagia scholar George Larsen, who had responded to an observation that patients who received help with their swallowing disorders could be released from the hospital sooner than those who did not. Since SLPs had extensive knowledge and expertise of the oropharyngeal/laryngeal structures as part of their training, it seemed only natural that these professionals would be the right choice to work with individuals with dysphagia.

At about the same time, Jeri Logemann was discovering during her work with Parkinson's patients coexistent issues with swallowing. Using video fluoroscopy, she could visualize the characteristics of the dysphagic swallow. Her subsequent text, *Evaluation and Treatment of Swallowing Disorders*, was published in 1983, and the role of SLPs in the treatment of dysphagia began to increase in both professionals' knowledge and SLPs' practice. It was only in the early 2000s, however, that the American Speech-Language-Hearing Association began to acknowledge this role and that universities began to require as part of their graduate curriculum a course in dysphagia.

National Dysphagia Diet Standard

Since that time, there have been increases in both knowledge of normal and impaired swallows and increase in the use of imaging studies such as the modified barium swallow study and fiberoptic endoscopic evaluation of swallowing, supplementing the clinical bedside swallow evaluation. Once a swallow has been diagnosed as impaired, the decision must then be made regarding appropriate treatment choices and/or whether to modify the diet.

In 2002, the National Dysphagia Diet standard was adopted by the American Dietetic Association (now called The Academy of Nutrition and Diets). This diet consists of the following food and liquid categories:

Regular Diet: All foods are acceptable. Foods may be hard and crunchy, tough, crispy and may contain seeds, skins, and husks. Persons on a regular diet can produce saliva and chew for as long as it takes for the food to form a cohesive "ball" (bolus) for safe swallowing. Mixed textures are no problem. (Internationally known as "7.")

Dysphagia Advanced Soft Diet: (Internationally known as "Soft" or "6"). Foods of "nearly regular" textures with the exception of very hard, sticky, or crunchy foods. This texture requires chewing and tongue control. Foods should be tender and easy to break into pieces with a fork.

Dysphagia Mechanical Soft Diet: (Internationally known as "Minced and moist" or "5"). Foods with a moist, soft texture. Ability to tolerate mixed textures needs to be assessed. Meats need to be chopped or ground. Vegetables need to be well cooked and easily chewed. Foods should be in small pieces (1/4" or 5mm). No hard, chewy, fibrous, crisp or crumbly bits. No husk, seed, skins, gristle or crusts. No "floppy" textures such as lettuce and raw spinach. No foods where the juice separates from the solid upon chewing, like watermelon.

Dysphagia Pureed: (Internationally known as "Extremely thick" or "4"). All food should be pureed to a homogenous, cohesive, smooth texture. Food should be "pudding-like" and hold its shape on a spoon. Contains no lumps. Not sticky. Pureed foods can be piped or molded and will not spread out if spilled. The prongs of a fork make a clear pattern when drawn across the surface of the puree.

Nectar Thick Liquids: Liquids coat and drip off a spoon like a lightly set gelatin. This consistency requires a little more effort to drink than thin liquid. It is easier to control throughout the swallow than thin liquid and can flow through a straw or nipple. (Internationally known as "Slightly thick" or "1.")

Honey Thick Liquids: Liquids thicker than "nectar thick"; it flows off a spoon in a ribbon, like actual honey. This consistency allows for a more controlled swallow. This consistency is difficult to drink through a standard straw. (Internationally known as "Mildly thick" or "2.")

Pudding Thick Liquids: Liquid stays on a spoon in a soft mass but will not hold its shape. It pours slowly off a spoon and is sip-able. This consistency is difficult to draw though a wide-bore straw. (Internationally known as "Moderately thick and Liquidized" or "3.")

Source: Used by kind permission of Laura Michael.

International Dysphagia Diet Standardization Initiative (IDDSI)

In 2015, an effort to standardize food and liquid modifications internationally—known as the *IDDSI* (see Figure 1)—was undertaken and has resulted in new globalized terminology and the development of eight levels of diet modification (Levels 0–7):

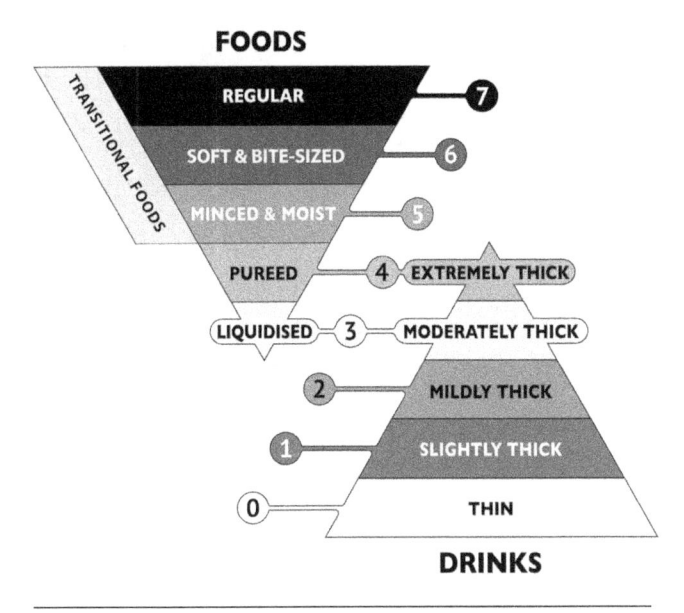

Figure 1 IDDSI framework and descriptors

Source: International Dysphagia Diet Standardization Initiative. Licensed under the Creative Commons Attribution Shareakike 4.0 Licence htts://creativecommong.org/licenses-by-sa/4.0/legalcode. © The International Dysphagia Diet Standardisation Initiative 2016 A http://iddsi.org/framework/.

- Level 0 (white): thin liquids
- Level 1 (gray): slightly thick liquids
- Level 2 (blue): mildly thick liquids
- Level 3 (green): moderately thick liquids (overlaps with liquidized food)
- Level 4 (yellow): extremely thick liquids (overlaps with pureed food)
- Level 5 (orange): minced and moist food
- Level 6 (purple): soft food
- Level 7 (black): regular diet

This work began by surveying individuals involved in dysphagia management worldwide to understand the state of professional use. The information gathered was used to construct the new diet modification framework: two inverted color-blocked pyramids (one for food and one for liquid) with a slight overlap of the two at the point where solids and liquids basically have the same flow properties. To simplify understanding, the levels were coded with colors and categorized by text inside the color blocks with a corresponding colored number written to the side. The diet structure was created with the aim of simplification of measurement methods and food/liquid characteristics such that they can be easily understood by clinicians, medical and academic professionals, patients, and caregivers. The IDDSI is being reviewed internationally and has received positive feedback. This international standardization of food and liquid modifications for swallowing disorders may advance the understanding and care the SLP community can provide to patients with dysphagia.

Karen E. Lynch

See also Swallowing Assessment; Swallowing Disorders; Swallowing Intervention

Further Readings

Chen, J., & Rosenthal, A. (Eds.). (2015). *Modifying food texture: Vol 2. Sensory analysis, consumer requirements and preferences.* Cambridge, MA: Elsevier.

Essential Purée 2016 The national dysphagia diet: Guidelines for purée. Retrieved from www.essentialpuree.com/national-dysphagia-diet-puree-guidelines

Groher, M. (2016, August 31). *The historical role of the SLP in dysphagia management.* Dysphagia Cafe. Retrieved from www.dysphagiacafe.com/2016/08/31/historical-role-slp-dysphagia

Logemann, J. (1998). *Evaluation and treatment of swallowing disorders* (2nd ed.). Austin, TX: Pro-Ed.

Rolfes, S. R., Pinna, K., & Whitney, E. (2015). *Understanding normal and clinical nutrition* (11th ed.). Boston, MA: Cengage.

Websites

International Dysphagia Diet Standardisation Initiative. Retrieved from http://iddsi.org

Modularity

Modularity, as a term in communication sciences and disorders, refers to a range of brain functions, but it is most often used in reference to theories of language and its representation in the brain. The basic idea of modularity is that mental functions are specialized and run separately from one another, in *modules*. Candidates for modular organization, in addition to language, include aspects of speech perception, theory of mind, and facial recognition. The opposite position would be to hold that higher order brain functions are managed by centralized processes. This entry provides an overview of modularity, including its history and relationship to language disorders.

History of the Modularity Construct

The idea that the brain is made up of separate components, each with its own particular job, dates at least to the earliest days of modern neurology, when Broca and Wernicke showed that damage to certain brain regions resulted in specific types of language impairments. But as understanding of the complexity of the brain has increased, simplistic ideas of "one structure, one function" are no longer tenable. While it is clear that certain brain regions have specializations, it is now understood that complex abilities such as language are widely distributed in diverse neural regions, within complex networks linking them. Thus, while modularity as a construct has a long history, in the decades since the 1980s, the term has been applied primarily to an abstract conception of mental processes rather than to highly localized brain regions with unitary functions.

The term *modularity of mind* stems from a work of that name by Jerry Fodor (1983); this work references neurology but is focused on philosophical argumentation as it pertains to psychology. Similar to theoretical linguists who used logic to develop nativist views of language, Fodor's work centered on logical argumentation to support his proposal that the mind is organized via modules, which exhibit *domain specificity*, that is, each has specific tasks (e.g., language processing). Specialized modules are argued to account for the mind's remarkable speed and smoothness in processing the array of complex information that constantly bombards it. Fodor further hypothesized that in order to achieve speed and efficiency, the modules would operate without conscious direction and automatically, with limited input from centralized processes. It is in this sense that Fodorian modules are "informationally encapsulated," meaning that they do not draw on other information in the system, operating only on their specialized inputs. He did argue that they have specific neural substrates, although not necessarily narrowly confined within a brain region.

Some of the arguments for (and against) modularity of mind draw on evolutionary theory. Some evolutionary psychologists argue that modular minds will operate more rapidly and hence increase survival fitness. The opposite view is that evolution does not support sudden development of a novel system, but rather new abilities such as language are built on older ones developed for other purposes (i.e., exaptations). From this perspective, language is unlikely to be a genetically endowed, informationally encapsulated, domain-specific system, contra the modularists' view.

Modularity and Language Disorders

Major arguments for modular organization of language relate to communicative impairments in development and in neurological disorders. So the fact that children with Williams syndrome have large vocabularies and elaborate sentence structure, but have visuospatial abilities within the range of moderate to severe intellectual disability, suggests a language *module* separate from their general cognition. Similarly, the pattern of language deficits seen in Broca's aphasia, where damage to a specific region results in specific types of grammatical deficits, is argued to reflect the modular nature of grammar. Both these interpretations of the data have been challenged; a major critic of modular accounts, Elizabeth Bates, argued that these clinical examples were misinterpreted and their true nature not carefully described. She pointed out that children with Williams syndrome do exhibit language delays, and their language profiles are not so much *spared* as significantly different from those of children with typical development. Similarly, the notion that Broca's aphasia results in specific impairment only in syntax is belied by findings that individuals with Broca's aphasia can make subtle grammatical judgments. Ultimately, arguments for modularity from populations with communicative disorders—so-called *double dissociation* where language is seen as separate from cognition and vice versa—have foundered when the complex nature of language and cognition in individuals with these disorders has been more carefully described.

Arguments against strict modularity align with many similar arguments against strict nativism. The notion that modular elements of mind are informationally encapsulated has been challenged; for example, there exist examples of phonological forms having meaning (e.g., onomatopoetic words like *click*, *buzz*, and *murmur*), showing that these two subsystems of language are not 100% walled off from one another. The *domain specificity* of language has also been challenged, where theorists subscribing to emergent accounts of language argue that language development draws on domain general (i.e., whole brain) processes and language itself is built on preexisting neural architecture. Annette Karmiloff-Smith's work on language development tried to bridge this theoretical divide by arguing that the infant's mind is not modular in its initial state, but as development proceeds, the human mind becomes modular as a matter of efficiency, as experience causes it to refine and optimize its operations. While there is wide consensus that humans are genetically endowed with neural architecture supporting language development, the notion that the mind is organized modularly in the manner proposed by Fodor continues to be highly controversial.

Lynne E. Hewitt

See also Aphasia; Cognitive Linguistics; Emergentism; Nativism; Psycholinguistics; Theories of Language Acquisition; Williams Syndrome

Further Readings

Bates, E. (1993). Modularity, domain specificity and the development of language. *Discussions in Neuroscience, 10*(1), 136–148.

Fodor, J. (1983). *The modularity of mind*. Cambridge: MIT Press.

Karmiloff-Smith, A. (1992). *Beyond modularity: A developmental perspective on cognitive science*. Cambridge: MIT Press.

Prinz, J. (2006). Is the mind really modular? In R. J. Stanton (Ed.), *Contemporary debates in cognitive science* (pp. 22–36). Malden, NJ: Blackwell.

MORPHEME

See Morphology; Mean Length of Utterance (MLU)

MORPHOLOGY

Morphology is the study of the grammatical (as opposed to phonological) makeup of words. Speech–language pathologists need to know about this area of study as they may encounter clients with morphological impairments, and, further, morphological units are often used as a measure of language development. This entry provides a brief overview of morphology, language classifications based on morphology, and the relationship between specific language impairment (now known as developmental language disorder) and inflectional morphology.

Overview of Morphology

Some units of morphology needed to understand the following discussion are *root* and *stem*. A root is the basic word form to which extra units can be added. So, in English, the word *help* is a root. The term *stem* is used when describing the addition of any extra units to a word. Thus, the stem of *helpful* is *help*, and the stem of *helpfulness* is *helpful*.

The unit of morphological analysis is the *morpheme*, which is considered the smallest grammatical unit of language. A morpheme cannot be divided into smaller grammatical units (though it can be divided into smaller phonological ones). For example, *cat* cannot be divided into smaller units of meaning or grammar; however, *catlike*, *catty*, and *cats* can all be further divided. This can be seen by analogy with other forms: *catlike* patterns with *toylike* (> "toy" + "-like"); "catty" patterns with "messy" (> "mess" + "-y"); and cats patterns with *pets* (> "pet" + "-s"). Therefore, it can be stated that while *cat* is a single morpheme, so are *-like*, *-y*, and *-s*.

These examples also illustrate two important distinctions in morphology. First, one can distinguish between *free* and *bound* morphemes. Free morphemes can be used by themselves (e.g., *cat*), and some can have one or more other morphemes added ("cats," "catty," "cattiness" [> "cat" + "-y" + "ness"]). However, some free morphemes cannot have other morphemes added to them (e.g., *and*, *the*). Bound morphemes cannot stand by themselves but must be attached either to another bound or to a free morpheme. Some come before the stem to which they attach ("un-" + "happy"), in which case they are termed *prefixes*; some can follow the stem ("happy" + "-ness"), in which case they are termed *suffixes*; others can be placed within the stem (not found in English), in which case they are termed *infixes*. The term *affix* is used to cover all these cases, whereas *adfix* is sometimes used to cover just prefixes and suffixes. Bound morphemes usually occur in combinations with free or other bound morphemes. However, there are in English a few bound morphemes that are found in only one, or very few, words, an example being *cran* that only occurs in the word *cranberry*.

Second, the examples illustrate the distinction between affixes that create a new word when added to a stem, and those that do not, but add extra grammatical information. So, whereas *catty* is a different word from *cat*, *cats* is not, but is the plural. The first type is termed *derivational*, the second *inflectional*. Adding derivational bound morphemes will often alter the word class; thus: *cat* (noun), > *catty* (adjective), > *cattiness* (noun); or *happy* (adjective), > *happiness* (noun), or *happily* (adverb); or *rich* (adjective), > *enrich* (verb). However, it does not always do so: thus *happy* (adjective), > *unhappy* (also adjective); *red* (adjective), > *reddish* (adjective). It is possible to have phonologically identical forms in different word classes, thus *walk* (either a verb or a noun); *green* (either an adjective or a noun). This is often called *conversion* with the converted form being that attested more recently. In the cases noted, *walk* as a noun is deemed converted from the verb form, and *green* as a noun from the adjective form. Conversion can also be termed *zero derivation*.

Adding inflectional affixes does not alter the underlying semantics of the stem but adds grammatical information; thus: *purr, purring, purred* all have the same basic meaning but indicate different tense and aspect types. English has a relatively small number of inflectional affixes. Nouns inflect for plural and for possessives; shorter adjectives for comparative and superlative; verbs for third person singular present tense, present participle, past tense, and past participle. Examples of these are: *cat* > *cats* or *cat's*; *big* > *bigger*, > *biggest*; *purr* > *purrs*, or *purring, purred*, (*has*) *purred*; *eat* > *eats*, or *eating, ate*, (*has*) *eaten*.

This last example illustrates that many morphemes have differing phonological forms. Sometimes variant pronunciations of a morpheme are phonologically conditioned, while in other cases, the variants are irregular with no obvious phonological conditioning. Thus, the possessive morpheme in English (denoted as {'s}) will be realized phonologically as /s/ when following a voiceless sound, as /z/ when following a voiced one, or as /ɪz/ when following a sibilant. This can be seen in the following examples: *cat's* /kæts/; *dog's* /dɒgz/; *fish's* /ˈfɪʃɪz/. These three variants are called *allomorphs* of the possessive morpheme. Some allomorphs are irregular, however. So, in English, the regular plural morpheme behaves as the possessive one just described, but a range of irregular plural allomorphs are found, as in words such as *children, feet,* and *mice*.

One problem in morphological analysis is *modification* (and *suppletion*, a subtype of modification). For example, the regular past tense morpheme in English is *-ed*, but in *strong* verbs modification is often used: *sing—sang, run—ran*. If *walked* is deemed to be bimorphemic, should *sang* and *ran* be also? Some irregular verbs use suppletion: *go—went*. Here again, it is debatable whether *went* is one or two morphemes. This debate has implications for morpheme counting in child language.

Languages usually have set orders of affixes. For example, in English, inflectional suffixes follow derivational ones. Thus, the now rare form *quicklier* has the inflectional comparative affix *-er* following the derivational adverbial affix *-ly*. The form *quickerly*, with the affixes reversed, is not attested. With derivational prefixes there is also a specific order, thus "un+pre+meditate" not *"pre+un+meditate." Inflectional affixes also show a set order, so in Swedish nouns the plural suffix precedes the definite one, which in turns precedes the possessive inflection: "katt+er+na+s," "of the cats."

Words can be categorized by their morphemic structure. Thus, a *monomorphemic* (or *morpheme*) word is one composed of a single free morpheme (*cat*), a *compound* word is composed of two or more free morphemes (*cat-door*), a *derived secondary* word contains one free and at least one bound morpheme (*cats, catty*), and a *derived primary* word contains more than one bound morpheme but no free morpheme (*receive, detain*). Traditional immediate constituent analysis of word types illustrates that related words may belong to different word types. Thus, a compound word such as *teapot* will be classed as a derived secondary word when in the plural (*teapots*), indeed adding affixes to roots in the monomorpheme, compound, or derived primary classes will convert them to derived secondary status.

Language Classifications Based on Morphology

Natural languages differ in how morphology is realized, and linguists have proposed classifications of languages in terms of their (especially inflectional) morphology. A basic distinction is between *analytic* and *synthetic* languages. Analytic languages use little inflectional morphology and rely on syntax to convey meaning relations. On the other hand, synthetic languages use inflectional morphology to a greater degree. Another classification system divides languages into *isolating* (i.e., a type of analytic language where the great majority of words are monomorphemic); *agglutinative* (i.e., a type of synthetic language where affixes are commonly used and tend to one basic meaning or function each); and *fusional* (i.e., a type of synthetic language where affixes fuse a variety of functions and meanings together). (Polysynthetic languages are a variety of agglutinative where entire sentences are constructed as single words with affixes.) Examples of these types include all varieties of modern Chinese as isolating languages (with no or virtually no inflectional morphology), Turkish as an agglutinative language, and Latin as a fusional language. The difference between these last two can be illustrated as follows. Turkish *evlerinizin* translates as "of your houses," composed of the following morphemes: "ev" ("house") + "ler" (plural) + "iniz" ("you," plural; one can plausibly divide this into "in" second person, + "iz," plural) + "in" (genitive). Latin *amer* translates as "let me be loved," with the suffix *-er* carrying the meanings first person, singular, present tense, passive voice, subjunctive mood.

That these classifications are not rigid can be seen in the case of English. English is clearly more at the analytic end of an analytic–synthetic cline due to its limited inflectional morphology and the importance of word order. On the other hand, what inflectional morphology it has is fusional in that, for example, the *-s* verb ending represents third person, singular, and present tense (and, arguably, active voice and indicative mood).

Inflectional morphemes may be in a paradigmatic relationship with each other in certain word classes in synthetic languages, for example, the affixes that denote particular noun cases, or those that denote different persons of the verb. Traditionally, these have been set out in paradigms. This can be illustrated with a noun *declension* and a verb *conjugation* paradigm.

Old English *stan* (meaning "stone") and *sorg* (meaning "sorrow"):

Singular	Nominative	stān	sorg
	Accusative	stān	sorge
	Genitive	stānes	sorge
	Dative	stāne	sorge
Plural	Nominative	stānas	sorga/sorge
	Accusative	stānas	sorga/sorge
	Genitive	stāna	sorga
	Dative	stānum	sorgum

French *porter* (meaning "carry") present tense and imperfect tense:

	present	*imperfect*
1st singular	porte	portais
2nd singular	portes	portais
3rd singular	porte	portait
1st plural	portons	portions
2nd plural	portez	portiez
3rd plural	portent	portaient

Languages may have paradigms for word classes other than nouns and verbs. For example, in Welsh, certain common prepositions conjugate to show person, thus *yn* means "in," but *ynof* (*i*) is used for "in me," with the other persons as follows: *ynot* (*ti*), "in you (sing)"; *ynddo* (*fe*), "in him"; *ynddi* (*hi*), "in her"; *ynom* (*ni*), "in us"; *ynoch* (*chi*), "in you (plur)"; *ynddynt* (*hwy*), "in them." (These are the standard written forms.) In Irish, there is a paradigm for the comparison of adjectives: *bocht*, "poor"; *boichte*, "poorer/poorest." In German, for example, the determiners inflect to show gender, number, and case, and many languages inflect pronouns (e.g., English *he*, *him*, *his*).

Specific Language Impairment/Developmental Language Disorder and Inflectional Morphology

Specific language impairment (SLI)/developmental language disorder is a disorder one of whose characteristics is difficulty with inflectional morphology (clearly only manifested in languages which have inflectional morphology). Therefore, knowledge of this aspect of morphology, and of the patterns of typical development of inflections, is important for the speech–language pathologist.

Another area where morphology is often used in speech–language pathology is in the calculation of mean length of utterance (MLU). MLU can be used to determine a child's language abilities as compared to typical development. Although MLU can be calculated in words, it is usual with English to calculate it via a morpheme count from a representative sample of the child's speech (of at least 100 utterances). Guidance on calculating an MLU in morphemes for English normally notes that both inflectional and derivational morphemes should be counted. It is here that problems arise in this metric. While it may be relatively straightforward to determine that a child has productive use of inflectional affixes, it is less so with derivational ones. So, for example, should the word *raspberry* be counted as one morpheme or two? Even if the child also uses *berry* separately, it is unlikely that the word *rasp* would be in the vocabulary of a young child. A circular argument seems to be used in this regard: Derivational morphemes are counted separately if the analyst thinks that a child of a particular age understands that they are affixes (rather than that the word is monomorphemic). However, MLU in morphemes is used to establish the ages at which particular numbers of morphemes are used in an utterance. Clearly, this is a metric that has to be used with care.

Martin J. Ball

See also Language Disorders in Children; Mean Length of Utterance (MLU); Phonology; Vocabulary

Further Readings

Bauer, L. (1983). *English word formation*. Cambridge, UK: Cambridge University Press.

Carstairs-McCarthy, A. (1987). *Allomorphy in inflexion*. London, UK: Croom Helm.

Matthews, P. (1991). *Morphology* (2nd ed.). Cambridge, UK: Cambridge University Press.

Stump, G. (2006). *Inflectional morphology. A theory of paradigm structure*. Cambridge, UK: Cambridge University Press.

Motherese

Motherese is a special way of talking to infants and young children. Its unique characteristics highlight what is important when adults speak, which in turn helps infants and children to develop speech and language. It is also known by the terms *infant-directed speech*, *child-directed speech*, *caretaker speech*, and *parentese*. When using motherese, speakers unconsciously use a higher pitch and a more exaggerated pitch contour (i.e., rise and fall). These serve to gain infants' attention, which is critical for learning speech. Infants actually show a preference for listening to motherese. It can be used by anyone speaking to an infant or young child. It is similar to how humans speak to their pets (*pet-directed speech*). Motherese use has been observed across various languages. Its use may be part of a more general phenomenon in which speakers accommodate their communication partner during an exchange. This entry provides an overview of the purpose and the characteristics of motherese, as well as related research.

Purpose

Caregivers do not teach children communication skills directly. Children acquire them through social interaction, so a child's contribution in an interaction is as important as the caregiver's. This interaction starts early in infancy and caregivers naturally use motherese in a way that aids language learning. Motherese serves four primary functions: (1) communicating emotion, (2) facilitating social interaction, (3) acquiring and maintaining infants' attention, and (4) facilitating language development. Motherese helps children to grow their vocabulary and to select appropriate social partners (i.e., those more likely to interact with them). It can cue infants to notice the faces of their caregivers. Perhaps because infants associate motherese with responsive expressions such as smiles from their caregivers, they attend to caregivers' faces more when spoken to via motherese, rather than via *adult-directed speech* (ADS). Motherese is an important part of emotional bonding between parent and child. It is also critical to emotional and cognitive development.

Characteristics

Motherese, in comparison with ADS, is shorter, simpler, and more redundant. It includes isolated words (e.g., *cup, go*) and phrases (e.g., *red ball*). It makes frequent use of questions and proper names (e.g., *Daddy, Suzy*). It also involves longer pauses, slower rate of speech, higher pitch, and a wider pitch range. Studies have shown that prosodic contours vary according to mothers' intentions. For example, rising contours were seen when asking yes/no questions, falling contours were seen for commands, and rising then falling contours were seen for statements. These cues about a speaker's intent are easier to recognize in motherese than in ADS.

Interestingly, both motherese and pet-directed speech are similar in terms of pitch changes and rhythm, but motherese has more vowels produced with exaggerated articulation. For instance a speaker might say *open* as *ooo-pen* with emphasis on the *o*. Therefore, motherese seems to be essential for communicating emotion and intentions. In addition to highlighting intention and emotion, it gives cues about grammatical units. Its cues may enhance aspects of speech that are seen and aspects that are heard.

Research

Studies support that motherese does play a crucial role in language learning as well as cognitive and emotional development. Studies suggest that it helps children with *segmentation* (i.e., identifying where words begin and end). Research has shown that children who develop language the fastest are those who get the most acknowledgment and encouragement following their productions of speech, who are given time and attention to speak, and who are asked questions. Three characteristics found in numerous languages are discussed in the literature: (1) use of pitch such as higher overall pitch, (2) words and forms taken from ADS such as use of third person instead of first or second person (e.g., *Baby is drinking*), and (3) specific vocabulary items (e.g., *potty*).

According to studies, motherese involves linguistic changes: shorter utterances, simpler vocabulary and grammar, diminutives, and repetitions. These features serve to help with comprehension, as well as language acquisition in general. Motherese also involves *supralinguistic* modifications. Supralinguistics are features that occur on top of the language used, such as using a rising pitch contour to make a statement into a question. In motherese, these supralinguistics include a higher pitch and wider pitch range, as well as exaggerated pitch contours. These changes in pitch (also known as changes of *prosody*) are thought to help in acquiring and maintaining infants' attention while aiding their language learning. Changes in how speech sounds are produced may help infants to tell the difference among vowels, categorize speech sounds, segment speech, recognize words, and learn grammar.

Research shows that motherese use differs according to factors (e.g., cultural, psychological, physiological) related to the caregiver and the infant (e.g., his or her level of reactivity). Factors affecting use of motherese may include socioeconomic ones, and whether or not the individual has siblings. Caregivers adjust their syntax level according to a child's language ability. They may increase their pitch when it seems to gain infants' attention. Studies have even shown that mothers increase use of motherese in response to perceived lack of communicative abilities in their child. The nature of motherese may vary according to the infant's gender as well.

Also, motherese usage follows a developmental course that is influenced by an infant's experience. From birth, pitch will be higher, peak when the infant is around 4–6 months of age, and then decrease gradually until the age of 2 years. The prosodic contours also vary with age. A *comforting* contour is prominently used between birth and 3 months, *expressing affection* and approval dominate at 6 months, and *directive utterances* are common at 9 months.

Infants' preference (as demonstrated by better attention, gaze, and responsiveness) for motherese does change over time, probably due to changes in their cognitive and emotional abilities and needs. Motherese does increase infants' alertness level and may cue a child to gaze at someone and hold that gaze, an important foundational skill for conversation. Motherese may also indicate to the child that someone is directing speech to him or her.

Jennifer S. Corie

See also Language Acquisition; Prosody; Segmentation of Speech; Suprasegmental Aspects of Speech

Further Readings

Durkin, K., Rutter, D. R., & Tucker, H. (1982). Social interaction and language acquisition: Motherese help you. *First Language, 3*, 107–120.

Fernald, A., & Kuhl, P. (1987). Acoustic determinants of infant preference for motherese speech. *Infant Behavior and Development, 10*, 279–293.

Kemler Nelson, D.G., Hirsh-Pasek, K., Jusczyk, P.W., & Cassidy, K.W. (1989). How the prosodic cues in motherese might assist language learning. *Journal of Child Language, 16*, 55–68.

Saint-Georges, C., Chetouani, M., Cassel, R., Apicella, F., Madhaoui, A., Muratori, F., . . . Cohen, D. (2013). Motherese in interaction: At the cross-road of emotion and cognition? (A systematic review). *PLoS One, 8*(10), e78103.

Motivation

The motivation to initiate, attend, and participate in treatment is one of many factors that mediates clinical success. Research examining the role of client motivation in speech–language pathology has been minimal and restricted to fluency and voice disorders. The unique influence of client motivation prior to, or during, treatment remains largely anecdotal. This entry discusses research regarding client motivation—with specific focus on individuals who stutter—within a broader clinical framework established in the field of psychology, namely, the transtheoretical or *stages of change* model.

Stages of Change Model

The motivational profile demonstrated by individuals considering treatment for stuttering may not be dissimilar from clients seeking other forms of behavioral intervention. James Prochaska and Carlo DiClemente's model for *stages of change* has been used to describe the readiness of clients to begin the therapeutic process for a wide range of diagnoses (e.g., anxiety disorders, phobia, weight control, smoking cessation). This model includes five stages through which clients progress prior to and during treatment, as follows:

Precontemplation stage: An individual is either unaware of the problem or aware but feels unable or unwilling to change it. Entry into treatment is unlikely, but if it occurs, may be due to (often well-intentioned) external pressures.

Contemplation stage: The desire to change is present but the drive to initiate the change process is absent (i.e., the *thinking but not doing* stage). This stage is often characterized by ambivalence, and individuals often experience both a fear of staying the same and a fear of change, resulting in general homeostasis. Entry into treatment, if it occurs, may be initiated by meaningful external events (e.g., job promotion, interview, marriage) or internal events (e.g., feeling of helplessness, just being *fed up*).

Preparation stage: The individual demonstrates the will to change and initiates the process of change. This may be evidenced by relatively small but critical attempts to modify behavior or recruit assistance (e.g., locating a therapist, changing speaking pattern in some fashion, reducing avoidance). Prochaska and DiClemente also characterize this stage by periods of self-liberation, or the client's brief realization that he or she can change despite the presence of internal or external pressures.

Action stage: The individual has begun to voluntarily employ specific changes in the observable behavior and/or the cognitive–affective aspects related to the behavior. The client becomes increasingly autonomous in the therapeutic process and emerges as an active participant in the change process both within and beyond the clinical setting.

Maintenance stage: The individual demonstrates actions taken independently to diminish the return of the undesired behavior. These include the client becoming his or her own clinician, positive attitudes toward lapses (rather than *re*lapses), and a strong sense of self-efficacy.

A client's readiness to change at the onset of intervention, and throughout, can help determine the level of guidance required to meet the client's individual needs. The cognitive and affective aspects of stuttering that often accompany the behavioral characteristics make this level of analysis an appropriate starting point of stuttering intervention. As noted by Prochaska and colleagues, progression through these stages is cyclical rather than linear, as the potential for failure will continue to exist, and should be expected, during the process of change. That is, the successful client can revert back to previous stages but with the hope that progression within and between stages decreases over time.

Although the constructs of Prochaska and DiClemente's model seem well suited for clients within speech–language pathology, and particularly for clients who stutter, application of this model in clinical research has been limited. With regard to voice disorders, research is available to support the use of Motivational Interviewing—a therapeutic approach to clinical interaction, which incorporates the five stages described in the model—to address treatment adherence. With regard to fluency disorders, a study, in 2007, by Jennifer Floyd, Patricia Zebrowski, and Gregory Flamme provided preliminary data from adolescents and adults who stutter using the Stages of Changes Questionnaire, a measurement tool based upon the constructs of the transtheoretical model. Findings suggest that while slight modifications to item content and terminology may be required, the measure appears valid and applicable to assess the overall readiness of clients to commit to the process of change. These authors also provide a modified version that incorporates specific concepts relative to stuttering (e.g., feelings toward clinician, parent readiness) to provide more discrete characterization of people who stutter.

Because stuttering often begins in childhood and can persist into adulthood, clinicians are likely to encounter clients who stutter across the life span. Obviously, the motivation of a young child to participate in therapy will differ from that of older clients who have a lifetime of experiences with stuttering and are largely independent in their decision to begin (or restart) the therapeutic process. The following sections discuss motivational considerations regarding initiation of treatment, and continued participation in treatment, for each age group.

Children Who Stutter

Like all children with communication or behavioral difficulties, initiation of treatment is decided by the parents. To date, no study has examined factors that may motivate or dissuade parents to seek therapy for the child's stuttering. Data borrowed from other childhood diagnoses suggest that a considerable number of families do not seek diagnosis or treatment for their child's behavioral differences. For example, a study conducted by the University of Florida, in 2003, found that of the high percentage of parents (88%) who recognized the symptoms of attention-deficit hyperactivity disorder in their child, only one out of three sought or received formal treatment. Perceived barriers to seeking treatment, as reported by the parents of untreated children, included (a) no perceived need (i.e., "the problem will go away on its own"; 66%), (b) negative expectations (i.e., "treatment doesn't help"; 45%), and (c) stigma-related barriers (i.e., "concerned what others would think"; 39%). Given the prevailing misconception that children will *grow out of stuttering* as well as the negative stereotype that parents are somehow responsible for the onset of stuttering, similar reports may be present for parents of children who stutter. However, direct investigation is necessary before this assumption can be verified.

Parental investment in treatment once it has commenced has received relatively greater attention in the stuttering literature. In the two most common treatment approaches to childhood stuttering—direct intervention and indirect intervention—parents play a pivotal role in clinical success. During direct treatment programs, such as the Lidcombe Program, parents are trained to *become the clinician* and administer treatment techniques at home. During indirect treatment, such as parent–child interaction therapy and family-focused treatment approach, changes in parental communication style and nonverbal interaction at home are central to the clinical outcomes. Across both approaches to treatment, parental motivation to participate in these activities, and readiness to change their own behaviors, is a critical consideration. Parental counseling may be necessary to shift parents' conception of the clinical process, and clear understanding of parent-centered goals throughout the course of treatment is advisable to reduce the risk of premature termination. More formalized measures of motivation such as the Stages of Changes Questionnaire or Motivational Interviewing for parents would provide greater insight into the readiness of family members to begin and maintain therapeutic goals.

Adolescents Who Stutter

During the adolescent years, when the client has surpassed the typical age of *spontaneous recovery* and grows more autonomous in his or her life choices, the motivation to initiate or participate in treatment will likely change. A series of studies by the Australian Stuttering Research Centre, as well as Patricia Zebrowski and Walt Manning, have focused on the unique profile of adolescents who stutter relative to younger or older clients who stutter. In general, adolescents who stutter often report (a) general lack of motivation to seek or participate in stuttering treatment, (b) general lack of knowledge about the nature or cause of stuttering, and (c) relative indifference about their own stuttering. This combination of characteristics is unexpected based on research that reports increased bullying of adolescents who stutter during middle school and high school and frequent description of middle school and high school years as the *most difficult* by adults who stutter. The lack of interest in treatment and overall reticence to discuss their own stuttering, despite environmental pressures, may distinguish adolescents who stutter as a unique clinical subgroup.

To the extent that adolescents can be considered a unique subgroup of clients who stutter, it is worth noting the similarity of these reported characteristics with those of precontemplators. As described in a review by Jackie Turnbull, precontemplators often maintain this status due to (a) lack of knowledge about the disorder, (b) failure to view change as possible, and/or (c) rationalization that the problem is not a problem for them. Floyd and colleagues identified respondents who met the criteria for precontemplation as a potentially distinct subgroup of individuals who stutter and perhaps less likely to progress through the stages of change in the manner demonstrated by non-stuttering clinical populations. The number of adolescents who stutter characterized as precontemplators has not been determined, and these traits are certainly not exclusive to clients in this age range nor shared by every child within this age range. Nonetheless, the overall indifference to change shared by adolescents and precontemplators suggests that transition from this stage may present a unique challenge to clinicians.

Adults Who Stutter

By the time a person who stutters reaches adulthood, the decision to initiate treatment may occur for a wide variety of reasons. Often, the beginning of new life experiences (e.g., job seeking or promotion, secondary education, marriage, children) may prompt entry into the clinic. Many clients may be motivated to seek treatment due to continued frustration when navigating day-to-day interactions. Some may be ready to try after many years of suffering in silence, while others are ready to try again after receiving unsuccessful treatment or treatment that was incongruent with their readiness to change. An equally important consideration is that adults who stutter may opt to not seek treatment because the disorder is not viewed to have substantial impact on their life choices or pursuit of personal goals. No empirical studies have focused on the reasons why adults do (or do not) choose to initiate stuttering treatment, and few have directly investigated preclinical motivation to post-treatment outcome. Nonetheless, when adult clients decide to enter treatment, it is important to consider the wide range of personal experiences that prompted action, and each will demonstrate different levels of readiness throughout the therapeutic process. A clinician should be cognizant of these varied levels of motivation on the part of clients and appraise their level of readiness from initial contact to select goals appropriate for *where they are* in the process of change.

Following the client's entry into the clinic, clinicians should continue to assess the client's level of motivation during the course of treatment, which, as Prochaska and DiClemente suggest, can be cyclical rather than linear in nature. As the client begins taking incrementally greater risks that push his or her comfort zone beyond its normal limits, moments of failure should be anticipated rather than feared. A growing body of data suggests that alliance between client and clinician can minimize the long-term impact of these temporary lapses. In a 2010 qualitative study, a number of adults who stutter were asked to identify factors that contributed to successful or unsuccessful treatment. A recurrent theme was that successful treatment was characterized by the traits of the clinician, such as perceived empathy, knowledge of the cognitive and affective aspects of the disorder, and the ability to foster self-efficacy in the client. These traits are consistent with client-related factors thought to predict the long-term success of treatment. In a review of the clinical data conducted in 1998, Ashley Craig found that positive change in cognitive and affective factors pre- and post-treatment reliably predicted the likelihood of relapse (as measured by stuttering frequency). These factors included greater locus of control by the client, more positive attitudes toward speaking, and greater self-help strategies demonstrated by the client. It is important to note that the status of cognitive and affective variables *after* treatment had ended almost doubled their predictive value, suggesting that positive change in these critical areas *during* the course of treatment had considerable influence on long-term clinical success. The ongoing motivation necessary to sustain these changes can be supported by the clinician via ongoing appraisal of client motivation and client–clinician alliance.

Final Thoughts

Although no formal measures of pretreatment motivation and clinical outcome have been conducted in this population, indirect evidence suggests that these basic motivational factors may hold particular relevance to the stuttering population. However, these findings should be viewed as general trends of clients who stutter as a group. The direct relationship between an *individual* client's motivational profile with his or her *individual* success in therapy will differ on a case-by-case basis and can be impacted by additional therapeutic or extratherapeutic variables. Nevertheless, the readiness of clients who stutter to change should be assessed formally or informally during intervention to help ensure clinical interactions provide the necessary support to promote long-term success.

Geoffrey A. Coalson

See also Counseling in Speech–Language Pathology; Fluency and Fluency Disorders; Locus of Control; Post-Treatment Relapse in Stuttering; Stuttering and Emotional Reactions

Further Readings

Craig, A. (1998). Relapse following treatment for stuttering: A critical review and correlative data. *Journal of Fluency Disorders, 23*, 1–30.

Floyd, J., Zebrowski, P. M., & Flamme, G. A. (2007). Stages of change and stuttering: A preliminary review. *Journal of Fluency Disorders, 32*, 95–120.

Manning, W. H. (2010). Evidence of clinically significant change: The therapeutic alliance and the possibilities of outcomes-informed care. *Seminars in Speech-Language Pathology, 31*, 207–216.

Manning, W. H., & DiLollo, A. (2007). Traditional approaches to treatment if stuttering in adolescents and adults. In E. Conture & R. Curlee (Eds.), *Stuttering and related disorders of fluency* (pp. 233–255). New York, NY: Thieme.

McFarlane, L-A. (2012). Motivational interviewing: Practical strategies for speech-language pathologists and audiologists. *Canadian Journal of Speech-Language Pathology and Audiology, 36*, 8–16.

Plexico, L., Manning, W. H., & DiLollo, A. (2010). Client perceptions of effective and ineffective therapeutic alliances during treatment for stuttering. *Journal of Fluency Disorders, 35*, 333–354.

Prochaska, J. O., & DiClemente, C. C. (2005). The transtheoretical approach. In J. C. Norcross & M. R. Goldfried (Eds.), *Handbook of psychotherapy integration* (2nd ed., pp. 147–171). New York, NY: Oxford University Press.

Turnbull, J. (2000). The transtheoretical model of change: Examples from stammering. *Counseling in Action, 31,* 13–21.

Zebrowski, P. M. (2007). Treatment factors that influence therapy outcomes of children who stutter. Stuttering and related disorders of fluency. In E. Conture & R. Curlee (Eds.), *Stuttering and related disorders of fluency* (pp. 23–38). New York, NY: Thieme.

Zebrowski, P., & Wolf, A. (2011). Working with teenagers who stutter: Simple suggestions for a complex challenge. *Perspectives on Fluency and Fluency Disorders, 21,* 37–42.

MOTOR SPEECH DISORDERS

Impairments of speech communication due to a dysfunction of the central and/or peripheral motor system are referred to as *motor speech disorders.* Actually, these abnormalities rather must be called *sensorimotor speech disorders* since the motor system is closely interconnected with somatosensory functions as well as—in case of speech—with auditory representations. Proper assessment and treatment of these syndromes, eventually, must draw upon the expertise of several disciplines, including speech–language pathology, phoniatrics, neurology, and the language sciences. This entry comprises (1) a brief outline of the mechanisms of speech motor control and (2) an attempt to classify and to further characterize the various kinds of motor speech disorders. Motor speech disorders must be separated, on one side, from higher order language deficits, that is *aphasias,* and on the other side, from articulatory or phonatory dysfunctions subsequent to acquired or innate structural anomalies of the vocal tract (e.g., glossectomy, cleft palate).

Speech Motor Control

The emergence of a monosynaptic neuronal pathway allowing for direct cortical control of the laryngeal muscles during sound communication, absent in other primates, appears to have been a necessary prerequisite for the development of speech articulation within hominin ancestors. Nevertheless, some basic mechanisms of speech production, apparently, build upon phylogenetically older brain networks engaged in sound communication, as can be observed, for example, in case of emotionally driven modifications of the acoustic speech signal (emotive or affective prosody). Such affective modulation of verbal utterances may be associated with changes in breathing patterns, voice quality, tone height, strength of articulation, and speech rate. However, a phonological–hierarchical speech code, assembling a set of elementary movements into coordinative structures and superordinate sequences in a highly automatized way, represents a unique trait—among primates—of our species. As a rule, speech sounds are generated by a source-filter mechanism that combines a sound source (i.e., airflow and air pressure–driven vibrations of the vocal folds or frictions at a narrow passage) with the acoustic filter characteristics of the supralaryngeal vocal tract, determined by the position and the movements of, especially, the velum, tongue, and lips. Thus, verbal utterances are built upon coordinated and largely automatized sequences of respiratory, laryngeal, and orofacial movement patterns.

A variety of brain structures are involved in the process of speaking, including (1) the primary motor cortex and its efferent pathways geared toward the brain stem and, ultimately, the vocal tract muscles; (2) posterior parts of the inferior frontal gyrus and the anterior insula, engaged, presumably, in higher order aspects of speech motor control (articulatory programming); (3) the basal ganglia, which, among other things, represent an interface between motor and affective/motivational brain systems, controlling, for example, the *dosage* of speech effort; (4) the cerebellum, engaged in the refinement of motor output with respect to articulatory–phonatory precision, speech timing, articulatory velocity, and automatization; and (5) the supplementary motor area (SMA), located rostral to the primary motor cortex at the medial surface of the frontal lobes, subserving superordinate control functions. SMA receives input from the cerebellum and the basal ganglia via the thalamus and supports, primarily, the initiation and—in case of error detection—the inhibition of speech utterances.

Besides these motor components, speech production encompasses forward prediction and sensory feedback mechanisms, allowing a speaker to monitor and adjust the ongoing flow of verbal communication in a highly flexible way. Although closely interwoven with higher order linguistic operations such as lexical access and language generation, speech motor control recruits—within some limits—separate computational mechanisms. For example, the syndromes of aphasia clearly differ from motor speech disorders.

Taxonomy of Motor Speech Disorders

Motor speech disorders may reflect behavioral abnormalities at the motivational/emotional level or arise from disruptions of the various movement control mechanisms, including motor planning, initiation of verbal utterances, or muscle innervation patterns, depending upon which stage of the processing chain *from the brain to the mouth* is compromised during speech production. On the basis of the clinical signs and symptoms, these impairments, thus, can be subdivided into *affective disorders*; *fluency disorders* (e.g., stuttering phenomena, speech arrest, temporary mutism); *apraxia of speech* (AOS) (e.g., erroneous motor programs, phonological errors, articulatory groping behavior); and the various syndromes of *dysarthria* (e.g., spastic, hyperkinetic, hypokinetic, ataxic, flaccid). In the following sections, some prototypical types of motor speech disorders will be characterized in more detail. It is important to note, however, that these disorders may pertain to more complex constellations, encompassing the disruption of more than a single processing stage. Furthermore, linguistic operations such as lexical access and syntax implementation cannot be considered fully independent of motor control mechanisms, and the same suggestions apply to some aspects of verbal working memory. Thus, the boundaries between aphasia, fluency disorders, AOS, and dysarthria may sometimes be blurred.

Dysfluency

Dysfluent speech is characterized by involuntary interruptions of the flow of verbal utterances, giving rise, among other things, to prolonged silent intervals, syllable repetitions, and the insertion of non-lexical materials (i.e., fillers) such as "eh," "uh," "ehm," or more or less meaningless words. In addition, difficulties of speech initiation, including restarted or repeated phrases, have been observed. Dysfluent speech may occur as a distinct disorder on its own such as persistent developmental stuttering. However, stuttering-like behavior can also represent a feature of more encompassing syndromes. For example, syllable repetitions as well as compulsive iterations of mostly utterance-final words or phrases (i.e., palilalia) have been observed in association with the syndrome of *hypokinetic dysarthria*.

A variety of etiological conditions may give rise to stuttering, but predominantly this constellation seems to reflect damage to basal ganglia-thalamocortical circuits due to, for example, focal lesions or dysfunctions of dopamine metabolism. The core pathophysiological deficit appears related to an impaired generation of timing cues at the level of the basal ganglia and/or their frontal target structures. The often-documented impact of emotional/affective conditions such as enhanced stress on stuttering behavior further supports the suggestion that these dysfluencies are related to impaired basal ganglia functions.

Apart from basal ganglia disorders, patients with left-sided SMA lesions may exhibit reduced spontaneous verbal behavior, associated with dysfluent, stuttering-like speech, in the absence of any elementary motor deficits at the level of the vocal tract muscles and any deterioration of superordinate language functions. These deficits of verbal communication following mesiofrontal disorders are often classified as a variant of transcortical motor aphasia, and SMA has been assumed to operate as a *starting mechanism of speech*. Since this mesiofrontal area represents an important cortical output region of basal ganglia circuits, the observation of dysfluent speech after SMA lesions dovetails with the model of a crucial contribution of basal ganglia-thalamocortical circuits to the initiation and maintenance of verbal utterances.

SMA is also densely interconnected with the anterior cingulate cortex, an adjacent area in rostral direction, which appears also to represent an interface of the central motor system with structures subserving emotional/motivational functions. Bilateral damage to anterior cingulate cortex may give rise to a syndrome of akinetic mutism, that is, a loss of spontaneous verbal communication.

During the second half of the 20th century, some authors proposed a fundamental distinction between (persistent) developmental stuttering and acquired neurogenic dysfluencies in terms of, for example, responsiveness to speech flow–enhancing conditions. However, more recent studies criticized this dichotomy because of, first, the large variability of neurogenic stuttering at the behavioral level and, second, the commonalities of the various types of fluency disorders, for example, with respect to the involvement of the basal ganglia and/or SMA.

Apraxia of Speech

The syndrome of acquired AOS is characterized by phonological errors, variable distortions of consonants and vowels, and a discontinuous speech flow including trial-and-error groping behavior. As a rule, basic motor functions such as the generation of muscle tone or force are largely intact, an observation that assigns AOS an intermediate status between aphasia, on the one side, and dysarthria, on the other. Psycholinguistic studies indicate an impaired capability of these patients to *plan* speech movements at the level of syllable-sized or even larger linguistic units prior to the specification and execution of single gestures during speech production. Especially, Broca's area and the anterior insula have been considered the specific neuroanatomic substrates of this constellation, but the exact morphological correlate is still a matter of dispute. AOS often occurs in combination with nonfluent aphasia characterized by word-finding difficulties, slow speech, and agrammatism.

At the beginning of the 21st century, a genetically defined form of developmental AOS entered the discussion on the evolution of spoken language. More specifically, a distinct variant of this constellation is caused by a deviant DNA sequence within a single gene (*FOXP2*). Interestingly, the interspecies variability of a homolog of this gene in birds is correlated with the ability of vocal learning. These data gave rise to the assumption that a mutation within the *FOXP2* gene was one factor enabling voluntary control over sound communication in the evolution of archaic hominines during the Pleistocene.

Foreign Accent Syndrome

The *foreign accent syndrome* (FAS) is characterized—similar to AOS—by largely intact elementary vocal tract motor functions. However, such patients exhibit abnormalities at the level, presumably, of speech motor programming, giving rise to the impression of a foreign accent. The changes in the surface structure of verbal utterances affect not only speech prosody (i.e., intonation and speech rhythm) but also the segmental level in terms of altered vowel durations, errors in the place and strength of consonantal articulation, or changes of the voicing or aspiration characteristics of speech sounds (e.g., voice onset time). As concerns the underlying etiology, FAS in adults is often caused by vascular brain lesions encroaching upon cortical components of the motor speech network of the left hemisphere. In addition, these abnormalities have been observed as well in patients suffering from temporoparietal lesions, dysfunctions of the basal ganglia, or damage to cortico-cerebellar pathways. Sporadically, even psychiatric disorders may give rise to FAS, in the absence of recognizable cortical lesions. Some authors consider this syndrome a subtype of AOS because of an eventual co-occurrence of phonetic speech errors. A particular subtype of FAS is the *foreign language syndrome*, that is, a compulsive tendency to use a nonnative language during everyday communication. This disorder seems to reflect deficits in superordinate control areas that are involved in language switching, such as the pre-SMA at the medial surface of the frontal lobes.

FAS may also occur as a developmental disorder in children, sometimes associated with autistic tendencies and/or impaired emotional processing capacities. Developmental FAS may be due to structural brain anomalies, result from a disruption of neural organization during brain development, or reflect compensatory as well as maladaptive cerebral plasticity, affecting simultaneously the speech motor control and the emotion regulation networks.

Dysarthria

The term *dysarthria* denotes speech disorders arising from impaired elementary vocal tract motor functions subsequent to damage to the central or peripheral nervous system, including focal lesions, neurodegenerative conditions, hereditary syndromes, and (neuro-)muscular diseases such as myasthenia gravis or polymyositis. Dysarthric deficits reflect a disruption of the respiratory, phonatory, and articulatory movement patterns underlying speech production, comprising the adjustment of loudness, height, and quality of the speaking voice and the direction, extent, and timing of articulatory movements. Dysarthria also encompasses central motor disorders often referred to as *neurogenic dysphonias*, including spasmodic dysphonia or essential voice tremor, affecting only the laryngeal or phonatory component of speech production. Since the various dysarthrias are associated with elementary motor deficits, such as a paresis of orofacial structures or rigidity of the laryngeal muscles, nonverbal activities of the vocal tract are often impaired as well, but at least, in some cases, considerable discrepancies between speech production and other vocal tract activities may be observed. What follows is a summary of prototypic disorders that are associated with distinct types of dysarthria.

Disorders of Primary Motor Cortex and Its Efferent Corticobulbar Pathways (Upper Motor Neuron)

Stroke patients may experience, among other things, damage to the face, mouth, and larynx areas of lower primary motor cortex and/or their efferent projections to the respective brainstem nuclei. As a rule, unilateral lesions yield mild and transient motor speech impairments only. In most cases, rapid speech restitution occurs, presumably, due to the largely bilateral innervation of the vocal tract muscles. Nevertheless, however, a subgroup of patients with unilateral cerebral infarction displays persistent but mild dysarthria. By contrast, bilateral lesions of lower motor cortex and the respective efferent pathways (as, e.g., in case of *pseudobulbar palsy*) may give rise to the, as a rule, more severe syndrome of spastic dysarthria, encompassing slowed articulatory gestures of a reduced amplitude, hypernasality, tongue retraction, increased constriction of the pharynx, and hyperadduction of the vocal folds. In its extreme, anarthria and/or aphonia may develop under these conditions (e.g., the Foix-Chavany-Marie syndrome). Brainstem reflex mechanisms and emotional vocal behavior such as laughter and crying remain intact in case of (near-)cortical lesions.

Disorders of the Basal Ganglia

In most cases, the etiology of hypokinetic dysarthria traces back to Parkinson's disease (PD) or Parkinsonian subtypes of multisystem atrophy. As a rule, these patients show a loss of motility (i.e., akinesia), slowed and *undershooting* movement excursions (i.e., brady-/hypokinesia), increased muscle tone (i.e., rigidity), impaired initiation and sequencing of motor patterns, and a distinct variant of tremor. Speech is characterized by articulatory impreciseness, reduced vowel space, fast rather than slowed syllable rate, short rushes (i.e., hastening) of verbal utterances, inappropriate silences (i.e., difficulty of initiation), harsh or breathy voice quality, monotonous speech production, shifts of pitch level, and a reduction of emphatic stress and affective prosody. Phonatory difficulties seem to precede supralaryngeal articulatory impairments during the course of PD. Stuttering-like dysfluencies (i.e., neurogenic stuttering) or compulsive repetitions of words or phrases (i.e., palilalia) have also been reported in association with hypokinetic dysarthria. As perhaps the most serious problem of speech communication, auditory self-monitoring mechanisms have been found compromised. Therefore, hypokinetic–dysarthric speakers are often not aware of the reduced intelligibility of their utterances. In some respects, disordered speech does not strictly parallel the pattern of motor impairments in other domains. Furthermore, the dysarthric deficits of PD patients have turned out less responsive to pharmacological therapy, and treatment-induced deterioration of speech production may be observed after deep brain stimulation. Besides PD, dysfunctions of the basal ganglia of a, for example, vascular, traumatic, or inflammatory origin have also been observed to cause hypokinetic dysarthria.

Huntington's chorea, an autosomal-dominant hereditary disease and a further distinct dysfunction of the basal ganglia, may be associated with a syndrome of speech deficits called *hyperkinetic dysarthria*. Perceptual speech evaluation revealed, among other things, fluctuations of pitch and loudness, involuntary vocalizations, and *overshooting* articulatory gestures. These signs reflect, presumably, *hyperkinetic* activity of vocal tract and respiratory muscles. Acoustic analyses of sentence utterances and kinematic recordings of lip movements during speech production point at a tendency toward slowed movement execution in these patients.

Dysarthric speech has also been noted in patients suffering from dystonia or essential tremor, two further distinct movement disorders assumed to be related to dysfunctions of basal ganglia circuitries. Spasmodic dysphonia, for example, a focal dystonia of laryngeal muscles, is characterized by harsh voice quality, and essential voice tremor may interfere with (i.e., interrupt) articulatory movements.

Disorders of the Cerebellum and Its Afferent and Efferent Connections

Dysfunctions of cerebellar networks typically give rise to a syndrome of *ataxia*, characterized, among other things, by slowed and imprecise movement execution as well as compromised coordination of multijoint motor patterns. The respective condition within the speech domain, known as *ataxic dysarthria*, has been observed in a variety of cerebellar disorders such as gunshot injuries, degenerative diseases (e.g., Friedreich's ataxia or subtypes of spinocerebellar ataxia), inflammatory conditions, or ischemic infarctions. These deficits are predominantly bound to lesions of superior parts of the cerebellar hemispheres and characterized by imprecise articulation, especially, irregular articulatory breakdown, a slowed *scanning* speech rhythm, harsh voice quality, and pitch fluctuations. Furthermore, kinematic analyses revealed a reduced articulatory velocity in relation to movement amplitude, indicating an impaired ability to generate adequate muscular forces under time-critical conditions.

Several investigations reported the dysarthric signs of degenerative cerebellar diseases to be limited to rather mild deficits, and the decline of speaking rate appears to plateau at about three syllables per second. In some instances of a cerebellar disorder, voice tremor of a similar frequency could be detected during sustained vowel productions.

Removal of a midline cerebellar tumor, especially, in children, may cause a temporary loss of spoken language (i.e., *transient cerebellar mutism*) followed, in a subgroup of patients, by ataxic dysarthria. Rather than a genuine cerebellar dysfunction, initial mutism might reflect reduced cerebral blood flow (i.e., hypoperfusion) in contralateral areas of the frontal cortex (crossed cerebello-cerebral diaschisis).

Cranial Nerves and (Neuro-)Muscular Diseases

The syndrome of *flaccid dysarthria* may arise in lesions of the peripheral nervous system or lower motor neuron system, characterized by weakness and lack of normal muscle tone, giving rise at the perceptual level to hypernasality, imprecise consonants, breathy voice quality, and nasal air emission during stop consonants.

Dependent upon lesion site, disorders restricted to a single cranial nerve cause dysphonia, velopharyngeal incompetency, impaired tongue motility, or oral-facial paresis. More extensive disease processes may encroach upon all cranial nerves supplying the vocal tract, for example, nasopharyngeal tumors, polyneuritis, or progressive bulbar palsy (i.e., a degenerative motor system diseases). In these instances, severe forms of flaccid dysarthria must be expected. Eventually, amyotrophic lateral sclerosis presents with a similar syndrome prior to its development into a mixed flaccid–spastic constellation. Abnormal articulation and/or phonation can also be observed in case of myasthenia gravis, that is, a disorder characterized by disrupted neuromuscular signal transmission. Furthermore, muscular dystrophies have been noted to impair orofacial, laryngeal, and/or respiratory functions.

Ingo Hertrich and Hermann Ackermann

See also Apraxia of Speech; Articulatory Phonetics; Dysarthria; Emotional Impact of Communication Disorders; Fluency and Fluency Disorders

Further Readings

Ackermann, H., & Brendel, B. (2016). Cerebellar contributions to speech and language. In G. Hickock

& S. L. Small (Eds.), *Neurobiology of language* (pp. 73–84). Amsterdam, The Netherlands: Elsevier.

Ackermann, H., Hage, S. R., & Ziegler, W. (2014). Brain mechanisms of acoustic communication in humans and nonhuman primates: An evolutionary perspective. *Behavioral and Brain Sciences, 37,* 529–604.

Ackermann, H., Hertrich, I., & Ziegler, W. (2010). Dysarthria. In J. S. Damico, N. Müller, & M. J. Ball (Eds.), *The handbook of language and speech disorders* (pp. 362–390). Malden, MA: Wiley-Blackwell.

Alm, P. A. (2004). Stuttering and the basal ganglia circuits: A critical review of possible relations. *Journal of Communication Disorders, 37,* 325–369.

Duffy, J. R. (2013). *Motor speech disorders: Substrates, differential diagnosis, and management* (3rd ed.). St. Louis, MO: Elsevier Mosby.

Krishnan, G., & Tiwari, S. (2013). Differential diagnosis in developmental and acquired neurogenic stuttering: Do fluency-enhancing conditions dissociate the two? *Journal of Neurolinguistics, 26,* 252–257.

McNeil, M. R. (2008). *Clinical management of sensorimotor speech disorders* (2nd ed.). New York, NY: Thieme.

Müller, N., & Ball, M. J. (Eds.). (2013). *Research methods in clinical linguistics and phonetics: A practical guide.* Malden, MA: Wiley-Blackwell.

Yorkston, K. M., Beukelman, D. R., Strand, E. A., & Hakel, M. (2010). *Management of motor speech disorders in children and adults* (3rd ed.). Austin, TX: Pro-ed.

Ziegler, W., Aichert, I., & Staiger, A. (2012). Apraxia of speech: Concepts and controversies. *Journal of Speech, Language, and Hearing Research, 55,* S1485–S1501.

Multidimensional Scoring

Multidimensional scoring is a psychometric method for quantifying and converting the test responses of subjects to scores. It takes into consideration the primary components that are necessary for the successful completion of a test task. Originally developed to overcome the shortcomings of existing test scoring methods used in the evaluation of patients with aphasia, the general principles for developing multidimensional scoring systems have been applied to a variety of human behaviors or activities. Constructing such a system requires that the dimensions or components of the behavior be specified and then ordered hierarchically according to their importance to satisfactorily carrying out the target behavior or activity. This enables the fabrication of a binary choice flowchart that allows the observer to make a series of choices as to the presence or absence of each dimension, going from the most important dimension to the least important. The features under each dimension are assigned a score, usually going from the lowest to the highest score as scorer proceeds through the binary choices. As long as the observer responds to the binary choice positively, the process can continue through the flowchart. If a negative choice occurs, the score at that feature quantifies the level of functioning on that particular item at that point in time. Since this kind of scoring is a forced-choice system, it tends to have very high test–retest and inter- and intrascorer agreement, provided that the conditions of the observations are standardized, so that they are replicable across all observers and subjects. This entry provides an overview of binary choice multidimensional scoring and the need for training on the part of its testers.

Historical Perspectives

World War II produced an abundance of brain-injured patients, which, in turn, stimulated attempts at the development of more formalized psychological assessment for localizing where in the brain the lesions had occurred. Brain scans had not yet been developed, and so the localization of the various brain functions that could be discovered through aphasia tests was of considerable interest.

In the 1960s, Norman Geschwind resurrected and formalized some of the early models proposed by Paul Broca and Carl Wernicke and others, and he developed a nomenclature for classifying aphasia. This led to the development of several tests to facilitate the localization process, although few of these were subjected to close psychometric scrutiny. The existing scoring methods in use included descriptive methods, plus-minus scoring, ratings of goodness of responses, and category scales that were subjective and lacking in capturing the specific nature of the response or not replicable across scorers and over time. In answer to this clinical need, Bruce Porch developed the concept of multidimensional scoring and, in 1966, published the Porch Index of Communicative Ability.

Binary Choice Multidimensional Scoring

After observing that a wide range of responses to a given test item could be considered accurate, as there were a variety of possible attempts at each item that were inaccurate responses, Porch concluded from a detailed analysis of innumerable responses that the primary dimensions were the following:

Accuracy: The degree of rightness and wrongness.

Responsiveness: Indicates whether additional information is needed from the tester or from the patient's first inaccurate attempt at the response, before successfully producing an accurate response. It includes self-corrections or getting a repeat of the item or a cue from the tester.

Completeness: An accurate response that is incomplete grammatically, syntactically, or pragmatically in terms of the test requirements.

Promptness: An accurate response that requires more than normal processing time to initiate or complete the response.

Efficiency: The motoric skill with which the patient is able to respond or the degree of distortion or slowness in the response.

These dimensions were applied to the quantification of all accurate responses, but for inaccurate responses, it was not clinically important to

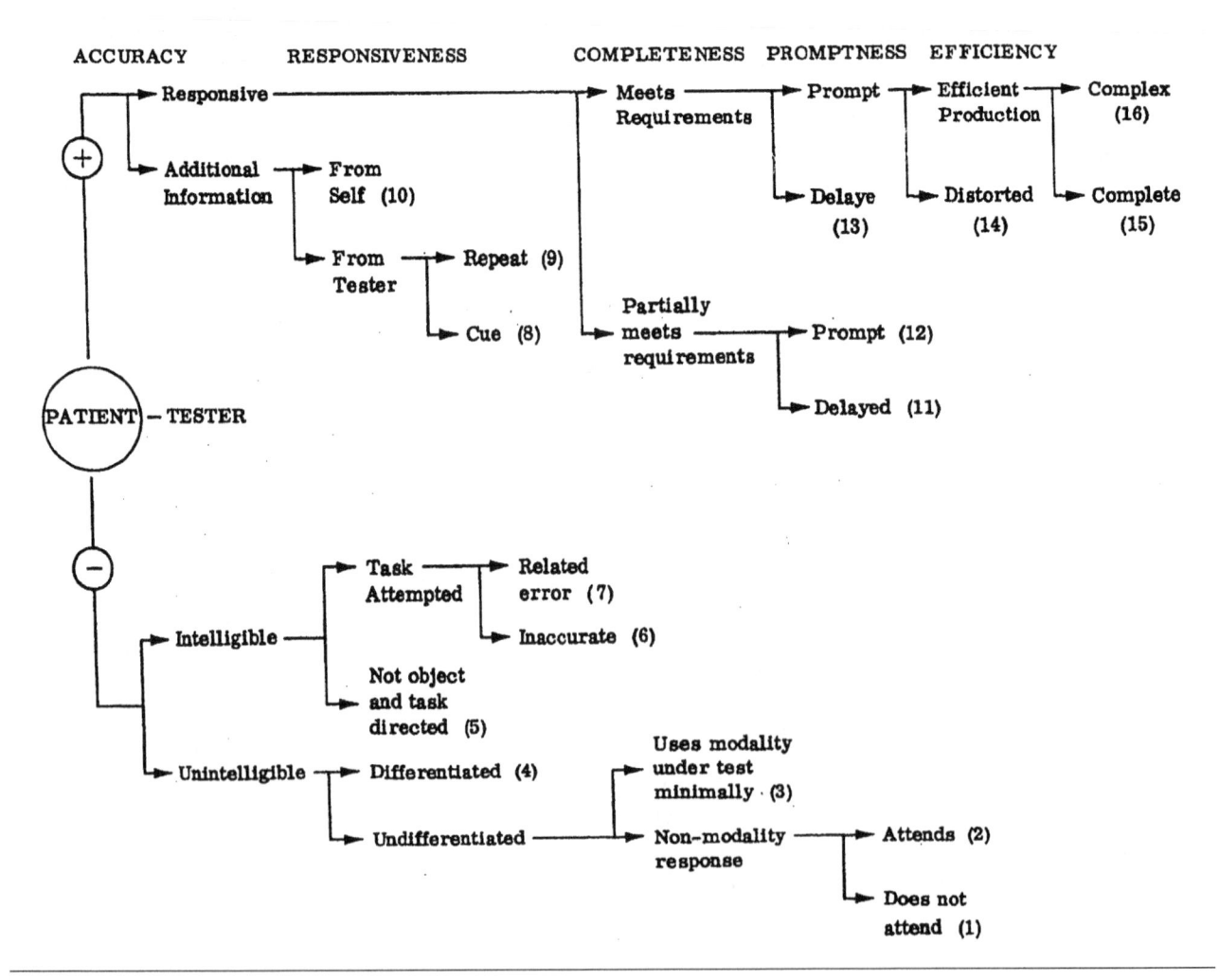

Figure 1 Multidimensional scoring as a binary choice style

Source: Porch (2001, p. 20). Copyright by Pica Programs. Reproduced with permission.

note whether the error was delayed or incomplete. That is, if a patient in trying to name a test object said "do-do-do," it wasn't significant if the patient took extra time to make a minimal response. However, it was important to document whether the patient could respond intelligibly or not, could attempt the task being tested, made an error that approached being correct, or was clearly wrong. Using this strategy, Porch was able to develop a binary choice multidimensional score system (see Figure 1).

The system involves 16 categories of response, going from the highest possible score of 16 for an accurate, responsive, complete, prompt, complex response down to the lowest possible score of 1, when the patient gives no response and does not attend to the test situation. The tester observes the patient's response on a given item and then thinks through the flowchart, asking whether the response included that dimension. If the decision is positive, the tester proceeds on to the next dimension. If the answer is negative, the tester decides why the response does not satisfy meeting the requirements of that dimension. This decision making leads to a score, which is then written on the score sheet. If a specific item is considered inaccurate, then, using the bottom half of the flowchart, the tester must decide how much credit must be given for the wrong response. The test must answer questions such as: Was the answer intelligible? Was it an attempt at the task? Was it partially accurate or completely inaccurate? Negative decisions lead to lower scores representing more severe degrees of processing problems.

Required Tester Training and Skill

The main difficulty with multidimensional scoring is that, although it is able to score the subtlest kinds of test behavior, the tester must be able to observe that behavior before applying the scoring system. For this reason, it is usually necessary to go through a training course that sensitizes the tester to all aspects of patients' behavior during their response. Once trained, the tester finds that the test behavior, which is now clearly recognized, is synonymous with the score. It also should be noted that once the multidimensional scoring is mastered, it may be applied to all other tests the clinician employs as well as to the treatment process.

Bruce Porch

See also Aphasia Assessment

Further Readings

Duffy, J. R., & Dale, B. J. (1977). The PICA scoring scale: Do its statistical shortcomings cause a problem. *Clinical aphasiology proceedings.* Minneapolis, MN: BRK.

Porch, B. E. (1971). Multidimensional scoring in aphasia testing. *Journal of Speech and Hearing Research, 14,* 4, 776–792.

Porch, B. E. (2001). *Porch index of communicative ability: Scoring and administration* (Vol. 2). Albuquerque, NM: Pica Programs.

Porch, B. E. (2008). Treatment of aphasia subsequent to the porch index of communicative ability (PICA). In R. Chapey (Ed.), *Language intervention strategies in aphasia and related communication disorders.* Philadelphia, PN: Lippincott, Williams & Wilkins.

Multilingualism

The use of many languages is known as multilingualism. Multilingualism is a communicative practice found in individuals or groups of individuals. On both the personal and societal level, multilingualism refers to knowing and/or using more than one language in the form of speech, gesture, writing, or reading. Multilingualism is an intersubjective notion in that an agreement is required between people regarding its exact definition, meaning, and practice. This is because any specific language may have many varieties, and there is variability across individuals and groups of individuals in terms of proficiency levels as well as the scope and extent of language usage. Despite this, multilingualism is a worldwide norm rather than an exception in language use. As part of the scientific study of language (i.e., linguistics), multilingualism is a major corollary of human communication sciences, which in turn also informs human communication disorders. This entry examines terms and definitions of multilingualism, its historical foundations, language statistics in the

21st-century world, and contextual factors and concludes with a discussion of the acquisition of multilingualism.

Terms and Definitions

The term *multilingualism* comes from Latin *multi* meaning "many, more than one" and *lingua* meaning "language, speech." *Plurilingualism* is a synonymous term with a similar structure, though less commonly used. *Polyglotism*, which comes from the Greek words *poly* meaning "many" and *glossa* meaning "language," is also used to refer to multiple language use that carries the extra connotation that languages are learned as a pastime rather than singly for communication. *Hyperpolyglotism* describes the use of many more languages than is normally expected in an individual's multilingualism. A *savant polyglot* is a developmentally disabled person whose exceptional multilingual capabilities surpass average performance.

A colloquial term used interchangeably with multilingualism is *bilingualism*. As justified by its etymology, however, multilingualism is an umbrella term encompassing subcategories including *bi-lingualism* (two-language use) and *tri-lingualism* (three-language use). Likewise, *bidialectalism*, *multilectalism*, and *diglossia* further fall within the scope of multilingualism. Bidialectalism refers to a person's ability to communicate in two distinct varieties of a specific language, one of which is usually the standard version and the other a regional dialect. The standard version of a language is a purposefully elevated variety used in public discourse that aims to preserve the political, cultural, and social unity of the nation that uses it. It is common for a language to have a standard version and many regional dialects. Nevertheless, some languages like Arabic, Chinese, English, French, Korean, Portuguese, and Swedish also have several standard versions and are known as pluricentric languages. In multilectalism, individuals in a society command a dialect proper that can be further broken down into basilects (rural variety) and mesolects and acrolects (urban varieties). An example of 21st-century bidialectalism is the use of both Standard Greek and Cypriot Greek on the island of Cyprus.

In diglossia, deriving from Greek *di* meaning "two" and *glossa* meaning "language," a single language community has access to both a low and high language variety. The low variety is the vernacular, that is, a mother tongue acquired since birth and spoken by ordinary people; the high variety is learned subsequently in educational settings, usually superposed by the social elite, and is reserved for use only in specific contexts such as literature, politics, and formal education. The high variety is very divergent, grammatically complex, and highly codified; it may originate from an older form of that language, may relate to a regional variety, or may be an altogether unrelated language. Examples of 21st-century diglossia are Standard German/Low German and the Baku/Gaul forms of Indonesian.

Since the early times of multilingual practice, however, a *lingua franca*, literally meaning "language of the Franks" to refer to Western Europeans, is a language systematically used for commercial, diplomatic, administrative, religious, cultural, and/or scientific purposes to facilitate communication between people with different native languages. Such examples include Greek used in the empire of Alexander the Great, Latin and Greek in the Roman Empire, Akkadian and Aramaic in the empires of Western Asia, and 21st-century English, Spanish, and so on. A lingua franca is a nation's official language whose range of use, however, extends beyond its geographical borders, and is practiced throughout the world or in certain regions of the world.

Historical Foundations

A well-known biblical story on the origins of multilingualism is that of the tower of Babel. According to the story a single language, called Adamic, existed in the beginning of humankind. The act of humankind to build a tower in Babel, with the ambition to reach heaven, enraged God and led to the fragmentation of human language into about 70 varieties, which hindered subsequent human communication and solidarity. Although there is no complete consensus on the origins of language, various types of evidence (e.g., genetic, archaeological, paleontological) suggest that language emerged some 200,000 years ago in the *Homo sapiens* who lived in Africa, below the Sahara region. Oral language began diversifying at least by 60,000 years ago as a result of the migration of

Homo sapiens to other areas. Interestingly, Africa is one of the most linguistically diversified geographical areas in the world; also, African indigenous languages have a relatively large number of phonemes compared with languages in other regions, such as Oceania, which was the last to be inhabited. Subsequent evidence of multilingualism is found in Mesopotamia (3rd millennium BCE), Asia Minor and Egypt (first 2 millennia BCE), and in the Roman Empire (1st century CE to 4th century CE). In the Middle Ages (5th to 15th centuries CE), invasions and settlements of new people around Europe instigated linguistic convergence and multilingualism in the area. It is estimated that between 30,000 and 500,000 languages created over the course of human history are now extinct. Among the few surviving for over 2,000 years are Basque, Chinese, Egyptian, Greek, Hebrew, Persian, Sanskrit, and Tamil.

Language Statistics in the 21st Century

Based on the information in the *2016 Ethnologue*, there are 7,016 living languages in today's world; about 6% are endangered. Adding sign languages to these estimates would almost double the number. Based on the number of native speakers, the first five languages worldwide are listed here in descending order: Chinese, Spanish, English, Arabic, and Hindi. There are 147 language families; the six major ones are listed here in descending order: Niger-Congo, Austronesian, Trans-New Guinea, Sino-Tibetan, Indo-European, and Afro-Asiatic. The distribution of oral languages by area of origin in decreasing order is as follows: Asia (2,303, 32.4%), Africa (2,146, 30.2%), Pacific (1,312, 18.5%), Americas (1,060, 14.9%), and Europe (285, 4%). The distribution of the number of speakers per area differs somewhat: Asia (59.9%), Europe (26.3%), Africa (12.9%), Pacific (0.1%), and Americas (0.8%). A point to note is that there are more speakers compared to fewer languages in Europe but fewer speakers compared to more languages in Africa. Asia exhibits the largest linguistic diversity and the largest number of speakers.

Changing distributions of human populations across the world influence the number of speakers of specific languages in different regions; migration increases the probability of language contact, which diversifies language use and leads to multilingualism in the society and in individuals. English, French, and Spanish are found commonly in use around the world (often as lingua franca). Central Asia is the sole geographical area where only local languages are spoken. Combining native and non-native speakers, English is the most commonly spoken lingua franca in the world, with over a billion second-language speakers, a figure subject to how mastery is assessed. Work by David Crystal has shown that of every four speakers of English, three are non-native.

Furthermore, based on information in the *World Factbook* (2016), it is deduced that 44% of the countries in the world have more than one official language and 30% have two official languages. India and South Africa have the most, 16 and 11, respectively, while China, Zimbabwe, and Spain follow up with 7, 5, and 5, respectively. Alongside official languages, countries may also have national languages; of these, Mali and Namibia have the most in the world with 13 national languages each.

Contexts of Multilingualism

A fact not widely recognized is that multilingualism has been a common phenomenon in human history. Although societal and individual multilingualism are clearly interlinked, there is a distinct difference between the two. For instance, in countries that are officially monolingual, there may be large populations that are multilingual, or multilectal; also, while many countries, like Canada, India, South Africa, and Switzerland, are officially multilingual, some of their residents are monolingual. There are situations wherein multiple languages coexist in a society but are used separately.

There is also difference of opinion regarding what constitutes language competence in a multilingual individual. The tendency in linguistics has been to identify multilingual with *perfect* linguistic competence in all languages, similar to the competence of educated native speakers. In reality, the norm in multilingual individuals is that of variable degrees of competence in each language: from oral and written fluency to basic oral or comprehension skills. For example, a multilingual individual may be fluent in two or three languages, communicating and translating between them, but that individual may only be able to identify written form in a fourth language or have comprehension (i.e., receptive language skills), though no literacy skills, in a fifth one. A multilingual person's competence and performance in the languages relates to a combination of factors, such as how a person has reached mastery in each language, what is the purpose of using each language, and the extent of the use of each language in a multilingual person's life span. Because of these factors, together with limitations in current census buildup that is not specialized enough to account for variability in multilingual use, accurate numbers on the populations of multilinguals in the world are not easy to determine.

Multilingual Acquisition

Multilingual development is not only feasible but often inevitable in humans. Multilingualism in the 21st century is reinforced globally by governments, educators, and parents for the cognitive, social, and economic benefits emanating from its practice. There are fewer children worldwide educated exclusively in a native language than there are children also educated in additional languages. Language acquisition in infancy/toddlerhood is more advantageous than later on because maturation constraints dominate after a *critical period* ending in childhood. Nevertheless, languages may be learned during a person's entire life span through education or natural exposure, or both. Differences in sociolinguistic contexts, the timing and length of exposure to each of the multilingual's languages, and individual differences in acquisition affect the acquisition patterns, rates, and ultimate proficiency in each language.

Language, like a living and perishable organ, is affected by a person's well-being and general life circumstances. Thus, the status of a language in multilingualism may change over time. To exemplify, though it is common for infants to be exposed to the heritage languages of their families or their caregivers' native or accented speech, languages acquired this way tend to be weak, or cease being used when formal instruction starts in the language of the majority. Less-than-perfect performance in a multilingual's languages is commonly evident in accented speech and weak literacy skills, and it is overwhelmingly associated with social stigma and subject to satire. This is the case reflected in native-speaker attitudes toward foreign-language speech or the speech of immigrant and marginalized groups in a society. Furthermore, irrespective of levels of mastery, the languages of a multilingual may atrophy if not sufficiently used, leading to incomplete acquisition and, in reverse fashion, to attrition or even loss of a language including the native one.

Lastly, given the need for human cognition to deal with more than one language, there is evidence of cross-linguistic influence in the multilingual individual's speech. This is manifest in patterns of language mixing, like code switching, in the course of conversations among multilinguals sharing the same languages. Also, during acquisition and beyond, the languages of a multilingual may interfere with each other. Previously acquired language(s) impact, both positively and negatively, subsequently acquired languages, and vice versa. The extent of cross-linguistic interaction depends on language status in terms of proficiency and use, and whether there is linguistic similarity between the languages.

As a direct consequence of such variables, measuring multilingualism in today's globalized reality and disentangling paths of multilingual acquisition present challenging tasks.

Elena Babatsouli

See also Bilingual Education; Bilingualism; Cognitive Linguistics; Communicative Competence; Critical Period for Language Acquisition; Expressive and Receptive Language; Indigenous Languages; Individual Differences; Language; Language Acquisition; Linguistics; Oral Language; Phoneme; Stigma

Further Readings

Andrews, E. (2014). *Neuroscience and multilingualism*. Cambridge, UK: Cambridge University Press.

Auer, P., & Wei, L. (2007). *Handbook of multilingualism and multilingual communication*. Berlin, Germany: De Gruyter.

Battle, D. E. (2012). *Communication disorders in multicultural and international populations*. St. Louis, MO: Elsevier.

Cenoz, J. (2013). Defining multilingualism. *Annual Review of Applied Linguistics, 33*, 3–18.

Crystal, D. (1997). *The Cambridge encyclopedia of language.* Cambridge, UK: Cambridge University Press.

Ethnologue: Languages of the world. (2016). Retrieved from https://www.ethnologue.com/

Franceschini, R. (2013). History of multilingualism. In C. A. Chapelle (Ed.), *The encyclopedia of applied linguistics.* New York, NY: Blackwell.

World FactBook. (2016). Retrieved from https://www.cia.gov/library/publications/the-world-factbook/

Multilingualism and Speech Sound Disorders

The majority of the world is multilingual and most children learn to speak the languages within their communities with adultlike competence. While there are a range of definitions of multilingualism, a broad definition from the International Expert Panel on Multilingual Children's Speech is that multilingual people can speak, sign, and/or understand two or more languages with at least a basic level of proficiency. Multilingual children are at the same level of risk for having speech sound disorders as monolingual children; however, for multilingual children, identification of speech sound disorders can be more complex given the multiple linguistic influences on speech production. According to the International Expert Panel on Multilingual Children's Speech (2012), "Children with speech sound disorders can have any combination of difficulties with perception, articulation/motor production, and/or phonological representation of speech segments (consonants and vowels), phonotactics (syllable and word shapes), and prosody (lexical and grammatical tones, rhythm, stress, and intonation) that may impact speech intelligibility and acceptability" (p. 1). Assessment and intervention should be based on the best available research evidence, as well as the preferences of the children and their families, and practice-based evidence from the professionals they work with. Key tasks for speech–language pathologists include differential diagnosis between children with speech sound disorders and speech differences (due to crosslinguistic transfer between languages/dialects) and creation of speech intervention techniques to support multilingualism and maintenance of home languages. The provision of equitable services for multilingual children with speech sound disorders may require additional funding, time, and resources compared to working with monolingual children who speak the dominant language of the community. This entry provides an overview of the complex issues surrounding assessment, diagnosis, and intervention for speech sound disorders in multilingual children, as well as addressing the importance of language maintenance.

Crosslinguistic Summary of Typical Speech Acquisition

By 4–5 years of age, most children are able to speak intelligibly to most people, even strangers, produce most vowels and consonants, put these sounds together into syllables, and use intonation, pausing, stress, and tones that are appropriate for their dialect/language(s). Vowels, nasals, and plosives are the earliest sounds to be produced by children. Children produce more sounds and greater articulatory variation as they grow older. Five-year-old children produce over 90% of consonants correctly. Most vowels are acquired by 3 years of age; however, in stress-timed languages, use of appropriate stress (especially unstressed vowels) is not correct until children are 7–9 years old. Tone acquisition is achieved by the age of 2–3 years. The consonant-vowel (CV) configuration is a universal is a universal syllable shape and is the earliest syllable structure to emerge. Although there are some similarities, common mismatches (i.e., errors) differ between languages. Systemic simplifications that occur in a range of languages include: backing, fronting, gliding/liquid deviation, stopping, devoicing, and voicing. Structural simplifications that occur in a range of languages include assimilation/consonant harmony, cluster reduction, initial consonant deletion, final consonant deletion, reduplication, and weak syllable deletion. Acquisition of stress is language-dependent with very early acquisition in languages that have consistent stress patterns (e.g., Israeli Hebrew) and later acquisition in languages with inconsistent stress patterns (e.g., Dutch and English). Children produce language-specific intonation between 1 and 2 years of age, but it is not fully acquired until 5;0. Perception continues to develop until children are 10–11 years of age.

Collaborating With Multilingual and Multicultural Families

Culture informs the way that people understand and interpret the world around them. This means that families will view a child's communication through their cultural lens to determine whether the child has difficulties communicating, and if so, what intervention is required to remediate the problem. In order to effectively assess, diagnose, and provide intervention for multilingual children with speech sound disorders, a respectful and reciprocal relationship with families is needed. Speech–language pathologists, audiologists, educators, interpreters, and cultural brokers may be members of the team to support multilingual children with speech sound disorders and should aspire to culturally competent practice. Collaboration with families is essential during case history (to gain a full picture of a child's context, strengths, and needs), assessment (to provide a model for target production), analysis, and intervention planning (to ensure that targets are relevant and motivating for the child and that intervention will be carried through to the home and community contexts).

Case History

When working with multilingual children suspected of having speech sound disorders, it is essential to gather comprehensive case history information to gain a holistic picture of the children and their environment. A case history should include information about the child's health and developmental milestones; family information (e.g., people living in the home, cultural background); concerns and expectations of parents, family, and the linguistic community; and a language profile. A language profile is a comprehensive map of a child's language learning experiences and environments. A comprehensive language profile includes the following information for each of the languages spoken by children suspected of having a speech sound disorder: the age they began hearing/speaking each language, who they hear/speak each language with (e.g., mother, father, grandparents, teacher, friends), where they hear/speak each language (e.g., at school, at home, in the community), how often they speak each language (i.e., hours per day/week), the children's preferred language(s), and the parents' preferred language(s). A language profile provides important information about a child's level of exposure and opportunity to learn each of the child's languages. This information will help in differential diagnosis between speech sound disorders and typical multilingual speech acquisition and can be used to guide intervention goals.

Assessment

In order to effectively detect the presence or absence of a speech sound disorder, it is necessary to assess all of the languages a child speaks. Assessment may include consideration of children's speech sound production in single words (to examine consonants, vowels, diphthongs, tones) and be connected speech (to assess intelligibility and prosody). It is also important to screen children's hearing, oromotor skills, language, fluency, and voice. A number of methods are used in the assessment of speech sound disorders in multilingual children. These include formal assessments, dynamic assessment, and parental contrastive analysis.

Formal Speech Assessments

Speech assessments are available in a wide range of languages. However, most single word speech assessments are designed for the assessment of monolingual children. Therefore, the normative data used to score these tests are based on typical monolingual acquisition of the speech sounds in that language and do not account for the diversity in acquisition patterns that may occur among multilingual speakers. As such, these tests can be useful in identifying a child's production in a single language, but the scoring using data from monolingual children cannot be used to diagnose speech sound disorders because assessing only one language does not provide comprehensive insight into a child's overall linguistic competence.

Dynamic Assessment

Dynamic assessment is used to assess children's capacity to learn about and produce speech sounds, rather than their current level of knowledge and production. Dynamic assessment involves a three-step pretest–teach–postest design: (1) the child's current knowledge or production of a target sound is assessed; (2) the child is explicitly taught about a target sound and given the opportunity to practice; and (3) the child is tested to see whether the child has acquired knowledge of the target sound.

Parental Contrastive Analysis

Parental contrastive analysis uses a parent (or other adult from the child's ambient language background) as a benchmark against which to rate a child's speech production. Given that parents often have similar linguistic influences as their children and are usually a primary language model from which children learn their languages, comparison with a parent's production of individual sounds and connected speech can assist in identifying the presence or absence of speech sound disorders. To undertake parental contrastive analysis, a speech sample is taken from both a parent and child in each language spoken by the child and then transcribed to compare their speech production. The samples may be produced using the same stimuli (e.g., a word list) for direct comparison, or they may be taken from a spontaneous speech sample to consider authentic conversational speech productions.

Analysis and Differential Diagnosis

Analysis of speech samples of multilingual children should take into consideration transfer between dialects and languages (i.e., different repertoires in each language overlap or transfer depending on the combinations of languages) in order to differentiate between difference and disorder as well as crosslinguistic knowledge about typical speech acquisition. Instrumentation (e.g., acoustic analysis, ultrasound, electropalatography) may also assist the speech–language pathologist in the analysis and diagnosis of speech sound disorder.

Intervention

Intervention for multilingual children with speech sound disorders should be undertaken in collaboration with the family and draw upon the principles of intervention for monolingual children with speech sound disorders. For example, intervention to reduce stopping can be undertaken in all of the languages the child speaks, drawing on examples of words containing fricatives from each language. Language-specific information is important for deciding whether some intervention techniques are appropriate. For example, minimal pairs intervention is appropriate for languages such as Cantonese, Vietnamese, Spanish, and English; however, there are no minimal pairs in multimorphemic languages such as Icelandic, so minimal pairs intervention is not appropriate. Intervention in one or both of the languages spoken by children has resulted in crosslinguistic improvements in speech production.

Language Maintenance

Multilingualism has many cognitive, academic, social, and community benefits to the individual and society. Speech–language pathologists and other communication professionals can encourage families to maintain their home language(s), while supporting their learning of the language(s) of the ambient community. Population-based research has demonstrated monolingual and multilingual children have similar academic and social outcomes in school, even if they are identified with speech and language difficulties in early childhood.

Sharynne McLeod and Sarah Verdon

See also Articulation (Phonetic) Assessment; Bilingual Children With Specific Language Impairment; Crosslinguistic Manifestations of Disordered Speech and Language; Delayed Phonological Development; Dynamic Assessment; Multilingualism; Second-Language Acquisition; Speech Sound Disorders

Further Readings

Fabiano-Smith, L., & Goldstein, B. A. (2010). Phonological acquisition in bilingual Spanish-English speaking children. *Journal of Speech, Language, and Hearing Research, 53*(1), 160–178. doi:10.1044/1092-4388(2009/07-0064)

Gildersleeve-Neumann, C., & Goldstein, B. A. (2015). Cross-linguistic generalization in the treatment of two sequential Spanish–English bilingual children with speech sound disorders. *International Journal of*

Speech-Language Pathology, 17(1), 26–40. doi:10.310 9/17549507.2014.898093

Hambly, H., Wren, Y., McLeod, S., & Roulstone, S. (2013). The influence of bilingualism on speech production: A systematic review. *International Journal of Language and Communication Disorders, 48*(1), 1–24. doi:10.1111/j.1460-6984.2012.00178.x

International Expert Panel on Multilingual Children's Speech. (2012). *Multilingual children with speech sound disorders* (Position paper, 1). Bathurst, Australia: Research Institute for Professional Practice, Learning and Education, Charles Sturt University. Retrieved from http://www.csu.edu.au/research/multilingual-speech/position-paper

McGregor, K. K., Williams, D., Hearst, S., & Johnson, A. C. (1997). The use of contrastive analysis in distinguishing difference from disorder: A tutorial. *American Journal of Speech-Language Pathology, 6*(3), 45–56. doi:10.1044/1058-0360.0603.45

McLeod, S., & Crowe, K. (2018). Children's consonant acquisition in 27 languages: A cross-linguistic review. *American Journal of Speech-Language Pathology, 27*(4), 1546–1571. doi:10.1044/2018_AJSLP-17-0100.

McLeod, S., & Goldstein, B. A. (Eds.). (2012). *Multilingual aspects of speech sound disorders in children.* Bristol, UK: Multilingual Matters.

McLeod, S., Verdon, S., & International Expert Panel on Multilingual Children's Speech. (2017). Speech assessment for multilingual children who do not speak the same language(s) as the speech-language pathologist. *American Journal of Speech-Language Pathology.* Advance online publication. doi:10.1044/2017_AJSLP-15-0161

Websites

Multilingual Children's Speech. Retrieved from www.csu.edu.au/research/multilingual-speech

Multimodal Communication

Human communication is multimodal by nature and includes linguistic and nonlinguistic modalities (with the term *modality* suggesting a particular means of expression). Linguistic modalities include language expressed and understood via speech (and its written equivalent) and manual sign languages; nonlinguistic modalities include natural kinesthetic systems (e.g., natural gestures, emblems, pantomime, facial expression, body orientation, or other embodied forms); visual-graphic systems (e.g., drawings, photographs, pictographics); proxemics (i.e., use of space during communication); and chronemics (timing of communication). Paralinguistic systems exist only as accompaniments to linguistic communication and include dimensions of prosody, rate, loudness, and stress patterns expressed in modality-appropriate ways. Terminology can be confusing because people use terms interchangeably; for example, the term *nonverbal communication* can mean nonspoken communication (i.e., the reference domain is the modality), or it can mean nonlinguistic communication (i.e., the reference domain is the symbol system). It is therefore important that the respective usage is clearly specified. Failure to differentiate usage can result in manual sign language losing its linguistic status as a communication modality. This entry provides an overview of multimodal communication from a variety of perspectives, focusing on its relationship to communication disorders.

Multiple Perspectives

Multimodal communication can be considered from multiple perspectives, each reflecting different historical frameworks. The term *modality* suggests a particular means of expression. The term *channel* suggests more of a means of reception, deriving from engineering. Particular modalities rely more on some senses than others: auditory-verbal versus visual-kinesthetic, or visual-graphic. Sometimes, the terms *channel* and *modality* are used somewhat interchangeably. These concepts may also be considered semiotic resources. The proliferation of terms used derives from the fact that researchers and practitioners come from vastly different backgrounds beyond linguistics and traditionally related areas and include the arts, cinematography, and burgeoning communication technologies.

Historically, the field of communication disorders concerned itself predominantly with linguistic modalities; initially, only speech and written language modalities were addressed, but manual sign language was eventually recognized in its own right. Nonlinguistic systems were treated as secondary means of expression. Anthropological, sociolinguistic, and social semiotic research has revealed the importance of nonlinguistic systems not only in everyday communication but also as part of compensatory systems that emerge secondary to a communication disorder. Conversational analysis has appropriated multimodality as a means of considering the role played by fine-tuned coordination of actions that accompany conversation and add richness of meaning.

The concept of multimodal communication must be distinguished from a related area, augmentative and alternative communication, despite the obvious overlap. The latter is a special case of multimodal communication because it describes a complex array of communication techniques used by people who cannot rely on natural speech for some or all of their communication needs. So, for these people, communication boards and displays or speech-generating devices serve as critical communication tools.

Underlying multimodal communication is some social system that shapes usage, whether in terms of individual modality usage or of larger, coordinated units. One cannot necessarily make sense of multimodal meaning without recourse to the communicator's social community. A second critical variable is context. Although linguistic systems have considerable capacity to transcend temporal, spatial, and interpersonal contextual barriers to reference, even they can lose meaning without context. Multimodal communication can be relatively context dependent. Whether this property is considered an advantage or disadvantage rather depends on the communicators: people whose ability to communicate relies heavily on the affordances of contextual support and may attain greater measures of success through multimodal means than strictly linguistic means.

Communication Disorders

Communication disorder professionals have a special interest in the dimensions of multimodal communication and their respective roles in the process of communication, because some? disorders may exert a negative impact on particular modalities/channels more than others. Understanding the role played by each modality in communication can help the professional develop compensation techniques for the affected person. Disorders such as autism spectrum disorder frequently are accompanied by particular deficits with the auditory-verbal channels of communication; thus, compensations can include use of visual-kinesthetic channels, which bypass the deficit area. Communication can remain linguistic, but it can be realized in a different way.

Multimodal channels of communication can be synchronous and asynchronous; that is, communication can happen in real time or with delays, respectively. Contemporary channels, such as text messaging, can occur in both ways. The chronemic factor can be manipulated to maximize communication strengths, while minimizing weaknesses in a communication profile. Text messaging can accomplish relatively immediate interaction, while affording communicators just a little more time to manage expressive or receptive demands of the situation.

An extended body of psycholinguistic research supports the notion that more meaning is actually communicated via nonlinguistic channels, as compared to linguistic channels. Studies vary in the stated proportions, but the finding is robust overall. The implication is that special attention to nonlinguistic communication is warranted. It follows that disorders affecting facial expression, body tone, and movement patterns (e.g., Parkinson's disease and other dyskinesias, cerebral palsy, or right hemisphere impairment) can exert a disproportionately negative impact on expressive communication. Disorders that impair ability to detect or interpret facial expression (e.g., some presentations of aphasia, Right Hemisphere Impairment, autism spectrum disorder) or paralinguistic codes can also disrupt communication, particularly communication of affect, where it is the speaker's *mood*, or disposition to the truth value of linguistic communication (e.g., figurative speech), that is important.

Final Thoughts

Multimodal communication in the 21st century forms a central focus for people working in communication disorders. Insights gained from diverse disciplines examining the transaction and construction of meaning by people of different cultures and age groups inform and shape therapeutic approaches that seek to compensate for deficits, whether they have an impact on one modality/channel, or many.

Judith D. Oxley

See also Augmentative and Alternative Communication (AAC); Autism Spectrum Disorder; Conversation Analysis; Nonverbal Communication; Parkinson's Disease; Semiotics

Further Readings

Bezemer, J. (Ed.). *Glossary of multimodal terms*. Retrieved July 13, 2015, from https://multimodalityglossary.wordpress.com/multimodality/

Goodwin, C. (2000). Action and embodiment within situated human interaction. *Journal of Pragmatics, 32,* 1489–1522.

National Centre for Research Methods. *Key readings: Introducing multimodality*. Institute of Education, University of London. Retrieved July 13, 2015, from http://eprints.ncrm.ac.uk/2239/1/MODE_Bibliography_multimodality.pdf

Norris, S. (2004). *Analyzing multimodal interaction*. London, UK: Routledge Falmer.

Muscle Tension Dysphonia (MTD)

Muscle tension dysphonia (MTD) is a voice disorder that is characterized by excessive and dysregulated muscle activity in the larynx and surrounding regions. Muscle tension dysphonia is classified as a functional voice disorder, which assumes a physiological misuse of the phonatory, respiratory, or articulatory systems during voice production. Functional voice disorders are differentiated from those voice disorders with structural or neurologic laryngeal pathology. MTD was first described by Murray Morrison and colleagues as a syndrome of musculoskeletal voice disorders that included primary and secondary subtypes. The term *primary muscle tension dysphonia* is used to describe the disorder variant that occurs in the absence of other organic or neurologic laryngeal abnormalities, in contrast to *secondary muscle tension dysphonia*, in which the dysphonia is considered to be a compensatory response to underlying pathology. Primary muscle tension dysphonia is among the most common disorders seen in voice clinics and is therefore important for speech–language pathologists. This entry provides an overview of the characteristics, etiology, assessment, diagnosis, and treatment of MTD.

Characteristics and Etiology

Auditory-perceptual, acoustic, physiologic, and aerodynamic characteristics of MTD have been studied to describe the disorder and assist in its differential diagnosis. Voice quality of those with MTD is often rough, strained, and effortful. Breathiness can also occur when hyperfunction results in incomplete adduction of the vocal folds. Abnormalities in pitch are frequently evidenced, with some patients showing elevated pitch that is atypical for their age or gender. Frequency-based acoustic measures that do not rely on the time-based waveform for their derivation are increasingly used in the management of voice disorders. These include measures such as the cepstral peak prominence, indicating the strength of the dominant harmonic energy relative to the overall signal, and spectral measures such as the ratio of low- to high-frequency energy. Mean values of cepstral peak prominence for patients with MTD are lower than normative values, but they may not differentiate MTD from other disorders such as benign vocal fold lesions or vocal fold atrophy. A useful distinguishing feature of MTD is the presence of *consistent* dysphonia severity across multiple speaking contexts, including sustained vowels, connected speech, and sentences loaded with either voiced or unvoiced consonants.

Several laryngeal configurations patterns have been established in people with MTD and reflect the intrinsic and extrinsic laryngeal muscle tension associated with the disorder. One such defining characteristic of MTD is elevated laryngeal position, which can co-occur with a reduction in space between the hyoid and thyroid cartilages. The overall elevation of the hyolaryngeal complex may negatively impact voice quality and speaking effort through changes in stiffness and tension of the vocal folds and surrounding structures. Subjective palpation assessments indicate that laryngeal elevation is present in many patients with MTD, and objective radiographic assessment has confirmed that laryngeal position is higher in people with MTD during phonation than in people without voice problems. It is thought that increased or imbalanced activation of the extrinsic laryngeal muscles contributes to these differences in hyolaryngeal position. However, results of surface electromyography studies in people with MTD have been mixed. Several prior studies indicated that elevated levels of extrinsic laryngeal muscle activity characterized patients with MTD relative to people without voice problems. However, studies in 2013 and 2017, which included carefully defined groups of patients with primary MTD, found that surface electromyography levels did *not* distinguish people with MTD from a comparative healthy control group. Many anatomic and instrumental issues affect the measured signal in electromyography and may therefore limit its utility in the diagnosis and treatment of MTD.

Classification schemes for MTD have included several distinct patterns of laryngeal configuration at the level of the true vocal folds and supraglottis. Lateral or medial contraction of the supraglottis can result in obstruction of the true vocal folds and when severe, ventricular phonation due to the approximation of the false vocal folds, producing an alternative sound source. The true vocal folds can also show over-adduction, often associated with strained voice quality. Anterior–posterior compression of the supraglottis involves the approximation of the base of the epiglottis to the arytenoid prominences and can contribute to overall laryngeal hyperfunction. In some patients, a nonadducted pattern of true vocal fold closure is evidenced during phonation, in which intrinsic and extrinsic laryngeal muscle tension stiffens the vocal folds and produces incomplete closure along the membranous margin or in the posterior commissure region. Although these patterns of laryngeal hyperfunction are commonly evidenced in endoscopic assessment of people with MTD, research has shown that supraglottic compression is not unique to MTD and can be evidenced in people with other voice disorders as well as those without voice problems.

Differing laryngeal configuration and stiffness of laryngeal structures associated with muscular overactivity can result in measurable differences in aerodynamic parameters associated with voice. Estimated subglottal pressure and phonatory airflow are higher for women with primary MTD, and individual patterns of laryngeal resistance, subglottal pressure, and airflow may vary according to the type of laryngeal constriction pattern shown by the patient. However, high variability between and within subjects for most aerodynamic measures limits their clinical utility in the differential diagnosis of MTD.

The causal mechanisms of MTD are not well understood. Excessive and imbalanced muscle activity presumably affects the intrinsic and extrinsic laryngeal muscles, producing a sequela of negative consequences to vocal fold vibration and the resulting voice. Several different causal categories are attributed to the onset of MTD and may co-occur in many patients. Consensus exists that physiologic misuse of the muscles and structures needed for voice production, including muscles of the respiratory, laryngeal, and articulatory systems, is a large causal factor in the onset and propagation of MTD. Typically, this physiologic muscle misuse occurs in conjunction with heavy occupational or social vocal demands when dysphonia is evident. Maladaptive voice production patterns involving muscle misuse may be inadvertently learned during or following an upper respiratory infection or illness, which is commonly reported as a preceding event in the onset of MTD. Another etiologic category is described as secondary MTD, in which laryngeal hyperfunction emerges as a compensation for other underlying structural or neurological laryngeal pathology that produces glottal insufficiency. The resulting hyperfunction occurs in an attempt to achieve better vocal fold closure. A third causal category relates to personality or psychological factors that may predispose certain individuals to laryngeal hyperfunction. Some studies have indicated that people with MTD show greater levels of introversion, neuroticism, anxiety, or stress reactivity relative to people with other voice disorders, which can affect tension in the muscles in and around the larynx. Finally, laryngopharyngeal reflux, which is a common diagnosis in people with MTD, may play a causal role in the disorder by altering the health of the laryngeal mucosal tissue and inducing subsequent maladaptive phonatory patterns.

Assessment and Diagnosis

Standard elements of a voice evaluation as well as specific tools and tasks are important in the assessment and diagnosis of MTD. The case history should include a thorough inventory of phonotraumatic vocal behaviors, which may contribute to the disorder, including habitual throat clearing, coughing, shouting, use of hard voice onsets, intake of dehydrating substances, smoking, and exposure to smoke or other environmental irritants. An inventory of typical phonation load is helpful for both the assessment and management plan and includes determining the time spent with sustained talking, loud talking, talking in noisy environments, and specific occupational and social voice needs. Medical history and potential contributory factors such as allergies and gastroesophageal reflux must be comprehensively determined, along with a history of the onset and progression of the dysphonia, co-occurring onset factors, and history of prior voice problems. Both for assessment and documenting change pre- to post-treatment, it is important to determine the degree of impact of the dysphonia on the patient using a standardized and validated tool.

Laryngeal videostroboscopy or digital high-speed video is important for determining laryngeal configuration patterns at the level of the vocal folds and supraglottis during phonation. The use of nasoendoscopy versus rigid endoscopy will reveal patterns present during connected speech, which is more representative of everyday speaking. Clinical assessment of MTD often includes palpation of the laryngeal and surrounding neck and jaw regions to subjectively determine areas with elevated muscular tension or tenderness as well as position of the hyoid and larynx. A few published laryngeal palpation scales are available to help standardize this assessment, but information on their validity and reliability is limited.

Several acoustic measures and speaking tasks may have clinical utility for differential diagnosis of MTD. The analysis of intra-word phonatory breaks in the acoustic signal can help distinguish MTD from a neurologic disorder with similar auditory-perceptual voice characteristics, adductor spasmodic dysphonia. Acoustic analyses are also effective in objectively demonstrating the consistency of dysphonia severity for patients with MTD across multiple speaking tasks, in contrast to patients with adductor spasmodic dysphonia who show a task-dependent variation in dysphonia severity. The inclusion of multiple speaking contexts such as sustained vowels, connected speech, sentences loaded with voiced or unvoiced consonants, and sentences that will elicit hard voice onsets is important in revealing the consistency of dysphonia severity that is typical in MTD. Variation in the fundamental frequency of a vowel that immediately follows a voiceless consonant (i.e., onset relative fundamental frequency) provides an additional objective acoustic measure that distinguishes MTD from healthy voice, and it may provide an indicator of vocal hyperfunction.

Intervention

MTD typically responds well to behavioral voice intervention, and a variety of voice treatment techniques are successful in improving the dysphonia. Manual manipulation of the laryngeal area to reduce extrinsic laryngeal muscle tension and stiffness of structures, to lower the laryngeal complex, and to facilitate improved phonatory patterns has been effective in improving multiple parameters in voice. Typically, these techniques are performed while the patient phonates in order to shape an improved voice output and to facilitate kinesthetic and auditory feedback for the patient, which can then be incorporated for improved self-monitoring and self-adjustment. Positive auditory-perceptual, acoustic, and articulatory changes in the voice have been documented following intervention with these techniques, with voice improvement often demonstrated in the first few treatment sessions.

Many other voice intervention techniques that have general applicability to voice disorders involving hyperfunction are effective for MTD. Vocal function exercises, easy phonation style including breathy and easy voice onset techniques, and resonant voice therapy techniques target improved phonatory patterns, while reducing excessive tension in and around the vocal folds, with some techniques addressing a stretching and rebalancing of intrinsic laryngeal muscles. Stretch-and-flow phonation targets the coordination of respiratory output with an altered laryngeal configuration that promotes low-effort phonation patterns. When differentiation of disorders with similar characteristics is difficult, such as with adductor spasmodic dysphonia and MTD, one to two sessions of trial voice therapy can be effective in supporting one diagnosis over the other. MTD is likely to respond well to behavioral voice intervention, whereas adductor spasmodic dysphonia is often less responsive or shows limited carryover of improvement to connected speaking contexts.

Soren Lowell

See also Dysphonia; Instrumental Assessment of Voice Disorders; Manual Circumlaryngeal Techniques in Voice Disorders; Voice Acoustics; Voice Quality; Voice Therapy

Further Readings

Gillespie, A. I., Dastolfo, C., Magid, N., & Gartner-Schmidt, J. (2014). Acoustic analysis of four common voice diagnoses: Moving toward disorder-specific assessment. *Journal of Voice, 28*(5), 582–588.

Khoddami, S. M., Talebian, S., Izadi, F., & Ansari, N. N. (2017). Validity and reliability of surface electromyography in the assessment of primary muscle tension dysphonia. *Journal of Voice, 31*(3), 386.e9–386.e17. doi:10.1016/j.jvoice.2016.09.010

Mathieson, L., Hirani, S. P., Epstein, R., Baken, R. J., Wood, G., & Rubin, J. S. (2009). Laryngeal manual therapy: A preliminary study to examine its treatment effects in the management of muscle tension dysphonia. *Journal of Voice, 23*(3), 353–366.

Morrison, M. D., & Rammage, L. A. (1993). Muscle misuse voice disorders: Description and classification. *Acta Otolaryngologica, 113*(3), 428–434.

Morrison, M. D., Rammage, L. A., Belisle, G. M., Pullan, C. B., & Nichol, H. (1983). Muscular tension dysphonia. *Journal of Otolaryngology, 12*(5), 302–306.

Roy, N. (2008). Assessment and treatment of musculoskeletal tension in hyperfunctional voice disorders. *International Journal of Speech Language Pathology, 10*(4), 195–209.

Roy, N., Mazin, A., & Awan, S. (2014). Automated acoustic analysis of task dependency in adductor spasmodic dysphonia versus muscle tension dysphonia. *Laryngoscope, 124*(3), 718–724.

Van Houtte, E., Claeys, S., D'haeseleer, E., Wuyts, F., & Van Lierde, K. (2013). An examination of surface EMG for the assessment of muscle tension dysphonia. *Journal of Voice, 27*(2), 177–186. doi:10.1016/j.jvoice.2011.06.006

Watts, C. R., Hamilton, A., Toles, L., Childs, L., & Mau, T. (2015). A randomized controlled trial of stretch-and-flow voice therapy for muscle tension dysphonia. *Laryngoscope, 125*(6), 1420–1425.

Myasthenia Gravis

Myasthenia gravis (MG), the most common of several diseases in which impairment has been localized to the neuromuscular junction, is an autoimmune disease that results in the defective transmission of nerve impulses to the muscles. Specifically, antibodies destroy, block, or alter the receptors for acetylcholine, a neurotransmitter. Without adequate acetylcholine, the muscle is unable to contract, and so individuals with MG present with physical and psychological impairments that impact daily functioning. Complaints include weakness without accompanying pain in the muscles that control eye and eyelid movement, swallowing, limb movement, breathing, and speech. If respiratory muscles weaken to a point where mechanical ventilation is needed to sustain life, an individual is considered to be in *myasthenic crisis*. The name, referring to *grave muscle weakness* (Latin and Greek origin), is actually a bit of a misnomer as therapies make MG a treatable neurological disorder. Thomas Willis is credited as being among the first to report on a patient with MG in his book, *De Anima Brutorum* (1672); he described a woman who talked freely except after long or laborious speaking tasks, which rendered her *mute* and unable to speak a word. After resting for an hour or two, the woman would regain her speaking competence. This entry provides an overview of demographics, diagnosis, and treatment as they relate to MG.

Demographics

MG most commonly affects adult women under the age of 40 years and men over the age of 60 years. However, MG can occur at any age, and one form is neonatal myasthenia, which often resolves 2–3 months after birth. Rarely, children may show signs of congenital myasthenia or congenital myasthenic syndrome. In these cases, the cause is defective genes that produce abnormal proteins rather than proteins that produce acetylcholine. Rare cases of juvenile myasthenia, with cause and symptoms mirroring that of adult MG, can occur. MG is not an inherited disease, although it may occur in more than one member of the same family.

The incidence of the disease is reported to range between three and 30 per million population annually, and the prevalence is reported to be approximately 200 per million population.

Diagnosis

MG can be challenging to diagnose. While there is no single test that definitively proves the diagnosis of MG, one key sign that points to a possible diagnosis of MG is improved muscle strength with rest. In addition to collecting a careful case history, medical practitioners interested in rendering a diagnosis of MG often recommend that patients participate in a series of tests.

For individuals with MG, an injection of chemical edrophonium chloride (Tensilon) results in temporary, sudden (often 30–45 s after injection) improvement in muscle strength lasting up to 5 min. Tensilon acts to block the enzyme that breaks down acetylcholine, thus making it available for the muscle receptors. Variations of this test include the use of neostigmine or Mestinon, again for the purpose of observing temporary improvement in muscle weakness. False positive results have been reported.

The most frequently used electrodiagnostic test for MG is repetitive nerve stimulation to assess the nerve's ability to send signals to the muscles. With repeated nerve stimulation, the anticipated response is a gradual progressive decrease in the compound muscle action potential. Repetitive nerve stimulation is positive in 75% of patients with generalized MG. Decremental responses can occur with other disease processes such as Amyotrophic Lateral Sclerosis (ALS), Lambert-Eaton, and myopathies.

Finally, blood tests can be used to detect the presence of immune molecules, acetylcholine receptor antibodies, or anti-MuSK antibody. Elevated levels of these antibodies are common in individuals with MG. Finally, blood tests can be used to detect the presence of immune molecules, acetylcholine receptor (AChR) antibodies, or anti-muscle-specific kinase (MuSK) antibodies.

Some individuals with MG have an abnormality in their thymus. Located behind the sternum and in front of the heart, the thymus is a specialized organ of the immune system. Thymoma, a tumor originating from epithelial cells of the thymus, can disrupt the normal functioning of the thymus. The connection between MG and abnormalities in the thymus is not fully understood. However, due to the relatively high number of individuals with thymoma and MG, chest computed tomography or magnetic resonance imaging is also often conducted to look for thymoma, when individuals are suspected of having MG.

Treatment

Symptom control of MG has remarkably improved since the 1980s, primarily due to the use of acetylcholinesterase inhibitors, corticosteroids, and/or steroid-sparing agents such as azathioprine and mycophenolate mofetil. For those with thymoma, surgical treatment is often considered as well. With medical management, most individuals with MG can live with few to no symptoms of the disease. However, there is a subset of individuals with MG (estimated to be about 10%) who are described as having *treatment-refractory myasthenia*. In these cases, individuals fail to respond or have adverse reactions to conventional treatments, require excessive amounts of agents that may become harmful, are unable to use conventional treatments due to comorbidities, and/or have frequent myasthetic crisis requiring mechanical ventilation and/or other rescue treatments.

Alana Mantie-Kozlowski

See also Motor Speech Disorders; Neurogenic Communication Disorders; Pharmacological Interventions in Speech and Language Disorders; Speech Mechanism Examination

Further Readings

Fujii, Y. (2013). The thymus, thymoma and myasthenia gravis. *Surgery Today, 43*(5), 461–466.

McGrogan, A., Sneddon, S., & deVries, C. S. (2010). The incidence of myasthenia gravis: a systematic literature review. *Neuroepidemiology, 34*, 171–183.

Silvestri, N. J., & Wolfe, G. I. (2014). Treatment-refractory myasthenia gravis. *Journal of Clinical Neuromuscular Disease, 15*(4), 167–178.

Willis, T. (1672). *De anima brutorum* (pp. 404–406). Oxford, UK: Theatro Sheldoniano.

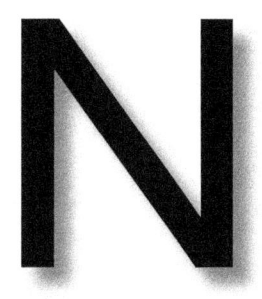

Naming

Naming is the process of associating a lexical (i.e., word) label to a concept or object and involves selection at the semantic, lexical, phonologic, and phoneme levels. Naming and concept formation depend on the cognitive process of association, in this case, between auditory stimulation (i.e., word label) and other types of stimulation that convey the concept, namely, visual or tactile.

In the process of lexical development, a child acquires the capacity to name an object by hearing its name and associating it with the visual and tactile stimuli he or she receives from the object, establishing an association between a sound, stored as a phonological form, and a meaning, stored as a semantic representation. Naming difficulties may show up in discourse as reformulations, unnecessary repetitions, fillers, circumlocutions, saying empty words (e.g., such as *thing* or *stuff*), long pauses, or target word substitutions (i.e., *paraphasias*). This entry provides an overview of naming tasks as well as factors that influence the ability to name and disorders related to it.

Naming Tasks

Naming tasks (i.e., assessing both accuracy and speed in naming words) are popular among speech–language pathologists to test language knowledge and performance in both adult and children populations, targeting dimensions such as lexical knowledge, lexical access, phonological knowledge, or articulation proficiency. Naming tasks are usually one of two types: visual confrontation and responsive naming. In visual confrontation, a picture of an object is shown, and one is expected to name the object. Contemporary models of visual confrontation naming assume it to be a multistage, dynamic process that includes at least three basic stages: a stage of visual processing of a stimulus to be named, a stage of semantic appreciation of the object, and a stage of phonological retrieval. In responsive naming, no visual stimulus is provided, and the word is retrieved from a characteristic of the object given as an auditory stimulus, for instance, an answer to a question: "What do we drink?" Rapid naming is also used as a naming task, by simply asking to name as many words as possible within a frame of time for each category (e.g., *animals*). Naming speed tasks are predictive of reading abilities.

If an answer is not given to a naming task, different cues can be provided, usually organized into a hierarchy. The cues can be an auditory or gestural stimulus, and, when auditory, they can be sound or meaning cues (i.e., cueing at the phonological or semantic dimensions of the word). Sound cues can be the first sound or sounds of the word. Meaning cues can provide words of the same semantic class or others suggesting different associative meanings, such as function, whole-part relations, antonymy, or characteristics of the concept (e.g., color, size, shape). Comparable to sound cues, when working on the written level, orthographic cues can be given, such as the first letter(s) or syllable(s) of the word to be named.

Related Factors

Factors that influence the ability to retrieve a word, in naming tasks, are word frequency and familiarity of the word in the lexicon, age of acquisition, imagability, concreteness, operativity and animacy of the concept, word length, phonological complexity, and lexical neighborhood.

Disorders

Disorders of naming are generally referred to as *anomia* and affect not the receptive but the expressive dimension of language performance; anomia is the inability to access spoken names for objects, actions of events, most often associated with elderly individuals experiencing cognitive communication disorders, or aphasia, namely the types that imply brain damage to the left hemisphere. However, naming difficulties may also affect children and young people with primary language disorders (also known as *specific language impairment*), with learning or reading disabilities, or with a suspected or a known brain lesion.

The failure to name something might be of different sources: either the individual does not recognize the object or does not associate it with a word label or he or she recognizes it but cannot recall the word from lexical memory or cannot initiate or program the necessary actions to utter a word he or she does recall.

In elderly people, naming difficulties, such as the inability to remember names of people, places, or things, may be an effect of cognitive impairments with a focus on semantic memory, as in the case of individuals with dementia of the Alzheimer's type.

Errors in naming by substituting a word with another are called paraphasias and may be classified according to the linguistic module they allude to: semantic paraphasias (also known as verbal paraphasias), when one produces a word that is semantically related, for instance, saying "cat" instead of "dog," and phonemic paraphasias (also known as literal paraphasias), when one produces a word that is similar in its sound shape, such as saying "fog" or "god" instead of "dog." Paraphasias can also take the form of an unrelated word (e.g., "window" instead of "dog") or a nonsense word (e.g., "fnog" instead of "dog"). The production of many paraphasic substitutions in one's speech, which may make it mostly unintelligible, is called *jargonaphasia*. Another common breakdown in aphasia patients that affects naming is perseveration: the recurrent or uncontrolled repetition of a word, in place of the appropriate target word. Naming deficits can be selective: They can affect only the word label selection but not the recognition of its meaning; they can be restricted to certain categories of nouns (e.g., colors or animals) or proper names; or they can be restricted to certain sensory modalities, such as visual or hearing.

Ana Castro

See also Anomia; Aphasia; Aphasia Assessment; Aphasia Intervention, Expressive and Receptive Language; Language Disorders in Children; Oral Language; Paraphasia; Semantic Disorders

Further Readings

Code, C. (2010). Aphasia. In J. S. Damico, N. Müller, & M. B. Ball (Eds.), *The handbook of speech and language disorders* (pp. 317–336). Oxford, UK: Wiley-Blackwell.

Goodglass, H., & Wingfield, A. (1997). *Anomia: Neuroanatomical and cognitive correlates*. San Diego, CA: Academic Press.

Messer, D., & Dockrell, J. E. (2006). Children's naming and word-finding difficulties: Descriptions and explanations. *Journal of Speech, Language, and Hearing Research, 49* (April), 309–325.

Nickels, L. (1997). *Spoken word production and its breakdown in aphasia*. Hove, UK: Psychology Press.

NARRATIVES

A narrative is how we as humans convey a sequence of events and the actors in those events in a way that reflects our culture, our perceptions and experience of the events, and our conceptualizations of the listeners. Narratives are one of the most natural and common forms of human communication. Understanding narratives is therefore fundamental to the field of Communication Sciences and Disorders. This entry explores the basic structure of narratives, followed by a description of how communication disorders can affect narratives. The role of narratives in assessment, intervention, and research is also described.

Types and Forms of Narratives

Narratives are whole performances of something that has happened to someone, along with the possible meanings of the events and the potential effects on listeners or others. Narratives are most commonly referred to as stories. One of the forms of discourse is narrative discourse, in which a story is told.

The specific components of narratives are generally agreed upon as time, characters, narrator, plot, and listeners, but all must work together to form a complete and coherent narrative. Every narrative is a description of a sequence of events and includes some aspect of temporality and the characters that are critical to that sequence of events. The sequence of events is told from a particular point of view, either the speaker or someone else. This telling from a particular point of view encapsulates cultural beliefs and assumptions and is how narrative contributes to the expression and formulation of the speaker's selfhood. The narrator will also be making assumptions or have beliefs about those listening to the story, and that will contribute to how the story is told. We have all probably told the same story about a particular life event on different occasions to different listeners, and each retelling varies somewhat. The changes across retelling do not reflect differences in the veracity of the sequence of events but rather show how the narrator interacts with the listeners in a particular way that is embodied in the narrative.

Most simply, narratives are structured with a beginning, middle, and end. These structures can be more specifically described as four important structures of a story. Exposition includes a description of the setting, including the place and time in which the story takes place. The conflict is the problem or challenge that initiates the sequence of events. The climax or turning point is followed by how the conflict is resolved. These structures relate to story grammar and its applications in assessment and intervention.

Narratives can be simple, but to be a narrative rather than a simple recitation of facts it should include an interpretation about what is happening.

In this example, two events are juxtaposed: "I walked to the parking lot. My tire was flat." In typical everyday conversation, a narrative around these two events would also include something about my experience of that event: "I walked to the parking lot, and I couldn't believe that my tire was flat. What a day! It took me 2 hours to change it." In this second example, one can find all of the basic structures of a narrative: exposition (parking lot), conflict (flat tire), climax (bad day), resolution (tire was fixed after long wait).

Narratives can vary in length, from quite short (as in the preceding example) to novel length. Narratives are used to accomplish a number of different kinds of storytelling goals. The narrative types of most interest to clinicians are autobiographical narratives, referred to as *personal narratives, life narratives,* or *life stories. Illness narratives* are stories about a person's injury or illness and typically include the background of the problem, what made the person seek medical help, how health-care professionals responded, and what treatment was sought. An illness narrative, like all other types of narratives, includes the teller's emotional reactions to the events, either explicitly or implicitly.

Illness narratives are considered a particular genre of story, and they link cultural and individual perceptions and beliefs about health, illness, disability, and coping. The seminal work of Arthur Frank in the importance of telling and casting illness narratives has led to an understanding of different types of illness narratives. The most frequently occurring type of illness narrative is the quest narrative, in which the person perceives the illness or disability as a journey, and some kind of meaning is sought and obtained. Restitution narratives are those that focus on the treatment or management of the illness or disability. Chaos narratives are the least frequent, perhaps because they are the least socially acceptable, and express the loss of control or life disruption that comes about as a result of injury or illness.

Narrative Skills: Milestones, Assessments, and Impairment

Typically developing children begin to use simple narratives by the age 2½–3 years. There is a sudden spurt in the complexity of narrative development around the age of 5 years, and by 6 years, the basic and complete, adultlike narrative structure is observed. Indeed, personal narratives make up between 50% and 70% of all conversation among young children aged 5 years and above. By the age 10–12 years, children are relatively good at judging whether their own narratives are "good stories."

Children with brain injuries are more likely to produce irrelevant or tangential information in their narratives. Children with language impairment show differences in narrative organization compared to typically developing children. Among adults, there may be some age-related changes in narrative production, including changes in quantity, density, or coherence of narrative among older adults compared to middle-aged adults. Adults with aphasia due to stroke or focal injury typically produce all of the basic narrative structural elements, with a reduction in complexity and quantity of words produced. Thus, the linguistic cohesion and the informativeness of narratives are affected by aphasia. Right hemisphere disorder, traumatic brain injury, and dementia can all affect the coherence, organization, relevance, and structure of narratives among adults.

Elicitation techniques will result in slightly different narratives, because narrative is embedded in context and listener sensitivity. Assessment of narrative skills, then, may be highly dependent on the assessment approach. It has been argued that the personal narrative is the most highly relevant to everyday living; however, for the clinician, it may be difficult to check personal details or accuracy of the narrative. Story generation, with or without pictorial support, is another possible context for narrative assessment. Story retelling, along with the presence of visual stimuli, reduces the cognitive linguistic load of story generation during the assessment task. Different assessment conditions tap different cognitive linguistic functions. Personal narratives may require greater access to episodic knowledge, but story generation or retell may depend more on the lexical–semantic system.

Narrative Therapy and Narrative Interventions

Narrative skill impairments have sometimes been improved by targeting specific linguistic forms that are needed for successful narrative production. For example, a focus on word-finding or sentence form production may generalize to improved narrative production, but this is not always the case. On the other hand, using and producing narratives during intervention has sometimes shown downstream transfer to other specific linguistic functions, such as word-finding. Providing visual supports for conversation, such as augmentative devices, assistive supports, memory books or wallets, or conversation books can also result in more elaborated narrative production.

Story retelling and story generation is one possible intervention for those with communication impairments that affect narrative skills. This has been sometimes called *narrative-based language intervention*. Narrative-based language intervention typically involves the production of oral narratives by the client, in the context of specific forms of modeling by the clinician. For example, structured, therapeutic practice formulating narratives in response to pictured, sequenced stimuli can improve the narrative abilities of adults with right hemisphere disorder, children with autism, and preschool and school-age children with language impairments, including the language impairments associated with hearing loss and cochlear implants. The outcomes of this type of therapy typically include improvements in the macrostructure of the narrative or improvements in the microstructure including sentence structures and word choices. There is limited evidence for these effects, however, and more systematic research is warranted before making a firm conclusion about the effects of narrative-based interventions.

Beyond cognitive, linguistic, or conversational functions, narrative—and especially personal narrative—may affect one's view of oneself and the ability to maintain or create one's identity. Narrative is the means by which people link events of the day and events of their lives cohesively and coherently. Narrative is linked to planning and organizing, and not just the planning and organizing of one's daily affairs, but also to the organization of thinking about one's own life.

Narrative therapy is a counseling approach in which the clinician helps the client to exchange one narrative about a problem with a different, more adaptive narrative. It is a process in which a new narrative about one's disorder and identity can be created. Individuals who have grown up with lifelong communication disabilities, such as stuttering or language–literacy disabilities, may experience a narrative about themselves in which the problem or disorder is central. The narrative that has been created by them and with input from the important others in their lives may be centered on the disability, rather than other abilities that they may possess. Through narrative therapy, these individuals may be able to reformulate that narrative to acknowledge that the communication disability is separate from themselves and from many of their other qualities and traits. The anticipated outcomes of this counseling intervention might include changes in self-efficacy, the belief that one can complete particular tasks, or perceptions related to self-esteem and communication confidence.

Narrative Medicine and Narrative Practice

Narrative Medicine, *Narrative-Based Medicine*, and *Narrative-Based Practice* are terms that all refer to the acknowledgment that a clinical interaction of any kind contains narrative elements and that a focus on these narrative elements can improve clinical care. Any clinical encounter is a temporal sequence of events that takes place between the clinician and the client. In addition, there may be other characters that play a role, such as other health-care workers or client family members. The clinical encounter is not just a sequence of events or pronouncements. Any event in the health-care context will be interpreted by both the clinician and the client, and influence their experience of future events. In this way, then, a clinical encounter—whether a single short visit, or a series of visits over a longer period of time—contains all of the elements of a story.

Indeed, the clinician will retell the *story* of any particular client in meetings, grand rounds, and case reports of all kinds. In many contexts, however, the report of a client may be relegated to a recitation of linked facts, omitting discussion of the human impact of these events on the person as a meaning-maker. An important part of clinical care is the recognition by the clinician that the story of the client's whole life, and not solely his or her illness, is relevant to effective care.

The client will also retell the *story* of his or her care to others in various contexts and on various occasions, because the encounter, whatever its purpose, will have an important meaning to the client. The client's retelling of the clinical encounter will almost certainly include his or her interpretation of what transpired and his or her emotional reactions and perceptions. The story of the clinical encounter may become part of the whole illness narrative of the client.

Narrative Forms in Research

Generally, there are two broad applications of narrative forms in research. Narrative researchers elicit stories from people and analyze them in order to learn about either (a) the production of the structure of the narrative or (b) the experiences and perceptions of the people who told the stories. A third development in the field of narrative research is to summarize a set of empirical studies into a broader narrative that can convey the meaning of the studies in a way that is more easily used.

Narrative researchers first collect stories through observational techniques or interviews. One goal of research may be to study the form, structure, or content of the narrative, asking why the story was told that particular way under those circumstances. To achieve those research goals, transcriptional approaches and conversational and discourse analyses may be used.

A second goal of narrative research may be to study the overall message or themes in the narratives, in order to address holistic questions about lived experience or perceptions of the storytellers. These techniques depend strongly on qualitative research methods, recognizing that the therapeutic process occurs not only during the clinical interaction but also outside that interaction during everyday life. In paradigmatic analysis, the researcher collects stories and then seeks to identify and describe common themes across these stories. In this case, the researcher moves from stories to common elements with the goal to develop general knowledge about a collection of stories. In narrative analysis, the researcher collects descriptions of events and configures them into a plot or story, moving from elements to stories. One of the strengths of narrative analysis is preserving or identifying the individuality of stories.

Narrative approaches focused on the overall theme or message of narratives can range from producing a narrative-based summary of a systematic review of the literature, to collecting life narratives from a group of individuals of interest, to using a personal narrative of the researcher. In each case, the source narrative and the researcher's own narrative are intertwined to varying degrees.

Rhetorical analysis is one way to analyze a synthesis of the literature and produce a usable narrative. A research team is formed that conducts an organized literature search on a specified topic. The research team reviews the relevant studies in a way that creates an overarching story about the state of the literature, including time, characters, narrator, plot, and listeners. The narrative that is produced is based on the team of researchers achieving agreement.

A *life narrative* is linked to other forms of research including *life history* or *narrative case study*. The life history is often generated from interviews but also participant observation in the field. A life history or life narrative is an opportunity to describe an individual's behavior, beliefs, and interpretations in the broader context of a culture. A narrative case study is a term also used to describe the detailed examination of an individual, family, or community within its context. *Ethnographic narratives* blend a life narrative or life history with the researcher's reactions to learning about the life narrative, thus explicitly acknowledging that the interview and resulting narrative are affected by the interaction with the researcher. Finally, *autoethnography* is a newer genre of narrative inquiry in which the researcher uses the self as a source, blending autobiography with ethnographic narrative. The self-narrative of the researcher's lived experience is blended with links to the relevant literature.

Narrative approaches in scientific inquiry serve to explore and generate hypotheses based on experiential phenomena. Narrative approaches can also provide a means to scientific dialogue about topics that might otherwise be difficult to address; these topics include highly specific contexts, issues of individual variability, or explorations of human experience that are not easily quantifiable. Narrative approaches can also help to set a client-centered agenda, in which the experiences of the clients that clinicians serve can be foregrounded. Although narrative approaches can have several important applications, there are also limits to these approaches, as with any other research tool. Narrative techniques do not generate the kind of weighty scientific evidence that is necessary for the creation of practice guidelines or standards, for example.

Jacqueline Hinckley

See also Conversation; Discourse; Discourse Analysis; Discourse Impairments; Ethnographic Approaches in Research; Language; Phenomenology; Qualitative Research

Further Readings

Bamberg, M. (2012). *Narrative development*. Hoboken, NJ: Taylor and Francis.

Charon, R. (2006). *Narrative medicine: Honoring the stories of illness*. New York, NY: Oxford University Press.

DiLollo, A., Neimeyer, R. A., & Constantino, C. D. (2014). *Counseling in speech-language pathology and audiology: Reconstructing personal narratives*. San Diego, CA: Plural.

Frank, A. W. (2013). *The wounded storyteller: Body, illness, and ethics*. Chicago: University of Chicago Press.

Greenhalgh, T., & Hurwitz, B. (Eds.). (1998). *Narrative based medicine: Dialogue and discourse in clinical practice*. London, UK: BMJ Books.

Hinckley, J. J. (2007). *Narrative-based practice in speech-language pathology: Stories from a clinical life*. San Diego, CA: Plural.

Hurwitz, B., Greenhalgh, T., & Skultans, V. (Eds.). (2004). *Narrative research in health and illness*. Malden, MA: Blackwell.

Petersen, D. B. (2011). A systematic review of narrative-based language intervention with children who have language impairment. *Communication Disorders Quarterly, 32*, 207–220.

Reese, E., Haden, C. A., Baker-Ward, L., Bauer, P., Fivush, R., & Ornstein, P. A. (2011). Coherence of personal narratives across the lifespan: A multidimensional model and coding method. *Journal of Cognition & Development, 12*, 424–462.

Wolter, J. A., DiLollo, A., & Apel, K. (2006). A narrative therapy approach to counseling: A model for working with adolescents and adults with language-literacy deficits. *Language, Speech, and Hearing Services in Schools, 37*, 168–177.

Nasalance and Nasometry

A key distinguishing perceptual characteristic of speech and voice is *resonance*. In speech production, resonance refers to the vibration of air within the cavities of the vocal tract that occurs along with an initial sound source (e.g., the sound produced by vocal fold vibration). In addition, resonance is also used to describe the relative balance of sound energy conducted via the oral versus nasal cavities. In this context, resonance may be judged as normal, hypernasal, or hyponasal. *Hypernasality* refers to excessive nasal resonance during vowel and semivowel production due to atypical coupling of the oral and nasal cavities and may be due to structural and/or neurological differences or learning deficits. In contrast, *hyponasality* refers to a reduction or absence of expected nasal resonance during the production of nasal phonemes (e.g., /m/, /n/, and /ng/ in English) and may indicate some degree of obstruction in the nasopharynx or nasal cavities.

An instrumental correlate of perceived nasality is *nasalance*. Nasalance (i.e., the ratio of nasal to oral-plus-nasal signal amplitude or sound pressure level) is a measure of the relative amount of oral versus nasal acoustic energy exhibited by a speaker. Nasalance is perhaps the most widely used instrumental, noninvasive measure that relates to the aforementioned perceptual judgments of hyper- and hyponasality. This entry provides an overview of how nasalance is measured as well as normative expectations and the clinical application of nasometry.

Operational Components of the Nasometer

The Nasometer 6200, manufactured by Kay Elemetrics Corporation, was initially introduced in 1987 and has been the most frequently used instrument for the measurement of nasalance. In the Nasometer 6200, the sound produced via the speech mechanism is artificially separated into nasal versus oral components via a sound-limiting separator plate fitted with directional microphones on either side. The microphone mounted to the superior surface of the plate may be referred to as the *nasal* microphone, and the microphone mounted to the underside of the plate, the *oral* microphone. Prior to patient testing, a calibration routine is conducted to assure that both nasal and oral microphones are of equal sensitivity.

During patient testing, the separator plate is suspended from an adjustable headgear (i.e., separator plate and microphones) such that the plate is held firmly against the face between the patient's upper lip and nose. During speech recording, the nasal and oral microphone signals are separately preamplified and fed to band-pass filters (center frequency = 500 Hz; ±3 dB bandwidth of 300 Hz) to capture the lower frequency region of the speech spectrum. The data acquisition routines in the Nasometer 6200 software sample the RMS amplitude of the nasal and oral microphone signals at a rate of 120 Hz at 8 bits of resolution. Nasalance is then computed using the following formula:

$$\text{Nasalance} = \frac{n}{n+o} \times 100$$

where n is the amplitude of the nasal signal and o is the amplitude of the oral signal. Nasalance is presented on a percentage scale, with strong oral productions (e.g., "Look at this book with us") expected to have very low nasalance values and strong nasal productions (e.g., "Mama made some lemon jam") expected to have high nasalance values.

In 2003, the Nasometer 6200 was discontinued and replaced with the Nasometer II 6400, manufactured by Kay Elemetrics/KayPENTAX. Although the headgear and the band-pass filtering procedure were maintained, the Nasometer II incorporated improved sampling rate (i.e., 11025 Hz per channel at 16 bits of resolution) of the oral and nasal microphone signals via an analog-to-digital sound card. In addition, changes in the microphone calibration procedures and the capability for signal playback were also incorporated into the Nasometer II 6400. A newer version of the Nasometer, Nasometer II 6450, transfers digitized data to the computer via an USB without the requirement for an additional data acquisition card.

Normative Expectations and Clinical Application of Nasometry

Normative nasalance data expectations have been reported for various versions of the Nasometer for three commonly used passages: the Zoo Passage (0% nasal content—often used to measure nasalance associated with hypernasality), the

Rainbow Passage (»11% nasal content—useful for observing rapid changes in nasalance), and the Nasal Sentences (35% nasal content—often used to measure nasalance associated with hyponasality). Expected nasalance values using the Nasometer II 6400/6450 are »11% for the Zoo Passage, »30% for the Rainbow Passage, and »60% for the Nasal Sentences. Standard deviations of these aforementioned expectations tend to range from »4% to 8%, with larger average variability observed during the Nasal Sentence productions.

Various studies have documented the potential clinical value of the Nasometer in the assessment of patients with resonance imbalances. Measures of nasalance have been used to document nasality characteristics in a variety of disorders including patients with velopharyngeal insufficiency in overt or submucus cleft palate, velopharyngeal incompetence in motor speech disorders, and cases of congenital hearing impairment. Other studies have used the Nasometer and measures of nasalance to obtain presurgical and postsurgical measurements related to nasality in speech. The use of nasalance scores may be beneficial in making clinical decisions regarding the various behavioral or surgical treatment options for hypernasality.

It should be noted that measures of nasalance may be influenced by extraneous factors other than the specific effects of disorder, which is the primary focus of the clinician. As examples, multiple studies have shown that females tend to have significantly increased nasalance versus males (attributed to factors such as increased nasal to oral-plus-nasal airflow ratios and longer velar movement and velopharyngeal closure time in females). In addition, dialectical variation may affect nasalance. Dialect-related differences in nasalance are most probably due to differences in vowel production since, in languages such as English, consonants tend to be produced in essentially the same manner, regardless of dialect. Dialectical variations that emphasize high front tongue positions may result in increased nasalance.

While a wide variation in measures of clinical sensitivity and specificity, as well as in strength of correlation between measured nasalance and perceived hypernasality, have been reported, measures of nasalance using instruments such as the Nasometer provide valuable, objective measures to augment the clinician's perceptions of characteristics such as hyper- and hyponasality. In addition, the ease of data collection and noninvasive nature of nasalance testing make this a beneficial clinical measure that may be utilized with a wide range of patients.

Shaheen N. Awan

See also Acoustics; Cleft Lip and Palate: Speech Effects; Motor Speech Disorders; Resonance Disorders

Further Readings

Awan, S. N., Bressman, T., Poburka, B., Roy, N., Sharp, H., & Watts, C. (2015). Dialectical effects on nasalance: A multicenter, cross-continental study. *Journal of Speech, Language, and Hearing Research, 58*(1), 69–77.

Awan, S. N., & Virani, A. (2013). Nasometer 6200 versus Nasometer II 6400: Effect on measures of nasalance. *The Cleft Palate Craniofacial Journal, 50*(3), 268–274.

Bressmann, T. (2005). Comparison of nasalance scores obtained with the nasometer, the nasalview, and the oronasal system. *The Cleft Palate Craniofacial Journal, 42*(4), 423–433.

Dalston, R. (2004). The use of nasometry in the assessment and remediation of velopharyngeal inadequacy. In K. Bzoch (Ed.), *Communicative disorders related to cleft lip and palate* (5th ed., pp. 493–516). Austin, TX: Pro-Ed.

Dalston, R. M., Warren, D. W., & Dalston, E. T. (1991). Use of nasometry as a diagnostic tool for identifying patients with velopharyngeal impairment. *The Cleft Palate Craniofacial Journal, 28*(2), 184–188; discussion 188–189.

Hardin, M. A., Van Demark, D. R., Morris, H. L., & Payne, M. M. (1992). Correspondence between nasalance scores and listener judgments of hypernasality and hyponasality. *The Cleft Palate Craniofacial Journal, 29*(4), 346–351.

Nellis, J., Neiman, G., & Lehman, J. (1992). Comparison of nasometer and listener judgments of nasality in the assessment of velopharyngeal function after pharyngeal flap surgery. *Cleft Palate Craniofacial Journal, 29*(2), 157–163.

NASALITY

Nasality is a term used to describe the addition of the nasal and paranasal spaces to speech sound production. Most speech sounds are oral, so they are produced with the velum (soft palate) elevated and the velopharyngeal sphincter (the soft palate and the nasopharyngeal aspect of the pharyngeal walls) closed. Nasal speech sounds are produced by lowering the velum and opening the velopharyngeal sphincter so that sound and airflow can enter the nose. Nasalization is a normal phenomenon in speech production. In contrast to normal nasality, pathologically excessive nasal contribution to speech sound production due to velopharyngeal sphincter dysfunction is called *hypernasality* (sometimes also referred to as *rhinophonia aperta*). The pathological absence of nasality in speech due to blocked nasal passages is called *hyponasality* (also called *rhinophonia clausa*). Nasal speech sounds are common in the overwhelming majority of the world's languages. Nasality can be added to speech in the form of nasal consonants, nasalized vowels, and nasalized consonants, which are the focus of this entry.

According to the Source-Filter Theory of Speech Production, the phonation generated in the larynx, which has a relatively linear spectrum, is filtered by articulatory movements in the vocal tract. The position of the articulators acts like a set of subtractive filters. As a result, different frequencies are attenuated, allowing the speaker to produce differentiated speech sounds. If the velum is lowered and the velopharyngeal sphincter is opened, an additional series of resonating chambers with different filter characteristics is added to the vocal tract. The largest of these resonating chambers is the nasal cavity, but it has been demonstrated that the paranasal sinuses also influence the resulting sound. Nasalized sound is characterized by an energy peak between 200 Hz and 1000 Hz. This low-frequency energy peak is also called the *nasal murmur*. The nasal passage acts as a side duct to the vocal tract. Compared to the relatively small nostrils, the nasal space is relatively large and branches off into different chambers. Because of these multiple side ducts, the nasal passage acts as a sound muffler and attenuates higher frequencies. This leads to a characteristic energy dip in the spectrum above the nasal peak. These energy minima in the frequency spectra of nasal sounds are called *antiresonances*.

In speech science and phonetics, the mechanism of speech production is commonly subdivided into different functional subsystems, including respiration, phonation, resonance, and articulation. Nasality is commonly attributed to the subsystem of resonance, especially by speech–language pathologists. However, in this case, the use of the term *resonance* is misleading because, technically, the sum of all frequency responses of the vocal tract spaces that together modify the sound from the phonatory subsystem is the resulting resonance of the speech sound produced. Nasality relates specifically to the oral–nasal balance in speech, which is just one aspect of the overall resonance.

Nasal Consonants

Nasal consonants are produced with complete occlusion of the oral cavity so that all sound and airflow are directed through the nasal passage. The location of the occlusion can be at different points in the oral cavity. Depending on the location, bilabial [m], labiodental [ɱ], alveolar [n], retroflex [ɳ], palatal [ɲ], velar [ŋ], or uvular [N] are distinguished in the International Phonetic Alphabet. Because of the occlusion of the oral passage, the nasal consonants are sometimes called *nasal occlusives* or *nasal stops*. Although it is well understood that nasal consonants are continuant sounds and therefore quite different from oral stops (such as /p/, /t/, or /k/) in their manner of articulation, this terminology is motivated by the fact that the transitions of vowel formants (i.e., the concentrations of acoustic energy) in the wideband spectrum before or after nasal sounds are similar to the formant transitions observed for the oral stop sounds in the same articulatory places (e.g., /n/ and /d/ will show similar formant transitions in adjacent vowels). Since the spectra for different nasal sounds are quite similar, the formant transitions for different oral places of articulation add acoustic clues to help the listener distinguish perceptually between nasal sounds. Most languages will use a small set of nasal sounds, such as the [m], [n], and [ŋ] that are found in English. However, some languages distinguish multiple nasal phonemes, such as Tamil, which has writing symbols for [m], [ɳ], [n], [ɳ], [ɲ], and [ŋ].

Nasalized Vowels

In the International Phonetic Alphabet, nasalization of vowels is denoted with a tilde symbol above the vowel in question, so that a nasalized [e] will be transcribed as [ẽ]. Historically, an ogonek diacritic [ę] was also used to indicate vowel nasalization in transcriptions.

Nasalization can affect vowels in different ways. It can be observed as a phenomenon of coarticulation (i.e., the assimilation of the phonetic place or manner of articulation between adjacent speech sounds); there can be allophonic nasalized vowels (i.e., the speaker can decide whether a vowel in a word will be nasalized, without affecting the meaning of the word), or nasalized vowels may be full phonemes. When nasalization is a feature of coarticulation, nasalization is carried over to the preceding or following vowel. The final part of a preceding vowel sound becomes nasalized during the opening phase of the velopharyngeal sphincter for the nasal consonant. In a vowel following a nasal consonant sound, the velopharyngeal sphincter closes during the beginning part of the vowel. These preceding or lagging opening and closing gestures of the velopharyngeal mechanism are estimated to be about 0.1 s in duration.

In some languages, vowels are nasalized without nasal sounds in their immediate phonetic neighborhood. Nasalized vowels can be allophonic. An example is North American English, which allows speakers to add nasal twang to vowels in some dialects, so that a word like [hɪm] (*him*) can be equally realized as [hɪ̃:m]. In other languages, the vowel nasalization can be phonemic so that its absence or presence will change the intended meaning. For example, vowel nasalization can result in a difference in meaning for the Brazilian Portuguese minimal pair [lã] (*wool*) as opposed to [lɑ] (*there*).

Nasalized Consonants

Like vowels, oral consonants can also be affected by nasalization. Assimilation to a nasal consonant can be observed to different degrees when this sound follows or precedes an obstruent (i.e., a speech sound formed by obstructing airflow, such as a plosive, fricative, or affricate). For some languages, it has been argued that the nasal and the obstruent are truly coproduced and that the resulting sound should be considered a single phoneme. If the nasal precedes the obstruent, this phenomenon is called *prenasalization*. This may be observed in languages such as Fijian. The transcription in the International Phonetic Alphabet indicates prenasalization either with a tie [n͡d] or by using superscript [ⁿd]. The mirror image of this is the nasal release of an oral stop in so-called post-stopped nasal consonants, such as [nᵈ], found in Zhongshan Cantonese, a Chinese dialect. Nasalized productions of other consonant sounds have been occasionally reported in the literature, such as the South Arabian nasalized fricative /z̃/. Languages in South Africa are known for their perceptually salient click sounds, and these clicks often have nasalized counterparts.

Nasal fricatives (i.e., consonants produced by audibly forcing air through the nasal cavity) can also be a feature of disordered speech. They can occur as phoneme-specific nasal emissions, meaning that the child has a normally developing phonological inventory but replaces sibilant sounds (i.e., fricative sounds such as /s/ and /S/ with spectral energy in higher frequencies) with nasal fricatives. In such a case, [s] is produced as a voiceless nasal air emission [n̥]. These sounds are also characteristic compensatory speech errors for patients with cleft palate.

Absence of Nasal Sounds

Only a very small percentage of the world's languages have been reported to have no systematic use of nasalization in speech productions. However, even in the very few languages, which are said to be devoid of nasal consonants, other forms of nasalization of vowels and consonants were described, so the phonological feature of nasality was still present.

In some languages, production of nasal consonants may be optional in specific phonetic contexts, which is called *nasal deletion*. For example, the French word *fin* ("end") is produced as [fɛ̃] with nasalization of the vowel but without the final alveolar nasal, which is still present in the orthography. In English, the word *sent* may be realized as [sɛ̃t] in connected speech.

The final concept that needs to be mentioned in this context is the diachronic process of denasalization. In the case of denasalization, a historically nasal sound may lose the nasality over time as a function of language change. Examples of this phenomenon of densalization are the word-initial [m] and [n] sounds in Korean, which can be realized as their voiced plosive cognates [b] and [d], respectively.

Tim Bressmann

See also Acoustics; Cleft Lip and Palate: Speech Effects; Motor Speech Disorders; Resonance Disorders

Further Readings

Dang, J., & Honda, K. (1996). Acoustic characteristics of the human paranasal sinuses derived from transmission characteristic measurement and morphological observation. *Journal of the Acoustical Society of America, 100*(5), 3374–3383.

Fant, G. (1960). *Acoustic theory of speech production.* Den Haag, The Netherlands: Mouton.

Hixon, T. J., Weismer, G., & Hoit, J. D. (2008). *Preclinical speech science.* San Diego, CA: Plural.

Ladefoged, P., & Maddieson, I. (1996). *The sounds of the world's languages.* Oxford, UK: Blackwell.

Miller, A. (2011). The representation of clicks. In M. van Oostendorp, C. Ewen, E. Hume, & K. Rice (Eds.), *The Blackwell companion to phonology* (Vol. 1, pp. 416–439). Oxford, UK: Blackwell.

Stevens, K. (1998). *Acoustic phonetics.* Cambridge: MIT Press.

NATIVISM

In all debates about human development, there is a continuum regarding how much can be attributed to nature (i.e., what is inherited) versus nurture (i.e., what is learned from the physical and social environment). In the debate regarding language acquisition, nativism is on the extreme nature end of the nature–nurture line. Noam Chomsky is most recognized for the modern nativism position of the mid-20th century, with variations of this view also proposed later by Jerry Fodor and Steven Pinker. Chomsky defines language as the unique human ability to use syntax, or word ordering rules, to build phrases, and morphology, or affix ordering rules, to build words. These properties enable a language user to understand and produce an infinite variety of sentences. This ability distinguishes it from all other animal communications. This entry discusses the nativist position, the proposed innate language acquisition device, supporting evidence, and viewpoints that counter nativist theory.

Solving the Language Learning Puzzle

The nativist view proposes that a syntactically generative language is a species-specific ability, hardwired into the brain at birth. Chomsky calls this the language acquisition device (LAD). The nativists suggest that neurophysiological properties of the LAD enable language to be learned very rapidly, without direct instruction, in a similar developmental order across cultures and languages. These are strong arguments that have been supported by considerable evidence. For example, despite its complexity, all grammatical structures and basic morphological forms of language are mastered before the age of 5 years. Adults learning a second language struggle with this challenge, while preschoolers easily acquire the complex language rules without using logical thought or knowledge of grammar. Roger Brown found language development progressed in predictable stages. New sentence elements, grammatical morphemes, or types of sentences emerge every 3–5 months. By the time children enter kindergarten, they are able to understand and use complex and sophisticated language. The nativists argue these rapid achievements would not be possible without a specialized module for acquiring language.

Further, language is acquired naturally during these early years. Except for a small percentage of children with language disorders, all children acquire language without lessons or corrective feedback. Instead, caregivers communicate meaningful ideas and respond to the truth-value of what children say. Errors such as *wented* or *goed* are not corrected. Even more remarkable, all children across cultures and languages acquire approximately the same forms and structures of language in the same sequence. This finding is true despite wide variations in language exposure and cultural practices. Children of poverty by 3 years of age are already far behind middle-class peers in vocabulary development, but they produce the same grammatical constructions and morphological forms as their more privileged peers. Some cultures do not encourage talking by children, while others engage them in highly interactive conversations. Despite these differences, children in all cultures follow the same pattern of language acquisition.

Chomsky claims cultural language differences are not important because the LAD is capable of abstracting rules of language from what he calls the *poverty of the stimulus*. Parents talk in sentence fragments, children hear incomplete and ungrammatical sentences, and parents do not correct children's grammatical errors, yet children develop adultlike sentence structures.

It is nearly impossible to stop language acquisition. Children with disabilities such as cerebral palsy who cannot produce speech may still learn perfect receptive language without instruction. Children who are blind and deaf exposed to sign language acquire language in the same developmental stages as typically developing peers. Children growing up in a mixed culture population where adults do not share a common language and resort to speaking a pidgin language with no consistent rules do not speak the pidgin but rather develop a creole language with consistent syntactic rules. Deaf children in Nicaragua who were not exposed to a deaf language developed their own sign language system that included syntactic rules. These findings suggest all children have an innate language acquisition ability, and that there appears to be a critical period of time when this mechanism is able to acquire rules of syntax. After puberty, the ability to acquire grammar may be lost. Nativists attribute this finding to an innate LAD.

The LAD

The speed and fixed sequence of language acquisition led Chomsky to propose that the child innately has the conceptual structure for language at birth. This LAD is endowed with a universal understanding of syntax that only needs to be fine-tuned through experience with a specific language. The major principles of language are in place, such as the need for a subject and predicate, a way to mark time distinctions, or ways to negate sentences or produce questions. The parameters within the LAD merely need to be set in accord with language input. For example, in English, the parameter would be set for adjectives to precede nouns, while in Spanish, adjectives would be set to follow nouns.

The LAD makes it possible to set parameters and induce syntactic and morphological rules of a specific language because the principles are innate. Even though every child is exposed to a unique history of sentences, the sequence of development is the same because of universal properties in the LAD that set the parameters in sequence. The LAD enables children to rapidly discover and use regularities in a specific language, as evidenced by errors such as *eated*. This error can only occur if the regular rules for past tense are applied to irregular forms. The principles of language found within the LAD do not favor any language but rather are universal principles common to all languages. Linguists have spent decades analyzing various languages to determine what comprises a universal grammar.

Universal Grammar

Universal grammar proposes that all languages have the same basic underlying structure. Although languages sound very different, these variations are only superficial. The underlying rules or principles guiding diverse languages are more uniform or universal. According to Chomsky, a principle is a grammatical element that is required by and applies to all languages. It may be expressed using word order (i.e., syntax) or word affixes or inflection (i.e., morphology). The generative grammar for each specific language is derived from the innate universal grammar. The principles of universal grammar constrain what can be combined or sequenced. These underlying principles are modified to correspond to the patterns of language to which the child is exposed. Chomsky delineated these principles further, originally in his theory of *transformational grammar* and subsequently with his work in *government and binding*.

Transformational Grammar

In his original theory, Chomsky proposed phrase structure rules that govern the underlying relations of words and phrases. Phrase structure rules are universal and apply to all languages. Transformational rules operate to translate these deep structure universal rules into the surface structure grammar of a specific language. With this finite set of phrase structure and transformational rules, an infinite number of sentences can be derived. The transformational rules also link phonology (i.e., rules for word pronunciation) and semantics (i.e., vocabulary and meaning). In this model, syntax generates sentences, while phonology and semantics are interpretive.

In later iterations of his theory, Chomsky moved away from deep structure and toward the central subtheories of *government* and *binding*. Government refers to principles used to assign grammatical function or case performed by a noun or pronoun within a phrase, clause, or sentence. Case indicates whether the noun functions as a subject or object and its relationship to the governing head (e.g., "the old man's hat" has a different interpretation if the head noun is *man*, in which case the man is old versus *hat*, in which case the hat is old). Binding deals with pronouns and the expressions to which they corefer (e.g., "Jane talked with her mom. She didn't want her to go"). These and other subtheories are considered as elements of universal grammar.

Criticisms

There are many criticisms of nativism, and many opposing viewpoints. Many perceive the theory to be too vague, with no explanation of where the LAD exists or how an innate grammar is coded in the genes. Defining language as syntax does not account for the semantic, pragmatic, and phonological aspects of language that are developing along with, and many would argue facilitating, the acquisition of syntax. The entire developmental period from birth to 2 years, when word-ordering strategies begin to be used, is discounted as unimportant for language. Yet, these are the years when infants and toddlers learn to interact, use gestures to communicate meaning, hone phonology to match the sounds heard in their language, and produce first words and word combinations to communicate different language functions such as requesting or informing. The nativist stance creates a strange disconnect between early communication and language since all attempts to explain early words and word combinations using a syntactic model failed. If the earlier accomplishments are not part of the LAD, then the child would need to abandon highly effective semantic and pragmatic strategies that had led to successful communication in favor of a syntactic strategy, and no evidence for this has been found.

Nativists argue that language acquisition occurs too rapidly to explain unless an innate grammar is already present at birth. Eve Clark countered that 5 years is really not that rapid, totaling 1,825 days and approximately 18,250 awake hours hearing and producing language.

Nativists also argue that children acquire adult-like grammar from impoverished input. The research of Catherine Snow and others showed that speech directed to the child is slow, clear, and very repetitive within and across routine activities. During activities such as storybook reading, adults isolate words and then place them back in a sentence context, often with the use of a general phrase such as "There's a ___" (e.g., "Look! Puppy. There's a puppy. Puppy goes *woof*"). Michael Tomasello proposed that these repetitive phrases provide early steps into syntax as children learn that many different words can be inserted into these phrases. Thus, children begin to find patterns in the words and word combinations used in common phrases, and patterns provide a means for children to discover additional patterns where the same words are used (e.g., "The puppy goes *night-night*" [noun phrase]. "The puppy goes *outside*" [prepositional phrase]).

Tomasello, Snow, and others argue that a unique mechanism for learning language is not necessary. Rather, more generalized cognitive mechanisms such as pattern finding and cooperative social–pragmatic behaviors can account for language development. These same cognitive mechanisms are generalizable across all cognitive domains, implying the brain acquires all information in a unified manner without the need for specialized modules.

Final Thoughts

The nativist view of language is one of the most debated theories in language acquisition. The proposed innate LAD accounts for many of the puzzling facts known about language development, such as a similar sequence of acquisition at approximately the same ages across children from different cultures speaking different languages. Other researchers have posited alternative theories to explain these observations, but they also have limitations (e.g., usage-based approach to language acquisition). A complete theory of language development has not been developed, but continued research will help solve the nature–nurture debate.

Jan Norris

See also Constructivism; Generative Linguistics; Grammatical Development; Language Acquisition; Syntax and Grammar; Theories of Language Acquisition; Universal Grammar; Usage-Based Approach to Language Acquisition

Further Readings

Brown, R., & Hanlon, C. (1970). Derivational complexity and order of acquisition in child speech. In J. R. Hayes (Ed.), *Cognition and the development of language*. New York, NY: John Wiley.

Chomsky, A. N. (1986). *Knowledge of language: Its origin, nature and use*. Westport, CN: Greenwood.

Clark, E. (2003). *First language acquisition*. New York, NY: Cambridge University Press.

Fitch, W. T. (2011). Unity and diversity in human language. *Philosophical Transactions of the Royal Society of London Series B: Biological Sciences, 366*, 376–388.

Pinker, S. A. (2007). *The language instinct: How the mind creates language*. New York, NY: Harper Perennial Modern Classics.

Snow, C. E., & Ferguson, C. A. (Eds.). (2013). *Talking to children: Language input and acquisition*. New York, NY: Cambridge University Press. [Original work published 1977]

Tomasello, M. (2003). *Constructing a language: A usage-based theory of language acquisition*. Cambridge, UK: Harvard University Press.

NEUROCONSTRUCTIVISM

Neuroconstructivism is a theoretical framework for the study of cognitive development, emerging from the work of several authors, including Mark Johnson, Annette Karmiloff-Smith, Denis Mareschal, Gert Westermann, and Michael Thomas, and articulated in two volumes published in 2007. The *neuro-* affix represents the theory's commitment to explaining the process of cognitive development within the context of human brain development. Neuroconstructivism advocates that theories of cognition should be constrained by but not wholly reduced to the neural substrate in which it is situated. *Constructivism* refers to the Piagetian perspective that mental representations (which reflect human knowledge and influence human behavior) progressively increase in complexity during development via experience-dependent processes.

Focus on Mechanisms of Change

Neuroconstructivism therefore describes the emergence of mental representations, which constitute patterns of neural activity in the brain that contribute to adaptive behavior. While much of developmental psychology has identified the abilities that a child exhibits at different ages, neuroconstructivism pursues an understanding of the mechanisms that allow these progressive transitions and the extent of their dependency on and interaction with the environment. Therefore, neuroconstructivism integrates research from multiple domains, including cognitive studies, computational modeling, neuroimaging, and developmental and evolutionary biology.

Foundations, Principles, and Mechanisms

Neuroconstructivism is based on three foundations: (1) encellment, (2) embrainment, and (3) embodiment. First, *encellment* refers to the emergence of collective patterns of brain activation that result in functionally defined areas. These task-specific areas develop collectively, gradually forming patterns of connectivity between cell assemblies.

Second, *embrainment* specifies that networks of functional brain areas emerge and are maintained within the context of existing patterns of connectivity between each other. This notion contrasts sharply with modular accounts that state functionally specific regions develop independently and do not exert or receive external influence. Embrainment is closely associated with Johnson's *Interactive Specialization* view that functional brain regions emerge through cooperative and competitive interactions. These exchanges gradually tune cortical regions to become specialized by being increasingly more responsive to specific stimuli. The adaptive capability of regions to adjust their responses is referred to as *plasticity* and reduces as functions become increasingly specialized. Regions with a high level of plasticity can adjust and accommodate new and existing knowledge quickly. Regions with low plasticity make smaller, more gradual adaptations. Although this seems to be disadvantageous, systems with low plasticity are more stable.

The third foundation, *embodiment*, refers to the view that the brain should be considered within the context of its environment: the body. This perspective is allied with the Gibsonian tradition of affordances, which suggests that certain properties of external environment infer particular actions. Therefore, the development of functional systems in the brain should be considered alongside the body and external environment. Consequentially, mental representations consist of information about the environment sufficient to support behavior and are not an internal replication of the external environment.

These foundations support the core principle of neuroconstructivism: *context-dependency*, which states that the emergence of representations should be considered within co-occurring neural, physical, and social contexts. This perspective differs significantly from David Marr's information processing view that the human cognitive system can be studied independently from its neural substrate, physical constraints, or social context. By contrast, according to neuroconstructivism, mental representations emerge as a process of development, which is influenced by the child's physical and social environment (which can also change over time). These environments interact with neural factors and patterns of gene expression, resulting in representations that are partial in that they are distributed across multiple brain regions.

The three mechanisms that shape the emergence of mental representations within the neuroconstructivist framework are (1) competition, (2) cooperation, and (3) chronotopy. *Competition* incrementally refines and stabilizes internal representations, while *cooperation* coordinates and integrates functionally interrelated representations. *Chronotopy* acknowledges time as a dimension of development, which influences patterns of gene expression and physical development. These mechanisms are underwritten by *proactivity* and *progressive specialization*. Proactivity acknowledges that the child initiates and selects interactions within his or her environment. Progressive specialization refers to the constructive element of neuroconstructivism, which is to build increasingly more complex representations, for example, that faces are made up of features like eyes, nose, and mouth, that words are made up of letters, or that plans are made up of actions. This process supports rather than limits further learning by providing a trajectory for subsequent cognitive development.

Application to Developmental Disorders

Neuroconstructivism has made a strong contribution to the study of developmental disorders by emphasizing that development follows a trajectory, which is shaped by multiple interactive factors, which may differ in the case of disorders (exemplified in work by Karmiloff-Smith and Thomas). Researchers supporting this view advocate the use of developmentally sensitive designs such as longitudinal studies or cross sectional developmental trajectories. These methodologies contrast dramatically with the adult cognitive neuropsychological model, which states that cognitive modules can develop independently of each other and which describes cognitive skills as either spared or impaired. Neuroconstructivism suggests that initially small differences during early development can have a cascading effect, with early low-level variations potentially resulting in the emergence of domain-specific impairments. This means that low-level impairments in neural processing may be the source of uneven profiles at the cognitive level.

Fiona M. Richardson and Michael S. C. Thomas

See also Brain Imaging; Cognitive Development; Cognitive Processes and Operations; Constructivism; Language Disorders in Children; Plasticity of Brain

Further Readings

Gibson, E. J. (1982). The concept of affordances in development: The renascence of functionalism. In W. A. Collins (Ed.), *The concept of development: The Minnesota symposia on child psychology* (pp. 55–82). Mahwah, NJ: Erlbaum.

Goswami, U. (2003). Why theories about developmental dyslexia require developmental designs. *Trends in Cognitive Sciences, 7,* 534–540.

Johnson, M. H. (2005). Sensitive periods in functional brain development: Problems and prospects. *Developmental Psychobiology, 46,* 287–292.

Karmiloff-Smith, A. (2009). Nativism versus neuroconstuctivism: Rethinking the study of developmental disorders. *Developmental Psychology, 45,* 56–63.

Mareschal, D., Johnson, M., Sirios, S., Spratling, M., Thomas, M. S. C., & Westermann, G. (2007a). *Neuroconstructivism: How the brain constructs cognition* (Vol. 1). Oxford, UK: Oxford University Press.

Mareschal, D., Sirois, S., Westermann, G., & Johnson, M. H. (2007b). *Neuroconstructivism: Perspectives and properties* (Vol. 2). Oxford, UK: Oxford University Press.

Marr, D. (1982). *Vision.* San Francisco, CA: WH Freeman.

Piaget, J. (1955). *The child's construction of reality.* London, UK: Routledge & Kegan Paul.

Thomas, M. S. C., & Karmiloff-Smith, A. (2002). Are developmental disorders like cases of adult brain damage? Implications from connectionist modelling. *Behavioral and Brain Sciences, 25,* 727–788.

Neurogenic Communication Disorders

Neurogenic communication disorders are a group of disorders that occur as a result of illness, damage, or progressive disease that affects the structure or function of the nervous system. The subsequent brain damage can affect a person's communication abilities including speech, language, and/or cognitive abilities. Neurogenic disorders that affect the linguistic system result in aphasia. Those that affect cognitive–language functions include right hemisphere disorder (RHD), traumatic brain injury (TBI), and dementia. Neurogenic disorders that impair speech output result in motor speech disorders. Speech–language pathologists (SLPs) work with individuals with neurogenic communication disorders and their families to rehabilitate or maintain communicative functioning.

Neurogenic Disorders of Language

Aphasia is a neurogenic language disorder resulting from focal lesion in the language centers of the left hemisphere of the brain. Damage to this area of the brain typically occurs due to stroke, tumor, or localized injury. Depending on the site and size of the damage, aphasia can impair all language modalities of verbal expression, comprehension of spoken language, and reading and writing abilities, to varying degrees. Damage to the left anterior portion (i.e., Broca's area) of the brain is involved in language output, and damage to the posterior portion (i.e., Wernicke's area) of the brain is involved in reception/comprehension of language. Aphasia can be classified into two major categories, nonfluent and fluent. Nonfluent aphasia may also be referred to as anterior aphasia, expressive aphasia, or motor aphasia. The three most common nonfluent aphasias are Broca's aphasia, Global aphasia, and transcortical motor aphasia. The speech of someone with Broca's aphasia sounds halting, effortful, and slow. Word-finding difficulties contribute to the halting nature of speech. Articulation of sounds may be imprecise. Syntax in sentences is simplified to mostly nouns. The length and amount of speech is reduced. Auditory comprehension of language is relatively spared. Reading and writing abilities are typically impaired to the same degree as the verbal skills. The person is typically aware of his or her deficits.

Transcortical motor aphasia has similar symptoms to Broca's except that the individual has surprisingly good repetition of language skills. Global aphasia is the most severe form of aphasia due to impairments in all language modalities. Damage occurs in the frontal, temporal, and parietal lobes. Speech and language deficits include minimal speech output, impaired auditory comprehension and reading comprehension, poor verbal repetition skills, and severely impaired naming abilities.

Fluent aphasia can be referred to as receptive aphasia, sensory aphasia, posterior aphasia, and semantic aphasia. The most common fluent aphasias include Wernicke's aphasia, conduction aphasia, anomic aphasia, and transcortical sensory aphasia. Impairment is due to lesions in the posterior left hemisphere where auditory comprehension is represented. Wernicke's aphasia results in deficits in auditory comprehension of spoken language. The speech output of someone with fluent aphasia is more fluid and less effortful compared to nonfluent aphasia. However, there may be a decrease in the use of real words or inappropriate word usage. There are generally four types of inappropriate word usages. Semantic paraphasias occur when one word is substituted for another similar word (e.g., "baby" for "sister"). Phonemic paraphasias occur when a sound in a word is changed (e.g., "toat" for "boat"). Circumlocutions are when descriptions are used to describe a target word (e.g., "the thing that you use to comb hair with bristles"). Jargon or neologisms are made-up words (e.g., "pege" for "pen"). Reading and writing are often impaired, with writing mimicking the errors produced in speech.

Transcortical sensory aphasia is similar to Wernicke's aphasia yet less severe. Characteristics of transcortical sensory aphasia can include fluent speech marked with paraphasias and neologisms, word-finding difficulties, and auditory comprehension deficits. Repetition of verbal speech is typically intact.

Conduction aphasia can result from a lesion to the arcuate fasciculus (i.e., the connection between Broca's and Wernicke's areas). Speech is characterized as relatively fluent with paraphasias yet may include frequent self-corrections. Repetition of verbal speech is impaired; however, there is relatively good auditory comprehension.

The predominant feature of anomic aphasia consists of difficulties related to word finding, which is more significantly impaired than any other language function. Auditory comprehension, morphology (i.e., sounds of words), and syntax are all relatively intact. Reading and writing may be affected depending on site of lesion.

The loss of language due to aphasia can be devastating for the individual and his or her loved ones. It can lead to isolation, depression, and reduced quality of life. The goal of aphasia therapy is to work on the damaged linguistic system, teach language compensatory strategies, and train communication partners of people with aphasia to facilitate communication.

Neurogenic Cognitive–Communication Disorders

Neurogenic disorders that affect cognitive–communication abilities include RHD, TBI, and dementia. RHD is typically a result of a focal lesion in the right hemisphere of the brain, most often from a unilateral stroke. The nature and severity of RHD varies widely. Potential deficits that influence communication include pragmatics, prosody, discourse, writing, and reading. Other cognitive factors present can include anosognosia, attention, memory, executive functioning, and visual processing.

Pragmatics refers to how we use language and communication in a social context. RHD can influence several aspects of pragmatics. During conversation, some individuals with RHD may have difficulty with the following: sustaining eye contact, expressing facial expressions, interpreting another person's facial expressions, using varying intonation levels, being abundantly talkative, not notifying a listener of the topic of conversation, or failing to understand the listener's point of view. Interpreting language too literally or understanding sarcasm can also be impaired. Aspects of humor may also be affected: The person with RHD may not be able to understand humor or may find something inappropriately humorous.

Prosody is the rhythm or pattern of speech that includes elements of intonation, tone, stress, rhythm, and loudness. As with facial expressions, understanding emotion conveyed in the prosody of someone's speech may be missed in a person with RHD.

Discourse is the combination of words and sentences that conveys thoughts and ideas. People with RHD can have difficulty producing or comprehending the main point of a story. Writing and reading deficits can also be present due to various factors such as impairments in visual processing or attention.

People with RHD can exhibit anosognosia, which is a lack of awareness of their disorder or lack of understanding of how the disorder affects their functioning. A lack of attentional resources necessary for cognitive–communication processing can be present. The most significant attentional impairment in RHD is neglect syndrome. There are numerous types of neglect, which can be manifested as the absence of attention or perception in a certain direction (e.g., the left side of body). Visual processing problems can be present and manifested as lack of understanding what or where an object is located in space. Different aspects of memory and executive functioning deficits have been recognized in people with RHD, including planning, problem solving, reasoning, and organization. SLPs work with individuals with RHD to address the disabling effects of the disorder and improve cognitive and communicative functioning for daily life.

TBI occurs when there is an abrupt blow to the head (e.g., a closed head injury such as in a car accident) or a piercing injury to the head (e.g., open head injury such as a gunshot wound). The primary causes of TBIs are due to automobile accidents, sports injuries, falls, or gunshot wounds. The symptoms can be similar to RHD since TBIs typically result in diffuse damage in the brain. Consequently, symptoms can be cognitive, physical, behavioral, and emotional and range in severity from mild to severe. Cognitive problems are more prominent than linguistic. Physical difficulties such as loss of consciousness, headaches, dizziness, vomiting, and reduced muscle strength may occur. Potential cognitive deficits may affect attention, reasoning, judgment, problem solving, executive function, memory, learning, and lack of awareness. Attention problems can be exhibited with all forms of attention—selective, alternating, divided, and sustained. Memory problems can be varied but working memory, episodic memory, and long-term memory are most susceptible to damage in a person with TBI. Deficits in executive functioning frequently include problems with reasoning and problem solving, poor planning and organization, disinhibition, and anosognosia. The effect on communication varies based on the site and the size of lesion. Similar to the effects of RHD, pragmatics and discourse production and comprehension are often impaired. For example, a person with TBI may have difficulty taking turns in a conversation, maintaining a topic, sequencing events in a story, and understanding figurative language. Other impairments can include production and comprehension of language; production of speech can be imprecise from muscle damage (i.e., dysarthria) or damage to motor programming for speech (i.e., apraxia). Behavioral changes can occur such as mood (e.g., impulsivity, irritability), agitation, anxiety, depression, and difficulty expressing emotion. Depending on the site of the brain damage, sensory deficits in all modalities may be affected. SLPs work with individuals and families of people with TBIs to increase their awareness of deficits and rebuild cognitive and communicative skills required for independent functioning.

Dementia is an umbrella term for a group of degenerative diseases or neurological illnesses that cause a decline in memory, language, executive function, perception, and personality to the extent that it impedes normal functioning in everyday living. The neuropathology of dementia typically includes the presence of b-amyloid plaques and neurofibrillary tangles in the brain. The most common form of dementia is Alzheimer's disease. The cognitive and language profiles of a person with dementia depend on the etiology. Severity also depends on the etiology and stage of progression of the disease.

All cognitive domains are affected in dementia. Memory impairment is found in the different forms of dementia but progresses at various rates. The final stages of most dementias include severe memory impairment. Executive functioning problems are present in the different forms of dementia (e.g., problems related to planning, decision making, responding to feedback, flexibility, and inhibition). Various types of attention can deteriorate with dementia, including sustained, divided, and selective attention, as well as processing speed. Language problems occur with dementia but vary based on etiology. Symptoms can include difficulty with word finding, object naming, grammar, comprehension of language, reading, and writing. The late stages of dementia include very little language output to the point of mutism. SLPs work with people with dementia and their families to maintain cognitive and communication functions in the face of progressive deterioration.

Neurogenic Disorders of Speech

Neurogenic disorders of speech are referred to as motor speech disorders, which are due to stroke or trauma that damages the part of the brain that controls muscles used for speech production. These disorders are classified as dysarthria or apraxia of speech (AOS). Dysarthria arises when there is impaired muscle control for the speech mechanism. The impairment can be manifested as paralysis or paresis, slowness or incoordination. Articulation (i.e., pronunciation of speech), prosody (i.e., intonation of speech), phonation (i.e., sound source of speech), resonance (i.e., quality of the perceived sound), and respiration (i.e., breath support for speech) may be affected. There are several types of dysarthrias that are characterized based on the damage to the underlying physiology. These include flaccid, spastic, unilateral upper motor neuron, ataxic, hypokinetic, hyperkinetic, and mixed dysarthria.

Flaccid dysarthria results from damage to the lower motor neurons in the cranial or spinal nerves that serve the muscles for speech. The damage causes weakness or paralysis to the muscles of speech. Muscles can become hypotonic (i.e., reduced tone) or atrophy (i.e., lose bulk). The effects on speech vary based on which cranial or spinal nerves are impaired.

Spastic dysarthria results when there is bilateral damage to the upper motor neurons. There is weakness of the speech muscles that causes articulation of speech to sound slow and labored. The voice typically sounds strained–strangled with little variation in pitch and loudness and can sound hypernasal.

Unilateral upper motor neuron dysarthria occurs when there is unilateral damage to the upper motor neurons that supply cranial and spinal nerves for speech production. The predominant symptoms are weakness of the facial and lingual muscles on the side opposite the site of lesion. Speech is characterized by imprecise articulation of consonants. This type of dysarthria is typically mild and/or temporary.

Ataxic dysarthria is a distinct form arising from damage to the cerebellum. Speech is characterized as slow with irregular breakdowns in articulation, excess or even stress patterns, harsh voice, and excess pitch and loudness variation. The speech of ataxic dysarthria has been likened to sounding intoxicated (i.e., having slurred speech).

Hypokinetic dysarthria results from damage to the basal ganglia control circuit (i.e., subcortical structures that control voluntary motor movements). This type of dysarthria is unique in that it only has one common etiology, Parkinsonism. Articulation sounds imprecise, and speech can have a variable rate—very slow or very rapid. The voice can sound harsh and breathy with reduced pitch and loudness. Respiration can sound shallow.

Hyperkinetic dysarthria is caused by damage to the basal ganglia, which results in unwanted involuntary movements that can disrupt speech. All aspects of speech can be disrupted, including articulation, phonation, resonance, and respiration. Hyperkinetic dysarthria can manifest differently based on the etiology.

Mixed dysarthrias can occur when there is a combination of two types of dysarthrias present. There is mixed spastic–flaccid, when there is damage to both the upper and lower motor neurons. One common etiology of this type of mixed dysarthria is amyotrophic lateral sclerosis. Another mixed dysarthria is spastic-ataxic. A common etiology of this type is multiple sclerosis that affects both upper motor neurons and the cerebellum.

AOS is a disorder that affects the ability to program and sequence muscle movements required for speech production. Contrasting to dysarthria, there is no muscle weakness, slowness, or incoordination. AOS can occur due to stroke, tumor, trauma, or degenerative disease that affects the basal ganglia, insula (i.e., deep cortical structure), or perisylvian area (i.e., region of the brain around the language centers) of the left hemisphere of the brain. Articulation and prosody are adversely affected. Speech is slow, labored, and halting. Struggle and groping of articulators can be observed. Sound substitutions are the most common error type. Inconsistent errors as a hallmark feature of AOS are debated. The rate of speech is slower than normal. There is equal stress on all syllables. Pitch and loudness ranges can be diminished. AOS is represented in a wide range of severities from mild with only difficulty on multisyllabic words to mute. SLPs work with individuals with motor speech disorders to address the speech deficits to improve communicative functioning.

Neurogenic communication disorders are all due to neurological damage or disease yet present with varied impairments to language, cognitive, and speech functions. All present challenges with communication. SLPs work with individuals with neurogenic communication disorders and their families to reduce the effects on communication.

Meghan Savage

See also Aphasia; Childhood Apraxia of Speech; Dementia; Dysarthria; Motor Speech Disorders; Right Hemisphere Cognitive–Communication Disorders; Traumatic Brain Injury

Further Readings

Bayles, K., & Tomoeda, C. (2013). *Cognitive-communication disorders of dementia: Definition, diagnosis, and treatment* (2nd ed.). San Diego, CA: Plural.

Chapey, R. (2008). *Language intervention strategies in aphasia and related neurogenic communication disorders* (5th ed.). New York, NY: Lippincott, Williams & Wilkins.

Duffy, J. (2012). *Motor speech disorders: Substrates, differential diagnosis, and management* (3rd ed.). St. Louis, MO: Mosby.

Guendouzi, J., Loncke, F., & Williams, M. (2011). *The handbook of psycholinguistic and cognitive processes: Perspectives in communication disorders*. New York, NY: Psychology Press.

Papathanasiou, I., Coppens, P., & Potagas, C. (2013). *Aphasia and related neurogenic communication disorders*. Burlington, MA: Jones & Bartlett Learning.

Neurogenic Stuttering

Stuttering is a speech disorder that is intermittently characterized by involuntary repetitions of speech sounds or syllables (including single-syllable words), sound prolongations, and audible or inaudible blockages. Two main types of stuttering are identified: *developmental stuttering*, which has its onset during early childhood, and *acquired stuttering*, which typically starts in adulthood in speakers with no prior history of a speech fluency disorder. Acquired stuttering, in turn, can be differentiated as acquired neurogenic stuttering (ANS) and acquired psychogenic stuttering. The latter form of stuttering is usually defined as being triggered by an emotional or psychological trauma in the absence of an identifiable neurological cause, and for this reason, it will not be discussed further here.

Since the late 1800s, many clinical case reports have been published of patients who suddenly or gradually showed stuttering-like symptoms following a variety of neurological diseases or traumas. Based primarily on clinical observations, Canter in 1971 suggested that ANS has seven unique characteristics that differentiate it from other fluency disorders: final consonant repetitions and prolongations; sound-specific stuttering, specifically on /r/, /l/, and /h/; no correlation with grammatical word class; an inverse correlation between severity and the propositionality of the text; no adaptation with repeated reading; no marked anxiety response; and no development of secondary coping behaviors. Since then, several other differential diagnostic lists have been proposed. However, the validity and usefulness of such generic lists have been questioned given the intra- and interindividual variability of speech fluency symptomatology in this patient population, which results in a less homogeneous clinical presentation. Furthermore, research has shown that specific speech fluency characteristics of patients with ANS may well depend on the nature of the underlying neurological disease or disorder. This recognition prompted some to suggest that proposed lists of differentiating features should be considered as rule of thumb rather than strong indicators of the disorder. This entry provides an overview of the incidence, etiology, and behavioral characteristics of ANS as well as its assessment and treatment.

Incidence and Etiology of ANS

Despite a relatively large volume of case studies, the real incidence of acquired stuttering is not well known. A longitudinal study by Catherine Theys and colleagues has provided a more systematic estimate to the true incidence of stroke-related ANS. They reported that 17 of 319 (5.3%) patients developed ANS, of which eight patients (2.5%) experienced stuttering that persisted for more than 6 months. Interestingly, these figures are strikingly similar to the incidence (5%) and prevalence (1%) typically seen in developmental stuttering.

The onset of ANS has been linked to a wide range of conditions that affect brain function, but the three main conditions are stroke, head trauma, and neurodegenerative disorders. In addition, ANS has been observed in a number of other health conditions, including brain tumors, HIV, epilepsy, encephalitis, and following surgical or pharmacological intervention, among others. While the precise link between each of these neurological conditions and the onset of stuttering is not well understood, research points to a disruption of the cortico-basal ganglia integrative speech network. In a study published in 2013, Theys and colleagues used structural neuroimaging and behavioral observation in an effort to investigate the role of this neural network in stroke patients. Lesion data from 20 stroke patients with ANS were compared with similar data from 17 stroke patients without ANS symptoms. All patients with ANS were observed to have stroke-related lesions in the speech-related cortico-basal ganglia network in the left hemisphere. Thus, the development of ANS may be the result of a disruption in the cortical and subcortical integrated neural network involved in speech articulation. Others have suggested that such a disruption could point to a breakdown in internal timing processes in the basal ganglia. In 1987, Christy L. Ludlow and colleagues investigated the site of lesion in 10 patients who developed ANS as a consequence of penetrating head wounds, then compared their data to those of patients without ANS as well as healthy participants. All but one of the patients with ANS showed unilateral lesions in either the left or right hemisphere, with lesions located in white matter (i.e., internal and external capsule and frontal white matter tracts) and subcortically in the caudate and lentiform nuclei. They suggested that while lesions in these brain structures did not necessarily lead to ANS, as some patients with lesions in these locations did not develop the disorder, variations in susceptibility for speech disorders and recovery might be linked to individual differences in neural organization for speech.

While the etiology of ANS is not yet fully understood, evidence suggests that its manifestation is linked to a disruption of integrated cortical and subcortical speech motor systems. Interestingly, these neural systems also appear to be involved in development stuttering, suggesting a possible causal link between the two fluency disorders.

Behavioral Characteristics of ANS

A number of authors have provided guidelines to assist clinicians in their differential diagnosis of ANS. While these guidelines are widely referred to in the clinical literature, even a cursory review of existing patients' case reports shows that these guidelines may not apply to all or even the majority of patients and that there is considerable variability and overlap between various diagnostic patient groups. As a result, caution has been recommended against a strict interpretation of these guidelines.

ANS is most prevalent in stroke patients and more so in males than in females with sound and syllable repetitions as the most common stuttering disfluencies. As is the case with developmental stuttering, these disfluencies are most commonly observed on initial sounds of a syllable or word, with some disfluencies occurring on medial sounds but only rarely on final sounds. Stuttering severity can vary widely from a low of less than 3% to more than 50% and tends to be higher during conversation than during either monologue or reading. Stuttering also tends to be more severe in patients who have other co-occurring aphasia or apraxia but not necessarily for other concurrent disorders such as dysarthria or cognitive problems. While reports have suggested that adaptation, which is observed in stuttering as a decrease in disfluency following repeated reading of the same text, is not commonly seen in patients with ANS, both a review of published case studies conducted by De Nil and colleagues in 2007 and direct observation do not seem to support this contention. At least for stroke patients, adaptation was observed in about 50% of the reported cases. Similarly, about half of stroke patients show clear signs of struggle or other secondary coping behaviors.

The second group associated with ANS consists of patients with neurodegenerative disorders, most commonly Parkinson's disease. Because stuttering characteristics often reflect the nature of the underlying neurological condition, stuttering in patients with Parkinson's disease has been described as consisting of rapid movements, articulatory blocking, and prolongations. In contrast, the stuttering speech in a patient with multiple sclerosis was said to be very slow with an abnormal prosody and consisting of excessive sound and syllable repetitions, possibly reflecting the movement discoordination and spasticity observed in these patients. Little systematic information is available about stuttering localization, severity, or other concomitant behaviors in these patients. As is the case for developmental stuttering and ANS in stroke patients, most stuttering appears to occur on word or syllable initial sounds with occasional disfluencies medially or on final word positions. Although the available data are quite limited, it is possible that stuttering adaptation is less present in these patients compared to stroke patients, suggesting that the stuttering adaptation may be one of the fluency characteristics that differentiates between patient groups.

The third main condition associated with ANS is traumatic brain injury (TBI). Published cases have described the onset of stuttering in patients with TBI from accidents or penetrating head wounds. In these patients, the onset of acquired stuttering is often reported soon after the injury, with speech that is described as intermittently and irregularly very fast with uncontrollable repetitions and prolongations and long struggle-free pauses. Again, most disfluencies occur in the word-initial position. Stuttering adaptation may be less likely in these patients, as are concomitant coping behaviors. Negative speech-associated attitudes, commonly seen in people with developmental stuttering, also are frequently observed in TBI patients. An important observation was that a number of TBI patients who developed ANS were initially diagnosed with psychogenic stuttering due to the absence of any readily observable neurological lesions. Such conditions only came to light as the condition progressed or following a more extensive clinical examination. Such reports highlight the need for a careful and multidisciplinary diagnostic workup in these patients before drawing conclusions about the neurogenic or psychogenic nature of the stuttering.

Assessment of ANS

Because of its complex nature and the multitude of potential underlying health conditions, the diagnosis and evaluation of ANS necessitates a multidimensional and multidisciplinary approach. As is the case for most individuals experiencing speech or language disorders, each person presents as a unique individual with his or her own history and communication characteristics. Such an assessment requires a multifaceted approach that tries to understand the multiple interwoven facets of the person's speech characteristics. This definitely is the case for patients with ANS. In addition, these patients often experience additional speech, language, motor, or cognitive disorders that affect their overall communication ability and thus need to be considered as part of the overall assessment.

In order to assist clinicians with this task, De Nil and colleagues in 2007 proposed an assessment battery that provides a comprehensive evaluation of the patient's overall communication ability. Each assessment needs to include a detailed case history and probing of the patient's medical and developmental background, including information gained from medical records. As part of the history taking, special attention needs to be paid to the time lapse between the onset of the underlying neurological condition and the onset of stuttering. In most but not all patients, the onset of stuttering closely follows the onset of the disease or trauma, often within days or a few weeks. The longer the time interval between the two events, the more difficult it will be to establish a clear link, and the clinician will need to consider the potential influence of other factors, including psychogenic ones.

A second important component of an assessment is a detailed analysis of the speech-fluency disruptions. This should be done based on speech samples that represent a variety of speech contexts (e.g., reading, conversation, varying speech complexity levels). Clinicians need to try to obtain a complete picture of the nature and extent of the stuttering, including the frequency of stuttering and other disfluencies, the type and location of such disfluencies, whether stuttering severity is influenced by factors such as the nature of the speech task or the context of the communication environment, whether stuttering is variable across time, the presence of concomitant behaviors such as avoidance or escape behaviors, and the attitude or perception the patient has about his or her stuttering.

Third, each assessment should include a thorough analysis of other speech, language, and cognitive capacities. This may include tests for word finding, apraxia, memory, executive functions, and other functions that are relevant to the patient being evaluated. As a result of the assessment, and in order to reach an appropriate differential diagnosis and plan the most effective intervention, the clinician strives to obtain a comprehensive picture of the various components, and their interactions, that make up the patient's communication deficit.

As part of the assessment, the clinician will need to consider whether the stuttering observed in the patient is truly a new manifestation of speech-fluency disruptions or a return or exacerbation of a previously existing stuttering problem. Several cases have been described in which a neurological trauma or disease led to the reoccurrence of aggravation of previously present developmental stuttering. While guidelines to assist clinicians in this differential diagnosis have been proposed, there is significant overlap between the way in which stuttering is manifested in these two speech-fluency disorders, and heterogeneity is the norm rather than the exception. For example, it has often been suggested that people with developmental and acquired stuttering can be differentiated based on their responses to fluency-enhancing conditions, but studies have raised doubt about the usefulness of that criterion. In most cases, of course, the presence or absence of premorbid stuttering is relatively easily available from reports by either the patients themselves or their relatives, especially after some targeted probing by the clinician. Knowledge of any preexisting stuttering will be important for the planning of fluency-intervention strategies. The patient's prior personal experiences with developmental stuttering, even if long ago, may well impact the perceptions of current stuttering. Also, prior history with perceived effective or ineffective treatment approaches will need to be considered as part of developing and engaging the patient in the most optimal intervention plan.

A second issue that needs to be addressed is whether the presenting stuttering is neurogenic or psychogenic in nature. While in many patients, the answer to this question may be relatively straightforward, especially if the onset of stuttering coincides with a well-defined neurological deficit, it can be challenging in other patients, and a conclusive answer may not always be possible. A number of differential criteria have been proposed, which can serve as a guideline for clinicians. Psychogenic stuttering is often diagnosed based on the absence of an identifiable neurological condition rather than the presence of positive identifiers. When there is no seemingly neurological cause, clinicians are more likely to look for signs of stress or other emotional or psychological conditions that could explain the onset of stuttering. A differential diagnosis between neurogenic and psychogenic stuttering may be further complicated by the fact that emotional or stress reactions can coexist with and indeed be triggered by neurological disease or trauma. In addition, a number of cases have been described where stuttering was initially labeled psychogenic but, in effect, was later found to be the first symptom of an as-of-yet undetected neurological condition.

Treatment of ANS

Not all patients who experience ANS will develop a chronic speech-fluency problem. Unfortunately, research on recovery from the condition is rather sparse, and little is known about possible predictors for recovery or chronicity. In a 2012 longitudinal study by Theys and colleagues, approximately 50% of the stroke patients with ANS were observed to recover, with the other 50% demonstrating stuttering lasting more than 6 months. Given that the chronicity of stuttering cannot yet be predicted, and patients often express distress over their speech disfluencies, early intervention is warranted in many cases.

A number of treatment approaches for ANS are available to clinicians. Most clinicians will at least initially use a behaviorally oriented intervention, similar to those typically described for developmental stuttering. This may include teaching-specific fluency-control techniques such as slowed speech, continuous phonation, and gentle onset. A number of reports have described or investigated the effectiveness of altered auditory feedback with varying levels of success as well as use of medication or surgical intervention.

Unfortunately, the effectiveness of various treatments has not been thoroughly investigated and, indeed, there may be a bias in the literature toward reporting treatment that has a beneficial effect for patients. Because evidence suggests that the nature of the stuttering disfluencies may be influenced by the underlying neurological condition, it is possible also that treatment will need to be tailored to specific patient groups and that types of treatment may be more or less effective for different groups. Some initial support for this comes from a 2008 survey study by Theys and colleagues of clinicians who were actively working with patients with ANS. As expected, the survey revealed a wide variety of intervention techniques that were being used mostly but not exclusively focused on teaching specific fluency-enhancing skills. Of the 23 stroke patients reported in the survey, 18 were said to have benefitted from treatment while only one was reported to have shown a full recovery. Among the patients with TBI, four of the eight patients showed fluency improvement, while four did not. In contrast, of the five patients with neurodegenerative disorders, only one was reported to have improved fluency following treatment.

Much work needs to be done to better understand the effectiveness of particular types of treatment in patients with ANS. While the presence of ANS in a patient may at times receive less clinical attention because of the presence of other medical, communicative, and cognitive problems, it is incumbent upon clinicians to be knowledgeable of ANS and identify its presence in the patients they work with in order to be in a position to provide appropriate intervention. ANS can and often does interfere not only just with a patient's ability to communicate but also with his or her overall perception of well-being and quality of life, and further basic and applied research is needed to better understand and treat the disorder.

Luc De Nil

See also Fluency and Fluency Disorders; Neurogenic Communication Disorders; Speech Production, Theories of

Further Readings

De Nil, L. F., Jokel, R., & Rochon, E. (2007). Etiology, symptomatology, and treatment of neurogenic stuttering. In E. G. Conture & R. F. Curlee (Eds.), *Stuttering and related disorders of fluency* (3rd ed., pp. 326–343). New York, NY: Thieme.

Ludlow, C. L., Rosenberg, J., Salazar, A., Grafman, J., & Smutok, M. (1987). Site of penetrating brain lesions causing chronic acquired stuttering. *Annals of Neurology, 22*(1), 60–66.

Theys, C., De Nil, L., Thijs, V., van Wieringen, A., & Sunaert, S. (2013). A crucial role for the cortico-striato-cortical loop in the pathogenesis of stroke-related neurogenic stuttering. *Human Brain Mapping, 34*(9), 2103–2112.

Theys, C., van Wieringen, A., Sunaert, S., Thijs, V., & De Nil, L. F. (2011). A one year prospective study of neurogenic stuttering following stroke: Incidence and co-occurring disorders. *Journal of Communication Disorders, 44*(6), 678–687.

Ward, D. (2010). Sudden onset stuttering in an adult: Neurogenic and psychogenic perspectives. *Journal of Neurolinguistics, 23*(5), 511–517.

Neurolinguistics

The origin of the discipline of neurolinguistics as a systematic study of brain–language relation can be traced back to the contribution of Franz Joseph Gall in the late 18th century and those who had debated his theory of modularity of mental functions and their representations in the human brain (Figure 1).

Subsequently, localization of mental functions, including the faculty of language, became a hot topic of research. In the late 19th century, ideas related to the importance of the left cerebral hemisphere for language and speech began to emerge, although not without dissenting voices. Initial attempts were made to localize language/speech in specific brain structures, for instance, in 1861 Paul Broca hypothesized that articulated speech was localized in the left posterior inferior frontal cortex. Another significant development during this period was a neural model of language processing known as the *association model* (of Carl Wernicke and Ludwig Lichtheim) that explained language-related functions and disorders in terms of lesions to language-related centers or disconnections between cortical centers. The decades that followed witnessed further development in theory/model building about the relation between the brain structures and language as exemplified in the neurodynamic model of language and higher mental functions proposed by a Soviet psychologist, Alexander R. Luria. Advances in several disciplines of knowledge such as neuroscience, linguistics, cognitive science, psycholinguistics, computer science, and cognitive neuropsychology began to shape the theoretical and methodological aspects of neurolinguistics. As a result, both theoretical and methodological aspects of neurolinguistics have become complex, making it hard to distinguish it from cognitive neuroscience and neurobiology of language. In contemporary

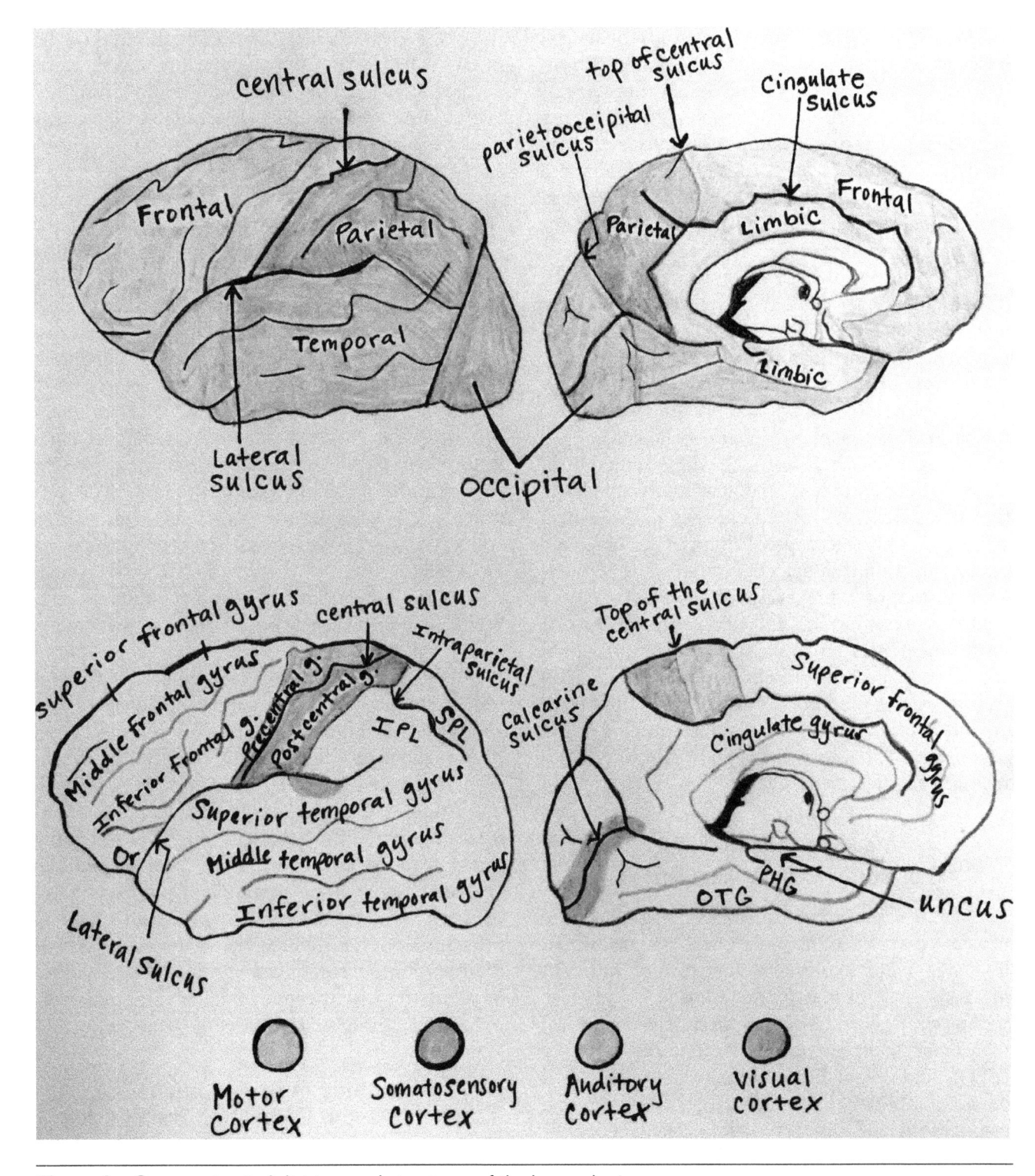

Figure 1 Gross anatomical divisions and structures of the human brain

neurolinguistic research, Gregory Hickok and David Poeppel's *dorsal and ventral stream model* of language processing represents the fusion of multiple disciplines listed previously.

Although neurolinguistic investigation made huge progress from the study of language impairments resulting from brain lesions, the object of study is not entirely restricted to clinical cases, and an equally important part is the study of neural bases of language processing in the normal population. In the past few decades, a number of experimental neuroimaging studies had explored language processing in normal subjects. It has become a standard practice in this discipline to seek converging evidence from both experimental and clinical research that favors a model or theory of neural representation.

The primary objective of this entry is to introduce readers to the field of neurolinguistics by way of discussing a few topics of contemporary research: (a) study of brain–language relation in the context of brain damage induced by stroke or other etiologies, as mentioned previously; (b) neural bases of language processing in normal population; (c) neural bases of language acquisition in infants and children; (d) geriatric neurolinguistics that deals with age-related changes in the neural structures and age-related changes in language communication in older populations; and (e) neurolinguistics of bilingualism that deals with the neural representations and processing of two or more languages in bilingual and multilingual speakers. As a point of departure, a brief description of the contemporary methods in neurolinguistics is offered to facilitate understanding of the description of the topics of neurolinguistics research that follows.

A Note on the Methods of Study in Neurolinguistics

The neural representation of language and the neural processes underlying the dynamic use of language were explored using several different methods such as the brain lesion-based clinicopathological correlation method, electrophysiological methods such as electro encephalography (EEG) and event-related potential (ERP), and hemodynamic methods such as positron emission tomography (PET) and functional magnetic resonance imaging (fMRI).

The clinicopathologic correlation (lesion) method, the oldest of all, seeks to establish correlations between the site and extent of lesion with the altered behavior (language/speech) to infer the role of the damaged area of the brain for the altered behavior. This method is still popular, and it is the basis of the classification of language disorders known as *aphasia* (an acquired disorder of language use through any or all modalities such as speaking, listening, reading, and writing). The lesion sites and extent of lesions can be easily detected using structural imaging techniques such as the computerized tomography and MRI.

The EEG method measures the electrical charges (amplitude and frequency bands) of the brain. It involves placing surface electrodes (embedded in a cap) on the scalp and recording the neural activity directly. It is used to detect clinical conditions such as epilepsy and sleep disorders by inspecting the fluctuations of the amplitude and frequency of electrical charges recorded from the electrodes. The ERP measurement involves an additional step of recording changes in the ongoing EEG, which are time locked to the presentation of external stimuli such as words or sentences. The magnitude of these changes is small compared to the amplitude of the background EEG; hence, it requires a number of trials to calculate the ERP-related changes. Language comprehension and speech production can be studied using ERP measures.

The PET scan measures the cellular-level metabolic changes occurring in brain tissue. The assumption behind the use of PET scan in cognitive/language task is that the area of the brain that is involved in processing specific type of stimuli will show increased metabolic changes. fMRI tracks the blood flow changes in the brain that are thought to be correlated with local changes in neuronal activity. This method calculates the ratio between oxygenated and deoxygenated blood in the brain tissue, which is known as *blood-oxygenation level-dependent effect*. The blood-oxygenation level-dependent effect is extensively used in exploring neural basis of language.

The Study of Brain–Language Relation in the Context of Brain Lesion

This section introduces three most salient neural models of language representation from a historical perspective without getting into the details of the intellectual context in which they have emerged. These neural models were based on lesion data or lesion data plus neuroimaging studies of language processing in speaker–hearers without brain lesions.

Wernicke's Model of Neural Bases of Language: Centers and Connections

In the late 19th century, Carl Wernicke, a German neuropsychiatrist, proposed a neural model of language processing (Figure 2) based on lesion data mainly from cerebrovascular disease.

According to this model, speech production and auditory comprehension are associated with the foot of the third frontal convolution of the left hemisphere (known as *Broca's area*) and the posterior superior temporal convolution (known as *Wernicke's area*), respectively. These two areas are connected by a major fiber tract called *arcuate fasciculus*. Performance on language-related tasks was supposedly supported by the centers and connections among them. Lichtheim, a student of Wernicke, had further expanded the Wernicke's model by adding two more syndromes, namely transcortical sensory and transcortical motor aphasia. An American neurologist, Norman Geschwind, expanded this model by adding more disconnection syndromes such as agnosias and apraxias (agnosia refers to an inability to recognize objects or faces following brain lesion; apraxia is a disorder of voluntary motor movements resulting from brain damage). Based on this updated model, Harold Goodglass and collaborators developed a psychometric approach for the identification of syndromes of aphasia following lesion to centers and/or connections between the centers via subcortical white matter (Table 1).

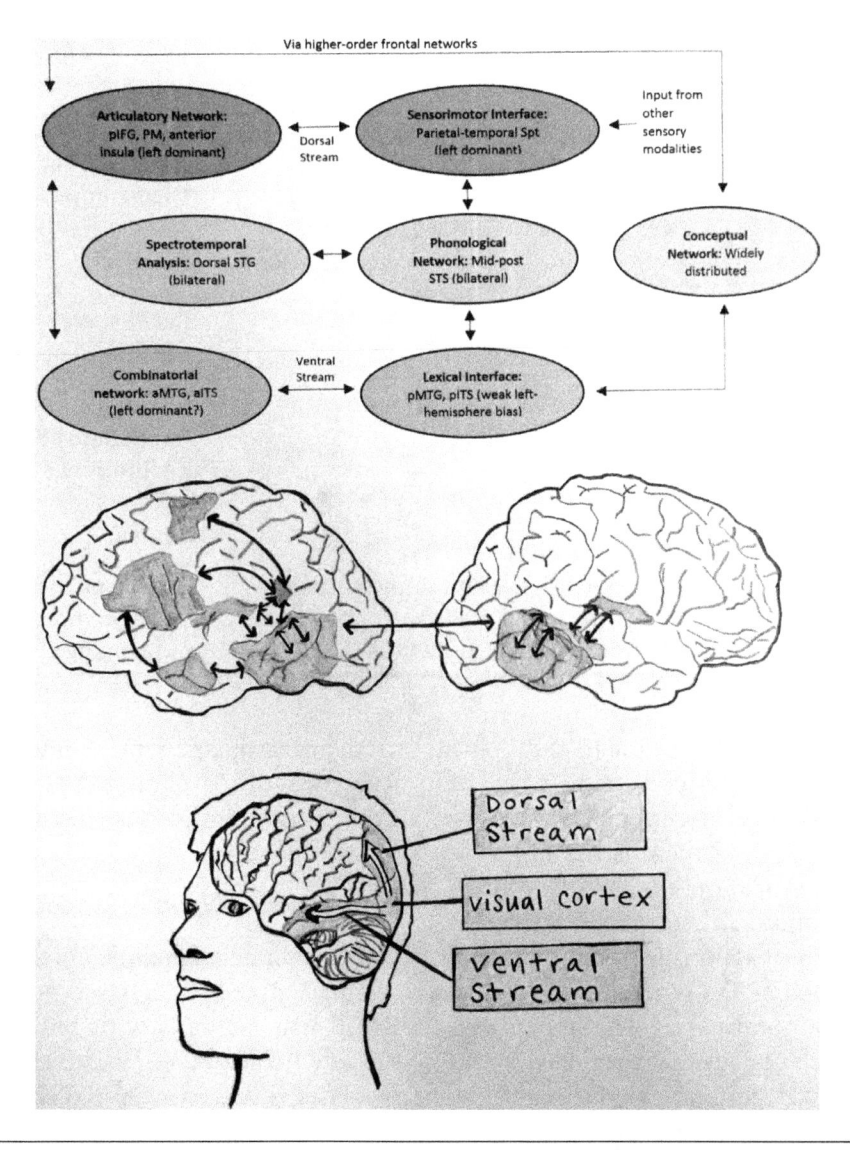

Figure 2 Dorsal and ventral stream model

Table 1 Boston Approach to Aphasia Classification

Aphasia Type	Most Typical Site of Lesion	Characteristics of the Aphasia Type
Anomic aphasia	Mostly not possible to localize Angular gyrus lesion was suggested in early research.	Fluent speech with intact speech comprehension and repetition but presents deficits in naming.
Broca's aphasia	Broadmann's areas 44 and 45 (also known as Broca's area)	Nonfluent speech with intact speech comprehension but presents deficits in repetition and naming.
Transcortical motor aphasia	Supplementary motor area	Nonfluent speech with intact speech comprehension and repetition but presents deficits in naming.
Wernicke's aphasia	Wernicke's area	Fluent speech with deficits in speech comprehension, repetition, and naming.
Conduction aphasia	Traditional literature identifies the causal lesion in the arcuate fasciculus, which interconnects Wernicke's and Broca's areas.	Fluent speech with intact speech comprehension but presents deficits in repetition and naming.
Transcortical sensory sphasia	Posterior parietal lobe	Fluent speech with intact repetition but presents deficits in speech comprehension and naming
Isolated speech area	Watershed areas	Nonfluent speech with intact repetition but presents deficits in speech comprehension and naming.
Global aphasia	Extensive lesion in the cortical and subcortical areas surrounding the Sylvian fissure	Nonfluent speech with deficits in speech comprehension, repetition, and naming.

Although this model is still popular and being used in medical school curricula, a number of shortcomings of this model were reported in clinical research. Chiefly among them is the observation that less than 50% of aphasics could be classified into syndromes. This approach attributes molar functions such as language comprehension to specific region such as the posterior portion of the left superior temporal gyrus. This model did not conceptualize language comprehension as consisting of subcomponents that might be distributed to other areas of the left hemisphere, an idea that is well articulated in the dynamic model of language representation proposed by the Russian neuropsychologist Alexander Romanovich Luria and his colleagues in the 1960s and 1970s.

Luria's Neurodynamic Model

Luria's neurodynamic model of language processing (Table 2) was based on data obtained from world war veterans with bullet-induced injury to the left hemisphere. Unlike the strict localization theorists, Luria conceptualized language production and comprehension as processes, each including component processes that are accomplished by

Table 2 Aphasia Classification Based on Luria's Neurodynamic Model

Aphasia Type	Most Typical Site of Lesion	Characteristics of the Aphasia Type
Afferent (apraxic) motor aphasia	Left postcentral area (parietal lobe), especially in the inferior portion	Phonological paraphasias. Attempts at self-correction do not improve articulation due to the lack of kinesthetic feedback from the articulators.
Acoustic-gnostic aphasia (sensory aphasia)	Lesions involving the superior parts of the left temporal lobe	It is a phonemic hearing disorder. No awareness of phonemic paraphasias (substitutions). Fluent speech with impaired comprehension.
Acoustic-mnestic aphasia	Inferior part of the left temporal area	Patients do not have phonemic hearing disorder. Difficulty remembering long sentences.
Amnestic aphasia (semantic aphasia)	Left posterior inferior parietal lobe	Disturbances in the semantic network of words. Semantic paraphasias (word substitution), difficulty with word retrieval, circumlocutions. Difficulty processing complex grammatical relations.
Dynamic aphasia	Lesions in prefrontal, premotor areas, sometimes extended medially	The structure of inner speech is altered. Absence of spontaneous speech. Repetition and naming skills are intact.
Efferent motor aphasia	Damage in the left premotor area (Broca's area)	Speech loses its smoothness of delivery (kinetic melody). Transitioning from one phoneme to the next is difficult resulting in pathological inertia or repetition.

several regions of the brain working together. In other words, comprehension is not localized in one small center of the brain; hence, comprehension disorder might occur due to lesions in different regions of the brain. This model is based on conceptualization of the human brain consisting of three functional zones working together to support language: limbic system and upper brain stem (zone 1); parietal, occipital, and temporal lobes (zone 2); and frontal lobe (zone 3). The limbic system and the brain stem maintain cortical tone to facilitate stimulus processing in the cerebral cortex. The postcentral lobes (zone 2), according to Luria, are involved in categorical (paradigmatic) organization of the phonemic, lexical, morphological, syntactic, and semantic units of language. The frontal lobes are involved in sequential (syntagmatic) organization of language. In addition, the frontal lobes also direct goal-directed behavior. The paradigmatic and syntagmatic organization of language in Luria's model reflects the influence of the linguistic theory of Roman Jakobson. As Levelt has lucidly stated in his work, *A History of Psycholinguistics: The Pre-Chomskyan Era* (2013),

Luria's neurodynamic model attempted to integrate modularity of faculty psychology with a network of functionally significant brain regions. He strongly believed in selective impairment of mental functions under discrete lesions, as his categories of aphasia clearly illustrate (see Table 2). Many of the advances made in the West in applying developments in linguistic theory of Noam Chomsky and cognitive science as well as the psycholinguistic theories and models in explaining aphasia were in tune with Luria's neurodynamic theory in terms of the basics, if not in details.

Dorsal and Ventral Stream Model of Language Processing

In the later part of the 20th century, advances in neuroimaging methods and neuropsychological studies of aphasia, and the application of linguistic theory and psycholinguistic models of language processing in aphasia research began to reveal that the neoclassical model (of Wernicke–Lichtheim–Geschwind) was clearly inadequate in explaining brain–language relation, in general, and aphasia symptoms, in particular. Poeppel and Hickok had succinctly summed up the problems with the neoclassical localization model; thus, it cannot account for a range of aphasic syndromes, and it is both linguistically and anatomically underspecified. To overcome these limitations of the neoclassical model, Poeppel and Hickok proposed a new model, namely, the dorsal and ventral stream (DVS) model of language processing (Figure 2). Poeppel and Hickok argue that the DVS model might explain the human brain's ability to produce and comprehend speech and language. Additionally, their model is also claimed to be theoretically sound, computationally explicit, and anchored in biology. However, it needs to be remembered that this model is also a framework that is in the early stage of development.

The DVS model is an extension of the Wernicke–Lichtheim model but analogically created following the DVS model of visual processing. Visual processing research identified a dual route for visual input: visual input leading to a conceptual system for object identification (function of ventral stream) and to a visually guided reaching and grasp (a dorsal stream function). Similarly, the Hickok and Poeppel model portrays the auditory input, after its early stage of bilateral cortical processing with a left hemisphere bias in the superior temporal gyrus, diverging into a dorsal stream and a ventral stream of processing: The dorsal stream proceeds dorsoposteriorly to the inferior parietal lobe and then onto the posterior frontal cortex. This stream supports auditory–motor integration function that maps the acoustic characteristics to articulatory representations of sounds. The ventral stream proceeds ventrolaterally through the middle and inferior temporal lobes and provides interface between sounds and meanings by mapping sounds onto widely distributed conceptual representations. Thus, the DVS model links the auditory input to motor production on the one hand, and comprehension of sound-meaning relation, on the other. The neural networks within both streams include an important feature called *bi-directionality*. For example, the dorsal stream network can also map motor speech representation onto auditory representation supporting the articulatory loop component of the working memory as conceptualized in Alan Baddeley's work. Similarly, the ventral stream networks could also mediate between sound and meaning for both production and perception.

This is a broad scheme that can explain a variety of clinical, experimental, and neuroimaging data. For instance, Hickok and Poeppel describe how the ventral stream disruption can result in deficits of word comprehension by compromising the interface between sound and concepts/meaning. The sound–meaning relation could be compromised in aphasic conditions such as transcortical sensory aphasia and Wernicke's aphasia. In illustrating word comprehension deficit, Hickok and Poeppel draw attention to the stages through which comprehension takes place and the neural underpinnings of these stages could vary. This approach, unlike the neoclassical model of language processing, does not localize complex functions such as word comprehension in one area of the brain. Instead, the comprehension task is analyzed into components and an attempt is made to identify the neural underpinning of each component. In this characteristic, it resembles the Lurian approach to language processing.

Undoubtedly, neurolinguistic models of language processing are the core of the discipline. However, a variety of topics of research related to language representation and processing in non-brain-damaged subjects using contemporary methods in neuroscience have also received considerable attention from researchers. As a matter of fact, results from such studies will carry implications for the neurolinguistic models.

Experimental Neurolinguistics: Neural Underpinning of Language Processing in Normal Subjects

Neurolinguists such as Poeppel and Hickok have cautioned about the search for the neurological bases of coarse categorization of language functions such as phonology, morphology, syntax, and semantics. These categories are too underspecified to be related to the brain structures. Similarly, functions such as lexical processing, syntactic parsing, and speech perception and speech articulation are also grievously underspecified to guide brain mapping. Hence, the basic questions regarding brain–language relation are necessarily more specific in nature: Which parts of the brain store concrete nouns and verbs? Are there separate neural bases for morphosyntactic (i.e., between-word consistency) and morphophonological inflections (i.e., inflectional features in sound patterns)? Can PET and fMRI anatomically differentiate functional and positional aspects of syntactic encoding? What are the components of the neural circuitry of the left hemisphere that subserve sentence comprehension? Similar questions can be raised at the levels of story production and comprehension. These research questions are always, or nearly so, based on psycholinguistic and cognitive models that usually identify levels of representation and processing. Thus, one could avoid the danger of underspecifying the object of inquiry in neurolinguistics research.

The answers to these questions are taken from related contemporary neuroimaging studies, and these answers are just examples, not an all-inclusive list. Neuroimaging studies offer support to the view that object concepts for tools are represented in the anterior intraparietal sulcus, supramarginal gyrus, and the ventral premotor cortex. Transitive verb (e.g., petted) processing depends on the posterolateral temporal cortex and the angular gyrus more than the intransitive ones (e.g., purred). When it comes to the question regarding processing of the two types of inflections, fMRI studies observe that two different aspects of Broca's area are engaged. Although a limited number of imaging studies support the view that Broca's area is engaged in syntactic processing, these studies could not tease apart the functional and positional levels of encoding. With regard to sentence comprehension, the cortical components of the network that support sentence comprehension include posterior mid temporal gyrus, superior temporal gyrus, posterior superior temporal sulcus and Broadman's area 39, and the inferior frontal gyrus, especially Broca's area.

Developmental Neurolinguistics: Neural Bases of Language Acquisition in Infants and Children

This section highlights the correlation between stages of postnatal (after birth) development of the nervous system and the emergence of stages of language development from birth till the teen years. The newborn baby's brain at birth shows completion of cell formation and migration. Around the same time, the left hemisphere bias for speech stimuli emerges. At about 9 months of age, long-range connections among the lobes will be established, and the child's brain metabolism will closely resemble that of adults. During this period, word comprehension and intentional communication will be present. Between 18 and 24 months after birth, a rapid increase in synoptic connections within and across lobes occurs. A corresponding increase in vocabulary development and early development of grammar occurs, followed by a rapid increase in grammatical development. When the child is 4 years of age, the brain metabolism reaches the peak level. At this age, grammatical development attains maturity and stabilizes. The period between 4 years and the onset of adolescence witnesses a slow decline in brain metabolism and synoptic connections. Language markers during this period include the use of complex grammatical rules. Also, the capacity for acquisition of a second language and recovery from childhood-acquired aphasia will decline.

Geriatric Neurolinguistics

The biological process of aging will bring about changes in sensory, cognitive, and language functions. These changes reflect the structural and functional decline of the nervous system in the elderly. The areas of decline that are pertinent to language and cognition include gyral atrophy in frontal and temporal lobes, most probably due to loss of mass in the white matter. In the old-old (i.e., those who are older than 75 years), there will be additional loss of gray matter. Age-related changes will be noticed in hippocampal gyrus as well. Frontal, temporal, and parietal lobes constitute a network of structures that support both language and memory. The vascular system that supplies the brain will also undergo age-related changes that might affect the continuous supply of oxygenated blood to the brain structures. Vascular diseases such as stroke can cause damage to the aging brain; depending on the area of damage, various linguistic and cognitive disorders may result. One such disorder is aphasia. Degenerative diseases will also afflict the elderly. Alzheimer's disease, for instance, through its stages of progression will result in impaired cognition and language. Neurolinguists are interested in exploring the nature of language loss in the normal aging process, in stroke-induced language disorder, and in degenerative diseases-induced (e.g., Alzheimer's and primary progressive aphasia) language loss. Varieties of linguistic theories and psycholinguistic models of language processing are being used to achieve a better understanding of the nature of language loss in these clinical conditions.

Neurolinguistics of Bi- and Multilingualism

Considering advances in technology, communication, and global trade, the incidence of bi- and multilingualism are on the increase. Population migration further contributes to the necessity for acquiring new languages. While neurolinguists and cognitive neuroscientists are in the process of inaugurating newer models of language representations/processing in monolinguals, for example, the DVS model discussed previously, a much more intriguing and challenging issue is at hand for researchers dealing with bilingual/multilingual brain.

In accounting for the representation of languages in the bilingual (and multilingual) brain, Ullman in 2001 has postulated two types of language knowledge: *Mental Lexicon* (ML) and *Mental Grammar* (MG). ML stores information about words (i.e., phonologic, orthographic, and semantic representation), whereas MG contains rules and operations that permit the combination of lexical forms into sentences. These types of knowledge are claimed to be managed by two different memory systems, as suggested by some theoretical models: ML depends on declarative memory processes that are biologically rooted in the neural structures of temporal lobe (the hippocampus and the surrounding structures), and the MG depends on the procedural memory rooted in the left frontal-basal ganglia circuits.

In late bilinguals, one way of conceptualizing neural representation of languages is as follows: MG in L1 depends on procedural memory and in L2 on declarative memory, if L2 was acquired in pedagogical environment.

The ML aspects of language representation in the bilingual brain are shared by L1 and L2, and they are neutrally represented in the neural structures that depend on declarative memory.

The issue of neural basis of bilingualism has been investigated in multiple scientific clinical and neuroimaging studies. Some clinical and experimental data seem to suggest that L1 and L2 are represented differently in the Left Hemisphere of the brain. Other studies have suggested that language is left lateralized for monolinguals, and in bilinguals, language is represented bilaterally. These and other such issues require further research.

Final Thoughts

The overarching goal of neurolinguistics is to develop a neural model (or competing models) that can account for the neural bases of monolingual and bilingual speaker–hearers' ability to produce and understand language through all four modalities of use (i.e., speaking, listening, reading, writing). Although critically important topics and issues have been touched upon, topics such as language evolution and clinical neurolinguistics need to be further explored.

Venugopal Balasubramanian

See also Aphasia; Cognitive Processes and Operations; Psycholinguistics; Stroke; Traumatic Brain Injury

Further Readings

Caplan, D. (1987). *Neurolinguistics and linguistic aphasiology*. Cambridge, UK: Cambridge University Press.

Embick, D., & Poeppel, D. (2015). Towards a computational (ist) neurobiology of language: Correlational, integrated and explanatory neurolinguistics. *Language, Cognition, and Neuroscience, 30*, 357–366.

Hickok, G., & Small, S. L. (Eds.). (2016). *Neurobiology of language*. London, UK: Academic Press.

Kemmerer, D. (2015). *Cognitive neuroscience of language*. New York, NY: Psychology Press.

Luria, A. R. (1976). *Basic problems in neurolinguistics*. The Hague, The Netherlands: Mouton.

Stemmer, B., & Whitaker, H. A. (Eds.). (2008). *Handbook of the neuroscience of language*. New York, NY: Academic Press.

Neurophonetics

Neurophonetics studies neural bases of speech production and perception. Speech production starts with a proposition that is transformed into a verbal message by a series of pragmatic and language-specific rules and constraints, to be finally articulated with the help of motor control mechanisms and auditory feedback loop and monitoring processes. Speech perception involves auditory encoding of phonological features as a step in lexical access and comprehension of the message within the perception–memory–action loop. Just as the boundary between the more general fields of phonetics and linguistics is blurry, the area where neurophonetics and neurolinguistics meet is gray and some overlap is to be expected. There seems to be general agreement that neurophonetics covers acoustic, phonetic, and phonological aspects of speech processing to the level of lexical access. Neurophonetic research has found application in areas such as speech acquisition, clinical phonetics, and bilingualism. This entry provides an overview of the methodology used in neurophonetics, then explores the neural bases of speech processing, and finally addresses issues related to bilingualism and neurogenic speech disorders.

Methodology

Until the advancement of modern technology, *neurological cases* were the only source of information about possible neural bases of speech processing (e.g., aphasics, split-brain patients). In spite of its limitations (e.g., absence of premorbidity data, effects of comorbidity, lack of insight into relevance of locations other than the ones affected by the condition, inappropriateness of testing situations, varying diagnostic tools), this vast body of evidence is still valuable in studying the neurophysiological underpinnings of speech.

Groundbreaking data have been collected from *electrostimulation studies* that provide direct recordings of brain surface activity during various tasks in awake patients, but for obvious reasons, this method is reserved for medically justified uses. In transcranial magnetic stimulation, areas of interest on the brain surface can be stimulated through the skull by means of an electrical coil. Stimulation effects are very brief and timing is crucial. Although it has been used on healthy subjects, it may cause seizures and possibly affect memory.

Event-related potentials (ERP) are one of the most widely used noninvasive *electrophysiological methods*. It is a derivative of electroencephalography and is based on the fact that each event evokes electrical responses in the central nervous system that can be measured (after multiple repetitions of the same stimulus that are necessary in order to separate the signal from the noise). Phonetic and phonological processes typically have latencies up to 200 or 250 milliseconds (ms). Latency of approximately 50 ms (P50) is characteristic of processing place of articulation. Periodicity and vowel height have been linked with the latency of 100 ms (N100). The so-called mismatch negativity is a response to deviant stimuli. Deviant vowels in an oddball design typically elicit a frontocentral response with the latency of 100–250 ms. Such response is also found when an incoming stimulus conflicts with the top-down processing or with information from another modality and has therefore been considered as reaction to error. ERP has good temporal but poor spatial resolution, and it is not suitable for studying perception of continuous speech. Magnetoencephalography is based on electromagnetic fields that form during neural activity and displays deflections comparable to those of ERPs. It also requires multiple presentations of the same stimulus but is less affected by surrounding tissue than ERP.

Neuroimaging methods provide information about metabolic activity in reaction to a stimulus. Functional magnetic resonance imaging, based on blood-oxygen-level-dependent response, positron emission tomography, based on positron-emitting tracers after injection/inhalation of a radioactive isotope, and functional near-infrared spectroscopy, based on the brain's permeability to infrared rays, are the most common ones. Functional near-infrared spectroscopy is applicable to populations less suitable for functional magnetic resonance imaging or positron emission tomography (e.g., infants). These methods share good spatial but poor temporal resolution. Another problem common to all these techniques is that increased blood flow is present when both excitatory and inhibitory neurons are active. Diffusion-weighted magnetic resonance imaging and the related method of diffusion tensor imaging, based on the diffusion of water molecules in tissue, are used for tracking white matter fiber bundles, which is relevant in connectivity research because it reveals not only connections among different regions of the brain but also their direction. Limitations of all of these methods include small sample size, artifacts, resolution issues, task restrictions, and neglecting nonstudied parts.

One of the most widely used *behavioral methods* is dichotic listening. In this method, two different auditory stimuli are presented to the left and right ears simultaneously and response time and/or accuracy are measured. It provides indirect indication of which hemisphere of the brain is more involved in processing various types of auditory information. Right ear advantage is typically found for speech stimuli, which is taken as evidence of greater involvement of the left hemisphere (LH). Contrary to this, nonspeech stimuli result in left ear advantage, suggesting greater activity of the right hemisphere (RH). Right ear advantage for syllables and left ear advantage for music stimuli have been found in 4-month-old babies. This method is closely related to divided visual field studies, which have revealed right visual field advantage for language stimuli and left visual field advantage for nonlanguage stimuli, indicating LH and RH dominance, respectively. Both methods are susceptible to attention manipulation/control and are suitable for very short stimuli.

Naturally, more *peripheral* methods—those that measure the outcome of actual perception/production rather than visualizing the underlying (central) neural processes (e.g., perceptual assessment, auditory and acoustic analysis, electromyography, glottography, ultrasound, electropalatography)—are widely used for studying speech production and perception.

The best and most reliable results are obtained by combining different methods and utilizing their individual strengths to yield converging evidence.

Neural Bases of Speech Processing

Speech production is predominantly an LH activity, especially in nonautomatic speech and more complex production (e.g., reciting poetry). Automatic speech (e.g., listing days of the week, swear words) is bilaterally or RH represented. In addition to areas essential for speech production (i.e., Broca's area, primary motor area and supplementary motor area, insula), basal ganglia and cerebellum as well as somatosensory and auditory feedback mechanisms constitute the intricate network involved in the process.

Speech perception seems to be less clearly left-lateralized and more widely distributed than production. This claim is partly based on the observation that in LH-injured patients, perception recovers faster than production. Bilateral activation of premotor areas has been recorded in tasks of syllable detection, subvocal repetition, and paying attention without overt response—which again suggests activation of motor programs consistent with the motor theory of speech perception and reveals neural bases of the phonological/articulatory loop in Alan Baddeley's working-memory model (involving numerous bilateral speech production and perception areas including Brodmann area [BA] 44, 33, 42, 40, supplementary motor area, insulas, cerebellum, and BA 1, 2, 3, 4).

LH is generally considered dominant for processing CV syllables (e.g., /pa/), but some studies report no significant asymmetry. With respect to individual *segments*, LH is predominantly activated during processing of stops and fricatives whose perception relies on transitions (e.g., /ð/, /θ/) as opposed to those that are characterized by noise cues (e.g., /s/, /ʃ/, /z/, /ʒ/). However, there are indications that place of articulation and voicing may be represented in LH and RH, respectively. Semivowels (e.g., /w/) and liquids (e.g., /l/) are less clearly left-lateralized than consonants, but still more so than vowels, that exhibit bilateral activity or inconsistent lateralization. However, in difficult listening conditions (e.g., noise, distortion), LH clearly takes over. Segmentation task activates LH inferior frontal gyrus/inferior frontal cortex. Sensitivity to phonetic contrasts is represented in inferior frontal cortex and in temporal regions. Encoding new speech categories activates bilateral middle frontal gyrus, indicating its involvement in learning sounds of nonnative, foreign language (L2). Some electrophysiological data suggest that RH is involved in segmentation and prosodic timing at syllabic level and in preprocessing of speech signals (at a prelinguistic level).

Positron emission tomography and functional magnetic resonance imaging studies have identified increased activity in superior temporal gyrus (STG) in response to frequency-modulated sounds in contrast to noise and in the area between STG and middle temporal gyrus in response to speech sounds in contrast to nonspeech stimuli. Both findings are taken as evidence that these areas are involved in spectrotemporal processing inherent in speech perception. Greater activity is usually recorded in the LH, but RH is active as well. This process is sublexical because it is found in words and pseudowords alike. The *phonological store* seems to be represented at the parietal–occipital–temporal junction in LH. It involves LH supramarginal and angular gyri and BA 40 bilaterally. Phonological working memory is represented in the inferior parietal cortex (roughly corresponding to BA 40). Phonological discrimination is represented in the LH planum temporale, and phonological word form representations seem to be stored in the LH anterior superior temporal lobe. Clinical and neuroimaging data clearly show that LH STG is crucial in speech processing because it houses general auditory systems and specialized networks for phoneme recognition. Areas involved in phonological access and storage partly overlap with general speech perception areas, but they are more strongly left-lateralized than speech perception.

Prosody is usually described as linguistic (i.e., intonation and accent position) or affective/emotional (i.e., emotional content, attitude, condition and mood of the speaker), and neurophonetic research is typically conducted along these lines. Brain-injured patients exhibit double dissociation in their ability to process prosody: LH-damaged patients have difficulty understanding words, with spared interpretation of emotional prosody; RH-damaged patients have intact comprehension of linguistically expressed meaning but are impaired in distinguishing among utterances on the basis of affective prosody (this extends to nonverbal expressions as well).

In tone languages, such as Thai or Mandarin Chinese, LH is dominant for lexical tones. However, speakers of one tone language do not process lexical tones of another in their LH by default. It is reserved only for language-specific tonal distinctions. In languages that use pitch accent such as Norwegian or Croatian, the little available data on laterality are inconclusive.

Research into neural bases of prosody has offered often contradictory answers. Although it is most frequently claimed that RH is dominant for affective/emotional and LH for linguistic prosody, it has been proposed that RH is dominant for all types of prosody or that the building blocks of prosody (i.e., duration, tone, and intensity) are lateralized differently or even that prosody may be a subcortical activity. However, it appears that production and perception of prosody require intact parts of RH that correspond to traditional speech/language areas in the LH.

Dual Processing Streams/Pathways

Acquisition and learning of speech sounds as well as their use in communication rely on connections between the auditory and motor areas of the brain. These connections enable associations between perceptual and motor representations as well as syntactic and semantic processing via two dorsal and two ventral pathways/streams. The (dorsal) pathway connecting dorsal premotor cortex with posterior STG/middle temporal gyrus via parietal cortex supports bottom-up auditory-to-motor mapping (as in speech repetition), and the pathway connecting BA 44 with posterior STG via arcuate fasciculus (AF) is in charge of complex syntactic processing (providing top-down prediction for the incoming input).

Immature model of interconnectivity has been found in children before the age of 6 years, and it is characterized by stronger connections between homotopic areas in the two hemispheres than between anterior and posterior regions. The mature pattern of connections between STG and inferior frontal gyrus is established between 5 and 18 years. However, this seems to be true of the *syntactic* connection (between STG and BA 44, probably due to not fully matured AF), whereas the *somatosensory* connection (between STG and premotor cortex) is present at birth and constitutes the basis for auditory-based phonological learning. This dorsal stream is crucial in speech acquisition.

The two ventral pathways are devoted to semantic and basic syntactic processing. The pathway connecting frontal cortex with temporal cortex, parietal cortex, and occipital cortex supports semantic processing and comprehension. The one that connects anterior inferior frontal cortex with anterior temporal cortex is in charge of local syntactic processing.

In the process of acquisition/learning, these pathways are important for recognition and perfecting movement patterns necessary for production, but it is also known that the primarily auditory areas are activated in speech production and that perceptual tasks activate the anterior language areas primarily associated with production. This (in addition to the discovery of mirror neurons in the 1990s) sheds new favorable light on the motor theory of speech perception since there is actual evidence that speech perception activates motor representations. However, higher level processes that involve comprehension (i.e., listening for meaning) seem to be independent of the speech motor system. It should be stressed that the initial enthusiasm in trying to relate the primate mirror neuron system to spoken language processing has been dampened by the findings that speech processing involves a much more complex network than predicted by hypothesis resulting from nonhuman primate studies.

Disorders

Some of the typical neurogenic speech disorders are dysarthrias, apraxia of speech (AOS), aphasias, and pure word deafness. Dysarthrias affect motor execution in some or all of the components of speech production: respiration, phonation, and articulation. Severity and type of dysarthria (which can be spastic, flaccid, ataxic, hypokinetic, hyperkinetic, or mixed) depend on the affected part of the nervous system: rolandic motor cortex, anterior cingulate cortex and supplementary motor area, upper motor neuron, brainstem, and basal ganglia or cerebellum, including its afferent/efferent pathways. Some of the characteristics include disorders of speech tempo, changes in voice quality, limited movement of articulators, and muscle weakness.

AOS does not involve motor execution problems, and the intended target (i.e., phonological form of the word) is preserved, but the problem lies in phonetic encoding (i.e., in transforming abstract representations of word forms into motor commands to articulators). It is characterized by segmental (e.g., phonetic distortions, phonemic paraphasias) as well as prosodic impairment (e.g., different kinds of dysfluencies) and inconsistent errors. Acquired AOS occurs after lesions to Broca's area and left anterior insula. Developmental AOS presents with similar speech production errors, but without consistent neuroanatomical basis, and is thought to have genetic origin.

Aphasias are generally described as language impairments, but phonemic errors in speech production (e.g., substitutions, omissions, additions, or combinations) are a common aphasic symptom. Absence of phonetic distortions distinguishes phonemic paraphasias in patients with aphasic phonological impairment from those suffering from AOS. Phonemic paraphasias are a result of faulty phonological encoding (i.e., incorrect selection or sequencing of phonemes). They extend to reading and writing, because reading/writing involve mapping from phonological to orthographic representations. Owing to this, failure to develop phonological awareness in children is an indicator of risk of dyslexia.

Severity and type of aphasia (which is commonly categorized on the basis of criteria of fluency, speech comprehension, and ability to repeat words/phrases) also depends on the affected brain areas. Damage to AF typically results in impaired speech repetition (characteristic of conduction aphasia), which supports the view that AF is crucial in auditory-to-motor mapping.

Pure word deafness (i.e., inability to understand speech in spite of normal peripheral hearing) occurs after lesions in the temporal lobe (mostly bilateral). The findings that it sometimes occurs after LH-temporal lesions but never after RH-temporal lesions support the notion that auditory processing of speech is left-lateralized. On the other hand, RH seems to be dominant for processing of music, environmental sounds, and speaker characteristics. A wider term, *auditory agnosia*, is used for such selective impairments. Like other types of agnosias, they are consequences of lesions in the so-called secondary cortical areas that are devoted to pattern/form recognition (*gestalts*), and as opposed to bilateral and modality-specific primary cortical areas, they are functional and lateralized. In other words, an auditory stimulus will reach primary auditory areas in STG in both hemispheres and then, depending on the type of the stimulus, it will be further processed in the hemisphere dominant for that type of stimuli (e.g., predominantly LH for speech, RH for nonspeech stimuli). Since the early 2000s, the more frequently used terms for primary, secondary, and tertiary/associative areas are *core*, *belt*, and *parabelt*.

Another way of looking at this is based on claims that the two hemispheres have different skills/priorities with respect to temporal and spectral analysis of auditory stimuli—LH having better temporal resolution and poorer spectral resolution abilities and RH having the opposite characteristics. This is in line with general LH-RH processing dichotomies, where LH is devoted to analytical, serial/sequential, and categorical processing; local representation; and high frequencies, whereas RH is devoted to holistic, parallel, and coordinate processing; global representation; and low frequencies.

Bilingualism

The key neurolinguistic question in studying bilinguals is nonnative, foreign language (L2) representation in comparison to native language (L1), and in that context the focus of neurophonetics has been on the representation of phonological store(s) and dealing with language-specific aspects. There is no evidence that L2 would involve a special module or structures not present in monolinguals, but the precise ratio of overlap and specificities is still under investigation. Due to neural plasticity, humans are able to master sound systems of languages different from their own even after L1 system is firmly in place, constituting a filter of sorts through which all novel sounds (and rules) are processed. Learning new criteria of categorical perception as well as learning to attach phonological relevance to tones in case of a tone L2, in addition to posterior speech areas (mostly STG and adjacent regions), activates frontal regions bilaterally. This bilateral activation does not necessarily mean that L2 prefers the RH; rather, it reflects the fact that unfamiliar tasks/materials increase processing demands, resulting in more neural tissue being engaged. It may also be an indication of employing other/additional strategies.

Final Thoughts

Neurophonetics also tries to address the question: Is speech special? In other words, is there a special module or network that is reserved exclusively for speech production and perception, or is speech just another function that relies on multipurpose structures and mechanisms? The *hardware* used for listening and speaking has other primary roles (e.g., determining the source and direction of sound or chewing, swallowing, and breathing, respectively). As for *software*, some clinical data, especially on agnosias, may suggest that speech processing engages a module/network of its own, but in light of other evidence, it seems more (or just as) likely that it is a matter of the signal's temporal and spectral properties. In terms of speech production, it is clear that there are motor control disorders that are characteristic exclusively of speech. However, neuroimaging data have not revealed any exclusively speech-specific modules/networks that would not be activated in a number of other functions as well. It seems that speech is not special from birth, but in the course of intense motor and perceptual learning during the period of speech acquisition, humans develop this innate ability to adapt general cognitive functioning to accommodate speech processing.

Neural basis of speech is best viewed as a comprehensive multimodal network distributed across and throughout the brain, with some focal and highly specific areas.

Vesna Mildner

See also Anatomy of the Hearing Mechanism and Central Audiology Nervous System; Anatomy of the Human Neurological System; Neurogenic Communication Disorders; Neurolinguistics; Speech Perception, Theories of; Speech Production, Theories of

Further Readings

Binder, J. R. (2008). *The neural bases of communication: Evidence from neuroimaging.* Retrieved July 20, 2017, from www.asha.org

Friederici, A. D., & Gierhan, S. M. E. (2013). The language network. *Current Opinion in Neurobiology, 23,* 250–254.

Hertrich, I., & Ackermann, H. (2013). Neurophonetics. *WIREs: Cognitive Science, 4,* 191–200. doi:10.1002/wcs.1211

Mildner, V. (2008). *The cognitive neuroscience of human communication.* Mahwah, NJ: Erlbaum.

Ziegler, W. (2011). Neurophonetics. In M. J. Ball, M. R. Perkins, N. Müller, & S. Howard (Eds.), *The handbook of clinical linguistics* (pp. 491–505). Malden, MA: Wiley-Blackwell.

NEUROPRAGMATICS

Pragmatics refers to the way people use and interpret language while considering context, situation, and social and psychological variables. The way our brain represents and processes phenomena of pragmatics is the domain of neuropragmatics. Subfields of neuropragmatics are nonclinical pragmatics that aims to establish the brain mechanisms underlying pragmatic phenomena and clinical pragmatics that focuses on pragmatic disorders in illness. Clinical pragmatics deals with pragmatic abnormalities or impairments such as psychiatric and neurological conditions in clinical populations. Pragmatic disorders can be acquired after damage to the brain caused by stroke, trauma, or brain disease (e.g., dementia, encephalitis) and can also accompany developmental disorders (e.g., autistic spectrum disorders, attention-deficit hyperactivity disorder). The field of neuropragmatics evolved from the study of patients with damage to the right hemisphere who, despite intact linguistic abilities (such as vocabulary and grammar), showed inappropriate pragmatic behavior in discourse and conversation (e.g., verbosity, inability to identify the main point of a discourse, inappropriate turn-taking). These patients also showed difficulties with interpreting figurative language, including metaphors, idioms, and jokes, and they behaved inappropriately in communicative situations. Subsequent research addressed the question whether it was only the right hemisphere that was involved in these difficulties, and an effort was made to elucidate in more detail the brain correlates involved in pragmatic disorders.

Brain Correlates

Numerous explanations for the observed pragmatic disorders have been advanced. Although they differ in many respects, they overlap in the view that an important aspect of the language production and comprehension process is our ability to reason and make inferences from and about the context and situation around us as well as about the people involved. An attempt has thus been made to describe the brain mechanisms underlying these inferences and reasoning processes. In this context, the hypothesis that has been investigated most frequently in terms of its underlying brain correlates is the Theory of Mind (ToM) Hypothesis, which refers to the ability to attribute mental states such as beliefs, intents, and desires to oneself and to others. It also involves the ability to understand that others have beliefs, intents, and desires that are different from one's own. Core regions in the brain considered to contribute to ToM tasks are the inferior parietal cortex (more precisely, the junction of the temporal and parietal lobe on both sides of the brain), the medial parietal cortex (precuneus), and the medial prefrontal cortex (see Figures 1 and 2). While most researchers agree that these brain regions are activated during ToM tasks, the exact role of these regions during mentalizing is, however, still a matter of debate. Some researchers have proposed that the core regions of communicative intent (including ToM) are part of an intention processing network in which the precuneus and the right

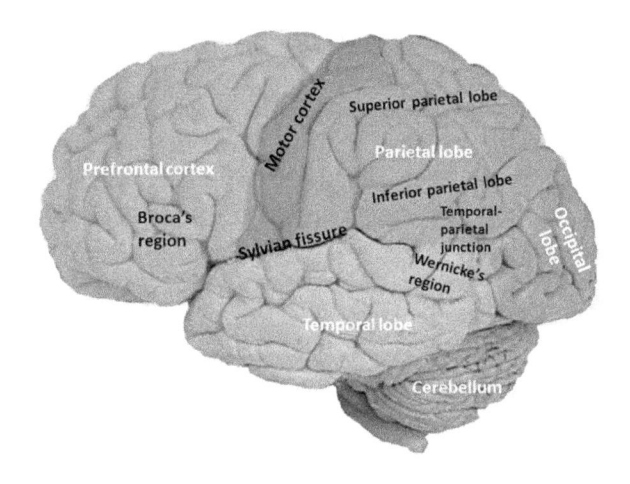

Figure 1 The left hemisphere of the brain looked at from the side, or in anatomical terms, a lateral view of the brain. Main brain divisions are printed in white. Note that the prefrontal cortex plus the region depicted as motor cortex make up the frontal cortex

Source: Author.

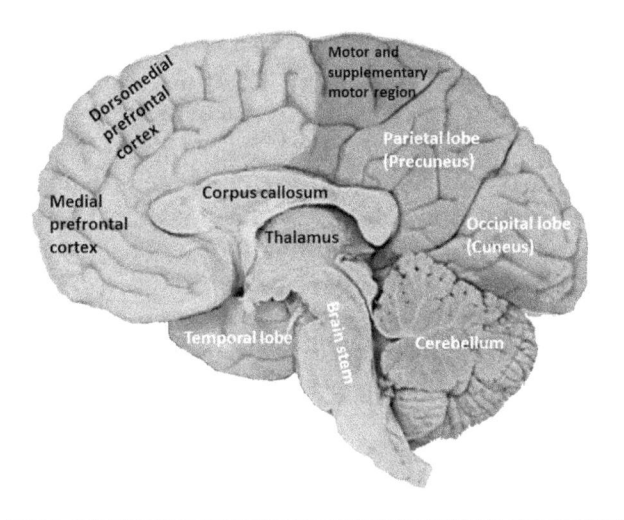

Figure 2 The right hemisphere of the brain looked at from the inside, or in anatomical terms, a medial view of the brain. Main brain divisions are printed in white

Source: Author.

temporo–parietal junction are recruited by private intentions, the left temporo–parietal junction by prospective social intentions, and the medial prefrontal cortex by communicative intentions. Others have criticized the ToM as an elusive concept that is multidimensional, ill-defined, and vague.

Other Questions Addressed

A question that has received particular attention relates to the contribution that each cerebral hemisphere makes to pragmatic behavior. While classical lesion studies with patients had pointed to a dominance of the right hemisphere, neuroimaging studies on text, discourse, and nonliteral and figurative language processing in healthy individuals report findings that range from only left hemisphere involvement and only right hemisphere involvement to an engagement of both hemispheres. While no consensus has as yet been reached, the picture that seems to be emerging is that a number of variables determine the degree to which the left and/or right hemisphere contributes to nonliteral and figurative language processing. These variables include contextual, situational, social, and cultural factors as well as specific characteristics of an individual such as attention, memory, language abilities, and emotional state.

Another issue addressed has been whether the brain regions implicated in the representation and processing of single words and sentences (i.e., lower level language processing) differ from those implicated in pragmatic processing. Neuroimaging studies investigating how language is represented and processed at lower level language have consistently reported brain activation in regions such as Broca's and Wernicke's regions as well as other specific brain regions including frontal, prefrontal, temporal, and inferior parietal cortex. Work that analyzed neuroimaging studies with regard to this question concluded that the brain networks involved in higher level language processing (i.e., discourse, figurative language) overlap with the brain network for lower level language processing (referred to as the default language network) but extend beyond these brain regions. This view is, however, not supported by all researchers. Some neuroimaging studies have indicated that communicative abilities and language abilities rely on different cortical systems, and patient studies have shown that pragmatic disorders can occur independently of language disorders (and vice versa). The question remains controversial.

Final Thoughts

One of the reasons that it is difficult to discern the neural underpinnings of pragmatic behavior relates to the control of the numerous variables contributing to pragmatic behavior. Another reason may be that, in cognitive neuroscience, pragmatic behavior has been viewed as a static rather than a dynamic concept. Viewed from a dynamic perspective, pragmatic behavior would result from brain operations at various levels of organization and thus emerge through the workings and interactions of local and more global brain networks. This view awaits further investigation.

Brigitte Stemmer

See also Neurogenic Communication Disorders; Pragmatics

Further Readings

Bara, B. G., Enrici, I., & Adenzato, M. (2016). At the core of pragmatics: The neural substrates of communicative intentions. In S. L. Small & G. Hickok (Eds.), *The neurobiology of language* (pp. 675–685). London, UK: Elsevier.

Stemmer, B. (2017). Chapter 23: Neural aspects of pragmatic disorders. In L. Cummings (Ed.), *Perspectives in pragmatics, philosophy, and psychology* (pp. 561–585). Cham, Switzerland: Springer. doi:10.1007/978-3-319-47489-2_21

Stemmer, B. (2017). Chapter 19: Neuropragmatics. In Y. Huang (Ed.), *The Oxford handbook of pragmatics* (pp. 362–379). Oxford, UK: Oxford University Press.

Willems, R. M., De Boer, M., De Ruiter, J. P., Noordzij, M. L., Hagoort, P., & Toni, I. (2010). A dissociation between linguistic and communicative abilities in the human brain. *Psychological Science, 21*, 8–14. doi:10.1177/0956797609355563

NOISE-INDUCED HEARING LOSS AND ITS PREVENTION

Hearing loss is defined by the International Organization for Standardization (ISO) as a deviation or a change for the worse of the threshold of hearing from normal, where "normal" refers to the median hearing threshold level (HTL) for an equivalent, representative population free from all signs or symptoms of ear disease, obstructing ear-canal wax and who have no history of exposure to noise, ototoxic substances or familial hearing disorders. Normative hearing thresholds are conventionally based on those of a typical 20-year-old population of males and females. Hearing thresholds can be expected to differ with respect to age and between sexes. The term *sound-induced HL* is sometimes used in order to be more inclusive of sounds that are not noise in the sense that *noise is unwanted sound*. *Noise-induced HL* (N-IHL) refers to damage to the auditory system caused by noise, usually continuous but sometimes impulsive. It is also frequently referred to as occupational HL. This entry provides an overview of the causes of HL, including workplace noise, the two main types of HL, the role of the audiogram in assessing HL, and methods for preventing HL.

Sounds That Cause Damage

Dangerous sound can be either impulsive or continuous. Impulsive sounds are of brief duration such as explosions and impacts. Such sounds are thought to cause injury if they are above a 130-dB C-weighted peak sound level (L_{Cpeak}). Continuous sounds are ongoing exposures, such as a motor running, music playing, or a series of impacts. Continuous sound above around 75 dB, over time, has the potential to cause injury or damage to hearing. In many jurisdictions, the exposure level ($L_{Aeq,8h}$) at which people working in noisy environments must be protected is 85 dB. Exposure is a function of the loudness of a sound (L_{Aeq}) and the exposure duration or time. An $L_{Aeq,8h}$ is equivalent to an L_{Aeq} of 85 dB for 8 hr. It is important to be aware that an exposure of 85 dB is not considered to be a *safe exposure* but rather an exposure of *acceptable risk*. There will be a HL over time for a percentage of the population at this level. The decision about whether a given exposure is dangerous for an individual is complex because it involves an interplay between the level of the sound, the length of exposure each day, the number of years of that amount of exposure, and intrapersonal factors such as vulnerability to noise.

Types of HL

N-IHL is typically measured using pure-tone audiometry. It has been described as having two forms: One is irreversible and has a permanent threshold shift (PTS) in hearing, and the other is a temporary threshold shift (TTS). A TTS will usually recover over a period ranging from hours to days depending on the level and duration of the original sound. In order to determine a PTS, a specified period of *quiet* is usually required prior to audiometric assessment in order to eliminate the presence of a TTS.

Both PTS and TTS occur due to the response to overstimulation of the auditory system. The human auditory system encodes sound energy via sensory hair cells in the cochleae. Two classes of mechanism lead to injury of this system by sound: mechanical and metabolic. Mechanical damage is caused by sound at very high levels, where the shock of the sound energy hitting the ear can rupture membranes or dislocate the ossicles of the middle ear. This is the primary characteristic of impulsive noise exposure. Metabolic harm is caused by chronic high-level noise exposure via oxidative stress. When the hair cells are overworked for prolonged periods, they become inefficient and release free radicals called *reactive oxygen species*. These charged molecules react with cells, membranes, and DNA in the cochlea, causing damage, which may lead to cell death. Damage due to high-level sound occurs at multiple sites including the sensory cells, particularly the outer hair cells, the stria vascularis, and the neurons of the spiral ganglion of the auditory nerve. The damage to the nerve affects the transmission of the signal along the auditory pathway to the brain. These injuries are permanent and result in PTS.

TTS results from adaptation of the auditory system. The auditory system reacts dynamically to ambient sound levels, thereby preserving its dynamic range (i.e., ability to respond to sounds at levels present in a given environment). In high-level sound, adaptation may occur at multiple sites, including the hair cells, their synapses, and throughout the auditory nervous system up to the level of the cortex, reducing the responsivity of the system. As a result, pure-tone audiometric thresholds tend to be poorer for some time after exposure to high-level sound. This is the result of physiological, not pathological, processes and is therefore temporary, hence the name TTS. It is quite possible for TTS and PTS to occur at the same time. The temporary portion of the loss would recover, but the permanent would remain.

Hidden HL

HLs may not be detectable using pure-tone audiometry. Some auditory nerve fibers tend to respond to lower level sounds, and others reserve their responsivity for higher noise environments. It is the latter group of fibers that is more likely to be destroyed by noise injury, and this gives rise to an inability to hear sound in a noisy environment despite having apparently normal hearing when it is quiet, such as during pure-tone audiometry. This phenomenon has been termed *hidden HL* and has the characteristic of normal or near-normal hearing thresholds but difficulty understanding speech in noisy situations. For this reason, it is important to note that pure-tone audiometry does not provide a direct measure of a hearing impairment, disability, or handicap.

Workplaces

HL due to workplace noise is also referred to as *noise injury* or occupational HL and is the second most common cause of HL after presbyacusis (i.e., HL due to aging). While HL due to noise exposure is completely preventable by reducing exposure to loud noise, its elimination has proved to be one of the most difficult aspects of *Workplace Health & Safety*. This is because except for cases of sudden, extreme noise exposure from impulse noise, the slow onset of HL through reduced hearing threshold levels typically lasts many tens of years. This means exposed individuals progressively adapt their behavior, before they realize they actually have a HL. Any communication difficulties arising from the loss are more likely to be experienced by family and friends before the affected individuals themselves.

The experience of HL after exposure to years of noise at work is sufficiently well understood as to be the subject of an International Standard (ISO 1999:2013), whereby an estimate of the expected HL (reduced threshold levels) can be assessed against a set of predictable population-based normative values. (Note: These results can only be applied to the population and not to the individual.) This Standard has an important place in the Workers' Compensation assessments in many jurisdictions around the world. The dose–response of noise exposure to HL is low for small exposures to noise but increases rapidly for increasing exposure levels over the first few years and then shows signs of a saturation effect if high levels of exposure continue for many years.

The Audiogram

The audiogram is regarded as the first evidence concerning hearing health. By definition, the situation of no HL is represented by a line on the audiogram with all points on or above 0 dB HL. Anything below 0 dB HL represents a HL. As part of a hearing health assessment, individual variation may show departures from 0 dB HL with the test and measurement process also introducing variations. Hence, *losses* of up to 15 or 20 dB may be assessed as normal or not significant.

As an individual ages, so does his or her hearing (presbyacusis). Hearing sensitivity starting with the higher frequencies begins to decline. It is as if the treble control is being turned down. From the perspective of an audiogram, the flat line starts to sag from the high frequencies (on the right-hand side) starting around 8 kHz (usually the highest measured frequency), then slowly progressing leftward along the curve to the lower frequencies. The rate of decline is dependent on age and sex.

N-IHL is frequently exacerbated by exposure to ototoxic chemicals such as organic solvents, heavy metals, and some therapeutic drugs. The effect may be synergistic or additive depending on the chemicals involved. Ototoxicity is an area requiring greater research and clarification since there is limited knowledge of specific dose–response effects. The main characteristic of ototoxic effects are early audiometric losses at high frequencies (i.e., 8 kHz and above).

The Noise Notch and Noise Exposure

In the literature concerning N-IHL, there will frequently be reference to the *noise notch*. This notch was thought to become apparent because the rate of decay of the frequencies in the range 4–6 kHz appeared to occur at a greater rate than that at 8 kHz, when individuals were exposed to long-term noise. This leads to a dip or notch in the audiogram in the 3–8 kHz region. Originating from work in industrial areas, this notch has often been regarded as a characteristic of long-term noise exposure. The location of the notch will vary among individuals, and for some individuals, even after many years of exposure, a notch may not be evident. The notch is a statistical construct and does not apply to the individual. While it may be observed in some groups and individuals, the literature is not clear that the notch is a defining characteristic as evidence or nonevidence of noise exposure. For example, in several comprehensive reviews of the literature, there is no universal agreement on how to define the notch, and as of 2018, there is no computerized algorithm that can reliably do so. Even experienced professionals may differ in their assessment. The clearest way to understand the state of an individual's hearing health is a detailed history of his or her workplace and leisure noise exposure.

Prevention of N-IHL

The prevention of N-IHL is as simple as the reduction, or preferably elimination, of noise exposure through a hierarchy of controls from the elimination of the noise through exposure control measures including buy-quiet purchases, administrative controls, engineering noise controls, and the use of personal protective equipment (PPE). In the late 1990s, the workplace methodologies to reduce noise exposure were addressed by the term *hearing conservation programs*. The stumbling block of the hearing conservation approach was that it tended to concentrate on regular workplace audiometry and the use of PPE (i.e., earplugs and earmuffs) rather than the minimization or elimination of the noise source(s). As a consequence, hearing conservation programs tended to simply document the progressive loss of hearing and noncompliance of individuals to wear their hearing protectors. Even with the use of electronic technology, ensuring individuals comply with PPE programs is very difficult.

The contemporary approach to workplace noise as a potential hearing health hazard concentrates on *occupational noise management* programs, where the elimination of the noise is of primary importance and the use of PPE is seen as the solution of last resort since it involves behavioral change, which is difficult even under the best of circumstances. Hearing-health promotion programs have traditionally focused on intrapersonal level training such as education about the process of N-IHL and the ability to adequately fit and use hearing protectors. Research suggests that multilevel interventions are important. Such interventions address the *social ecology* of the system including the intrapersonal but also interpersonal (looking out for other workers), organizational (managers encourage good behavior), cultural (broader awareness of hearing-loss and the devastating effect it has), and policy (laws and regulations).

Hearing Protectors

Even though the use of hearing protectors to reduce noise exposure is considered a last resort, hearing protectors can and do have an effective role to play in reducing the harmful effects of noise exposure. It must always be remembered that when hearing protectors are worn, the individual is still exposed to the noise, albeit in a state of *protected exposure*, and the other harmful effects, such as fatigue and distraction, may still occur. The biggest difficulty with hearing protectors, plugs, or muffs is the variability in attenuation. This variability is due to factors such as inter- and intraindividual variations in anatomy, device aging (i.e., wear and tear), device fitting skill, and protectors becoming dislodged during active work. All are factors that can impair effectiveness.

There are many different hearing protector *rating* systems in use around the world. These were usually developed regionally but share basic common characteristics. All are based on the subjective, laboratory testing of groups of hearing protector users under controlled conditions and are intended to indicate the devices' expected performance in the field and account for possible variations among and between users. It must be remembered that this means that the performance figure is a statistical measurement and represents the expected performance (i.e., attenuation of noise-related damage) and hence does not represent the performance for an individual. This uncertainty in individual performance represents one of the greatest difficulties in trying to predict the noise exposure for individuals using hearing protectors to control their exposure to noise.

The most commonly seen hearing protector rating systems include:

Single Number Rating: most common in Europe;

Noise Reduction Rating: originally a single number rating (U.S. based) but later extended into a more detailed presentation of hearing protector attenuation information, now quite complex if fully utilized;

SLC$_{80}$—Sound Level Conversion: a single number system used in Australia and New Zealand designed to provide the attenuation expected to be provided for 80% of hearing protector wearers;

Class System: a five-category rating system designed to simplify hearing protector selection into five noise exposure ranges, extensively used in Australia and New Zealand;

High–Medium–Low: a three-number system, common in Europe, provides three attenuation estimates for *high frequency* noise, *medium frequency* noise, and *low frequency* noise, to match the characteristics of the noise spectrum of interest; and

Octave Band Method: similar to the *High–Medium–Low* but intended to match the attenuation of the hearing protector to the acoustic spectrum of hazardous noise by providing attenuation values in seven appropriate octave bands, more complex to apply, utilized worldwide.

All of the above rating systems have their characteristic advantages and disadvantages. They are all an approximation of what the individual user can expect to achieve in practice. Except for the Octave Band method, there is no universally agreed hearing protector rating system. (For those interested in the hearing protector rating system that applies in their jurisdiction of interest, they should find further details from a specialized source.)

Some rating systems require a minimum attenuation rating. The use of hearing protectors is usually mandated when the noise exposure equals or exceeds a declared limit, such as an equivalent A-weighted, free-field level (L_{Aeq}) of 85 dB for 8 hr ($L_{Aeq,8h}$). However, the attenuation rating is usually applied to the C-weighted, unprotected, exposed, free-field noise level in order to estimate the expected A-weighted equivalent, free-field noise exposure experienced by the individual when wearing the protectors. It is also quite common for the use of hearing protectors to be required, when the L_{Aeq} equals or exceeds 85 dB irrespective of the time the L_{Aeq} remains greater than the 85 dB.

Warwick Williams and David Welch

See also Anatomy of the Hearing Mechanism and Central Audiology Nervous System; Deaf Culture; Diagnostic Audiological Assessment; Hard of Hearing; Hearing Disability and Disorders

Further Readings

Berger, E. H., Royster, L. H., Royster, J. D., Driscoll, D. P., & Layne, M. (2000). *The noise manual* (5th ed.). Fairfax, VA: American Industrial Hygiene Association.

Dobie, R. A. (2015). *Medical-legal evaluation of hearing loss* (3rd ed.). San Diego, CA: Plural.

Goelzer, B., Hansen, C. H., & Sehrndt, G. A (Eds.), (2001). *Occupational exposure to noise: Evaluation, prevention and control*. Dortmund, Germany: Federal Institute for Occupational Safety and Health (Geneva, Switzerland: World Health Organization).

International Organization for Standardization 1999:2013. (2013). *Acoustics—Estimation of noise-induced hearing loss*. Geneva, Switzerland: International Organization for Standardization.

International Organization for Standardization 7029:2017(E). (2017). *Acoustics—Statistical distribution of hearing thresholds as a function of age and gender*. Geneva, Switzerland: International Organization for Standardization.

Kujawa, S. G., & Liberman, M. C. (2009). Adding insult to injury: Cochlear nerve degeneration after "temporary" noise-induced hearing loss. *Journal of Neuroscience, 29*(45), 14077–14085. doi:10.1523/jneurosci.2845-09.2009

Nondahl, D. A., Shi, X. Y., Cruickshanks, K. J., Dalton, D. S., Tweed, T. S., Wiley, T. L., & Carmichael, L. L. (2009). Notched audiograms and noise exposure history in older adults. *Ear and Hearing, 30*(6), 696–703.

Sataloff, R. T., & Sataloff, J. (1987). *Occupational hearing loss*. New York, NY: Marcel Dekker.

Nonlinear Phonology

Nonlinear phonology encompasses a number of theoretical perspectives on the organization of phonological (i.e., speech) systems. Phonological theories prior to the mid-1970s focused on speech sounds or segments (i.e., consonants and vowels) as they occur in contiguous *linear* sequences made up of a single line of discrete nonoverlapping elements. However, it became clear that some phonological features (e.g., high or low tone or place of articulation) last for longer or shorter periods than a single segment and that segments are grouped into higher units such as syllables; both of these properties cause problems for *linear* theories. Nonlinear phonological theories in contrast posit multiple lines of elements that last for different periods of time that are shorter (e.g., the feature [Labial]) or longer (e.g., syllables and feet). Elements on each line or *tier* are independent of elements on other tiers, but they are linked together in such a way that some elements occur at the same point in time, while others occur in sequence. Nonlinear phonology has led to a very different way of viewing assimilation, dissimilation, consonant deletion, and position in the word, among other things. Since the late 1980s, clinical applications of nonlinear theories have provided evidence-based frameworks for analyses of phonological systems as they pertain to goal setting and strategies for intervention. Independent of nonlinear phonology, but assuming many of its tenets, constraint-based theories (such as Optimality Theory) have further enhanced explanation and description of phonological patterns. This entry provides an overview of constraint-based nonlinear phonological perspectives and clinical application.

Overview of Nonlinear Phonology

In the 19th and early 20th centuries, phonologists noted alternations in speech sound systems. For example, plurals in English can be pronounced as [s], [z], or [əz], depending on the final consonant of the singular form: *cat/cats* [kʰæt + s], *dog/dogs* [dɑg + z], and *bus/buses* [bʌs + əz]. Structuralist theories (of Jan Baudouin de Courtenay, Ferdinand de Saussure, Nikolai Trubetzkoy, and Roman Jakobson) started to account for such alternations by positing distinctions between the pronunciation of a speech sound and its more abstract *underlying* form, the *phoneme*, an indivisible composite of smaller units (i.e., features). These features reflected a phoneme's place of articulation in the vocal tract, its manner of articulation (e.g., sound class as stop, fricative, nasal), and voicing (i.e., presence or absence of laryngeal vibration). Thus, in the preceding English examples, words ending in voiceless stops (or certain fricatives; e.g., [t] or [f]) generally showed plural [s]; words ending in most voiced consonants (e.g., [d], [n], [v]) showed plural [z]; but words ending in other sibilants (e.g., [s], [z], [ʃ]) showed plural [əz]. By assuming that one form was the base form (in this case /z/) and that others reflected influences of contiguous segments, such patterns could be explained. However, linear theories cannot account for all phonological patterns. Consider Labial Harmony in child phonology, such as where the English word *tip* is pronounced *pip*; the feature (Labial) in the word-final consonant is assimilated onto the word-initial consonant, skipping over the vowel in between, and linear theories do not account for the characteristics of such phenomena very well. Furthermore, there are iterative patterns; for example, a tone can spread to a long string of vowels following the original location of the tone. John Goldsmith and others in the 1970s and 1980s developed phonological theories that they called *autosegmental* (with each feature having segmentlike properties) or nonlinear (though *multilinear* is more accurate). These theories posit that phonology is organized hierarchically. Elements at one level of the phonological hierarchy are independent domains with their own set of conditions and operations. The elements in one domain can be associated with (i.e., link to) elements on other *tiers* (i.e., levels) in the system that are not necessarily neighbors on the surface. In a case such as *pip* for *tip*, the consonants can be considered contiguous neighbors for consonant place because the intervening vowel has only vowel place features and so can influence one another.

The phonological hierarchy comprises, starting at the lowest level, phonological features, with progressively larger *higher* units: the segment, syllable, foot, prosodic word, and prosodic phrase (see Figure 1).

Starting at the level of phonological features, phonologists posit slightly different sets of features and groupings. Table 1 shows feature-consonant correspondences for English, based on Bernhardt and Stemberger's 1998 publication

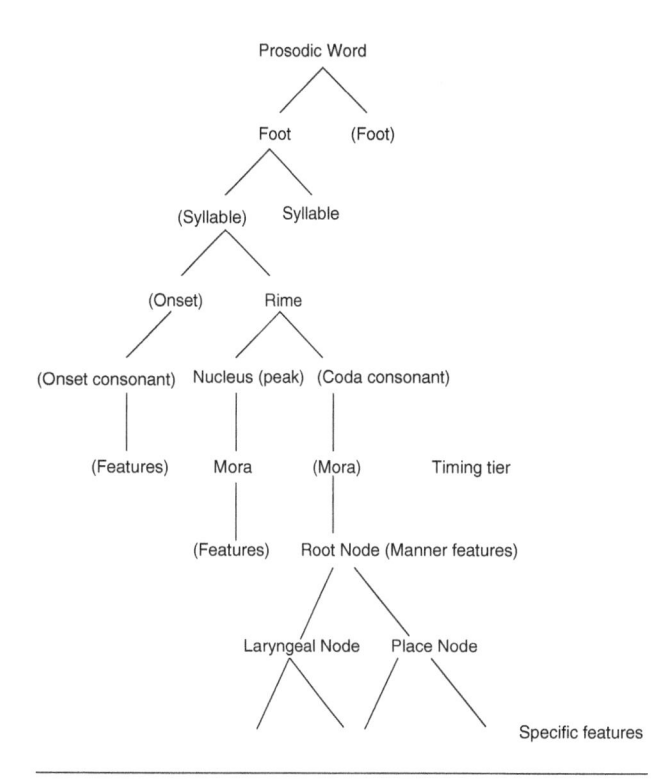

Figure 1 Phonological hierarchy

Handbook of Phonological Development. Feature geometry assumes a set of *grouping* nodes (i.e., Root, Laryngeal, and Place), around which more specific features are organized. The Root node links all features to the prosodic structures above; the Root node essentially creates the segment. Manner features are associated directly with the Root. The Laryngeal node subsumes the voicing features [voiced], [spread glottis], and [constricted glottis]. The Place node dominates the major place features ([Labial], [Coronal], [Dorsal], and arguably [Pharyngeal]), which in turn dominate more specific features; for example, [Coronal] dominates [anterior], distinguishing dental and alveolar consonants such as [s] from consonants produced with the tongue tip or blade farther back, such as [ʃ]. Each segment (consonant C or vowel V) is a composite of independent manner, place, and laryngeal features as seen in Table 1.

Early nonlinear theories posited that each segment has its own *timing unit* (which gives it a basic duration), with long vowels or consonants having two timing units, and some segments (such as in short diphthongs in some languages) sharing one timing unit (and so being quite short). These

Table 1 Feature-Consonant Correspondences in English

		Adult target features	English adult consonant
Manner		Glides: [–consonantal] ([+sonorant])	j w ɹ h ([ʔ])
		Flap [+consonantal] [+sonorant]	ɾ
		Liquid: [+lateral]	l
		Nasals: [+nasal]	m n ŋ
		Stops: [–continuant] (& [–nasal])	p b t d k g ([ʔ])
		Fricatives: [+continuant] (& [–sonorant])	f v θ ð s z ʃ ʒ
		Affricates: [–continuant]-[+continuant]	tʃ dʒ
Place		Labial	p b m f v w (ɹ)
		[+labiodental]	f v
		Coronal [+anterior]	t d n ɾ θ ð s z l
		[–anterior]	ʃ ʒ tʃ dʒ ɹ j
		[+grooved]	s z ʃ ʒ tʃ dʒ
		[–grooved]	θ ð
		Dorsal	k g ŋ j w (ɹ)
		Coronal-Labial (onset)	ɹ
Laryngeal		[–voiced]	p t k f θ s ʃ tʃ
		[+voiced] (stops and fricatives)	b d g v ð z ʒ dʒ
		[+spread glottis]	h pʰ tʰ kʰ f θ s ʃ tʃ

timing units correspond to slots in Gary Dell's connectionist model and in Peter MacNeilage's frame/content theory. They are referred to in child phonology as *wordshapes* and written CVC (*red*), CCVC (*bread*), CVVC (*ride*), CVCV (*yucky*), and so on. They are useful for highlighting, for example, the potential competition between the /s/ and /p/ of *spot* if only one consonant is allowed in the onset. Nonlinear theories since the 1990s posit that only some segments have timing units, referred to as *moras*: vowels (one mora for short, two for long), long consonants (one extra mora), and at least in some languages (including English), the first consonant in a coda (i.e., consonants of a syllable following the vowel).

Timing units (or moras and nonmoraic Root nodes) are grouped into syllables, which are made up of an obligatory nucleus (the most prominent unit, usually a vowel), an optional (but usually present) onset (one or more syllable-initial consonants), and an optional (and often missing) coda (one or more syllable-final consonants). The nucleus and optional coda form the *rime* of the syllable.

Syllables are grouped to form feet, which have different patterns of prominence. A left-prominent (trochaic) foot is stressed on the first syllable (e.g., *BA*-ker, *BAL*-co-ny), a center-prominent (amphibractic) foot on the middle syllable (e.g., pe-*TU*-nia), and a right-prominent (iambic) foot on the final syllable (e.g., ba-*ZAAR*). In some languages, words can have more than one foot. English words with two feet can be right prominent (e.g., *KAN*-ga-*ROO*) or left prominent (e.g., *HE*-li-*COP*-ter), with the less-prominent foot containing *secondary* stress.

Just as timing units can have varying impacts in the system (weighted or not weighted), it has been observed since the 1930s (most notably by the Russian linguist Nikoloai Trubetzkoy) that the relative status of similar elements may differ. In nonlinear phonology, the assumption of hierarchical organization implies that certain elements will be more dominant than others due to their very position in the hierarchy, for example, manner features versus specific place features. In addition, frequent elements may be considered *unmarked* or act as *defaults* and less frequent (or more complex) elements marked or nondefaults. In terms of structural forms, unmarked elements include monosyllabic words or left-prominent (trochaic) disyllabic words, singleton consonants and vowels (vs. clusters or diphthongs), nuclei, and onsets (vs. codas). Thus, in English, a CV syllable or word and a CVcv word are considered the least marked forms. Marked or nondefault elements include codas, clusters, and right- or center-prominent feet. Thus, a word such as *prepare* (ccvCVC) contains a number of marked characteristics. At the feature level, languages can differ in markedness/default status, although stops are generally the default manner category; [Coronal, + anterior] (dental or alveolar place) the default place and [-voiced] [-spread glottis] (voiceless unaspirated) the default laryngeal values; in most languages, [t] would be the default consonant.

Developmentally, unmarked defaults often appear early in children's phonologies, with more marked elements appearing later. However, individual children may produce more marked elements before less marked ones, depending on individual learning paths or input frequencies; for example, a child may show [ka] as the default syllable or split one segment into two segments as a less common way of realizing multiple features within a segment, for example, changing a word-final /d/ to [nt] by shifting [+voice] from the stop and creating a nasal consonant to carry the voicing.

As in linear theories, nonlinear phonology continues to assume that elements that are immediate neighbors (adjacent elements) can affect each other in phonological alternations (as seen for the preceding English plurals). Elements group together in certain ways across the hierarchy, however, and these groups can act as units in phonological patterns. For example, all features dominated by the (Oral) Place node may be deleted, yielding a *placeless* consonant either [h] (if the target consonant is [+continuant]) or [ʔ] (if the consonant is [-continuant], or as a general default). Further, patterns at individual levels may or may not affect or be affected by patterns at other levels. For example, if a syllable is deleted, generally what is below that level will also be deleted, for example, *basket* /ˈbæːskət/ as [ˈbæː]. Alternatively, deleted content at one level may become linked elsewhere (move) either in whole or part: for example, *tip* as [pɪ], where the [Labial] feature of the deleted word-final stop remains and migrates to the word-initial stop (replacing the target feature [Coronal]); or *basket* as [gæ], where the /k/ of the deleted syllable replaces the word-initial /b/. A feature such as [Labial] is independent of the segment in which it originally appeared, and a segment such as /k/ is independent of the syllable in which it originally appeared. Nonlinear phonology accounts for such migration of segments or features because elements on each individual level of representation (e.g., the Labial tier) can act independently of the elements in the same segment on other tiers. Some patterns reflect hierarchical organization, and others reflect the autonomy of individual elements. It has also been noted that elements in *weak* (i.e., marked, less frequent) positions may develop later; a child may have mastered affricates or consonant clusters in the onsets of stressed syllables in words such as *jail* and *crate*, while not yet being able to produce them in the onset of word-initial unstressed syllable such as *giraffe* and *create*.

Constraints and Phonological Patterns

Prior to the positing of phonological constraints, alternations were described with rules or processes. Constraint-based theories, however, especially Optimality Theory, posit that output (i.e., pronunciation) alternations result from competition between phonological constraints. The concept of competition is closely related to principles within connectionist models of language processing. In connectionist models, the various domains of language (i.e., phonology, morphology, syntax, semantics, discourse) and cognition (e.g., attention, memory) interact in a system, where an equilibrium must be established between activated elements. Early in development, elements that have a high activation level (including high-frequency elements) may be accessed, at a time where elements of low activation (including low-frequency elements) are often not accessed. Inaccessible target elements may simply disappear or may be replaced by more accessible elements. Hence, children use shorter and less complex structures (e.g., one syllable rather than two; C rather than CC) and less marked segments (e.g., stops rather than fricatives). Optimality Theory encodes accessibility in terms of a conflict between faithfulness constraints (which require that lexically specified elements must be produced) and markedness constraints (which rule out marked elements); if faithfulness is ranked higher, an element is accessible; if markedness is ranked higher, an element is inaccessible and may be replaced by a more accessible, higher frequency, less marked element. In both connectionist and optimality approaches, as activation levels or rankings are altered to more closely match the adult system, first there is variability between old and new child forms, which gradually stabilizes as the new form; different elements in the adult pronunciation may be mastered at different times. This view interacts with nonlinear phonology in a number of ways. Early systems may have extreme limitations on complexity at hierarchical levels above the segment (e.g., only CV syllables are possible or only one stressed syllable [i.e., foot]); this may lead to deletion or migration or two competing consonants coalescing into a new segment (e.g., /sp/ as [f], combining [+continuant] from /s/ and [Labial] from /p/). Early systems may also have extreme limitations on what features are accessible, leading to the deletion of specific features independent of other features in the segment and possibly the assimilation or insertion of other features. For example, if the feature [Dorsal] is not possible, but a single onset consonant cannot be deleted, then *keep* /ki:p/ may surface as [tʰi:p], with the feature [Dorsal] deleted and the highly accessible unmarked place features [Coronal, +anterior] filled in; or it may surface as [pʰi:p], with [Labial] assimilated from the word-final consonant. In rule- or process-based analysis, this would be *Velar Fronting* or *Labial Harmony*, terms which (originally) implied active manipulation of form, rather than a more passive output, due to the interaction of the impossible with the possible, based on what must occur (a segment where one is lexically specified), what cannot occur (dorsals), and what can easily occur (coronals and labials). Depending on the relative importance of the various constraints in the system, a number of outputs are possible for a given input. If an onset consonant can be deleted (lower activation), and [Dorsal] is impossible, an alternative production of *keep* could be [i:p], which has the advantage of not outputting anything that is not present in the adult pronunciation, at the cost of losing manner and voicing features that the child has mastered. Such *non-minimal repairs* occur at a fairly low frequency in child speech.

Assessment and Intervention

The clinical application of nonlinear phonology encompasses both assessment and treatment. Assessment involves sufficient elicitation of words whose pronunciations span all aspects of the phonological system of the adult language (both single-word and connected speech), from the feature up to the prosodic phrase. Analysis identifies both strengths and needs across the phonological system (high activation/low activation and high faithfulness/high markedness) for word structures (i.e., word length, feet, stress, syllables, and timing units [e.g., CV sequences]) and segments and features by word and stress positions. Particular attention is paid to the possible influences of foot and syllable structure strengths and needs on segment production. Some clients may show needs primarily in prosodic structure, and others primarily in individual segments or features. Others may show needs across the phonological system but still have certain strengths somewhere in the phonological hierarchy. An intervention plan is devised that exploits strengths at one or more levels of the system to address needs elsewhere in the system. Thus, new segments and features are addressed in existing word structures and vice versa. Generally, both word structure and segment/feature goals are considered for goal selection, with nondefaults giving priority as targets where possible. Research studies, including those by Barbara Bernhardt, Susan Rvachew, Daniel Bérubé, and Angela Ullrich, have confirmed the utility of nonlinear phonology in assessment and intervention. Generally, studies have shown faster gains in word structure development (higher level form) than specific feature development, confirming the influence of hierarchical structure.

*Barbara May Bernhardt and
Joseph P. Stemberger*

See also Connectionist Models; Optimality Theory; Phonological Disorders; Phonological Treatment; Phonology; Speech Sound Disorders

Further Readings

Bernhardt, B. (1990). *Application of nonlinear phonological theory to intervention with six phonologically disordered children* (unpublished PhD thesis). University of British Columbia, Vancouver, BC Canada.

Bernhardt, B., & Stemberger, J. P. (1998). *Handbook of phonological development: From the perspective of constraint-based nonlinear phonology.* San Diego, CA: Academic Press.

Bernhardt, B. M., & Stemberger, J. P. (2015). University of British Columbia (free tutorials and test materials). Retrieved from phonodevelopment.sites.olt.ubc.ca

Bernhardt, B. M., Stemberger, J. S., & Charest, M. (2010). Speech production models and intervention for speech production impairments in children. *CJASLPA, 34,* 157–167.

de Lacy, P. (2007). *Cambridge handbook of phonology.* Cambridge, UK: Cambridge University Press.

McCarthy, J. J. (1989). Linear order in phonological representation. *Linguistic Inquiry, 20,* 71–99.

Nonpulmonic Consonants

Whereas most consonants in natural language are produced on a pulmonic egressive airstream, there are nonetheless some classes of consonants that are produced using other airstreams. All of these classes are also attested in speech sound disorders even from speakers of languages where nonpulmonic consonants are not found as target sounds. This entry provides an overview of the main classes of nonpulmonic sounds and their presence in disordered speech.

Classes of Nonpulmonic Sounds

There are three main classes of nonpulmonic sounds in natural language: ejectives, implosives, and clicks. These are produced using two different initiators: the glottalic and the velaric. The glottalic initiator uses the upward or downward movement of the larynx with a closed or partially closed glottis to alter the sub- or supraglottal air pressure, thus causing an inward or outward flow of air. The velaric initiator uses air trapped between the tongue and the palate, set into motion by altering oral air pressure through a downward and backward movement of the tongue releasing the trapped air.

As can be seen by these descriptions, only small amounts of air are used by these initiators; thus, languages where nonpulmonic sounds occur use them as single sounds set in syllables, where the neighboring sounds are pulmonic egressive, for example, [iːk͡ǃáːk͡ǃa] *iqaqa* "polecat" (Zulu), where [k͡ǃ] is an alveolar click.

Ejectives

Ejectives are made on a glottalic egressive airstream. The extrinsic laryngeal muscles move the larynx upward and, if the glottis is closed (i.e., the vocal folds are tightly shut), this will cause an increase in air pressure in the supralaryngeal vocal tract, thus causing the amount of air in the supralaryngeal tract to flow outward. As the glottis is closed, only voiceless consonants can be produced on this airstream. The main obstruent types—oral stops, fricatives, and affricates—can all be produced as ejectives. Ejectives are comparatively common in natural language, occurring in languages of Africa and Asia and in Native American languages (among others). The following examples are all taken from Amharic (a language of Ethiopia): [tʼərrəgə] "he swept," where [tʼ] is an ejective stop; [sʼafə] "he wrote," where [sʼ] is an ejective fricative; and [tʃʼərrəsə] "he finished," where [tʃʼ] is an ejective affricate. As can be seen from the examples, ejectives are transcribed by adding an apostrophe after the relevant symbol. It is not unknown for English speakers to use ejectives for target voiceless plosives utterance finally when emphasizing a word. Also, speech–language pathologists have a tendency to use ejectives when modeling a target [k] in isolation, for example.

Implosives

Implosives are to some extent the reverse of ejectives. The extrinsic laryngeal muscles jerk the larynx downward, thus causing negative pressure in the supralaryngeal tract and therefore an ingressive airflow. However, such *reverse ejectives* are faint sounds and occur rarely in natural language. They can be transcribed by [ɓ, ɗ, ʄ, ɠ, ʛ], although the International Phonetic Alphabet now only recognizes the use of the voiceless diacritic added to implosive symbols [ɓ̥, ɗ̥, ʄ̊, ɠ̊, ʛ̥]. Implosives (as opposed to these reverse ejectives) are voiced. This comes about because the vocal folds are not held tightly shut in the production of implosives, and some of the pressurized subglottal air from the lungs leaks through the descending glottis causing vocal fold vibration. Thus, implosives are hybrid sounds in terms of the airstream mechanism: partially glottalic ingressive and partially pulmonic egressive. In natural language, only stoplike consonants occur as implosives; they are transcribed with the following symbols: [ɓ, ɗ, ʄ, ɠ, ʛ]. Implosives occur in several languages of Africa, India, South East Asia, and the Amazon basin. The following examples both come from Lendu (a language of the Democratic Republic of Congo): [ɓ̥àɓ̥à] "attached to," where [ɓ̥] is a voiceless bilabial reverse ejective, and [ɠð] "follow," where [ɠ] is a voiced velar implosive.

Clicks

Clicks are made on a velaric ingressive airstream. The back of the tongue forms a contact with the velum, and there is another contact further forward. If the body of the tongue is moved downward, the air trapped above it is rarefied so, when the articulatory stricture is released, air moves inward to equalize the intraoral pressure. Because clicks are made within the oral cavity, other airflows can co-occur. Thus, for example, clicks can be produced with concomitant nasal airflow (both ingressive and egressive), with voiced phonation, with aspirated or affricated release, among several others. Khoi-San languages of southern Africa and some southern Bantu languages, namely Zulu and Xhosa, are the only languages that use clicks linguistically, though speakers of many languages may use some clicks extralinguistically to express annoyance or encouragement. The International Phonetic Alphabet symbols of clicks are [ʘ, ǀ, ǃ, ǂ, ǁ] for bilabial, dental, alveolar, postalveolar, and lateral, respectively. Some click accompaniments are shown as follows (plain, nasal, voiced, and aspirated): [k͡ǃ, ŋ͡ǃ, ɡ͡ǃ, k͡ǃʰ], although it is also possible to transcribe the click symbol first in these combinations.

Disordered Speech

All of these nonpulmonic sounds have been reported in disordered speech. Ejectives of different types (i.e., stops, fricatives, affricates) have been reported in the speech of persons who stutter, of people with hearing impairment, and of cochlear implant users. These last two populations have also been reported as using implosives, although voiceless implosives (termed here reverse ejectives) have been reported in the speech of three clients with cleft palate.

Clicks are perhaps the most commonly reported nonpulmonic sounds in disordered speech. They have been reported in the speech of those with repaired cleft palate and other forms of velopharyngeal incompetence, the speech of a child with Down syndrome, and as an unusual example of phonological disorder.

It is important that speech–language pathologists are able to recognize and describe nonpulmonic consonants and be aware that remediation involves a change of airstream mechanism, not just place and manner of articulation.

Martin J. Ball

See also Articulation (Phonetic) Assessment; Articulatory Phonetics; Atypical Speech Sounds; Consonants; Phonetic Transcription; Pulmonic Ingressive Speech; Speech Sound Disorders

Further Readings

Ball, M. J., & Müller, N. (2005). *Phonetics for communication disorders*. Mahwah, NJ: Erlbaum.

Ball, M. J., & Müller, N. (2007). Non-pulmonic egressive speech sounds in disordered speech: A brief review. *Clinical Linguistics and Phonetics, 21,* 869–874.

Ladefoged, P., & Disner, S. F. (2010). *Vowels and consonants* (3rd ed.). Chichester, UK: Wiley-Blackwell.

Laver, J. (1994). *Principles of phonetics*. Cambridge, UK: Cambridge University Press.

Nonverbal Communication

The term *nonverbal communication* refers to communication effected by means other than words, for example, eye contact, facial expression, or gesture. These nonverbal behaviors can express meaning, and when they do so, they create nonverbal communication.

Nonverbal communication is carried out with varying degrees of control and awareness. When someone gives a thumbs-up gesture or winks, that person is more than likely doing so consciously, having planned to communicate a particular meaning. But nervous mannerisms and unguarded facial expressions usually happen outside a person's awareness and control, even though they can also communicate meaning. When awareness and control are high, as in the first example, the nonverbal behavior is done with intention, and so this kind of communication is referred to as intentional.

Intentional communication is when a person communicates with a purpose and with an awareness of the effect on someone else. Although many people would argue that both intentional and unintentional expressions of meaning through nonverbal behavior are instances of nonverbal communication, others would argue that there is a difference between nonverbal communication and nonverbal behavior more generally. The hallmark of nonverbal communication in the latter viewpoint is that it is intentional—the meaning the behavior communicates was intended by the person carrying out the behavior. In this entry, the nonverbal communication being described is intentional behavior. This entry discusses some of the different types of nonverbal communication described in communication research: It outlines the development of nonverbal communication skills in childhood and summarizes the evidence from investigations of nonverbal communication in communication disorders.

Development of Nonverbal Communication Skills

At around 1 year of age, there is significant development in the cognitive and communication abilities of young children. One important development in this period is the acquisition and consolidation of nonverbal communication skills. At this stage, nonverbal skills, such as the capacity to point in order to direct the attention of others, are key abilities that underpin the development of language. The development of nonverbal communication skills is thought to be important to language for two main reasons.

First, these skills appear to reflect core cognitive processes such as representational thought, which is the capacity to picture something in one's mind. Other fundamental cognitive processes underpinning nonverbal behavior include being able to plan movements and sequences of movements, to inhibit other movements, and to adapt planned behaviors in response to the reaction of others. These cognitive processes are part of a set of processes referred to as executive functions. Nonverbal behaviors such as pointing provide evidence that these executive functions are developing even before one sees them being used for language.

Second, the development of nonverbal communication skills reflects the development of core sociocognitive skills, which are the emotional and interpersonal skills needed for processing and applying information about other people and social situations. Nonverbal communication is social behavior; and because nonverbal communication develops before verbal communication, it provides the earliest evidence that a child's sociocognitive skills are developing. It has been argued that the development of nonverbal communication skills results from the application of cognitive capacities to the specific context of problem solving in social interactions. For example, smiling is a very early form of nonverbal communication, and as soon as it is under the awareness and control of the infant, it can be used to solve interpersonal problems such as how to attract and keep the attention of an adult. Pointing is also an early nonverbal behavior, and this can be used to solve problems such as how to communicate the particular object that the child wants even before the child can speak. The social–cognitive processes inherent in nonverbal communication therefore provide a foundation that supports or facilitates subsequent language development.

Types of Nonverbal Communication

Eye Contact, Eye Gaze, and Joint Attention

Eye contact between a newborn child and his or her caregivers begins from the earliest hours of a child's life and continues to be an important source of contact, communication, and development in the first year of life. Initially, the adult leads in this nonverbal behavior, but from around 6–10 weeks, the infant begins to direct his or her gaze more intentionally and can initiate and maintain eye contact with caregivers. From about 8 months of age, a child is able to follow the line of regard of a parent if the adult first establishes eye contact and then turns his or her head. This ability to follow the gaze of another person allows the child to share attention with him or her, for example, to share attention on a particular object. This ability is called joint attention, and it is a crucial foundational ability underpinning language development.

Joint attention is the process of sharing one's experience of observing an object or event, by following gaze or by the use of pointing gestures. At 12 months of age, a child can correctly locate target objects that adults look at, without the clue of a head turn. When both caregiver and infant are looking at the same object and the caregiver names or describes the object, the connection between a sight and a word is established. Also at 12 months of age, children begin to expect joint attention to lead to communicative act. This ability to share joint attention therefore allows a child to match a spoken word to the correct object rather than anything else in the room. Joint attention is a critical nonverbal skill underpinning social, cognitive, and language development.

In the first year of life, children also develop the ability to direct the attention of others, using eye contact, eye gaze (sometimes called eye pointing), and pointing. At 4–5 months of age, infants develop an interest in looking intently at objects and people; when another person notices this attention, it can lead to joint attention between infant and caregiver on the object of interest. As infants develop and extend control over their eye gaze between 5 and 8 months of age, to the point where they can follow the line of regard of other people, they also notice and benefit from the communicative effects of joint attention. As an example, there is evidence to show that children have a basic understanding of repeatedly used words (like *mommy*, *daddy*, *teddy*, *car*, *socks*) even at the young age of 6 months, and this is likely because these are the people and objects that were named or talked about as the child share attention on them with a caregiver. As the child begins to develop control over their own eye gaze, they also begin to use it to not only share joint attention but also to initiate joint attention, for example, by directing an adult's attention to a particular object. This ability to direct the attention of others allows children to set up a situation in which they might hear the word for the desired object and also to nonverbally communicate their desire for it.

Gesture

As well as eye gaze, children learn to direct attention and to communicate using pointing. This is a very important gesture, which children start to use themselves just before their 1st birthday and which is widespread across diverse cultures. It means something like "If you look there, you'll know what I mean" and can therefore be used in an almost infinite variety of communicative situations. Pointing can be used to request an object but can be used to nonverbally communicate more complex meanings as well. For example, pointing toward a door can be used to communicate that child wants to go outside or can be used as a question about where Daddy has gone; or as part of regular morning routine in which Mummy gets ready to leave for work, it can be used to indicate that the child is aware of what happens next.

Although pointing is perhaps the most important gesture for the support of language development, it is only one of a set of nonverbal communicative gestures that emerge between 9 and 16 months of age. At 9 months, children's earliest gestures begin to develop from their actions and the reactions of others. Children first learn to take an object and then, as they develop more control over their hand movements, to release and drop it. They also learn from the experience of a caregiver holding out his or her hand to catch fallen or dropped objects. Through these combined experiences, they learn to give which, alongside directing attention with eye gaze, is often the first intentional nonverbal communicative act.

During this time, children also learn to shake their head to indicate *no*. This behavior most often emerges during mealtimes when children first turn away from food they do not like and then, by looking back to see their caregiver respond by moving the undesired food away, they learn the communicative effect of their action.

Soon after, at around 10 months of age, children learn to communicate through reach. Their reaching behaviors develop from noncommunicative reaching to take an object to the communicative nonverbal behavior of reaching to signal to someone that they want an object and reaching to request to be picked up. As they learn to anticipate the reactions of others, infants will learn to use a reach gesture as a communicative signal. Interestingly, there is evidence to show that there is a particular developmental sequence in the developing of reaching behavior from a noncommunicative action to a nonverbal communication: First, an arm is used to reach for something; then, an arm is used with the open hand facing up, to indicate a request; and finally, two arms are raised to ask to be picked up.

At 11 months of age, children learn to hold up and show objects to get others to look and notice what they're interested in. Children of this age are motivated to share their interests with others, and this showing behavior is an extension of the attention directing communicative behavior they earlier began to develop with eye gaze. They are also motivated by the social experience of greeting in everyday routines where special people are coming and going. They learn that their body movements attract caregiver attention, and as their awareness and control over their body develops, they learn to intentionally use them to greet and to direct attention in other ways. Recognizable greeting behavior begins to emerge between 9 and 11 months of age, with a more fully developed waving gesture developing later.

At 12 months of age, children point with an open-hand point with the fingers spread, and they may also tap with the fingers together as an indicative gesture for drawing the attention of others to objects of interest. At this stage, children's gestures all become more clearly intentional and so can be more definitively categorized as forms of nonverbal communication. As development continues, forms of nonverbal communication expand to also include head nodding, thumbs-up, and hand-up gestures so that at around 15 months of age, children are using gestures as symbols that are like words in the way they communicate meaning. This resembles the ways older children and adults use gesture for nonverbal communication. Gestures are now intentional acts of communication, indicating nonverbally not only what children are thinking about but also that they know they are sharing ideas with others.

There are some interesting links between the development of gesture skills and language development. Research shows that the amount of gestures a child uses at around 1 year of age predicts his or her level of verbal language development at around 3.5 years, and there is also evidence to suggest that encouraging gesture use in children improves their language development. Although gesture and language development are known to occur at the same time, it is not known how these two communication systems interact with one another. Some people think that gesture and spoken language are two separate communication systems and that gesture simply facilitates spoken communication. Others have suggested that gesture and spoken language are part of the same communication system.

Imitation as Nonverbal Communication

Imitation refers to copying behavior, when someone reproduces an action that he or she has observed someone else carry out. Imitation can be used as a form of nonverbal communication and is a feature of child development. Imitation behavior depends on cognitive processing, including the ability to perceive, map, recode, and reproduce observed stimuli, and so a range of skills are thought to be involved, including perceptual and attentional skills, memory, motor planning and execution, and the ability to understand the intentions behind the action that is being copied. The social function of imitation serves the purpose of engaging socially with others in shared activity and allows a child to practice social communicative strategies in interactions with others, for example, by imitating a funny face.

From the research, it is clear, then, that infants gradually learn that other people have thoughts and a focus of attention different from their own, and they gradually increase their ability to share a focus of attention with others. They develop various combinations of looking, moving, gesturing, and vocalizing to assist them in directing another person's attention toward what they are interested in. These attention-directing behaviors become acts of intentional communication and lay the foundation for both nonverbal and verbal communication in later years.

Nonverbal Communication in Communication Disorders

Nonverbal as well as verbal communication falls within the domain of communication disorders and within the scope of practice of speech and language clinicians. Clinicians often use nonverbal methods of communication in their interactions with children and adults with communication disorders in order to maximize the potential for communication. This means using eye contact, eye gaze, pointing, gesture, and imitation alongside verbal communication. Clinicians may use nonverbal communication as a compensatory strategy when the comprehension of nonverbal communication is a strength for someone because it can be used by the clinician and other conversation partners to circumvent limitations in the comprehension of verbal language. Nonverbal communication can also be encouraged as a communication strategy for people, both children and adults, with a language disorder, to compensate for limitations in verbal communication skills. At other times, clinicians may work on remediating difficulties in nonverbal communication itself, when working with people who have difficulty communicating by any means.

Remediation Work for Nonverbal Communication Skills

The direct remediation of nonverbal communication difficulties is appropriate for people with cognitive difficulties that affect their communication skills, for example, children and adults with learning difficulties. Not all people with a learning disability have communication difficulties but the majority do, and around half have significant difficulties with both expressing themselves and understanding what others say. The aim of working to improve both verbal and nonverbal communication is to develop communication skills for independence, choice, inclusion, and individual rights, as well as for the maximization of communicative, social, and cognitive abilities. This aim requires a clinician to consider that the means of communication ensures people can express themselves (and understand when others communicate with them), and that opportunities for communication are addressed. In this context, nonverbal communication skills are specifically recommended or taught. Clinicians are tasked with finding the best ways of helping someone to be a competent, or more successful, communicator and this will often require several different methods of nonverbal communication and incorporate both unaided and aided methods.

There is also evidence that nonverbal communication skills are affected by autism. Children with autism show different patterns of nonverbal communication relative to typically developing children in a number of ways related to their cognitive profile. Young children with autism are more likely to use nonverbal communication to request objects or actions (using reaching gestures) and less likely to use it to direct attention (using eye gaze or using showing or pointing gestures). Conversely, typically developing children over 18 months of age are more likely to use eye gaze and pointing and showing gestures than reaching.

Use of Nonverbal Communication as a Compensatory Strategy

Other groups of people with language disorders benefit from being encouraged to use nonverbal communication as a compensation for their talking difficulties. Examples of such people include children born with speech and language difficulties, and adults who suffer speech and language difficulties following a stroke. Both groups are routinely encouraged to gesture alongside their attempts at talk, as part of their speech and language remediation. The aim is to provide an alternative nonverbal means to convey words or extend utterances.

Interestingly, there is also debate about whether this compensatory process is as straightforward as it seems for people with a language difficulty. As explained previously in this entry, some people have suggested that nonverbal and verbal communication might be part of an integrated system. This would suggest that people with language difficulties might be impaired in both verbal and nonverbal communication. It is also the case that the use of nonverbal communication (e.g., gesture) is a complex skill that requires the integration of social, cognitive, and motor skills, and it may be that people with language difficulties also have related difficulty with some of these skills.

Final Thoughts

Nonverbal communication is the intentional use of nonverbal behavior to convey meaning to someone else. The ability to communicate nonverbally develops in early childhood, ahead of and alongside spoken language development. The foundation for this development is laid by various attention-directing behaviors (e.g., looking, moving, and gesturing) that develop to become acts of intentional communication. There are links between the development of gesture skills and language development that raise questions about how these two communication systems interact with one another. Nonverbal communication is helpful in the remediation of communication disorders, although questions remain about whether nonverbal communication skills can fully compensate for language disorder.

Lucy T. Dipper

See also Aphasia; Attention; Gaze; Language Acquisition; Language Disorders in Children

Further Readings

Caselli, M. C., Rinaldi, P., Stefanini, S., & Volterra, V. (2012). Early action and gesture "vocabulary" and its relation with word comprehension and production. *Child Development, 83*(2), 526–542.

Dipper, L., Cocks, N., Rowe, M., & Morgan, G. (2011). What can co-speech gestures in aphasia tell us about the relationship between language and gesture? A single case study of a participant with conduction aphasia. *Gesture, 11*(2), 123–147.

Feyereisen, P., & Seron, X. (1982). Nonverbal communication and aphasia: A review: II. Expression. *Brain and Language, 16*(2), 213–236.

Goldin-Meadow, S. (2007). Pointing sets the stage for learning language—and creating language. *Child Development, 78*(3), 741–745.

McNeill, D. (2008). *Gesture and thought*. Chicago, IL: University of Chicago Press.

Owens, R. E., Jr. (2015). *Language development: An introduction*. London, UK: Pearson.

Watt, N., Wetherby, A., & Shumway, S. (2006). Prelinguistic predictors of language outcome at 3 years of age. *Journal of Speech, Language, and Hearing Research, 49*(6), 1224–1237.

NORMAL AGING

See Age and Aging

NOUNS AND PRONOUNS

The noun is a word, such as *girl*, *garden*, *diner*, or *chair*, that refers to a class of people, places, events, or things (common noun), or to name a particular thing from these classes (proper noun). It is the most fundamental grammatical category in all languages of the world, together with verbs. The core semantic properties of nouns are similar in all languages. Nouns are mastered by children from the earliest age, and all children with language disorders can use nouns, although they may not be able to master complex noun constructions. The pronoun is a word, such as *you* or *it*, that is used to refer to someone or something. Actually, pronouns are defined as any small set of words that may be substituted for nouns or noun phrases and whose referents are named or understood in the context. A pronoun is a complex and diverse category and contains various subtypes of elements, which are not all present in all languages. The complexity and abstractness of pronouns make them prone to create difficulties in young children's language and in children with language impairment. Although pronouns are strongly related to nouns (as they often, but not always, stand for a noun), their properties are very different from that of nouns. For this reason, this entry clearly separates the presentation of nouns, in the first part, from pronouns, in the second part.

Nouns

Nouns are defined by their form and their meaning (i.e., function), as is the case for all word categories. The dual definition (form and meaning) of nouns underlies widely different linguistic approaches, formalist or functionalist.

Nouns are first defined by their meaning: A prototypical noun is a word that refers to an object or a person. For example:
This is a book. This is Peter.

In these utterances, *book* and *Peter* are nouns. They refer to objects or people in the world. The ability to refer is fundamental to what a noun is. In these examples, *Peter* does not need any more information to be understood: this noun, a proper noun, has a clear unique reference in a given context. *Book*, on the contrary, comes with a determiner *a*. Other determiners can be used, which would induce different meanings, even in the same context. For example, using *the book* instead of *a book* suggests that *the book* refers to a specific book and that *the book* was already known in some way or another.

There are two fundamental types of nouns: proper nouns and common nouns. Proper nouns are names of specific people, places, days, months, and so on. In most cases, they denote unique referents, which makes it possible to avoid the use of any grammatical markers, unlike common nouns. Also, as they are unique, and they are not ambiguous, their grammatical category is lexically defined. Proper nouns can be extended to be used as common nouns, in which case they are accompanied by a determiner such as common nouns. The specific grammatical features of proper nouns are not present in all languages. There are languages where proper nouns have the same syntactic properties as common nouns but different semantic properties.

Common nouns have a generic meaning. They can denote one specific element, several elements, a whole set, a substance, or a quality. To differentiate the various uses, markers can be found on the noun (such as determiners). These markers and the position of the noun in a sentence also define the form of the noun category. Every word that has these markers will be a noun, regardless of whether it refers to an object or a person, or something else.

The fact that nouns can be identified on the basis of the form is fundamental in language because this makes it possible to extend the reference of prototypical nouns to things that are not objects or persons. This explains how it is possible, for example, to extend the meaning of a verb to that of a noun. Another use is that a noun can refer to abstract principles, to actions, to elements in language, to qualities, and to feelings, even when there is no actual thing that can be pointed at, as it is possible for an object or a person. In this case, the notion of reference is maintained, and common agreement within a linguistic community around a shared word form helps to define new meanings and new concepts.

The form of nouns (especially common nouns) is specific to each language, as the way nouns can be marked varies from one language to another. For example, in English, nouns can carry number and are preceded by a determiner and adjectives. There is a different form to mark count nouns and mass nouns. Count nouns are used to refer to elements that can be denoted as individual items, for example, *a book, two books, ten books*. Mass nouns correspond to a substance or quality, for example, *information, some information*, but not *two informations*. In Spanish and French, nouns have gender, but there is no systematic difference between count nouns and mass nouns. In German, nouns carry gender and number, but also case, which indicates the relationship between a noun and the verb it accompanies in an utterance. In Chinese, nouns do not carry any marker but can be accompanied by classifiers similar to those that exist in English for mass nouns. For example,

一本书 (yì běn shū), which means "one book," corresponds to *one (yì) volume (běn) of book (shū)*. The structure is similar to *a loaf of bread* (*of* is not necessary in the Chinese construction), but it is used for all words, not only for mass nouns. There is no specific construction for count nouns in Chinese.

Language Acquisition

Nouns are among the very first words understood and produced by young children. The first two words produced by 8-month-olds are *mommy* and *daddy*, two nouns. In this case, they should be considered as proper nouns. By the time children reach the age of 12 months, words produced by more than 10% of children are either onomatopoeias, interjections, communicators (e.g., *bye, hi, uh, oh, baa baa, yum yum, grrr, woof woof, vroom, night night, ouch, thank you, quack quack, peekaboo*), or nouns (e.g., *mommy, daddy, ball, dog, baby, bottle, kitty, duck, banana, cat, grandma, shoe, bird*). The frequency of nouns in early child vocabularies has been explained by a bias toward whole objects since whole objects and, consequently, names for whole objects (i.e., nouns) are cognitively simpler. The bias found for English-speaking children exists for many other languages. However, there are languages where this bias is not as strong, especially languages where verbs are more frequent and morphosyntactically less complex than nouns (e.g., Korean and Mandarin).

The advantage for nouns also exists when children learn to use words productively with adequate syntax. They are able to do so in English earlier for nouns than verbs.

Pronouns

As the etymology of the word indicates (from Latin *pronomen*: *pro* "stands for," and *nomem* "noun"), pronouns stand for nouns. However, as it is often the case in linguistics, the reality is more complex. There are several sets of pronouns (called *representing pronouns*) that can be used in the place of a noun (called the *antecedent*), which avoids repetition of the noun. For example, "A sparrow is a kind of bird. It can fly." Here *it* refers to *sparrow*. But not all pronouns correspond to a noun. Other pronouns (called *nominal pronouns*) refer to people or objects, but not directly to previous nouns. For example, "I cannot fly." Here *I* refers to the speaker but not necessarily to any previous noun. In this case, pronouns do not represent a noun, but they are used in a syntactic position where a noun phrase can occur and they express meanings that cannot be expressed using nouns. Also, in some cases, pronouns can be used to express a merely formal subject (such as *it* in *it rained*), which is called *impersonal use*.

When taking the place of a noun, pronouns have the same semantic value not only as the noun, but usually as the whole noun phrase. The reference is semantic and preserves the gender and the number (for languages where these categories exist). However, the reference does not take into account the syntactic position of the antecedent. The pronoun will have a syntactic form that is independent from the syntactic form of the antecedent. The pronoun can take the position of any verb argument or any adverbial. This explains why pronouns are often marked for case. For example:

He gives it to him.

He, *it*, and *him* are pronouns. *He* is in the nominative case, *it* in the accusative case, and *him* in the dative case, and here more specifically the recipient. *He* is marked both by the position (before the verb) and lexically (*he* is always nominative). However, *it* and *him* are marked only by their position in the sentence, as they would have other cases if they were in another position in the sentence.

Some pronouns do not refer to nouns. This is the case for the first person (the speaker) and the second person (the addressee). This is also the case in speech when the antecedent is semantically or pragmatically obvious, or when language is accompanied by gesture, pointing, and stance. In these situations, third person pronouns or demonstrative pronouns are used.

Pronouns are traditionally divided into classes according to their syntactic role or their semantic value: personal, possessive, demonstrative, relative, interrogative, and indefinite.

Personal Pronouns

These pronouns refer to the grammatical person (i.e., first person, second person, and third person). In some languages, personal pronouns can have different lexical values depending on their grammatical case. For example, in English, *I* is the first person personal pronoun for the nominative case, whereas *me* is the first person personal pronoun for other cases.

In some languages, there is a subset of personal pronouns, clitic pronouns, which have to be used with a verb as they express the arguments of the verb. For example, this is the case in English for *he*. Other pronouns such as *him* can be used as clitics (e.g., "he thanks him") or independently (e.g., "Who is it? Him!"). In other languages, for example, Spanish, there is no clitic nominative personal pronoun because the verb form contains a marker that refers directly to the subject (which corresponds to the nominative). Thus in Spanish, *hablo* means "I speak" and *I* corresponds to the suffix -o. This form is different from the second person and third person so clitic pronouns are unnecessary to discriminate persons. Clitic pronouns are important as they can create difficulties in language development and in children with language disorders.

Possessive Pronouns

These are pronouns that contain semantic information about something owned by someone or something. For example:

Look at this hat. It is mine.

In this example, *mine* is a possessive pronoun that, as a pronoun, refers to *this hat* and as a possessive pronoun refers to the speaker herself.

Demonstrative Pronouns

These are pronouns with deictic reference, which depends on the context shared by the speaker/writer and the hearer/reader. The reference can be to an object in a conversation or some shared knowledge. For example:

Look! This is a famous painting.

Here *this* is a demonstrative pronoun that refers to an object in the real world or discourse context but not to a noun or an antecedent.

Relative Pronouns

These are pronouns that link and organize relative clauses with respect to the main clause. For example:

This one is *The Mona Lisa*, which is a famous painting.

In English, relative pronouns are *that, which, who, whom, whose,* and the zero form (*that* can be omitted). In English, their syntactic position is to introduce relative clauses. Relative pronouns can have a syntactic function of subject, complement, adverbial, postmodifier, prepositional complement, or object in the relative clause, irrespective of their position as the first word of the clause.

Interrogative Pronouns

These are, in English, similar to the relative *wh*-pronouns, with the addition of *what*. However, they do not refer to an antecedent, but on the contrary they are used for requesting information which was not previously known. This category of pronouns is a good example of the dual role of many pronouns, which is to refer to previous language or to be used in a syntactic position where a noun or a noun phrase can be found and used in this case with semantic values that are more generic than nouns.

Indefinite Pronouns

These pronouns are used to refer to people or things without saying exactly who or what they are, instead of having a specific reference, unlike other pronouns. In English, these pronouns are *everybody, somebody, anybody, nobody,* and similar sets built around *-one, -thing,* and *-where*. Indefinite pronouns are a good example of how pronouns can be used to express new meanings where no specific word (or noun) can apply.

Language Acquisition

There is a lot of variation in the mastery of pronouns in language acquisition because the category contains many elements that vary hugely in terms of phonological complexity, frequency, and grammatical complexity. The main results in the acquisition of pronouns by English-speaking children could be described as follows. When children start to combine words in their second year, they will often use their own name or a term such as *baby* rather than *I* or *me*. This often reflects the way adults speak to the child and is an echo of child-directed speech. The first pronoun used productively is *it*, which is used for objects. The second pronoun used productively is one with first person reference, such as *me, my, mine,* or *I*. Some confusion is observed in the use of pronoun cases, especially for subject pronouns. Similar confusion also occurs for object pronouns; for example, *me, him, her, us,* and *them* can be used even where they are not used by adults. Plural pronouns occur later than singular forms, and second person pronouns occur later than first and third person forms. By age 3, typically developing children produce 71% of correct third person singular forms, and 98% by age 5.

Language Disorders

As for language acquisition, there is a large variety of behavior in children with language impairment when they are handling pronouns. Children with developmental language disorder have considerable difficulties with morphosyntactic markings, complex phonological patterns, and complex grammatical constructions. They are usually efficient when using simple constructions that underlie basic linguistic interactions. For instance, they are usually efficient in using constructions acquired by young children but have difficulties when handling the linguistic structures acquired when children are older. This is confirmed by various research findings on different languages. Weak stressed forms such as subject pronouns are difficult for children with developmental language disorder, as compared to mean length of utterance–matched typically developing children. Not all studies confirmed the existence of difficulties when comparing language-matched children, but the difficulties with personal pronouns were confirmed when comparing age-matched children.

Another example of specific difficulties with pronouns is the case of accusative clitic pronouns in Romance languages. For example, in French-speaking children, the accusative clitic production remained weak long in adolescents with developmental language disorder, no matter what the cause of the developmental disorder was. This suggested that the computation involved in the production of these elements places a particularly heavy load on performance systems. Similar results and explanations are suggested for another Romance language, Portuguese.

*Christelle Maillart and
Christophe Parisse*

See also Adjectives and Adverbs; Determiners; Grammatical Development; Language Disorders in Children; Morphology; Syntactic Disorders; Syntax and Grammar

Further Readings

Baker, M. C. (2003). *Lexical categories: Verbs, nouns and adjectives*. Cambridge, UK: Cambridge University Press.

Croft, W., & Cruse, D. A. (2004). *Cognitive linguistics*. Cambridge, UK: Cambridge University Press.

Gentner, D. (1982). Why nouns are learned before verbs: Linguistic relativity versus natural partitioning. In S. A. K. II (Ed.), *Language development*, vol. 2. Hillsdale, NJ: Erlbaum.

Goldberg, A. E. (2006). *Constructions at work: The nature of generalization in language*. Oxford, UK: Oxford University Press.

Gopnik, A., & Choi, S. (1995). Names, relational words, and cognitive development in English and Korean speakers: Nouns are not always learned before verbs. In M. Tomasello & W. E. Merriman (Eds.), *Beyond names for things: Young children's acquisition of verbs* (pp. 63–80). Hillsdale, NJ: Erlbaum.

Moore, M. E. (2001). Third person pronoun errors by children with and without language impairment. *Journal of Communication Disorders, 34(3),* 207–228.

Tomasello, M., Akhtar, N., Dodson, K., & Rekau, L. (1997). Differential productivity in young children's use of nouns and verbs. *Journal of Child Language, 24,* 373–387.

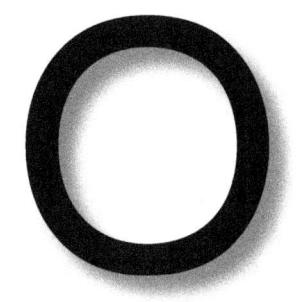

OBSERVATION

In its 21st-century manifestations, observation may be defined as an assortment of methods for systematically collecting; describing; and/or measuring the behaviors, events, and products exhibited in authentic environments. However, observation as a data collection technique is as old as human investigation. As far back as Thales of Miletus in the 6th century BCE, observation was the key to the establishment of the scientific philosophy. The advancement of science was often predicated on observation of nature and, according to the paleontologist and essayist Stephen Jay Gould, the observational format solidified positivism as the epistemological standard in science until the last quarter of the 19th century. A further indication of its influence is the concern researchers have expressed about how to conduct observation. As early as 1775, Jean Senebier published a two-volume book on the art of observation (*L'art d'observer*) and advocated various observational techniques within the natural philosophies; even in the 20th century, there were numerous suggestions in the social sciences instructing students on how to conduct observations of social phenomena.

Viewed from a wide perspective, observation has been touted in three major fields of inquiry: the natural sciences, the social sciences, and the psychological and educational sciences. This entry provides an overview of the role observation plays in these fields and then explores direct observation in particular.

The Natural Sciences and Scientific Observation

The Greek philosophers, particularly Plato and Aristotle, recognized the value of science over mythology, when attempting to explain the world. Crucial to explanation, however, was the observation of the natural world and trying to understand those observations. Even during the time of these Greek philosophers, there was a debate about whether observation was pure and uncompromised or influenced by one's preconceived ideas when interpreting the data; however, the data itself, collected by observation, were taken for granted. Throughout the modern era, observation has been the primary data collection technique when conducting natural science. Whether focusing on the observation of the heavens as in astronomy, the natural world as in biology, or observations of experimental results as in chemistry, the necessary and crucial skill is observation. During the 17th century, the scientific method was formulated and advocated in the natural sciences. Although there is disagreement as to who formulated this method as it is known (Francis Bacon, Johannes Kepler, or Galileo Galilei), observation is crucial to the process, including its five procedural steps: (1) *observing* a phenomenon and asking questions about it, (2) formulating a hypothesis, (3) making predictions about the logical consequences of the hypothesis, (4) testing predictions by experimentation and/or *observational* study, (5) and formulating conclusions based on the data collected. Although these observations may be made using one's own senses or employing various instruments (e.g., telescopes, microscopes, computers) to aid one's senses, *scientific observation* is ubiquitous.

The Social Sciences and Participant Observation

With the rise of the social sciences in the 20th century (especially anthropology and sociology), observation became the premier form of data collection, especially in the form of *participant observation*. As the term suggests, if one enters the targeted context with the intention of both observing what is occurring and participating in (at least) some of the events or activities, even while observing, then it is participant observation. The anthropologist James Spradley discussed six differences between an ordinary participant and a participant observer. First, the participant observer enters the scene with the dual purpose previously mentioned: participating appropriately in the activities in that scene and observing the activities within the scene. Second, unlike the ordinary participant who often engages in activities but who operates without complete conscious awareness, the participant observer is required to be explicitly aware of those things usually blocked out as routine. Third, the participant observer must be oriented to approach the scene and its social actions with a wide-angle lens so that a much broader range of information can be observed. Fourth, rather than experiencing the social situation only in a first-person, subjective manner that makes him or her an insider during any experiences, the participant observer must strive to experience from both the insider (subjective) stance and the outsider (objective) stance. The fifth difference is that while ordinary participants tend not to constantly assess or ponder their experiences, the participant observer must be very introspective about what is occurring and what is observed. In effect, introspection helps the participant become a research instrument due to the degree of reflectivity and attempts to understand the activities at a higher state of awareness. Finally, unlike ordinary participants who act and react and then let observations and emotions dissipate, the participant observer keeps a detailed record of experiences, observations, and emotions. While these records may only be recorded after the fact later in the day, keeping an ethnographic record is essential.

There are other aspects of participant observation, including the types of participation (ranging from passive participation to complete participation) and the progressive use of three different foci during the observations (i.e., descriptive, focused, and selective observations), but this entry will concentrate on the third observational application.

The Psychological/Educational Sciences and Direct Observation

While it is true that the disciplines within this third field of inquiry can (and sometimes do) employ both scientific and participant observation, especially when conducting research, the disciplines more often use several versions of *direct observation*. Defined as observation with a modicum (or absence) of interaction or participation with the events, people, or objects that comprise the setting under investigation, the functions of direct observation are honed to the needs of the pedagogical disciplines. Within direct observation, assessment of an individual, an environment, or an event is one of two major functions; descriptions of educational or remedial events or contexts to determine their effectiveness and to suggest modifications if needed is the second major function. There are numerous terms used to categorize direct observation; regardless of which terms are employed, however, there are two major divisions—*focused observation* and *open observation*.

Focused Observation

Focused observation involves using a well-researched tool that directs the focus of the observation to key behaviors or processes. Also referred to as *systematic* or *structured* observation, as the instruments employed should have well-documented reliability and validity indices, these instruments require: (1) a defined procedure to use during observations, (2) examples or definitions of the key behaviors to anchor the observations to some reference point, and (3) a set way to quantify the phenomena under investigation. For example, as discussed by Paul Yoder and colleagues in *Observational Measurement of Behavior*, the observer can use count-coding (i.e., documenting the occurrence of each instance of a targeted behavior or the duration of each instance) within a set time period while observing communicative interactions; in this process, specific behavioral indices related to communication are the focus of the data collection. The defined indices can be quantified using a straightforward frequency of occurrence or a duration of occurrence, or the indices can be documented using a rating scale, checklist, or protocol format. Examples of focused observational instruments are Bruce Porch's *Porch Index of Communicative Abilities*, Dorothy Bishop's *Children's Communication Checklist*, Mabel Rice's *Social Interactive Coding System*, Carol Prutting and Diane Kirchner's *Pragmatic Protocol*, Jack Damico's *Systematic Observation of Communicative Interaction*, Jenny Gibson and colleagues' *The Manchester Inventory for Playground Observation*, and Reinie Cordier and colleagues' *Pragmatic Observational Measure*.

Open Observation

Open observation is the second division of direct observation. Within this observational scheme, the observer enters the context with limited preconceived ideas about what to observe. That is, the observation is oriented to an open stance so that the behaviors, events, and actions emerge or reveal themselves within the targeted context. Although the observer is guided by a general purpose (e.g., language assessment, documenting adverse reactions, describing teaching strategies), the actual behaviors, actions, or events emerge and are identified and documented through both descriptive statements and some form of quantification (e.g., frequency of occurrence, duration of behavior). Unlike focused observations, the indices of social activity are not predetermined nor is there a set procedure for how the data are collected. Within open observation, the observer can enter the targeted context him- or herself and conduct the observation (primary observer), or he or she can have others collect observations-as-anecdotes (secondary observer).

The anecdotal method proceeds with the investigator or assessor asking individuals involved with the person, event, or actions targeted for observation to simply continue interactions within the observational context, but when that secondary observer notices an experience that *catches their eye* or *grabs their attention*, it directs the observer to document the behavior, usually as an anecdote on a clipboard. After a week of such observation, the investigator and this secondary observer review the anecdotes, and they are expanded to more fully understand what transpired.

When functioning as the primary observer, the investigator enters the observational context and observes with the intention of identifying, describing, and/or quantifying the emergent behaviors or events. This observer typically functions as a passive participant who merely observes and records; consequently, there is the opportunity to write descriptive passages and/or count behaviors within a sampling frame. The observational corpus is then summarized to provide evidence pertaining to the original purpose of the observation.

Tips for Open Observation

From a clinical perspective, the instruments used for focused observations guide the procedural affairs of the observer; these instruments are designed to provide the methodologies for observing in the context(s) of interest. With open observation, the observer can follow general guides that have been designed over time and across the pedagogical disciplines.

- *Let the stated purpose of the observation initially guide your observational frame.*
  Although no predetermined behaviors-as-indices are employed in open observation, the purpose of the observation will help determine what will be observed. For example, for assessment purposes, the concerns of the referral agent should help focus attention during the observation.
- *Engage in careful planning before initiation of the observation.*
  Since authenticity is valued, arrange for the observation to occur in the context(s) of greatest concern and meet with those in charge to ensure that you are unannounced when entering the context and that the activities observed will be as typical and natural as possible.

- *Employ strategies to reduce the potential for the observer's paradox.*
  Since there is a tendency for people to change their behavior when they are observed, don't focus excessively on the target while observing. Rather, employ scanning that enables you to focus on your target, on others for comparison purposes, and on the context and materials that may also play a significant role within the observed social actions. Additionally, observation over several periods of time will help triangulate your results for verification purposes.
- *Collect the observational data so that comparisons can be made.*
  Even in the open observational format, it is often necessary to make comparisons between the targeted individual or event and others so that some sort of anchor to a reference point can be employed. This is especially important during observational assessment, when the target of your observation is evaluated. Within the context of interest, this is not possible unless comparable data is available for others who are considered typical. Additionally, if quantification is employed, there must be a sampling frame to make comparisons across time, opportunities, or turn cycles (e.g., 30 min, 20 turns, 5 pages of text read).
- *Employ procedures that increase the effectiveness and efficiency of your observations, coding, descriptions, and interpretations.*
  When first learning open observation—and as you proceed—allow yourself to fall into comfortable work and coding (even idiosyncratic) patterns that you can easily employ and that place observation as the primary activity. When entering the scene and observing, be flexible so that you allow the data to take you where you need to go and continue to observe until you can see patterns of behaviors or activities emerging. Finally, once you are finished with an observation, verify the representativeness of the observational context with participants (not your target).

Final Thoughts

Observation's long-standing primacy across the various fields of inquiry is a verification of its effectiveness. Just as it has informed the sciences over the centuries as a data collection technique, observation can play a significant role in research and in clinical matters. Well-conceived and implemented observations can provide greater flexibility in data collection and a deeper understanding of the various aspects of human communication sciences and disorders.

Jack S. Damico

See also Anchored Assessment; Descriptive Assessment; Diagnosis of Communication Disorders; Functional Assessment; Pragmatics; Qualitative Research

Further Readings

Bishop, D. V. M. (2003). *The children's communication checklist* (2nd ed.). Oxford, UK: Pearson Assessment.

Damico, J. S. (1992). Systematic observation of communicative interaction: A valid and practical descriptive assessment technique. *Best practices in school speech-language pathology* (Vol. 2, pp. 133–144). San Antonio, TX: ProED.

Daston, L. (2008). On scientific observation. *Isis, 99*(1), 97–110.

Gould, S. J. (2000). The sharp-eyed lynx, outfoxed by nature. In *The lying stones of Marrakech: Penultimate reflections in natural history* (pp. 27–52). New York, NY: Harmony Books.

Hintze, J. M. (2005). Psychometrics of direct observation. *School Psychology Review, 34,* 507–519.

Kawulich, B. (2012). Collecting data through observation. In C. Wagner, B. Kawulich, & M. Garner (Eds.), *Doing social research: A global context.* London, UK: McGraw-Hill.

Prutting, C. A., & Kirchner, D. M. (1987). A clinical appraisal of the pragmatic aspects of language. *Journal of Speech and Hearing Disorders, 52,* 105–119.

Spradley, J. P. (1980). *Participant observation.* New York, NY: Holt, Rinehart, & Winston.

Yoder, P. J., Lloyd, B. P., & Symons, F. J. (2018). *Observational measurement of behavior.* Baltimore, MD: Brookes.

Occupation-Related Dysphonia

Dysphonia is the medical term for disorders of the voice. It is multifactorial, including anatomofunctional, psychoemotional, and environmental aspects. Occupation-related dysphonia is a behavioral voice disorder related to the use of voice at work. The use of voice in professional activities has gained great importance in several occupations, including teaching, acting, singing, and selling, among others. The voice is used to educate individuals, to transmit information, to facilitate learning, and to motivate teams. The lack of vocal training combined with adverse environmental quality may contribute to the development of occupation-related dysphonia. Although there is no consensus regarding which vocal disorders are typically associated with an occupation, the literature suggests that laryngeal tissue reactions, the so-called vocal fold or cords nodules, are benign lesions predominantly associated with working situations. The scenarios that facilitate the appearance of an occupation-related dysphonia are complex, and contributing factors include occupational voice risks, higher than normal voice usage, lack of vocal training, poor room acoustics, and little attention to prevention. Biological, psychological, social, and environmental factors may play different roles and must be considered as causal, and multicenter epidemiological studies need to be developed to obtain reliable causal information. This entry provides an overview of the complexities surrounding the multifaceted nature of occupation-related dysphonia, particularly its effects, assessment, and treatment.

Development of the Human Voice

The human voice is present since birth and develops throughout adulthood. Its full potential is reached between 25 and 45 years of age. Voice is the product of phonation and resonance. The vocal folds are two structures of muscle and mucosa, located inside the larynx, whose vibration produces the basic sound of the voice. This acoustic material is amplified as it travels through the vocal tract from the larynx to the mouth and nose. Combining the vibration of the vocal folds with the resonating cavities of the mouth, nose, and head results in the voice that is heard.

Laryngeal development is a long process that undergoes significant changes during puberty, especially in the males. Similar to all body functions, the larynx and voice also age. The consequences of aging on the voice, known as *presbyphonia*, are unique to each individual and usually perceptible after the age of 60. The vocal quality is based on biological characteristics, and it is influenced by psychological factors, professional demands, environmental conditions, as well as the presence of vocal training.

Voice as Tool and *Abnormal* Voice

The voice is the main tool for several professional activities and may directly impact performance. Teachers, singers, actors, radio announcers, and telemarketers are usually identified as voice professionals. However, aerobics instructors, sport coaches, sales representatives, lawyers, leaders, receptionists, and clergy also rely on optimal voice use. The impact of a voice deviation on the professional performance depends on the vocal quality required. A mild alteration can be devastating for a lyric singer but can easily be managed by a sales representative. There are no objective measures that define what make a voice normal or abnormal. The perception of normalcy is subjective and can be influenced by factors as the culture in which one lives. A binary classification does not exist for voice. In other words, a voice could be perceived as *normal* by a listener even though acoustic and physiological measures and the physical exam might indicate pathology exists. Moreover, a voice could be perceived as *abnormal* despite the absence of laryngeal malfunction. The individual's perception of his or her own voice is influenced not only by the presence of vocal symptoms, such as changes in the sound of voice, but also by the perception of fatigue or discomfort while speaking. Self-evaluation typically uses questionnaires to measure impairment, limitation in daily activities, and even disability. Teachers represent the professional category with the highest occurrence of vocal problems related to work. Their vocal impairment is caused by a complex interaction of factors including long-term voice usage without rest, high vocal intensity, high number of students per class, noisy environment, poor acoustics, and lack of vocal training and often no access to amplification equipment. Also, teachers tend to seek help only when their symptoms are already severe and impact substantially on their teaching activities. Other professionals who need an aesthetically superior voice quality (such as classical singers) or a supranatural voice (as in the case of a radio announcer) usually seek help from health professionals early in the process.

Voice Assessment

Voice assessment is multidimensional and comprises self-perception, auditory perceptual analysis, acoustic evaluation, and laryngeal examination. Laryngeal examination is essential for medical diagnoses. Laryngeal endoscopy can reveal many types of impairments such as those affecting the muscles, tissues, or the neurological system. It may also identify inadequate vocal tract adjustments during voice production. The most common diagnoses associated with occupation-related dysphonia are glottic insufficiency (i.e., inadequate or incomplete glottal closure) and benign mass lesions, such as vocal fold nodules, polyps, or cysts. Following a laryngeal examination, acoustic analysis is done to measure frequency, intensity, harmonics, and noise components. It seeks to quantify deviations in vocal quality and establishes the baseline of an individual. The diagnosis is the result of a complex process that often includes the evaluation by an otorhinolaryngologist (or phoniatrician), the speech–language pathologist, and the occupational physician. Frequently, a clinical diagnosis is not enough to confirm such a condition. Dysphonia related to working conditions is frequently employed as a synonym for occupational dysphonia. However, there is no consensus about this. This diagnostic label is frequently used to refer to voice problems experienced by teachers. Changes in the vocal quality, hoarseness, breathiness, strain, difficulties in vocal projection, vocal tract discomfort, excessive throat clearing, sore throat, irritated larynx, sensible throat, *lump* in the throat, and odynophagia (i.e., pain to phonate) are the main symptoms of a voice problem related to work. These symptoms are not exclusively related to working conditions; however, occupational activities can increase the risk of developing a voice problem.

Risk and Causality

Risk and causality regarding voice disorders at work are more complex than they seem, and there are no clear guidelines available to manage these cases. As mentioned previously, clinical diagnosis in these cases is not enough to attest to the association between occupation and voice disorder. Theoretically, it is the employer's responsibility and duty to prevent such health hazards. Unfortunately, there are no longitudinal or interventional studies attesting to the possibility of vocal risk reduction. Some progress deserves attention, such as the inclusion of vocal fold nodules under the number 2.503 of the European List of Occupational Diseases (see 2.5 Diseases caused by physical agents; 2.503 Nodules on the vocal chords caused by sustained work-related vocal effort). However, other vocal conditions such as fatigue and discomfort during speech production are not listed. Moreover, there is no uniformity regarding systems of evaluation. Financial compensation, when existent, varies from country to country.

Ideally, a teacher should have a pleasant voice, an adequate volume to be heard in a classroom, variable prosody to keep students' interest, and vocal endurance to face long periods of use. Having a healthy voice is especially important, as it relates to the longevity of the career and the students' quality of learning. Children whose teacher has a voice disorder may face learning difficulties. Moreover, individuals with voice problems are generally judged as less competent and reliable, which may impact professional performance, including during job interviews. In the case of telemarketers, the voice is fundamental to effective information transmission and good interaction with clients. Dysphonia in these cases not only affects job performance but also contributes to emotional stress. Since telemarketing is a modern profession, there are many laws and guidelines that take into consideration comfort, safety, health, and performance, including postural approaches, use of phone and microphone, and periods of voice rest during working hours. Health protection of telemarketers is currently more progressive than policies that benefit teachers.

Legal Protection and Reasonable Accommodations

The Americans with Disabilities Act of 1990 is an important document that also deals with the protection of individuals who use their voice at work. Speaking and communicating are listed on the document as major life activities. Therefore, individuals exhibiting vocal difficulties are legally protected in the United States. Even though the majority of voice disorders do not impair such tasks as walking, bending, reasoning, independence, and other major life activities, they can have a disastrous effect on emotional health and professional life for the individual who uses the voice as a main working tool or artistic expression. Economic losses can be huge in the case of artists such as actors and singers.

Professionals with voice problems who do not have adequate working conditions can face many more difficulties than what might be expected. Moreover, such challenges often have a negative effect on their mental health and contribute to the development of common mental disorders. Reasonable accommodations may improve the quality of life. These may include individual amplification systems for teachers and sales professionals, break times for vocal rest, hydration, performing vocal exercises for teacher and telemarketers, and installation of noise reduction panels in noisy areas. Some of these simple changes can improve health and reduce frustration at work.

Even if worldwide research data indicate a commonality regarding voice problems among teachers, there are currently no global public policies to modify this situation. One of the major limitations to the development of protective labor legislation is that voice problems frequently do not prevent the individual from working. Furthermore, vocal fold lesions are not exclusively related to the professional voice use, and they may occur in any situation where the individual has to use his or her voice.

Challenges That Remain

Finally, a voice disorder is usually multifactorial and can include an anatomical predisposition as well as psychoemotional factors, which are not easy to assess. There are differences among countries regarding medical insurance coverage and the guidelines to identify cases of occupation-related dysphonia, to evaluate the impairment, and to financially compensate the individual. Medicolegal assessment is not well structured for voice cases. The variable and sometimes unpredictable progression of some vocal impairments (such as functional and muscle tension dysphonia) often makes the legal assessment even harder and more complex. The role of voice behavior patterns, stress management, coping mechanisms, and self-regulation strategies must be better understood. The majority of nonartistic professional voice users keep working even when they present with a significantly altered voice quality and symptoms of vocal fatigue. Thus, it is more challenging for epidemiologists to track dysphonias related to work.

To prevent occupation-related voice problems, vocal hygiene strategies should be implemented for future professional voice users during their education and training. These include vocal training while in a university, strategies to improve vocal endurance, and awareness of voice conservation measures. Periodically monitoring those professionals in their work environment may also contribute to early diagnostic and adequate intervention.

The management of occupation-related dysphonia must be multidisciplinary and may involve physicians, speech–language pathologists, occupational medicine doctors, and acoustic engineers. Efforts should be made to increase the knowledge of dysphonia in all vocally demanding professions.

Mara Behlau and Fabiana Zambon

See also Dysphonia; Epidemiology of Communication Disorders; Vocal Hygiene; Voice Disorders

Further Readings

EU: European List of Occupational Disease [Internet]. (2003). Retrieved from http://eurlex.europa.eu/LexUriServ/LexUriServ.do?uri=CELEX:32003H0670:EsN:HTML Google Scholar

Giannini, S. P., Latorre Mdo, R., Fischer, F. M., Ghirardi, A. C., & Ferreira L. P. (2015). Teachers' voice disorders and loss of work ability: A case-control study. *Journal of Voice*, 29(2), 209–217. Retrieved from https://www.ncbi.nlm.nih.gov/pubmed/25499521

Hazlett, D. E., Duffy, O. M., & Moorhead, S. A. (2009). Occupational voice demands and their impact on the call-centre industry. *BMC Public Health*, 20(9), 108.

Isetti, D., & Eadie, T. (2016). The Americans with Disabilities Act and voice disorders: Practical guidelines for voice clinicians. *Journal of Voice*, 30(3), 293–300.

Rantala, L. M., Hakala, S., Holmqvist, S., & Sala, E. (2015). Associations between voice ergonomic risk factors and acoustic features of the voice. *Logopedics Phoniatrics Vocology*, 40(3), 99–105.

Roy, N., Merrill, R. M., Thibeault, S., Parsa, R. A., Gray, S. D., & Smith, E. M. (2004). Prevalence of voice disorders in teachers and the general population. *Journal of Voice, 47*(2), 281–293. Retrieved from https://www.ncbi.nlm.nih.gov/pubmed/15157130

Vilkman, E. (2004). Occupational safety and health aspects of voice and speech professions. *Folia Phoniatrica et Logopaedica, 56*(4), 220–253.

Zambon, F., & Guerrieri, A. C. (2012). Epidemiology of voice disorders in teachers and nonteachers in Brazil: Prevalence and adverse effects. *Journal of Voice, 26*(5), 665. e9–e18. Retrieved from https://www.ncbi.nlm.nih.gov/pubmed/?term=Roy%20N%5BAuthor%5D&cauthor=true&cauthor_uid=22516316

OPERATIONALISM

The theory of operationalism grew out of the work of Percy Bridgman, a Nobel Prize–winning American physicist, who was looking for a way to create operational awareness in his laboratory. Operationalism theory holds that concepts should be determined by the operations that create scientific understanding. Bridgman needed a way to measure the increasing pressure from the experiments he was conducting. He was concerned that, as his expertise in his field grew, he would not be able to measure or understand his results. His book *The Logic of Modern Physics* (1927) was intended to be a reflection on his personal physics experiments and to give meaning to the scientific method. Bridgman was seeking a way to rid physics of the metaphysical concepts of the time as he found them to be unreliable and unstructured.

Bridgman's goal was to define operational terms a scientist could witness and transform into observations giving value, rigor, and validity to the scientific method. Operations are a *unit of analysis*, which include actions or events as compared to theories, statements, or beliefs. This unit of analysis allows for a framework of understanding to be constructed. Bridgman believed concepts did not have meaning without measurement, and this included both physical and mental operations. This entry provides an overview of the historical development and principles of operationalism, those scientists who influenced the field, and examples of operationalism in research and theories.

Historical Overview

Some physicists adopted the theory of operationalism, but it did not become an accepted method in the field. However, Bridgman's theory influenced scientists from the external fields of philosophy and behavioral psychology, despite the fact Bridgman never meant for his theory to be used outside of physics and even argued it should not be used. Bridgman especially did not comprehend the use in psychology because he thought the results should be private, about the thoughts and observations of the scientist alone. Bridgman also did not see the purpose of using the theory to interpret behavior. However, the behavioral psychologists saw it as a way to combat the traditional introspective models of current psychological trends.

In 1935, Harvard behavioral psychologist Edwin Boring adapted the term *operationalism* to *operationism*, and his student Stanley Smith Stevens understood operationism as a way to increase rigor within the realm of psychology. Stevens believed this increased rigor was possible due to the *concrete operations* since the method recorded everything used in operations/procedures. Operationalism assumes science is empirical and translates into observations. So, behavioral psychologists understood this to mean operations were public, objective, and verifiable. This meaning was in stark contrast to Bridgman, who believed operations were the private observations of scientists.

Simultaneously with the advances of operationism in the field of behavioral psychology came the theory of positivism in the field of philosophy. Herbert Feigl traveled to Harvard in 1930 to learn from Bridgman. However, the field of philosophy rejected operationalism over two fundamental differences. The first was that logical positivists were opposed to science being private; they maintained scientific data were public. The second was the need for precise definitions of scientific terminology. Bridgman believed all terms could be defined and if not, they were *nonsense*. Positivists did not think all terms could be defined. Feigl set forth the requirements of operationism in his 1945 article "Operationism and Scientific Method" as (a) logically consistent; (b) sufficiently definite; (c) empirically rooted; (d) naturally, and preferably, technically possible; (e) intersubjective and repeatable; and (f) aimed at the creation of concepts that will function in laws or theories of greater predictiveness. After Feigl's arrival at Harvard, B. F. Skinner became aware of Bridgman's work on operationalism, and by 1935, mainstream psychologists had created a philosophy of science named operationism, which had critical differences from Bridgman's original intent and meaning for the philosophy of science.

Principles of Operationalism

The main principles of operationalism state:

(1) Operations (unit of analysis) are explicitly defined with the understanding that two scientists using the same term would yield the same results.

(2) Operations can be defined in any way as long as there is enough information to replicate the conditions.

(3) Terms used within operations must be verifiable.

Influencers on Field

Edward C. Tolman

Tolman used operationism to support his theories in the area of operational behaviorism. He asserted that behaviors were the result of cognitive activities instead of redefinitions of the actual cognitions as Bridgman detailed. Tolman ran experiments with rats to assess hunger by withholding food and having the rats run across an electrified grid to gain access to food. Two problems run counter to operationalism, which are the experiment was not just measuring food demand but the intersection of hunger and tolerance of shock. The second was to determine hunger; there is no reason for the shock unless one is trying to investigate an internal process. So, Bridgman's use of operations was to rid science of metaphysical concepts, and Tolman's use of operations was to measure expressions of the metaphysical, which are imperfect and not observable. A significant contribution was his cognitive theory of learning that held that learning was a process of *interacting with* the environment and not as a *response to* the environment.

B. F. Skinner

Skinner conceptually disagreed with Tolman and his views on operational behaviorism. What was essential to Skinner was whether a concept facilitated efficient analysis of the content, not whether the content was verifiable through intersubjectivity. He saw private and public events as different only in accessibility. The two were distinguishable not in a physical/mental path but only in a physical dimension. This view was a fundamental change in the field of psychology, and concepts changed from being *based upon* or defined regarding operations to the definitions coming from the operations themselves. Skinner brought a scientific investigation to a simultaneous intersection between the environment and behavior that changed the view of the scientist as a passive participant in the experiment to an active participant in observation and analysis. B. F. Skinner's 1945 book, *The Operational Analysis of Psychological Terms*, defined operationalism as the practice of talking about (1) one's observations, (2) the manipulative and calculation procedures involved in making them, (3) the logical and mathematical steps that intervene between earlier and later statements, and (4) *nothing* else. His belief supported the idea that environment changes behavior as behavior changes the environment, creating an interaction between the two. He is known as the "father of operant conditioning," meaning to change behavior based on the desired response.

B. L. Whorf

Around the same time that Skinner determined scientific exploration is an active process, B. L. Whorf, an American linguist, came to a similar conclusion. His work founded the premise that to fully understand scientific experimentation, one needs to investigate the scientific vocabulary. Whorf's research was in conducting a comparative qualitative analysis of Western and non-Western languages. His epistemology focused on how those who use knowledge come to learn, reason, and resolve meaning. He focused on *how* word choice in vocabulary is constructed and not *what* word choice is constructed. For example, Whorf's research is on the Hopi linguistic system. Their system does not distinguish between the subject and the object; the Hopi are part of the acts, instead of originating them. So in the Western languages, Whorf explained that terms like *stars*, *mountain*, and *river* are considered distinct things like a rug or a plate, where in reality, they should not be thought of as individual and separate objects. This idea aligns with the behavioral psychologists' work as they learn what their subjects *have* (internal) and not what they *are*. To observe and analyze what the subject possesses, the psychologists need to have clear, established operations, which can be more clearly understood whether the environment and behavior are not thought of as separate entities.

Stanley S. Stevens

A student of Skinner, Stevens thought that operationalism could create a validity and rigor in psychology, which was absent. Stevens wrote a primer of operational analysis for the field of psychology entitled "Psychology and the Science of Science" (1939). In this work, Stevens presented the idea that true operation is based on perception. In contrast to Bridgman, who did not give one operation more dominance than another, Stevens contended operations had a hierarchy, and for research to be valid, the relations between the operations were important. Stevens conceived operationalism as the relationship between objects and events, while Bridgman thought of operationalism in terms of how words are used in isolation from theory or a research practice.

Clark L. Hull

Hull's scientific philosophy regarding operationism was patterned after the philosopher John Dewey and aligned with Tolman's work. Dewey's writings gave Hull a practical perspective enabling him to create a framework of a quasi-operational analysis. Hull, when referencing Bridgman, focused operations on how observations and measurements occur. Hull shifted his focus to what is observed during operations, reminiscent of what positivists like Feigl did. Hull thought his theory would be able to explain *all* behavior of all organisms. He introduced objective measurement to quantify his results rather than only observation. Hull also introduced drive theory, which is based on a stimulus–response but included the drive of the subject.

Operationalism in Research

Process

To conduct research in the social sciences, there needs to be a conceptualization and then operationalization. During the conceptualization process, the abstract concept must be defined by a dictionary definition. Then operationalism, which defines how the abstract concept will be measured, occurs. This definition comes from the researcher and gives enough information for the study to be understood and replicated.

Abstract Concept	Conceptual Definition	Operational Definition
Academic achievement	Student's success	• Test scores • Reading level • Turning in homework • Good grades
Behavior issues	Expression of emotional or interpersonal maladjustment	• Expulsions • Suspensions • Calls/notes home
Family/home support	Help from family/home	• Attendance at conference • Support with homework • Communicates with school

Sample Research Questions

(1) Can children have *compassion* for their classmates?
- Conceptualization
    - Compassion—having sympathy for another person and taking action to improve his or her situation.
- Operationalism
    - Helping other students at a school.

(2) Does *socioeconomic* status affect academics?
- Conceptualization
    - Socioeconomic status—a combination of education, income, and occupation.
- Operationalism
    - Mathematical formula—taking education, income, and occupation into account.

(3) Is there *racial discrimination* in the schools?
- Conceptualization
    - Racial discrimination—being treated unfairly because of one's skin color or identification with a racial/ethnic group.
- Operationalism
    - Having negative things about one's race said about one's self.

Operationalism Theories

Cultural Understanding

Whorf's research demonstrated how cultures influence language and then how this language shapes reality and the world. He teamed up with Edward Sapir to create the Sapir–Whorf hypothesis, which stated that language impacts and forms an individual's cultural truth by restraining his or her thought development. An example found in American culture would be that Americans only have one word for *snow*, but the Inuit have multiple words, so they can be more precise about the type of snow. Another example is that when conducting a color memory test, the subject's perception is affected by his or her vocabulary and the number of words his or her culture has to distinguish between colors.

Behavior Modification

Skinner's research was in the area of learning behaviors. He believed, as many behaviorists did, that people were a blank slate and that all behavior could be modified. He looked to outward signs of learning and believed that by observing behavior, one could determine the best way to modify the behavior. For example, if a teacher is trying to get students to follow directions, there are two methods the teacher can try. After the teacher gives directions, he or she can reward those who followed the directions with a sticker or candy. Then, the teacher can give the instructions again to see whether those who did not follow the directions the first time will follow, in hopes of getting the reward. The second method would be for the teacher to give the directions and then punish those students who did not follow the directions. Then, the teacher could try again and see whether those noncompliant students follow directions the second time around, in hopes of not being punished.

Heather Stone

See also Cognitive Behavioral Therapy; Metacognition; Outcome Measurement; Qualitative Research; Research; Validity

Further Readings

Bridgman, P. W. (1945). Some general principles of operational analysis. *Psychological Review*, 52(5), 246–249.

Chang, H, "Operationalism", The Stanford Encyclopedia of Philosophy (Fall 2009 Edition), Edward N. Zalta (ed.), URL = <https://plato.stanford.edu/archives/fall2009/entries/operationalism/>

Feigl, H. (1945). Operationism and scientific method. *Psychological Review*, 52(5), 250–259.

Green, C. D. (1992). Of immortal mythological beasts. *Theory & Psychology*, 2(3), 291–320.

Hackenberg, T. D. (1988). Operationism, mechanism, and psychological reality: The second-coming of linguistic relativity. *The Psychological Record*, 38(2), 187.

Langfeld, H. S. (1945). Symposium on operationism: Introduction. *Psychological Review*, 52(5), 241–242.

Skinner, B. F. (1945). The operational analysis of psychological terms. *Psychological Review*, 52(5), 270–277.

Stevens, S. S. (1939). Psychology and the science of science. *Psychological Bulletin*, 36, 221–263.

Optimality Theory

Optimality theory (OT) is a constraint-based theory of grammar that was introduced in the early 1990s by Alan Prince and Paul Smolensky in their seminal work *Optimality Theory: Constraint Interaction in Generative Grammar*. The theory represents a radical departure from the generative rule-based theories that have dominated linguistics since the 1960s, and the subsequent research that has emerged from OT investigations has yielded answers to several long-standing questions, especially in the domain of phonology and acquisition.

One of the nagging questions that had eluded a satisfactory answer is why different, seemingly unrelated languages exhibit many of the same phonological processes. An equally perplexing question has been why children in the course of acquisition exhibit phonological processes that are not evident in the target language. OT addressed questions of this sort by adopting a novel architecture that employs universal constraints, eliminating any appeal to rules. The constraints of the theory are violable, and they can conflict with one another. Conflict is resolved by language-specific rankings (or weighting) of the constraints. The constraints evaluate all potential output candidates in parallel for any given input (underlying) representation and assign violation marks to candidates who violate a constraint. The output candidate who best satisfies the constraint hierarchy (i.e., incurs the least serious violations) is selected as optimal. The constraints are of two fundamental types: markedness and faithfulness. Markedness constraints impose well-formedness restrictions on potential output (surface) structures and are formulated exclusively in terms of output properties. Notions of naturalness are incorporated directly in the markedness constraints and are based on typological properties of language. Some examples of well-supported markedness constraints along with their definitions are given in (1).

(1) Markedness constraints

*Coda: Coda consonants are banned.

*CC: Consonant clusters are banned.

*Fricatives: Fricatives are banned.

Faithfulness constraints, on the other hand, demand identity between an input (underlying) representation and a corresponding output representation. Such constraints are the antithesis of rules, militating against changes between underlying and phonetic representations. There are, of course, many different ways that input and output representations might differ from one another. The constraints in (2) represent just two examples of the many faithfulness constraints that can limit the difference between the two levels of representation.

(2) Faithfulness constraints

MAX: Every input segment must have a corresponding output segment (no deletion).

IDENT: Corresponding input and output segments must be identical (no change in feature specification).

The notions of conflict and violability can be illustrated by considering the role of the two conflicting constraints *Coda and MAX for those many children who omit word-final consonants in the early stages of acquiring English. While final consonant deletion is not a process that any of these children would have observed in English, the process follows naturally from *Coda being ranked over MAX. Focusing on two potential output candidates for an English word ending in a consonant (i.e., one with and the other without a final consonant), the target-appropriate (faithful) candidate incurs a fatal violation of the top-ranked constraint *Coda and is eliminated from the competition. On the other hand, the child's erred phonetic output is selected as optimal because it complies with *Coda and only violates lower-ranked MAX, making its violation less serious. For these children, it is more important to comply with the markedness constraint *Coda than it is to be faithful to the input representation. This underscores another important assumption of OT, and that is, that markedness constraints by default dominate faithfulness constraints in the early stages of acquisition. Acquisition, thus, proceeds by the child's phonetic representations becoming more and more faithful (target-like) over time. This means that markedness constraints will be gradually demoted below faithfulness constraints based on the positive (observable) evidence in the language to which children are exposed. MAX will eventually come to outrank *Coda, resulting in target-appropriate productions and the loss of final consonant deletion.

Other common error patterns in early acquisition such as stopping of fricatives and cluster reduction receive a similar account, following from *Fricatives and *CC being ranked over IDENT and MAX. The loss of these error patterns follows from the reverse ranking of these constraints.

The universality of constraints and the default ranking of markedness over faithfulness (i.e., the OT essentials of acquisition) also explain why many of the same phonological generalizations hold crosslinguistically for fully developed languages. For example, Samoan and many West African languages retain the ranking of *Coda over MAX, disallowing coda consonants (i.e., all syllables are open). Similarly, the persistence of the default ranking of *Fricatives over IDENT results in those many languages that disallow fricatives in their phonetic inventories (e.g., Kiribati, Hawaiian). Finally, those languages that disallow consonant clusters within a syllable (e.g., Korean, Chinese) retained the default ranking of *CC over MAX.

OT also offers a solution to another longstanding problem, namely the occurrence of phonological *conspiracies* in both developing and fully developed languages. A conspiracy arises when two or more phonological processes in a language function together to effect different repairs in response to the same illicit class of sounds or sound sequences. For example, consider the case of a young child who employs one process that replaces fricatives with stops in all contexts, except when they are in a consonant cluster. In that more restricted context, the child instead deletes the fricative. Earlier theories miss the unifying generalization behind the co-occurrence of these processes, namely that both repairs are driven by the higher order need to avoid fricatives. OT captures the generalization behind this and other conspiracies in a single hierarchy of crucially ranked constraints. Of these constraints, the top-ranked is a markedness constraint that prohibits a particular class or combination of sounds (e.g., a ban on fricatives, clusters). The next two constraints are different faithfulness constraints such as MAX and IDENT that are also ranked relative to one another. Each of the faithfulness constraints yields a different repair for the banned structure. On the one hand, MAX preserves the segment when it is a singleton, and the violation of the lower-ranked IDENT allows the retained segment to change to a stop. When the fricative is in a cluster, it is deleted because changing it to a stop would still violate the higher-ranked ban on clusters.

Ongoing OT research continues to build on these and other advances by evaluating and refining its claims through descriptive analyses and computational modeling.

Daniel A. Dinnsen

See also Language Acquisition; Linguistics; Markedness; Phonology; Universal Grammar

Further Readings

Dinnsen, D. A., & Gierut, J. A. (2008). *Optimality theory, phonological acquisition and disorders.* London, UK: Equinox.

McCarthy, J. J. (2002). *A thematic guide to optimality theory.* Cambridge, UK: Cambridge University Press.

Prince, A., & Smolensky, P. (1993/2004). *Optimality theory: Constraint interaction in generative grammar.* Malden, MA: Blackwell.

ORAL LANGUAGE

Language is used to communicate ideas, needs, and emotions through a symbolic coded system. It is a human faculty, universal, that requires linguistic exposure to be acquired, as opposed to written language, which is learned.

Oral language is a modality. To be functional, it requires grammaticality, performed by a modular organization. Phonemes and morphemes combine themselves, coherently with the specific characteristics of each language system, in order to correspond to the lexicon (phonology and morphology). Words construct clauses and sentences (morphology and syntax); words have different meanings, sentences create different senses and intentions (semantics and pragmatics), and all of these infinite statements may concern the present, the past, or the future, establish different spatial relations with the interlocutors, and reflect cultural differences (semantics, morphology, syntax, and pragmatics). In short, the five modules that organize language are responsible for the management of its sounds, its structure and grammatical content, and its use, regarding personal, temporal, and spatial contexts.

Neuropsychologically, mind concepts have a phonological form. This relation assumes a physiological process in the sense that sounds are transmitted in the brain by impulses to the organs involved in the articulatory process, in order to produce acoustical waves that are received by a hearer and converted to mental representations of concepts. In a simple view, these processes represent the circuit of processing, namely the one related to perception and comprehension and the one related to production and expression.

The physical realization of production is articulation. Speech articulation is fast, is accurate, and involves a coordination of about 100 muscles. In reverse, there is the perceptive and receptive/comprehensive circuit of processing, started by the auditory process, which allows understanding the transmitted message. Oral language is therefore associated with articulatory processes—through which sounds are produced—and acoustic ones—through which the sounds produced are perceived—in order to interpret them as a linguistic material. The amplitude of this statement contributes to understanding why both circuits of processing cannot be exclusively described as peripheral competences but must also be described as systemic ones. The perception of phones and their permutation to phonemes, meanings, and intentions suppose a conversion of phonetic units to linguistic units, that is, from speech to language. That is the reason for the double naming of the output circuit: Although *production* corresponds to a vast concept—from phonemes to discourse—it is a term mainly used for speech issues, and *expression* is the one exclusively used for language aspects. *Production* is essentially used to describe processes that start with phones and phonemes. *Expression* is the term used for productions that start at the semantic module and emerge in discourse. Along these lines, *perception* is the term corresponding to the perceiving

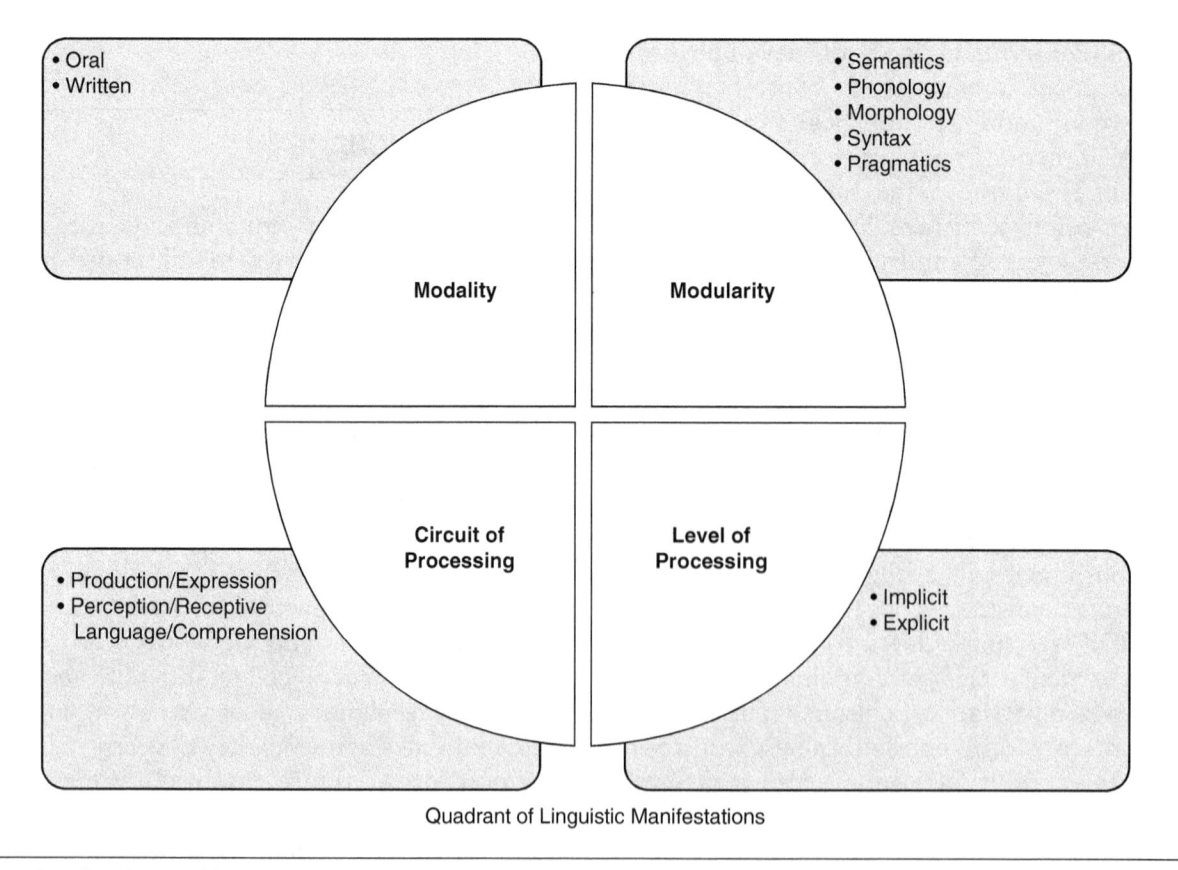

Figure 1 Quadrant of Linguistic Manifestations

Source: Dina Caetano Alves

process of phones and phonemes, and *comprehension* is the one used for the other linguistic modules. *Receptive language* is the equivalent term of *comprehension*, because this one may include the concept of *perception*.

Overall, the terms applied correspond to the lexical or sublexical levels of the linguistic unit involved in the circuit of processing: *production* and *perception* for the sublexical level (e.g., for phonemes) and *production* or *expression* and *comprehension* or *receptive language* for the lexical level (e.g., for words).

As to the nature of processing, it is unconscious whenever the linguistic manifestation is performed implicitly. When linguistic material is explored explicitly, however, speakers or listeners engage in reflections about language as an object.

Considering all aspects described thus far, language can be explained according to a conceptual quadrant, as illustrated in Figure 1.

In sum, each linguistic manifestation (1) assumes an oral and/or written modality; (2) recruits different modules—semantics, phonology, morphology, syntax, and/or pragmatics; (3) uses a specific circuit of processing; and (4) occurs on an implicit or explicit level of processing.

As for production, the ability to perceive speech and comprehend language involves aspects as sociocultural factors, properties of the linguistic material, frequency of words, and expressions to be processed and such aspects as the listener's health status, age, and language mastery.

The acquisition of oral language assumes clinical, cognitive, and linguistic prerequisites. There is widespread agreement that human growth and experience affect language development. In order to support and promote a proper linguistic acquisition, babies and children have to present a typical evolution in terms of global development; vocal tract; auditory system; and physical, sensorial, cognitive, and emotional skills, within a stimulating environment. Oral language development implies the acquisition of the rules for producing and understanding sounds, words, sentences, and conventions for their socially appropriate use in the linguistic system of the community into which children are introduced.

Milestones of communication acquisition, such as first words by 12 months, word combinations by 24 months, and sentences by 36 months, are often used to monitor language development in children and to guide family and professionals in determining whether a child is showing signs of disturbance. In some cases, children may not begin talking at the appropriate time just because people have distinct developmental rhythms and the environment presents different conditions. However, in other cases, the absence or disturbance of certain linguistic manifestations has to be interpreted as warning signs.

Adult population can also reflect language disturbances, typically in terms of the neurocognitive conditions of use. Language processing depends on different brain regions located in the right and left hemispheres. There are two relevant language areas in the brain: the Broca's area, located in the inferior frontal gyrus, and the Wernicke's area, located in the superior temporal gyrus. The Broca's area is responsible for the processing and production of speech and language. The Wernicke's area concerns linguistic comprehension. When neurological issues affect these areas, language disorders emerge.

Oral language disturbances are observable in both children and adults, resulting in persistent difficulties in acquiring or using language, respectively, when a developmental problem is detected or a brain injury occurs. These disorders can affect, globally or selectively, different linguistic modules (phonology, morphology, syntax semantics, and pragmatics) and/or different levels of processing (implicit and explicit) and/or different circuits of processing (production and perception/comprehension/receptive language). They may also arise independently—primary difficulty—or in association with other disorders—secondary difficulty.

Language impairment (LI) is the expression that designates a developmental language pathology, in which language skills are significantly delayed comparing with other children of the same age and excluding bilingual or multilingual factors. A bilingual or multilingual child may present with LI, and this would affect the languages concerned. LI diagnosis takes into account the results of formal assessment, the linguistic performances observed, and the clinical reasoning. LI is often described as being either primary or secondary. The primary one assumes that the cause of the language problem is unexplained although comorbid conditions such as behavior or hearing problems may be observed. Secondary LI occurs when the child's difficulty is associated with a clinical broader condition such as cerebral palsy, autism, Down syndrome, and other such diagnoses.

When language difficulties are not related to other disturbances, the diagnosis attributed is *specific language impairment* (SLI). The fact that this oral language pathology can affect different linguistic modules justifies the different proposals of SLI's classification, available in the literature. In this disorder, linguistic difficulties can affect one or both of the linguistic processing circuits—production and perception/comprehension/receptive language—and at the implicit and/or explicit level. The diagnosis is made by exclusion and assumes the absence of hearing impairment, the absence of a general development delay (children with SLI have a typical intelligence quotient), the absence of any neurological impairment—such as perinatal bleeds or cerebral palsy—and no autism. Children with SLI do not present oromotor disorders or hearing impairments (physiological and/or neurophysiological issues) although they may demonstrate difficulties on perception and production of speech (neurocognitive and/or psycholinguistics issues).

Considering the perspective of different researchers, SLI is considering a subtype of LI, and both affect oral language.

On the other hand, as explained above for the adult population, a brain injury may damage oral language performance, in terms of skills for production or understanding, in different linguistic domains, in both implicit and explicit levels, and even in written language. In this case, the diagnostic hypothesis is aphasia. This disruption is the result of an injury commonly located in the left hemisphere, assuming an acquired character. Excepting oral language, cognitive ability can remain intact, including memory and executive functions. There are several classification criteria that lead to discrimination between the different types of aphasia. The most common criterion is based on the interpretation of the language disorder characteristics that can be observed through naming, fluency, and comprehension. In aphasia, naming disorders are always present (anomia) and contribute negatively to the meaning access process of words and to the production or understanding of sentences and discourses, interfering significantly in the communicative ability of the subject.

The establishment of diagnosis should go through a rigorous assessment process of oral language, and the recommendation is that the assessment should include both the standardized and nonstandardized formats. The standardized one permits the classification of language skills as correct or incorrect, in order to achieve results, converted to numbers, comparable with other elements of the community. The nonstandardized format is not prepared and, consequently, not predefined; however, it is not conditioned and permits flexibility in the conduction of the assessment.

All modules of language should be evaluated to achieve a proper and detailed interpretation of the linguistic profile of the patient, in order to describe his or her language deficits and the areas of preserved function; then to plan a suitable intervention in terms of needs, identification of the enabling strategies to achieve communication, and/or goals that have to be prioritized; and to give a correct expectation to the patient and his family.

Intervention for subjects diagnosed with oral disorders supposes a set of practices, specifically designed to promote oral language development and/or to remove barriers to participation in society that arise from persons with this disturbance. Intervention may be carried out directly by specialists in language pathology themselves or through proxies such as family. It can be delivered at a health clinic center, at a hospital, through private or public education, at rehabilitation centers, at school, or even at home.

The goal of intervention is to reestablish linguistic behaviors that can be adopted by the subject in order to preserve communicative functionality. Commonly, intervention on oral language is based on approaches related to different theories, usually related to the natural process of language acquisition and development. The cognitive–interactionist theories describe the effect of social relations in the development of language, as with so-called, motherese. Behaviorism emphasizes the role of the environment. Nativism assumes that some aspects of children's language knowledge are present from birth, and generativist theory describes children's knowledge of grammar as consisting of knowing rules and operations that apply to linguistic categories and structures. (Socio-)constructivist theories defend that language structures emerge as a result of the continuing interaction between child's current level of cognitive functioning and environment.

Globally, the therapy chosen is based on the linguistic profile of the subject, the values and/or priorities identified during the assessment process, and considering the theory more suitable to the analysis of these factors.

Dina Caetano Alves

See also Aphasia; Articulatory Phonetics; Auditory Processing; Cognition; Comprehension; Expressive and Receptive Language; Meaning; Modularity; Morphology; Naming; Perception; Speech Production, Theories of

Further Readings

Coppens, P., & Patterson, J. (2018). *Aphasia rehabilitation: Clinical challenges.* Burlington; MA: Jones & Bartlett Learning.

Goldstein, G., Puente, A., & Bigler, E. D. (Eds.). (1998). *Human brain function—Assessment and rehabilitation.* New York, NY: Plenum Press.

Goldstein, S., & Naglieri, J. A. (Eds.). (2011). *Encyclopedia of child behavior and development.* New York, NY: Springer.

Hoodin, R. B. (2011). *Intervention in child language disorders—A comprehensive handbook.* Ontario, ON: Jones & Bartlett Learning.

Kreutzer, J., DeLuca, J., & Caplan, B. (Eds.). (2010). *Encyclopedia of clinical neuropsychology.* New York, NY: Springer.

Lust, B. (2006). *Child language: Acquisition and growth.* Cambridge, UK: Cambridge Textbooks in Linguistics.

Riper, C. V., & Erickson, R. L. (1996). *Speech correction: An introduction to speech pathology and audiology.* Needham Heights, MA: Allyn & Bacon.

Schwartz, R. G. (Ed.). (2009). *Handbook of child language.* New York, NY: Psychology Press.

Origins of Language

Language is a communication system. Human language is a particular example that is characterized by the use of a limited set of articulate sounds (phonemes) that can be combined in different ways to create meaningful units (morphemes and words). In turn, these meaningful units are combined into larger units (sentences). The relationship between different words in a sentence is provided by the grammar; grammar refers to the set of rules that govern the construction of phrases (syntax) and words (morphology) in a particular language. Consequently, any explanation about the origin of human language must consider the origins of phonology, vocabulary, and grammar. The characteristics of human phonological production are a direct result of the specific idiosyncrasies of the vocal tract, whereas vocabulary and grammar are a consequence of human neurologic organization.

Historically, the first reference to this question is found in Herodotus (484–425 BCE) in the second volume of his *Histories*. According to this Greek historian, the Egyptian Pharaoh Psamtik (664–610 BCE) wanted to know which language was the original one. To solve this question, he selected two babies and gave them to a shepherd with the instruction to care and feed them, but that nobody should speak to them. When these children were later observed, one of them said something that sounded like *bekos*; it was concluded that Phrygian language should be the original language because that sound was similar to the Phrygian word for "bread."

The interest in understanding how human language emerged and evolved continued during the following centuries; references to this question are found at different times and in different countries. During the 19th century, the discussion about the origins of human language became so complex and agitated that, in 1866, the Linguistic Society of Paris banned any debates on this question. The idea that this question was nearly impossible to solve remained for decades.

Currently, this question is approached from the perspectives of different disciplines, including linguistics, anthropology, neuroanatomy, archeology, comparative psychology, and genetics.

Initial Interpretations

During the 19th century, different hypotheses were presented in an attempt to explain the origin of language from the lexical point of view, that is, how words were created. Although some authors argued that these proposals were just simplistic speculation, they became popular and have continued to be used even in the contemporary literature. Some of these hypotheses were the following: (a) Language began as imitations of natural sounds, which implies that words are created from onomatopoeias (for instance, *splash*); (b) language began with interjections, emotive cries, and emotional expressions; consequently, yelling, screaming, and so on represented the elements of origin for the creation of new words. This type of emotional expression is frequently used in long-distance communication; (c) gestures are at the origin of language; initially communication depended on bodily movements; spoken language simply represents the use of oral gestures, whose origin lies in hand gestures. A number of authors currently support this point of view; (d) rhythmic chants and vocalisms created by individuals engaged in communal labor lie at the origin of human language; (e) language began with the syllables easiest to articulate attached to the most significant objects (e.g., /*ma*/); (f) it has been observed that there is a significant correspondence between sounds and meanings. Words describing small, sharp, referents tend to include high front vowels in many languages (e.g., *little*), while those denoting big, round, low things tend to have rounded back vowels (e.g., *large*). This is often referred to as *phonetic symbolism*; (g) it has also been also proposed that human language comes out of play, laughter, cooing, courtship, emotional mutterings, and the like; it suggests that language is derived from social activities; and (h) taking into consideration that there is a need for interpersonal attachment and contact, it has been proposed that language may have begun as sounds to signal both identity (Here I am!) and belonging (I'm with you!).

All these hypotheses may be partially true, and all these factors may have contributed to the creation of new words. Furthermore, these hypotheses attempt to explain how the initial communication systems (observed in animals) evolved to a second stage: the development of a lexical system, which can potentially be transmitted to the offspring, but these hypotheses do not account for the development of grammar. Grammar indeed represents the core distinguishing feature of human language.

Different Stages in Language Evolution

Some authors argue that human language developed across qualitatively different stages. Language evolution is consequently not just a matter of extending the number of elements that are used in communication; it also includes qualitative changes. This means that different linguistic abilities likely appeared at different historical moments. Departing from this perspective, different stages in language evolution have been proposed, including (a) initial communication systems using sounds and other types of information such as gestures, similar to the communication systems observed in other animals, including nonhuman primates; (b) primitive language systems using stereotyped combination of sounds (words) but without indication of the potential relationships among the words, that is, language as a lexical system. This type of language could be similar to the holophrastic period in language development, observed in children around 12–18 months of age; and (c) communication systems using grammar, in other words, indicating the relationships existing among different words, that is, language as a grammatical system. During a child's language development, it is observed that the use of grammar is found after the holophrastic period, which simply refers to a more advanced and complex stage. In developmental psychology, it has been observed that by the end of the second year, children begin to combine two or more words into simple *sentences*. Initially (around 24–30 months of age), two-word utterances without connecting elements are produced, resulting in the so-called *telegraphic speech* (e.g., *other cat* and *baby eat*). This simply means that language initially emerges as a collection of words (lexicon) and, only some time later, as a system indicating the relations among different words in sentences (grammar).

It has been argued that a simple protolanguage including only isolated words must have preceded the full-fledged syntax of today's discourse. This protolanguage probably appeared with the first hominids but became progressively more elaborate by increasing the number of words. This lexical language probably existed for thousands and even millions of years.

Larynx Position: The Origins of Human Phonology

Human articulatory ability has been related to the specific position and configuration of the larynx. The human larynx descends during infancy and the early juvenile periods, and this greatly contributes to the morphological foundations of speech development. This developmental phenomenon is commonly believed to be unique to humans.

This descent is completed primarily through the rapid descent of the laryngeal skeleton relative to the hyoid, but it is not accompanied by the descent of the hyoid itself. It contributes physically to an increased independence between the processes of phonation (vibration of the vocal folds) and articulation (shaping of the vocal tract to change the resonance of the laryngeal sound signal) for vocalization. Thus, the descent of the larynx and the morphological foundations for speech production must have evolved in part during hominoid evolution and has allowed producing the human speech sounds (phonemes) used in natural languages. Humans have the ability to produce more than 100 different speech sounds.

Neurology of Language Evolution: Intraspecific Communication

It has been observed that in monkeys, the brain's temporal lobes are involved in recognizing the sounds and calls of their own species. Human sounds and calls are evidently at the origin of spoken communication. Nonhuman primates, such as chimpanzees, have population-level leftward asymmetries for both surface area and gray matter volumes of the temporal lobe. These asymmetries seem to be related to a left temporal lobe specialization for an intraspecific communication system. Nonetheless, differences between humans and nonhuman primates relate to the volume of the temporal lobe. Overall, volume, surface area, and volume of white matter in the temporal lobe have been observed to be significantly larger in humans than predicted for an ape of human size and total brain volume. The greatest difference is observed in the temporal lobe's white matter.

This increase in the temporal lobe's surface area and white matter volume observed in humans probably reflects a reorganization of the temporal lobes associated with an increased complexity in the intraspecific communication.

Continuity Versus Discontinuity

It is not completely clear whether human language simply evolved from prelinguistic systems existing in nonhuman primates (continuity theories) or whether language represents a unique human ability that cannot be compared with the communication systems existing in nonhuman animals (discontinuity theories). This last point of view has been supported by such prominent linguists as Noam Chomsky; he considers that the emergence of human language could be linked to a mutation. This means that human language is not only quantitatively but also qualitatively different from other animals' communication systems. Nonetheless, these two points of view are not mutually exclusive.

Derek Bickerton emphasizes that there are only two most central issues in language evolution: (1) How did symbolic units (words or manual signs) evolve? (2) How did syntax evolve? He considers that symbolic units (i.e., lexicon) and syntax (i.e., grammar) are the only real novelties in human communication systems. That means, to understand the origin of human language, two different questions have to be considered: How to explain lexicon evolution? And how to understand grammar evolution?

Nonetheless, these two language levels (lexicon and grammar) may have followed different patterns of evolution: Whereas lexical evolution probably represents a continuation of prehominid communication systems (beginning several million years ago and continuing to the present day), grammatical evolution could represent a qualitative change.

Gestural Theory

An interpretation of language evolution that has been particularly influential during the last decades is the gestural theory. It simply states that human language developed from gestures; therefore, gestures represent the initial type of communication.

Authors supporting this point of view argue that gestures are found in nonhuman primates, such as chimpanzees, as a basic communication system. It has been speculated that spoken language simply represents the use of oral gestures, originating from physical bodily gestures. Gestures (praxis) and spoken language have a close brain representation in the left hemisphere.

Michael Corballis has pointed out that humans as well as nonhuman primates such as chimpanzees tend to move their hands when producing oral sounds: Chimpanzees move their mouths when performing different motor tasks. These close relationships between hand and mouth movement may have played an evolutionary role in enabling the development of intentional vocal communication as a supplement to gestural communication.

Language and Cognitive Evolution: The Emergence of Grammar

The evolution of grammar represents the most complex and poorly understood question in language evolution. It is noteworthy that human languages—regardless of the diversity in their details—present profound structural similarities in all regions of the world (i.e., there exists a kind of core syntax or universal grammar), suggesting an original grammar or at least some universal principles for expressing ideas resulting from the human brain's idiosyncratic organization.

Some proposals have been offered to account for the historical origins of grammar. Some authors have proposed that a mutation in the human species may have occurred about 50,000 years ago, accounting for the full human language (i.e., grammatical language). The rationale behind this claim refers to the fact that human culture significantly accelerated shortly afterward, resulting in a rapid increase in the number of produced elements, including the first symbolic artifacts (e.g., statuettes and cave paintings). This acceleration in cultural development may have been related to the development of the so-called *metacognitive executive functions* (such as planning, abstracting, problem-solving ability, and temporality of the behavior). Metacognitive executive functions are strongly linked to the internal representation of actions, the use of verbs, and the development of a grammatical language.

Grammar begins with the ability to combine words to create a new, higher level unit (a *syntagm*—two or more linguistic elements that occur sequentially in the chain of speech and have a specific relationship). This means that in order to create a syntagmatic relationship between two or more vocabulary words, different word categories have to be distinguished, specifically nouns (objects) and verbs (actions). To create a simple phrase, only two types of elements are indeed required: nouns (corresponding to the so-called nominal phrase) and verbs (corresponding to the so-called verbal phrase). The crucial point in emerging grammar is not just the complexity of the lexical/semantic system. What is really important is to have words corresponding to different classes that can be combined to form a higher level unit (syntagm, phrase, and sentence). One of the words has to refer to an object (noun); the other is an action (verb). A sentence has to contain a subject (noun) and a verb, indicating that two different word categories are required.

It has been suggested that verbs, grammar, and speech praxis appeared simultaneously in history. Interestingly, grammar, speech praxis, and the ability to use verbs are simultaneously impaired in cases of damage to Broca's area, suggesting a common neural activity. Accordingly, the origin of grammar is directly linked to the ability to use verbs and the ability to produce certain articulatory movements. The development of a grammatical language unquestionably had a significant impact on the evolution of human complex cognition.

Pidgins, Creoles, and Infantile language

Derek Bickerton developed the idea that a protolanguage must have preceded the full-fledged syntax of today's discourse. Echoes of this protolanguage can be observed, he argued, (a) in pidgin languages, (b) in the first words of infants, (c) in the symbols used by trained chimpanzees, and (d) in the syntax-free utterances of children who do not learn to speak at the normal age. Bickerton considers that such a protolanguage existed already in the earliest *Homo* (about 2.3–2.4 million years ago) and was developed owing to the pressure of the behavioral adaptations faced by *Homo habilis* (2.3–1.4 million years ago).

Pidgin refers to a communication system developed among people who do not share the same language but need to talk because of whatever reason. A *creole* language is a pidgin that has undergone development and become the native language of a community. There are many examples of creole languages of English, French, Spanish, and so on. Pidgin and creole represent in consequence two steps in the same process.

Pidgins are simple languages with a limited lexicon and rudimentary grammar; they usually include words with referents (nouns, verbs, and adjectives), along with a limited number of grammatical words (such as prepositions and articles). As in pidgin languages, quite probably, human language was initially composed basically by content words with a limited number of grammatical words.

It is also observed that when pidgin languages become creole languages and are spoken for generations, they become increasingly complex. Interestingly, creole languages present evident similarities in grammar, suggesting a fundamental human grammar, as proposed by Chomsky and other researchers.

Recent Language Evolution: Writing and Computers

Wall painting represents the direct antecessor of written language. It appeared during the Paleolithic era, some 30,000–35,000 years ago. Across Europe, particularly in France and Spain, cave paintings dating from the Paleolithic age have been found. Writing begins with concrete pictograms that reflect realities accessible to the senses, particularly to vision. These pictograms further evolved and became abstract, progressively separating from the concrete representation. This situation was observed in Sumer (contemporary Iraq) about 53 centuries ago, and it is usually regarded as the beginning of writing in human history. Symbols (graphemes) referred to the meaning of words; therefore, these original writing systems are regarded as logographic. Graphemes representing sounds (syllables) appeared later, about 4,000 years ago in Phoenicia, and graphemes representing phonemes appeared even later in Greece.

Language has consequently continued its evolution through the invention of written language, and written language has continued its evolution to the present day. This can be observed in recent years, with the use of massive storage and the use of verbal information, using automatically controlled systems, particularly computers, cell phones, and other technological communication advances. Using a computer is somehow akin to a new reading system. Obviously, there is no specific brain area related to using computers, just as there is no brain area related to reading and writing. These are cultural and technological elements recently developed in human evolution.

Alfredo Ardila

See also Executive Function and Communication; Language; Language Acquisition; Lexicon; Oral Language

Further Readings

Ardila, A. (2008). On the evolutionary origins of executive functions. *Brain and Cognition*, 68(1), 92–99.

Ardila, A. (2009). Origins of the language: Correlation between brain evolution and language development. *Foundations of Evolutionary Cognitive Neuroscience*, 153–174.

Berwick, R. C., Friederici, A. D., Chomsky, N., & Bolhuis, J. J. (2013). Evolution, brain, and the nature of language. *Trends in Cognitive Sciences*, 17(2), 89–98.

Bickerton, D. (2007). Language evolution: A brief guide for linguists. *Lingua*, 117(3), 510–526.

Botha, R. P. (2003). *Unravelling the evolution of language* (Vol. 19). Amsterdam, The Netherlands: Elsevier.

Chomsky, N. (2004). Language and mind: Current thoughts on ancient problems. Part I & Part II. In L. Jenkins (Ed.), *Variation and universals in biolinguistics* (pp. 379–405). Amsterdam, The Netherlands: Elsevier.

Christiansen, M. H., & Kirby, S. (Eds.). (2003). *Language evolution*. Oxford University Press. Oxford, UK.

Corballis, M. C. (2009). The evolution of language. *Annals of the New York Academy of Sciences*, 1156(1), 19–43.

Fitch, W. T. (2010). *The evolution of language*. Cambridge University Press. Cambridge, UK.

Foley, R. A., & Lewin, R. (2013). *Principles of human evolution*. John Wiley & Sons. Hoboken, NJ.

Hauser, M. D., Chomsky, N., & Fitch, W. T. (2002). The faculty of language: What is it, who has it, and how did it evolve? *Science, 298*(5598), 1569–1579.

Lieberman, P. (2007). The evolution of human speech. *Current Anthropology, 48*(1), 39–66.

Nowak, M. A., & Krakauer, D. C. (1999). The evolution of language. *Proceedings of the National Academy of Sciences, 96*(14), 8028–8033.

Tallerman, M., & Gibson, K. R. (2012). *The Oxford handbook of language evolution.* Oxford, UK: Oxford University Press.

OROFACIAL MYOFUNCTIONAL DISORDERS

Orofacial myofunctional disorders encompass a number of different conditions and behaviors involving inappropriate oral and/or orofacial movements and configurations. Potential consequences from such postures and patterns can include abnormal tongue positioning within the oral cavity, inadequacy of lip closure, irregular chewing and swallowing performance, abnormal facial tension, dental malocclusion, and issues with speech production. This entry provides an overview of the possible causes, presentation, structural involvement, effects on speech, and multidisciplinary treatment of orofacial myofunctional disorders.

Possible Causes

Orofacial myofunctional disorders may be caused by a single factor or a combination of factors, which may be congenital, developmental, or behavioral in nature. Factors may include a restricted nasal passageway (such as that caused by allergies or enlarged tonsils or adenoids) resulting in open-mouth breathing, atypical sucking or chewing behaviors, development of biting or clenching and grinding habits, prolonged use of pacifiers and hard-spouted sippy cups, structural abnormalities such as a short and thick lingual frenulum (tongue-tie), neurological deficiencies, and genetic predisposition.

Presentation

Individuals with orofacial myofunctional disorders may present in a variety of different ways that can negatively affect orofacial muscle performance, such as that required for speech and swallowing. One of the most reliably recognized orofacial myofunctional disorders is tongue thrust (i.e., the forward carriage of the tongue to the extent to which it may protrude between or rest against the teeth). A component of orofacial myofunctional disorders is the mismanagement of the open space within the oral cavity in terms of the movement and positioning of involved structures. Consequently, an additional presentation is simply an open resting posture of the mouth, resulting in mouth breathing and its accompanying issues, such as detrimental effects on the teeth, gums, and the growth and development of the jaw. Other behaviors associated with orofacial myofunctional disorders may include excessive thumb and finger sucking, clenching or grinding of the teeth, noisy chewing and swallowing, and other maladaptive oral habits. Left untreated, orofacial myofunctional disorders can have negative long-term effects on healthy and habitual nasal breathing, oral development, teeth alignment, and speech production. Unaddressed orofacial myofunctional disorders can detract from the benefits of orthodontic treatment.

Structural Involvement

In addition to the anterior carriage of the tongue as seen in tongue thrust, other structural abnormalities may be associated with orofacial myofunctional disorders. These can include delayed or atypical eruption of teeth, malocclusion or misalignment of teeth, lip incompetence, a short lingual frenulum, or enlarged tonsils or adenoids.

Speech

Effects on speech from orofacial myofunctional disorders can include distortions of sounds and production of sounds with an altered place of articulation, particularly those sounds that involve the musculature of the tongue body. For example, the alveolar fricatives [s] and [z] may be subject to articulatory distortions, but they can also be substituted by the more anteriorly produced interdental fricatives [θ] and [ð] in a phenomenon recognized as lisping. Other potentially affected sounds include the alveolar stops [t] and [d], the alveolar liquids [l] and [ɹ], the alveolar nasal [n], the postalveolar fricatives [ʃ] and [ʒ], and the postalveolar affricates [t͡ʃ] and [d͡ʒ]. Distortions that can affect these sounds due to orofacial myofunctional disorders may include fronting and dentalization. The speech–language pathologist may work with the patient on increasing awareness of the face, mouth, and tongue muscles and postures, as well as improving coordination, production of speech sounds, and patterns of swallowing. The speech–language pathologist must take care to attend to the possibility of coexisting phonological disorders (e.g., rule-based error patterns such as simplification of consonant clusters); apraxia of speech, which may be characterized by groping behaviors or difficulty with consistent production of complex words; or even other articulation impairments not related to an orofacial myofunctional disorder, all of which can contribute to speech impairment and complicate evaluation, diagnosis, and treatment.

Interdisciplinary Professional Collaboration

An individual presenting with an orofacial myofunctional disorder may benefit from having a number of different professionals involved with evaluation, diagnosis, and treatment. Depending upon the etiology of the condition, appropriate professionals may include a physician, an orthodontist, a dentist, an otolaryngologist, an allergist, a speech–language pathologist, and a professional trained in orofacial myofunctional therapy.

Recommended Treatment

While treatment from a physician or an orthodontist can address structural abnormalities related to orofacial myofunctional disorders and treatment from a speech–language pathologist can address affected speech production, treatment from a professional trained in orofacial myofunctional therapy can help to counter maladaptive habits and establish productive, healthy postures and behaviors. It can be initiated in children as young as 4 or 5 years of age when thumb or finger sucking is involved, even if limited to being preventative in nature. Therapy is highly individualized according to contributing factors, with the objective being to retrain the muscles of the face and mouth to create and maintain appropriate, productive oral configurations for rest, swallowing, and speech.

Treatment goals frequently target the positioning of the lips and tongue while at rest and the establishment of an appropriate closed-mouth breathing posture. A potentially effective strategy in working toward such goals may be to incorporate electropalatography, which is a biofeedback tool that provides a visualization of the placement and timing of the contact between the tongue and the palate. It may be necessary for the orofacial myofunctional therapist and other involved professionals to work closely in regard to the timing of treatment of structural abnormalities and orofacial myofunctional therapy, as orofacial myofunctional disorders involve many interrelated structures and functions. Addressing one aspect without the other may result in a slow or complete absence of progress, and long-term consequences may even involve a regression to previous maladaptive behaviors. Parental involvement for pediatric patients is encouraged and can be integral to the success of a treatment plan.

Sarah Lockenvitz

See also Anatomy of the Human Articulators; Articulation Therapy (Phonetic Intervention); Electropalatography (EPG); Tongue Thrust

Further Readings

Mantie-Kozlowski, A., & Pitt, K. (2014). Treating myofunctional disorders: A multiple-baseline study of a new treatment using electropalatography. *American Journal of Speech-language Pathology, 23*, 520–529.

Mason, R. M. (2008). A retrospective and prospective view of orofacial myology. *International Journal of Orofacial Myology, 34*, 5–14.

Orofacial Myofunctional Disorders. (2017). American Speech–Language–Hearing Association. Retrieved from http://www.asha.org/SLP/clinical/Orofacial-Myofunctional-Disorders/

Orofacial Myofunctional Disorders. (2017). International Association of Orofacial Myology. Retrieved from http://iaom.com/

Otitis Media

Otitis media is a pathology of the middle ear space characterized by inflammation and is the most common cause of conductive hearing impairment.

Its prevalence is impacted by the positioning (slope) and size (length) of the eustachian tube. Beginning at the birth up until the age of 7 years in children, the eustachian tube increases in length from approximately 13 to 35 mm, and the position alters from a 10° slope to approximately 45°. This accounts for the increased likelihood of dysfunction leading to otitis media for children 6 years of age and younger. The incidence of otitis media also decreases as an individual ages. The onset and duration of symptoms are used to categorize the disease as acute, recurrent, or chronic. These categories have implications for speech and language development that health-care providers need to be aware of, especially due to the incidence of otitis media in young children. This entry provides an overview of otitis media, its characteristics and clinical course, its risk factors and complications, and its audiological implications.

Overview

The range of categories of otitis media can be explained by the typical pathophysiology of the disease as well as the function of the middle ear space. Understanding the function of the middle ear space is integral to the diagnostic testing used by health-care professionals to determine the presence and implications of otitis media.

Otitis media most often occurs secondary to eustachian tube dysfunction and is also known to commonly occur secondary to an upper respiratory tract infection. The eustachian tube's opening into the middle ear is located in the inferior, protympanum portion of the cavity and transverses into the nasopharynx. The eustachian tubes are closed at rest, and they dilate either actively or passively. When an individual opens his or her mouth or swallows, muscles (i.e., tenor veli palatini and levator veli palatini) actively dilate the eustachian tube, whereas passive dilation occurs in response to atmospheric changes in pressure. Active dilation of the eustachian tube serves the primary function of allowing air to infiltrate the middle ear space from the nasopharynx; secondary functions include both clearance of middle ear secretions and protection of the middle ear cavity from the nasopharynx. If eustachian tube dysfunction inhibits dilation, the middle ear is prevented from properly equalizing internal pressure to atmospheric pressure. When this dysfunction occurs, eventually the air within the middle ear space will be absorbed, and the pressure in the middle ear cavity will become negative. Such negative pressure can cause tympanic membrane retraction and lead to otitis media if unresolved. Both the retraction of the tympanic membrane and the presence of otitis media disrupt the function of the middle ear.

The middle ear space primarily functions to transfer energy from acoustic to mechanical energy (outer ear to middle ear) and then from mechanical to hydraulic energy (middle ear to inner ear). This energy transfer is due to the impedance mismatch between the mediums; sound must travel through from a source to a listener. Acoustic energy travels through air (gas medium) and is collected by the human pinna (outer ear lobe). Unlike the outer ear and middle ear, which are air-filled, the inner ear is filled with cochlear fluid (fluid medium); therefore, most of the acoustic energy would be lost if the auditory system could not transfer it to hydraulic energy. The middle ear is necessary to transfer and amplify sound from the environment to the cochlea. This transfer function is dependent on the tympanic membrane's response to sound (acoustic energy) striking it. The vibration of the tympanic membrane causes ossicular chain movement (mechanical/vibratory energy), which results in the stapes directly displacing the oval window (pushes in or out) causing compression and rarefaction waves in the cochlear fluid, respectively. If the middle ear space is subject to pathology, and this transfer function is disrupted, a conductive hearing loss can manifest. The term *conductive hearing loss*, therefore, refers to the reduction of energy transfer from the outer to the inner ear and does not include hearing loss involving sensory (cochlea) or neural (auditory nerve) function.

Characteristics of Otitis Media

Otitis media can be described based on fluid type, onset/duration of symptoms, or the combination of both. There are four types of fluid: *serous* (i.e., watery and clear fluid), *mucoid* (i.e., thick fluid), *suppurative* (i.e., infected fluid), and *hemotympanum* (i.e., presence of blood in the fluid). The type of fluid depends on how the fluid manifests in the middle ear space (secondary to eustachian tube dysfunction or barotrauma) and the stage of the clinical course. The three main categories of onset/duration for otitis media include *acute* (known as a sudden onset), *chronic* (i.e., fluid present for more than 3 months), and *recurrent* (i.e., fluid present at least 50% of the time over 6 months). Therefore, a person can present with any combination of fluid and duration. For example, an individual can be afflicted with chronic serous otitis media or acute suppurative otitis media. As such, it is helpful to understand the clinical course of otitis media to better differentiate its clinical subtypes.

Clinical Course of Otitis Media

Otitis media's pathophysiology has four main stages: inflammation, suppuration, complications, and resolution. There are some newer theories that flip the sequence of inflammation and suppuration; however, traditional medical descriptions of the clinical course still refer to Stages 1 through 4. These stages typically progress secondary to either eustachian tube dysfunction or an upper respiratory tract infection; the dysfunction of the eustachian tube prevents the middle ear from properly equalizing.

Stage 1, inflammation, occurs when an obstructed or dysfunctional eustachian tube causes negative middle ear pressure and retraction of the tympanic membrane. This negative pressure irritates and inflames the mucosal cells due to absorption of nitrogen and oxygen and transudates serous fluid. See Figure 1 for a visual representation of middle ear cross section where otitis media is present (Stage 1). As mentioned previously, serous fluid or effusion is basically sterile fluid. Though sterile, this fluid can be associated with pain, swelling, and impaired hearing sensitivity. Medical treatment during this stage is typically observation *watch-and-wait* as it is common for fluid to resolve without medical intervention. Medical management during Stage 1, when no infection is present, may include the use of analgesics to reduce pain and swelling and/or nasal decongestants to help resolve fluid. Additionally, surgical intervention can be implemented if the fluid does not resolve during the monitoring period. If the fluid is present long enough to be considered chronic or recurrent, a *myringotomy* (i.e., incision in tympanic membrane) can be performed and is often accompanied by the placement of a *pressure equalization tube*. The myringotomy relieves the pressure and removes substantial fluid, while the pressure equalization tube allows ventilation of the middle ear space.

In Stage 2, suppuration, the serous fluid becomes infected, pus accumulates, and tension builds on the tympanic membrane. This occurs as opportunistic bacteria (i.e., bacteria that take advantage of *specific* immune weakened circumstance) colonize in the middle ear fluid, which leads to infection. The most common types of bacteria that lead to suppurative otitis media are *Streptococcus pneumonia*, *Haemophilus influenzae*, and *Moraxella catarrhalis*. Patients may experience fever, anorexia, otalgia, aural fullness, and irritability and notice a decrease in their hearing sensitivity. Treatment at this stage typically includes the use of oral antibiotics; the most commonly prescribed in the first round are penicillin derivatives, such as amoxicillin. If there is a tympanic membrane perforation or patent pressure

Otitis Media

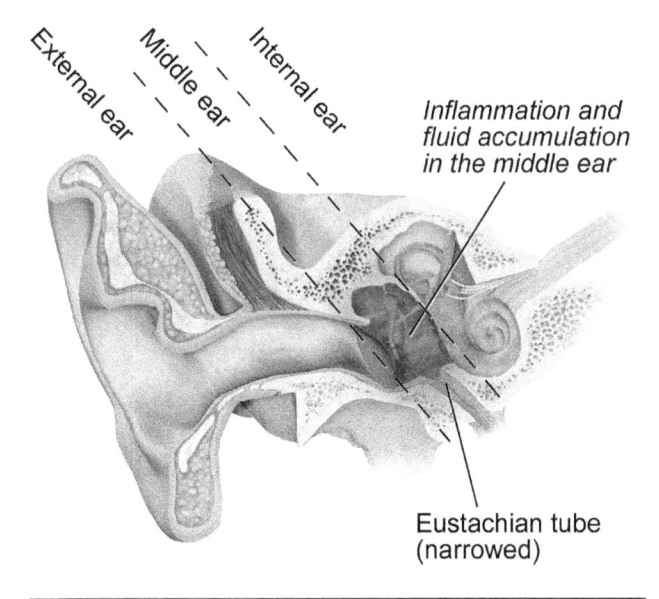

Figure 1 Schematic representation of middle ear cross section: Otitis media Stage 1

Source: Bruce Blaus/Wikimedia Commons, https://commons.wikimedia.org/wiki/File:Otitis_Media.png, Licensed under Creative Commons License Attribution-Share Alike 4.0 International (CCBY), https://creativecommons.org/licenses/by-sa/4.0/deed.en

equalization tube, antibiotic drops increase the concentration to the infection site and are preferred. If the infection is treated, but the fluid does not resolve, the patient returns to Stage 1; however, if the infection does not resolve, as expected with antibiotics, otitis media may progress to Stage 3, complications.

Stage 3 is complication, and depending on the source, this can include a continuum of issues ranging from a tympanic membrane perforation to a brain abscess, which can lead to death. Generally, complications refer to when the infection spreads to surrounding structures, which is why there is some debate regarding in which stage a perforation would occur. A *tympanic membrane perforation* can either fall into Stage 2, suppuration, or be considered a complication. When a perforation occurs, the patient might feel an initial sense of relief due to pressure release and think the otitis media has resolved. However, if the infection continues, it can spread to neighboring structures or potentially lead to the formation of a *cholesteatoma*.

If infection spreads to the inner ear labyrinth, it is considered labyrinthitis, or if the infection spreads to the air cells of the mastoid, it is referred to as mastoiditis. If the spread of infection to neighboring structures occurs, the patient's pain can return, and as the infection becomes more serious, he or she can experience cognitive impairments. Mastoiditis can lead to serious complications due to its proximity to the brain. Complications following, or in conjunction with mastoiditis, include *meningitis* (infection of the meninges) and potentially a *brain abscess*. While all complications of otitis media require medical management, meningitis and a brain abscess are life-threatening and require quick intervention. Treatment for this stage usually requires a combination of drug treatment (e.g., analgesics, broad-spectrum antibiotics, steroids) as well as surgery to drain and/or repair the structures involved. Not all cases of otitis media will progress to Stage 3 or include all of the complications indicated. Otitis media resolves (Stage 4) when the infection and fluid subside and any complications are treated or heal without intervention. Resolution can occur following any of the previous stages.

Risk Factors and Complications

The clinical course, and therefore complications, of otitis media depends on multiple factors. This includes patient characteristics/risk factors, the characteristics of otitis media (i.e., the type of fluid and onset/ duration), stage of otitis media (progression) when it is discovered/diagnosed, the treatment recommendations, and patients' compliance with medical recommendations.

Risk Factors for Otitis Media

Some factors increase an individual's likelihood of developing a case of otitis media. As indicated earlier, children under 6 years of age are more likely to develop otitis media than adults. Environmental factors including exposure to smoke, low socioeconomic status, and children in group day care settings increase the likelihood of developing a case of otitis media. Individuals are more at risk if they have barotrauma, allergies, upper respiratory tract infection, and craniofacial or middle ear anomalies (e.g., cleft palate and Down syndrome). Additionally, an individual with a medical condition that results in a weakened immune system (e.g., HIV/AIDS) or chronic inflammatory disease (e.g., tuberculosis) is more likely to develop otitis media.

Common Complications of Otitis Media Subtypes

When comparing the characteristics of otitis media, acute versus chronic, and serous versus suppurative, different patterns of complications will arise. Chronic otitis media is more likely to result in a long-standing perforation, erosion of the ossicles in the middle ear, middle ear adhesion, and/or a cholesteatoma. Cholesteatomas are more likely to develop if an atticoantral (i.e., posterosuperior regions of the tympanic membrane involving the pars tensa or pars flaccida) perforation develops. The location of an atticoantral perforation causes the healing process to be more difficult; marginal perforations can allow squamous epithelial cells of the outer ear to migrate into the middle ear cavity, which can develop into a dangerous cholesteatoma.

Conversely, acute serous otitis media is less likely to progress to complications (Stage 4) after initial medical treatment compared with chronic serous otitis media. Acute serous otitis media, which is more likely to occur following barotraumas—often caused by a hydrostatic pressure change—may be

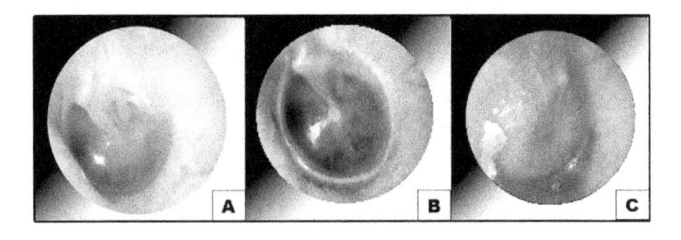

Figure 2 Otoscopy of normal and abnormal tympanic membranes. Panel (A) displays normal tympanic membrane and abnormal tympanic membranes due to serous otitis media panel (B) and acute supportive otitis media panel (C)

Source: (A) Michael Hawke, MD/Wikimedia Commons, https://commons.wikimedia.org/wiki/File:Normal_Left_Tympanic_Membrane.jpg, Licensed under Creative Commons License Attribution-Share Alike 4.0 International (CCBY); (B) Michael Hawke, MD/Wikimedia Commons, https://commons.wikimedia.org/wiki/File:Adult_Serous_Otitis_Media.jpg, Licensed under Creative Commons License Attribution-Share Alike 4.0 International (CCBY); (C) Michael Hawke, MD/Wikimedia Commons, https://commons.wikimedia.org/wiki/File:Acute_Otitis_Media_Stage_of_Resolution.jpg, Licensed under Creative Commons License Attribution-Share Alike 4.0 International (CCBY).

associated with trauma at onset. However, once treated, it is not expected to become recurrent or chronic (i.e., having persistent complications), whereas chronic serous otitis media, often secondary to allergies or structural anomalies (e.g., enlarged adenoids), is more likely to progress to Stage 3 over time.

Medical recommendations for both acute and chronic otitis media often include observation (i.e., watch and wait) for a 3-month period. However, in chronic cases, concerns for speech and language development or academic performance in the pediatric population may result in surgical intervention (i.e., myringotomy and pressure equalization tube placement). Surgical intervention may also be recommended if the fluid becomes mucoid over time.

Audiological Indications

Otoscopy

Otitis media is associated with abnormal appearance of the tympanic membrane (i.e., middle ear space visualized through the tympanic membrane), and often symptoms can expand laterally (outward) to the external auditory meatus (i.e., ear canal). During an otoscopic inspection, common symptoms include discoloration of the tympanic membrane (often red), swelling of the tympanic membrane, discharge in the ear canal, and/or fluid behind the tympanic membrane. Additionally, otoscopy may reveal fluid bubbles, a meniscus (i.e., fluid line), a tympanic membrane perforation, or dullness of the tympanic membrane. For reference, Figure 2 displays normal tympanic membrane (A), abnormal tympanic membranes due to serous otitis media panel (B), and acute supportive otitis media panel (C). If pneumatic otoscopy is available, a trained healthcare professional can determine whether air is present in the middle ear space. Therefore, pneumatic otoscopy is a key diagnostic tool for identifying otitis media or middle ear effusion. Otoscopy, however, is not able to determine the degree of hearing impairment caused by middle ear effusion or otitis media.

Conducting a comprehensive audiological evaluation provides diagnostic insight to determine the stage of otitis media as well as the degree of resulting hearing impairment. The degree and type of hearing impairment reflect how much the middle ear function is impeded. A comprehensive audiological assessment includes otoscopy, immittance testing, pure-tone air and bone conduction audiometry, and speech audiometry. A subtest of acoustic admittance audiometry, tympanometry, will most likely measure an abnormally large tympanic width in cases of otitis media.

Acoustic Admittance Testing

Dependent on the stage of otitis media, tympanometry can also be consistent with no measurable tympanic membrane compliance, reduced compliance (with large tympanic width), or negative middle ear pressure. If the tympanogram is a Jerger Type B, often referred to as a flat tympanogram, there is either sufficient fluid-prohibiting compliance or the presence of a tympanic membrane perforation. Jerger Type A_s tympanograms may indicate that compliance is reduced to some extent by fluid in the middle ear space with abnormally large tympanic width. Additionally, significantly negative middle ear pressure, a Jerger type C tympanogram, is suggestive of eustachian tube dysfunction. As there are multiple pathologies that can produce these tympanogram types,

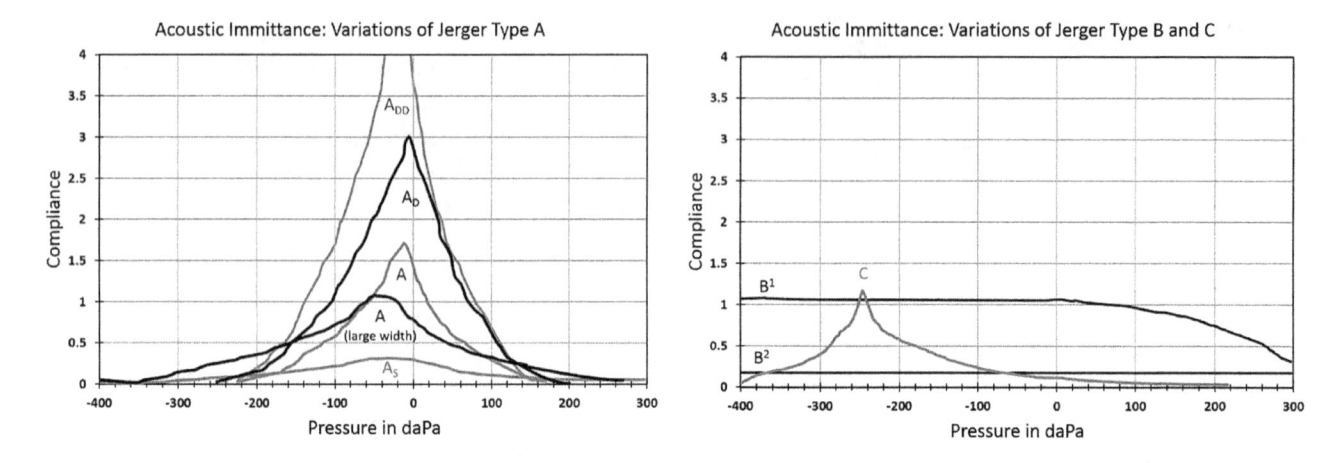

Figure 3 Tympanograms. The left panel displays the Jerger Type A classification system (Type A, A$_S$, A$_D$) with two additional variations of the (Type A with large tympanic width and Type A$_{DD}$). The right panel displays Jerger Type C and two variations of a Type B tympanograms B[1] and B[2]

Source: Author's own work.

additional audiometric assessment aids a healthcare professional in determining the probable pathology producing abnormal tympanograms. For instance, the degree and type of hearing loss are typically determined by pure-tone air and bone conduction audiometry. See Figure 3 for examples of tympanogram classification types.

Audiometric Testing

Pure-tone air and *bone conduction* audiometry is measured to determine an individual's hearing sensitivity. Pure-tone air conduction tests the air conduction pathway, which assesses how sound travels from the outer ear through the middle ear and inner ear. If hearing loss is present, air conduction thresholds determine the severity (i.e., degree of loss) and configuration of the loss. The configuration, or shape of the audiogram, indicates the degree of loss across frequencies of hearing. If hearing loss is present, bone conduction audiometry is necessary to determine the type of hearing loss (i.e., conductive, sensorineural, or mixed). Bone condition thresholds directly assess the inner ear by vibrating the mastoid surrounding the cochlea. This stimulation of the mastoid bypasses the outer and middle ear and therefore indicates the sensitivity of sensory hearing without regard to the air conduction pathway.

Hearing loss caused by otitis media is most commonly a mild-to-moderate conductive hearing

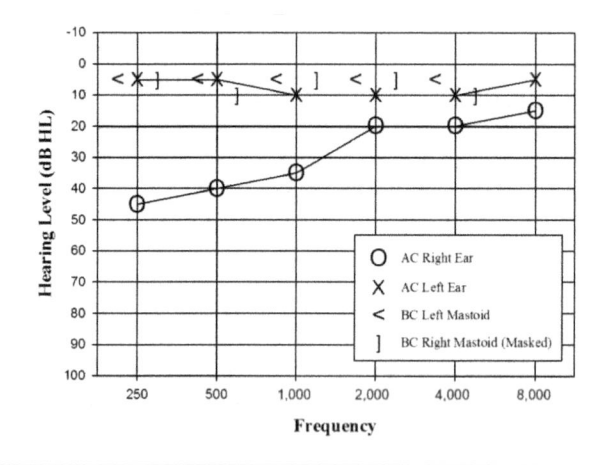

Figure 4 Audiogram reflecting a rising conductive hearing loss in the right ear, typical of otitis media with effusion in the right ear, and hearing within normal limits in the left ear

Source: Author.

loss and typically has a slightly rising audiometric configuration (see Figure 4). This means that *bone conduction thresholds* are obtained within normal limits, while air conduction thresholds are obtained with a mild-to-moderate degree of hearing loss. However, this configuration may be impacted by the complications associated with otitis media and any other comorbid hearing impairment. *Speech recognition thresholds* are expected to be in good agreement with the *pure-tone average* (i.e., the mean of air conduction thresholds at 500, 1,000, and 2,000 Hz). *Word recognition scores* reflect the accuracy with which an individual recognizes speech presented at *suprathreshold* levels. Individuals with otitis media and no comorbid sensory or neural hearing loss are expected to have excellent word recognition scores. This reflects the nature of the hearing loss, as suprathreshold presentation levels compensate for the conductive component without negatively impacting the clarity of sensory processing.

Audiological Management of Otitis Media

The course of otitis media pathophysiology can result in serious complications, as discussed previously, often leading to middle ear surgical treatments. Many patients will not pursue audiological management if medical treatments are successful. However, patients may choose not to pursue traditional medical management (e.g., middle ear reconstruction) or may have hearing loss following medical intervention. A patient's candidacy for a traditional hearing aid or a bone-anchored hearing aid will depend on the audiological test results. As word recognition is typically excellent in these patients, amplification that compensates for the conductive hearing losses typically has successful outcomes. Audiologists should select a product that is appropriate for a patient who could continue to have fluctuating loss, due to chronic middle ear effusion and active drainage.

Aurora J. Weaver and Megan M. Barnett

See also Acoustic Admittance; Air and Bone Conduction; Anatomy of the Hearing Mechanism and Central Audiology Nervous System; Conductive Hearing Loss and Its Treatment; Hearing Aids; Physiological Basis of Hearing; Pure-Tone Audiometry; Speech Audiometry; Speech Recognition

Further Readings

Bluestone, C. (1998). Anatomy and physiology of the Eustachian tube. In C. Cummings, J. M. Fredrickson, L. A. Harker, C. J. Kraus, M. A. Richardson, & D. E. Schuller (Eds.), *Otolaryngology: Head and neck surgery* (Vol. 3., pp. 3003–3025). St. Louis, MO: Mosby.

Musiek, F., Baran, J., Shinn, J., & Jones, R. (2012). *Disorders of the auditory system.* San Diego, CA: Plural.

Payne, E. E., & Paparella, M. M. (1976). Otitis media. In J. L. Northern (Ed.), *Hearing disorders.* Boston, MA: Little, Brown.

Proctor, B. (1967). Embryology and anatomy of the eustachian tube. *Archives of Otolaryngology, 85*(5), 503–514.

Sandler-Kimes, D., Siegel, M. I., & Todhunter, J. S. (1989). Age-related morphologic differences in the components of Eustachian tube/middle ear system. *Annals of Otology, Rhinology, and Laryngology, 98*(11), 854–858.

Zemlin, W. R. (1998). *Speech and hearing science: Anatomy and physiology* (4th ed.). San Diego, CA: Academic Press.

OTOACOUSTIC EMISSIONS (OAE)

The ear not only receives sound but also emits sounds of its own. These faint acoustic signals, referred to as *otoacoustic emissions* (OAEs), originate as backward propagating waves within the structures and fluids of the inner ear and are transmitted via the middle ear to the ear canal, where they can be recorded with a sensitive microphone. Whether measured in response to sound or in the absence of an evoking stimulus, OAEs are considered to be by-products of the active and vulnerable outer hair cell (OHC)–mediated processes that underlie cochlear sensitivity and frequency selectivity. OAEs therefore provide an invaluable window onto the mechanics and function of the cochlea and of OHCs in particular. This entry provides an overview of how OAES are generated, measured, and classified.

The precise details regarding how OAEs are generated and propagate out of the cochlea are still under active investigation. Nevertheless, the understanding of their biophysical origins is mature enough to allow OAEs to be widely utilized as an objective, noninvasive, and highly sensitive assay of OHC function in both humans and laboratory animals. Clinically, OAEs are used to screen hearing status in newborns, currently done universally in some countries, and to ascertain cochlear function in other populations, such as those seriously ill, for whom obtaining a voluntary, behavioral response to sound is problematic. OAEs are also used to monitor cochlear health in individuals exposed to noise or ototoxic pharmaceuticals (e.g., cisplatin, which is used to treat various cancers of the head and neck). In combination with other tests, such as behavioral audiometry, tympanometry, and the auditory brainstem response, OAE measurements can help to determine the site (e.g., middle or inner ear) and more precise etiology (e.g., sensory or neural) of an individual's hearing loss.

Measuring OAEs in the laboratory and clinic is accomplished using a small probe inserted into the ear canal. The probe contains the microphones used to record the OAEs and sometimes also includes built-in speakers used to deliver sound stimuli. In cases where external speakers are used, they are connected to the probe through plastic tubes. The stimuli played through the speakers are generated by a sound card or a device capable of converting digital commands from a controlling computer into analog voltage. This device also converts the analog voltage from the microphone into digital signals that can be analyzed by the controlling computer. Signal processing techniques such as the fast Fourier transform are commonly used to examine the spectral content of the ear canal recordings, so that the amplitude and signal-to-noise ratio of the response can be determined. Clinically used OAE-recording devices are either desktop models with an external probe connected to the main machine or all-in-one handheld devices with a few buttons to operate the machine and a small screen to view the results. Laboratory systems, on the other hand, are often custom-built using high-end audio devices, speakers, and microphones, often permitting OAE measurement over a wider frequency range and with a lower measurement noise floor than is achieved clinically.

OAEs are most commonly evoked by stimuli such as clicks or tones. OAEs evoked by tone bursts or clicks, referred to as *transient-evoked OAEs*, are often sufficiently delayed in time relative to the short stimulus, such that the response can be directly appreciated in the time domain. However, spectral analysis is also used to quantify the frequency content of the response, which typically resembles that of the stimulus. In addition, commonly measured are *distortion product OAEs* (DPOAEs), which are evoked by a pair of tones presented at closely spaced frequencies and measured at frequencies mathematically related to those of the stimuli. As the frequencies of the stimuli and response are different, DPOAEs are easily observable in the frequency domain following the spectral analysis. OAEs can also be evoked by single tones, which are termed *stimulus-frequency OAEs*. However, complex measurement paradigms must be used to separate the response from the stimulus, as they occur at both the same time and the same frequency. For this reason, stimulus-frequency OAEs are not as commonly utilized as transient-evoked OAEs and DPOAEs. Lastly, OAEs may also occur spontaneously, without purposeful stimulation. These *spontaneous OAEs* are evident as tone-like signals occurring at idiosyncratic frequencies in the spectrum of the ear canal signal obtained in quiet. However, the utility of spontaneous OAE measurements is somewhat limited, as they are not present in all ears with normal hearing.

While OAEs are commonly classified in terms of the nature of the response or the evoking stimulus (as above), a parallel classification system makes distinctions based instead on the underlying generation mechanism. Two primary mechanisms have been proposed: (1) reflection of stimulus-driven waves off mechanical irregularities located along the cochlear partition and (2) nonlinear distortion, likely imparted by the processes involved in OHC transduction. Emissions resulting from these mechanisms can be differentiated by how their phases change with frequency: The phase of "reflection-source" emissions varies rapidly, while that of "distortion-source" emissions varies little. Under this framework, evoked OAEs may receive contributions from both generation mechanisms, though it is generally accepted that transient-evoked OAEs and stimulus-frequency OAEs primarily arise from reflection, at least at low stimulus levels, while DPOAEs elicited under common recording conditions are dominated by distortion sources. The potential clinical value of unmixing OAEs into their different components is under active investigation.

In addition to examining the clinical utility of OAEs and addressing questions regarding their physical origins, researchers have also employed OAEs to address more basic questions about peripheral auditory function. For instance, OAEs have been used to compare cochlear frequency selectivity across species and to examine cochlear development, maturation, and aging in humans. OAEs have also proved to be a convenient tool for assessing the function and potential role of top-down efferent control over cochlear mechanics (neurons of the medial olivocochlear system project from the brainstem to the OHCs, providing inhibitory control that may be important for hearing in noise or protection from acoustic trauma). As understanding of the biophysics underlying OAEs improves, so will their utility in both clinical applications and basic science research.

James B. Dewey and Sumitrajit Dhar

See also Age-Related Hearing Loss; Cochlear Hearing Loss; Diagnostic Audiological Assessment; Distortion; Hearing Disability and Disorders; Hearing Screening; Hearing Tests

Further Readings

Abdala, C., & Dhar, S. (2012). Maturation and aging of the human cochlea: A view through the DPOAE looking glass. *Journal of the Association for Research in Otolaryngology, 13,* 403–421.

Joris, P. X., Bergevin, C., Kalluri, R., McLaughlin, M., Michelet, P., van der Heijden, M., & Shera, C. A. (2011). Frequency selectivity in old-world monkeys corroborates sharp cochlear tuning in humans. *Proceedings of the National Academy of the Sciences, 108,* 17516–17520.

Kemp, D. T. (1978). Stimulated acoustic emissions from within the human auditory system. *Journal of the Acoustical Society of America, 64,* 1386–1391.

Poling, G. L., Siegel, J. H., Lee, J., Lee, J., & Dhar, S. (2014). Characteristics of the 2f1-f2 distortion product otoacoustic emission in a normal hearing population. *Journal of the Acoustical Society of America, 135,* 287–299.

Shera, C. A., & Guinan, J. J. (1999). Evoked otoacoustic emissions arise by two fundamentally different mechanisms: A taxonomy for mammalian OAEs. *Journal of the Acoustical Society of America, 105,* 782–798.

Ototoxicity

The cochlea is a sensitive, highly metabolically active, and fragile organ that is easily, adversely affected by injury, leading to sensorineural hearing loss. The challenges may be noise, infection, or the attrition of hearing due to age (i.e., presbyacusis), but there are also several drugs that can instigate ototoxicity, causing cochlear dysfunction and resulting in hearing loss and tinnitus. Many of these drugs, particularly those that are strongly ototoxic, are only prescribed in cases of extreme need, such as chemotherapy for cancer, or severe infection, although others that have a less common or strong effect are in use for less life-threatening/limiting conditions such as arthritic pain and muscle cramp. This entry reviews the most commonly used ototoxic drugs and details the known mechanisms, impact, and possible strategies for the treatment and prevention of ototoxicity.

Platinum-Based Chemotherapy Drugs for Cancer

The use of chemotherapy drugs based on platinum for the treatment of cancer has vastly improved survival rates and outcomes since their introduction in the 1970s. The discovery of the cytotoxic properties of platinum was serendipitous, when platinum-containing instruments were used in a microbiology experiment involving the bacterium Escherichia coli: When the platinum electrodes were used, all the bacteria died. Platinum-based chemotherapy drugs are commonly used in the treatment of brain tumors in children and in adults in the treatment of testicular, ovarian, and breast cancers. Unfortunately, the powerful anticancer action of this family of drugs is accompanied by ototoxicity, leading to significant amounts of cochlear hearing loss, tinnitus, and, in some cases, vestibular dysfunction.

The most powerful, most commonly used, and also the most ototoxic drug in this category is cisplatin, which was also the first to be discovered and used. A similar yet distinct drug, carboplatin, is less ototoxic. New variants of platinum-based chemotherapy drugs, oxaliplatin for example, have been developed, but the issues of ototoxicity remain a challenge.

The pattern of ototoxic hearing loss associated with cisplatin in particular is of an initial bilateral high-frequency sensorineural hearing loss progressing to the low frequencies and progressing in severity with cumulative dose. The loss is permanent and irreversible, and it involves impaired auditory discrimination as well as the reduced detection of quiet sounds. The onset may lead a patient to be unconcerned about hearing loss until the situation is well established. The vestibular labyrinth may also be affected via similar pathways that affect the cochlea.

Vestibulotoxicity caused by platinum-based chemotherapy has been relatively poorly researched due to its lower reported incidence compared with hearing loss. The patient-reported incidence is less than 10%, but this figure is higher in specific screening programs designed to detect vestibular dysfunction. This may be in part due to its insidious onset. The patient's symptoms are vague imbalance rather than dizziness or vertigo and as such can be easily attributed to the possible anemia, loss of appetite and nutrition, or the effects of various other drugs that a cancer patient will be prescribed.

The prevalence of ototoxic hearing loss following treatment with cisplatin is significant, and while reports vary based on the definitions of hearing loss, dose, and adjunct treatments in conjunction with the chemotherapy, approximately 20% of adults and 50% of children experience significant hearing loss. While 40% of adults report significant tinnitus following cisplatin treatment, for children the prevalence is unknown.

The mechanisms of ototoxicity associated with platinum-based chemotherapy involve apoptosis (i.e., the triggering of programmed cell death) rather than necrosis. Multiple and complex pathways are involved, but a major role for reactive oxygen species (ROS) has been identified.

As of the early 21st century, any intervention that protects the cochlea from ototoxic hearing loss also protects the cancer, although many different agents are under investigation.

Aminoglycoside Antibiotics

The family of antibiotics that includes streptomycin, tobramycin, and gentamycin is highly effective in treating severe bacterial infection, with a mode of action including the inhibition of protein synthesis within the bacterial ribosome. They can also be ototoxic, with a similar mode of action to the chemotherapy agents described previously, triggering cochlear hair cell apoptosis with increased ROS. However, rather than the repeated dosing over extended periods of time used with chemotherapy, aminoglycoside antibiotics tend to be used in high dosages for short periods of time to treat life-threatening infection, and so the associated bilateral hearing loss can be sudden and severe. It can be accompanied by bilateral vestibular hypofunction, for which visual and proprioceptive systems of balance are imperfectly able to compensate, which can lead to bobbing oscillopsia, wherein walking movements can lead to the visual field moving up and down as the head moves. The entry of the drug and the damage to the vestibular system are poorly understood. In addition, vestibulotoxicity occurs with various forms of aminoglycoside administration including through topical ear drops, as well as intravenous, intraperitoneal, and inhalation routes. It seems toxicity is unrelated to dose or serum concentrations.

A genetic predisposition to ototoxicity associated with aminoglycoside antibiotics has been identified, involving mitochondrial DNA, and is more prevalent in some South American populations. Those with this mutation can experience an abrupt and catastrophic loss of hearing and balance functions following the use of these drugs, and screening for this susceptibility has been proposed, although is not yet in widespread use.

The ototoxic properties of gentamycin can be utilized therapeutically in patients with Ménière's disease that is refractory to medical treatment. While the mechanisms of this disorder are imperfectly understood, the unilateral involvement of the vestibular end organ is clear, and the function of the vestibular labyrinth can be ablated by intratympanic infusion of gentamycin, which spares cochlear function in most cases.

Loop Diuretics

Loop drugs are used to treat high blood pressure and edema associated with kidney disorders or heart failure; the most commonly used diuretic is furosemide. The mode of action is the prevention of sodium, potassium, and chloride resorption in the kidney. Associated cochlear hearing loss is often preventable, and hearing often returns to normal when diuretic use is discontinued. Furosemide is sometimes used in combination with either aminoglycoside antibiotics or platinum-based chemotherapy, and in such cases, the hearing loss is permanent and more severe than would be expected from either drug alone, indicating a possible synergistic impact. The mechanisms of diuretic ototoxicity are multiple and complex, but involvement of the stria vascularis, which is the metabolic hub of the cochlea, has been identified.

Salicylates and Nonsteroidal Anti-Inflammatory Drugs

Both salicylates and nonsteroidal anti-inflammatory drugs can cause cochlear hearing loss and tinnitus. In the case of salicylates, this is reversible, and function returns when the drug use is discontinued. However, permanent ototoxicity can be seen in very high dose of aspirin use, although now that this is an infrequent method of attempting suicide, this is rare. In nonsteroidal anti-inflammatory drug use, the hearing loss can be reversible or permanent, and tinnitus can be persistent. Mechanisms of outer hair cell dysfunction and of microvascular constriction have been proposed.

Quinine

At one time, quinine was widely used as an antimalarial, but this has been superseded by more effective medications, and so the drug is only in use in patients with debilitating cramp. In such persons, a reversible cochlear hearing loss can develop, with high-frequency tinnitus, which can persist when quinine use is discontinued. The possibility of permanent dysfunction of the vestibular labyrinth has also been identified. Various mechanisms of ototoxic action have been proposed, including microvascular constriction, and of potassium channels in the stria vascularis. Some patients with preexisting tinnitus and hearing loss may fear that the quinine present in some traditional tonic waters may worsen their symptoms; however, the dose involved is insufficient for that to occur even with the consumption of large quantities.

Impact and Treatment

Despite being the subject of extensive research, regeneration of inner ear hair cells following injury is not yet possible in mammals, and so when ototoxic hearing loss, tinnitus, and balance dysfunction have occurred, physical repair or restoration is not feasible, while in some of the clinical situations described previously, such as cancer, and severe bacterial infection, ototoxicity may seem a reasonable price for survival. However, in some patients, the impact of hearing loss, tinnitus, and balance dysfunction can be so debilitating that the quality of life in survivorhood can be poor, and more awareness of this potential impact is needed.

In view of the high prevalence of ototoxicity in patients treated with platinum-based chemotherapy, or aminoglycoside antibiotics, programs to monitor hearing thresholds have been implemented. Some of these involve the testing of very high frequency thresholds (i.e., 10–16 kHz) as it is these frequencies that are generally affected first. There are some challenges in monitoring ototoxicity: In the case of aminoglycoside antibiotics, administration is often in an emergency basis, and baseline audiometry is not possible. Patients undergoing chemotherapy are often very unwell, and concentration during a hearing test may be a challenge. In addition, audiology units are traditionally housed with Departments of Ear, Nose, and Throat and may be inconvenient or inaccessible for patients. The uptake of monitoring hearing, even when ototoxicity is expected, is low.

Monitoring vestibular dysfunction suffers from similar challenges. Measuring the level of dysfunction often requires specialist equipment and personnel, which further prohibits universal screening. A significant proportion of vestibulotoxic patients have signs that can be picked up in an outpatient clinic; these symptoms include nystagmus (i.e., jerking eye movements) and decreased vestibulo–ocular reflex. The simple, but effective Halmagyi headshake test is an acceptable screening tool for vestibular dysfunction along with a balance dysfunction questionnaire. Treatment with targeted vestibular function exercises will provide some degree of improvement in most patients.

Treatment for hearing loss involves hearing aids and, in severe cases, cochlear implants. Modern technology is such that the majority of patients with hearing aids and cochlear implants can achieve effective communication and are able to listen to and perform music. Interventions and support for troublesome tinnitus include information, counseling, and sound therapy and relaxation therapy, with moderate success in many cases. In patients with bilateral vestibular hypofunction, the other senses that contribute to maintaining equilibrium, namely vision and proprioception, can be trained to compensate and substitute for vestibular function, but this is often unsatisfactory. Improving any coexistent hearing loss will also aid in overall balance functions.

Once ototoxicity has occurred, it can lead to permanent reduction in hearing and balance functions, resulting in reduced quality of life. While some treatment strategies do exist, some patients may benefit from psychological support to deal with a sense of loss that may persist.

Prevention

Work toward the prevention of ototoxicity associated with platinum-based chemotherapy and aminoglycoside antibiotics has focused upon the role of ROS and investigated the administration of free radical scavengers as potential otoprotectants. An alternative theme has been the use of drugs that inhibit or prevent the production of ROS. The results have been meager to date, and several attempted otoprotective interventions have carried their own risks, but a large international research effort is underway in this regard.

David M. Baguley and Anand V. Kasbekar

See also Cancer of the Head and Neck; Cochlear Hearing Loss; Hearing Aids; Hearing Tests

Further Readings

Landier W. (2016). Ototoxicity and cancer treatment. *Cancer*, 22(11), 1647–1658.

Lanvers-Kaminsky, C., Zehnhoff-Dinnesen, A. G., Parfitt, R., & Caimimboli, G. (2017). Drug-induced ototoxicity: Mechanism, pharmacogenetics, and protective strategies. *Clinical Pharmacology and Therapeutics*, 101(4), 491–500.

OUTCOME MEASUREMENT

Outcome measurement refers to the ability to determine the effect of a procedure or an intervention. It has become increasingly important to gather such information in a reliable and valid fashion using measures with robust psychometric properties to ensure that public and private investment is appropriate. The most successful speech and language therapy services are the ones that recognize the multifaceted nature of the services they provide and make every attempt to deliver across all dimensions of quality provision. This includes providing evidence-based practice, safe services, and excellent service user experience while balancing budgets. Having a clear understanding of how people are helped by therapy services is an essential feature.

While the term *outcome measurement* has been used in research since the 1990s, it is becoming increasingly required in clinical services as part of quality assurance. This is primarily due to the developed understanding that certain procedures may not deliver the purported benefits. Furthermore, the increasing financial demands on health and care services related to changes in demography, developing technologies, and increased expectations of the population have led to a focus on the importance of investing in treatments and procedures with known worth and maximum benefit to the population. This entry provides an overview of the principal types of approaches to examining the quality of service provision: patient-reported outcome, patient-reported experience, clinician-led outcome, and therapy outcome measures (TOMs).

Patient-Reported Outcome Measures (PROMs)

PROMs aim to assess the health benefit the service users have gained from their own perspective using surveys or questionnaires before and after they have received a health intervention/treatment. PROMs may determine, for example, whether the individuals feel that they are able to walk further following surgery, experience less pain, or feel less depressed. While the patients' own view of their health and any health benefits gained from a service is essential, it is also important to consider the confounding factor of "response shift" when using PROMs. Patients measuring their own health-related quality of life can be problematic. Findings are frequently unstable because of personality differences or changes within people regarding internal standards, values, or conceptualization of health-related quality of life. Furthermore, PROMs can be unstable because individuals may be comparing themselves within different time points within their recovery, which may not be explicit. For example, individuals reporting comparing their quality of life immediately after a trauma with that later may be different from a comparison of quality of life between two later points in their recovery. These "response shifts" can affect standard psychometric indices, such as reliability and validity. Furthermore, response shift theory can be particularly problematic for people with disabilities and may confound function, health, and causal indicators such as environment. However, the views of patients when it comes to their own situation, health, and well-being and whether they feel that a benefit of some kind has been received from a service should always be sought by a health-care professional.

Patient-Reported Experience Measures

PROMs should not be confused with patient-reported experience measures, which aim to determine the experience that patients have had during their contact with a service (e.g., whether they felt comfortable, informed, and at ease). These are often examined through surveys and questionnaires but do not review the actual health benefit of the patient. Studies have found that there is often a relationship between patient experience and patient outcome. An approach that has been used successfully is the one question that patient-reported experience measure asks patients or their relative whether there was anything that would have improved their experience with a particular service. This can be a valuable component of quality assurance.

Clinician-Led Outcome Measures

There are pros and cons to outcomes determined by a clinician. Among the advantages is that a clinician can analyze the disorder, function, and well-being of an individual as compared to other individuals with similar problems and thus determine the degree of challenge, severity, and change. This is only appropriate if the measure has been found to be valid and reliable, particularly considering intrarater reliability. One of the major disadvantages of a clinician-mediated outcome measure is the possibility of the professional's view being colored by his or her own expectations and relationship with the client. To guard against this, it is necessary to consider whether a change can be observed by another individual, that is, whether there has been an "arms-length change." A difficulty arises when a clinician is aware of a small change, which he or she feels is significant, but the measure is unable to reflect that change. For different outcome measures to be reliable, they may not be as sensitive as clinicians would like, as there is a trade-off between reliability and sensitivity.

Speech and language therapists frequently use psychometrically robust assessments before and after interventions to determine progress or otherwise. However, it is clear that in clinical practice, these robust assessments are often amended, altered, or abridged for use in a clinic, and these adaptations undermine the psychometric properties. This would be particularly inappropriate if the same measure is being used to determine a difference, or otherwise, before and after treatment but that measure is not being used consistently. Furthermore, interventions often aim to have an impact on a broad range of difficulties experienced by the patient, and the chosen robust assessment may only be gathering information on one or two of these. Thus, for example, if an assessment of dysarthria is being used before and after treatment, it will be able to determine (if used in the correct fashion) whether that impairment has been modified, but it would not determine whether patients are more confident in their speaking and happier in themselves, which may also be positive outcomes to the intervention by the speech and language therapist and may well occur with little change to the actual speech impairment.

The TOM

The TOM was developed to overcome these challenges. Following an analysis of the objectives of a broad range of allied health practitioners and nurses working in different settings with different patient and client groups, it was found that the goals of intervention could be grouped into four separate areas: impairment, activity restriction, social participation, and well-being of the individual and sometimes the main caregiver. For some, the purpose of the health intervention was to identify, reduce, or resolve the disorder (i.e., impairment), while in other cases the main focus would be to improve functional independence and activity (i.e., activity restriction) by means of, for example, improved communication. In some cases, the purpose of therapy would be to improve social involvement (e.g., access to education, recreation, or employment [social participation]).

Furthermore, a frequent objective of the professional would be to support individuals or their caregivers to improve their well-being and ability to cope. (The first three of these domains map directly onto the International Classification of Functioning developed by the World Health Organization [2001].) Thus, the TOM aims to reflect the challenges in those four domains that an individual has at the beginning of an intervention and at the end of an episode of care. Health-care professionals can use their preferred assessments, knowledge of the client, and observations to judge the TOM rating on these domains using an 11-point ordinal scale that is supported by six best-fit descriptors clarifying the ambiguous definitions of profound, severe, moderate, and mild.

The third edition of the Therapy Outcome Measures for Rehabilitation Professionals (2015) incorporates 47 adapted scales that aim to assist with improving the reliability of different health professionals working with different client groups. Reliability and validity have been established with the use of this measure in a research undertaken by others as well as the authors.

Final Thoughts

Whatever outcome measure one chooses to implement, it is important that the data generated are used to improve services as part of the quality assurance cycle. Thus, collecting the data is not sufficient. It is essential that these data stimulate reflection on the strengths and weaknesses of the service. This can be extended by similar services comparing outcomes of their patients in benchmarking exercises. Such activity will give some assurance to service users, funders of services (e.g., governments and insurance companies), and managers that the value of the service is being critically appraised.

Outcome measurement can identify strengths and weaknesses of services and practitioners, informing investment of resources, focusing continuing professional development, stimulating service developments, and contributing to evidence-based practice.

Pamela M. Endeby

See also Evidence-Based Practice

Further Readings

Browne, K., Roseman, D., Shaller, D., & Edgman-Levitan, S. (2010). Analysis & commentary measuring patient experience as a strategy for improving primary care. *Health Affairs, 29*(5), 921–925.

Dawson, J., Doll, H., Fitzpatrick, R., Jenkinson, C., & Carr, A. J. (2010). The routine use of patient reported outcome measures in healthcare settings. *BMJ, 340,* c186.

Enderby, P., & John A. (2015). *Therapy outcome measures for rehabilitation professionals* (3rd ed.). Croydon, UK: J and R Publishing.

Schwartz, C. E., Andresen, E. M., Nosek, M. A., Krahn, G. L., & RRTC Expert Panel on Health Status Measurement. (2007). Response shift theory: Important implications for measuring quality of life in people with disability. *Archives of Physical Medicine and Rehabilitation, 88*(4), 529–536.

World Health Organization. (2001). *International classification of functioning, disability and health* (ICF). Geneva, Switzerland: Author.

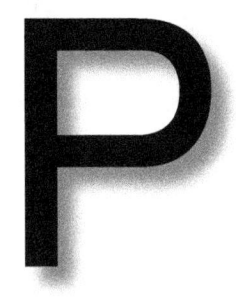

Paradoxical Vocal Cord Dysfunction (PVCD)

Paradoxical vocal cord dysfunction (PVCD) is a laryngeal (i.e., voice box) disorder, characterized by abnormal closure (i.e., adduction) of the vocal folds or cords during breathing, resulting in respiratory distress usually in the form of "noise" during inhalation or exhalation. This noise is called *stridor* and is very distressing to the patient and the family. Usually, these abnormal vocal cord behaviors and the stridor come and go in "episodes," and the patient will have periods of time when the breathing is quiet. The abnormal behavior can be triggered by exercise, odors, emotions, illness, and sometimes what appears to be for no reason at all. PVCD has also been called paradoxical vocal fold dysfunction, paradoxical vocal fold motion, vocal cord dysfunction, and even laryngeal asthma. This entry provides an overview of the possible causes, symptoms, assessment, and treatment for PVCD.

Etiology

The cause of PVCD is often difficult to determine. The most widely reported cause of PVCD has been laryngeal hyperresponsiveness, which is also called *laryngeal hypersensitivity*. This may be due to swelling which can be related to numerous causes such as gastroesophageal reflux (i.e., reflux and gastroesophageal reflux disease). There have also been cases of neurological PVCD when there is known brain damage and some cases where the belief is that it is a psychological disorder (also called a *conversion disorder*). The primary biological function of the larynx (i.e., voice box) is to protect the lower airway (i.e., trachea and lungs) from foreign bodies. There is one nerve that controls the sensations and movements of the larynx: the vagus nerve (also called *cranial nerve X*). The superior laryngeal nerve, one branch of the vagus, detects noxious stimuli in the larynx and transmits the signal to the brain, which then triggers a motor movement in the voice box, for example, closing the vocal cords inappropriately. It is not understood why the vocal cords choose this behavior instead of a throat clear or a cough. Research has demonstrated that irritants may trigger these vocal cord dysfunctions to occur by overstimulating the vagus nerve's sensory functions. Irritants such as reflux material in the larynx, smoke, alcohol, caffeine, chemical fumes, dust, and dry air can trigger an attack. There is little research as to why a person would develop this symptom as a part of a psychological disorder.

It is possible for a PVCD episode to be triggered by exercise or other strenuous tasks. Laryngeal structures serve as pathways for air during breathing (i.e., inhalation and exhalation). The sensory system helps the lungs to maintain a balance of pressure. This balance is maintained by "constriction" or "dilatation" of the vocal folds (and the surrounding structures) depending on respiratory demands. During intense exercise, the lungs have an increased need for air, and this alters the resistance to airflow. This imbalance in the resistance could lead to "spasms" and cause inappropriate adduction of the vocal folds during breathing.

Symptoms

The primary symptom typically found in individuals with PVCD is respiratory distress, characterized by stridor (i.e., noisy breathing). People will call it wheezing, but wheezing actually comes from within the lungs, not at the level of the vocal cords. This acute shortness of breath is often intermittent but can become chronic in severe cases. Some individuals develop a chronic cough as a symptom instead of the episodes of stridor and shortness of breath. PVCD is often thought at first to be asthma or chronic cough because of the similarity in symptoms. Patients will also report throat clearing, throat mucus, hoarseness, "something sticking in the throat," heartburn/chest pain, and difficulty swallowing as additional symptoms. These are also symptoms associated with asthma and chronic cough, which makes PVCD diagnosis difficult.

Assessment

Laryngeal Examination

If a patient is suspected of having PVCD, most of the time the care begins with pulmonology because patients are often referred to the pulmonologist first when there is any sign of breathing difficulty. Now that PVCD is better known, many patients are initially referred to an otolaryngologist for evaluation of the vocal cords as well. The otolaryngologist will examine the larynx using an in-office procedure called *laryngoscopy*. Using a flexible endoscope, usually through the nose, the otolaryngologist may directly observe the abnormal vocal cord behavior during the respiratory cycle. It is best for the physician to examine the patient during an attack so that the paradoxical vocal fold motion can be observed; however, patients are examined in between attacks too, and diagnosis can be made based on case history information and what the patient reports. Patients can be examined after inducing the abnormal vocal cord behavior by running, jogging, or exposure to noxious stimuli. Some paradoxical vocal fold adduction could occur when patients are asymptomatic as well.

Voice Characteristics

At times, the patient demonstrates a hoarse voice along with the paradoxical vocal cord dysfunction. The hoarseness, more appropriately called *dysphonia*, is not always present. Production of voice involves an intricate balance and coordination of the respiratory and voice production systems. PVCD interferes with appropriate functioning of this coordination, thus negatively impacting voice. Voice problems in these individuals can oftentimes be overlooked in attempts to manage their respiratory issues. Although the effects of PVCD are obvious when patients experience respiratory distress, often the paradoxical adduction occurs even when patients are asymptomatic, thereby affecting voice production. Research has demonstrated that even if a patient has a relatively good sounding voice, a clinician may be able to identify that he or she is likely to have PVCD based on a perceptual evaluation of the voice. Research is starting to document that these individuals have abnormal voice production even though it is barely detectable to the naked ear.

When using acoustic evaluation programs (via computer), researchers have documented abnormal voice characteristics in these individuals as well. Measures that demonstrate stability (or instability) of vocal cord movement often document the vocal cord abnormality. For example, a significantly higher percentage of jitter (i.e., the cycle-to-cycle changes in frequency in a voice signal) and significantly shorter maximum phonation time (i.e., the maximum time an individual can hold out a sustained phonation, e.g., "ahhhh . . .") than control subjects have been documented. Another measure called *harmonics to noise ratio* has also distinguished individuals with PVCD from individuals who do not have it. The pitch of the voice is not typically affected by PVCD, and research has confirmed that finding.

Treatment

Treatment for PVCD usually focuses on teaching the patient how to control the larynx again through a series of breathing exercises. The exercises are designed to increase pressure above the vocal cords so that pressure at or below the vocal cords can decrease and thus "relax" the system. Speech–language pathologists who treat these patients will talk about these exercises helping to "open the airway," and in fact, maintaining an open airway is the major goal of the therapy. More specifically, treatment for PVCD frequently focuses on respiratory retraining therapy, which involves teaching patients to increase their awareness of their symptoms and use techniques that include diaphragmatic breathing and exhalation against light resistance such as exhaling on a fricative such as /s/ (which is a high-pressure sound). Speech–language pathologists may teach patients to trigger their symptoms as part of therapy to increase their own awareness and to practice respiratory retraining techniques in the context of an attack. The techniques of respiratory retraining therapy ease respiration during attacks, establishing the patient's sense of control and reducing emotional distress. Other focuses of treatment for PVCD include vocal hygiene, cough suppression strategies, and psychoeducational counseling.

Because PVCD often occurs in conjunction with other disorders, treating co-occurring conditions is an important aspect of treating PVCD. Speech–language pathologists may be able to treat co-occurring disorders, as in the case of PVCD and chronic cough, or such disorders may require a multidisciplinary approach. For example, managing reflux with medicine from a physician while treating PVCD with respiratory retraining therapy would likely improve treatment outcomes. In the case that PVCD may be related to psychological or emotional factors (i.e., conversion disorder), patients may also seek psychological assessment and treatment. Medical management including desensitization to triggers has been proved useful in many patients. In severe cases or neurological cases, patient distress may be exceptionally high, and a tracheotomy may be the only way to provide easy breathing. This "hole" in the neck bypasses the larynx and allows the patient to breathe without the interference of the vocal cords.

A complex disorder, PVCD, is best diagnosed and treated through a multidisciplinary approach in which all medical and health-care professionals collaborate to ensure the best possible outcome for the patient.

Kathleen Treole Cox and Balaji Rangarathnam

See also Chronic Cough; Dysphonia; Voice Disorders

Further Readings

Boyer, N., Morris, M., & Kemp, K. (2014). Retrospective validation of screening studies to detect vocal cord dysfunction. *Chest, 146*(4_MeetingAbstracts), 906A–906A.

Cukier-Blaj, S., Bewley, A., Aviv, J. E., & Murry, T. (2008). Paradoxical vocal fold motion: A sensory-motor laryngeal disorder. *The Laryngoscope, 118*(2), 367–370.

Deckert, J., & Deckert, L. (2010). Vocal cord dysfunction. *American Family Physician, 81*(2), 156–159.

Dunn, N. M., Katial, R. K., & Hoyte, F. C. (2015). Vocal cord dysfunction: A review. *Asthma Research and Practice, 1*(1), 1–8.

Hicks, M., Brugman, S. M., & Katial, R. (2008). Vocal cord dysfunction/paradoxical vocal fold motion. *Primary Care: Clinics in Office Practice, 35*(1), 81–103.

Hull, J., & Panchasara, B. (2015). The larynx and exercise. In *Laryngeal and tracheobronchial stenosis,* Sandhu, G.S. & Reza Nouraei, S.A. (Eds.) (pp. 409–424) San Diego, CA: Plural Publishing.

Morris, M. J., Allan, P. F., & Perkins, P. J. (2006). Vocal cord dysfunction: Etiologies and treatment. *Clinical Pulmonary Medicine, 13*(2), 73–86.

Murry, T., & Sapienza, C. (2010). The role of voice therapy in the management of paradoxical vocal fold motion, chronic cough, and laryngospasm. *Otolaryngologic Clinics of North America, 43*(1), 73–83.

Røksund, O. D., Heimdal, J. H., Olofsson, J., Maat, R. C., & Halvorsen, T. (2015). Larynx during exercise: The unexplored bottleneck of the airways. *European Archives of Otorhinolaryngology, 272*(9), 2101–2109.

Treole, K., Trudeau, M. D., & Forrest, L. A. (1999). Endoscopic and stroboscopic description of adults with paradoxical vocal fold dysfunction. *Journal of Voice, 13*(1), 143–152.

Paralinguistic and Prosodic Impact on Stuttering

Speech production requires the integration of segmental properties (i.e., sounds within words) and suprasegmental properties. Suprasegmental properties include the *prosodic* characteristics of speech production (rhythm, pitch, stress, tone, tempo, rate, loudness) and the *paralinguistic* characteristics of speech production (emotional state, speaking style, vocal quality). The examination of suprasegmental information in stuttering research has focused primarily on the role of syllabic stress in syllable-timed or stress-based languages. Historically, stuttered speech has been observed to co-occur with syllabic stress. This observation has prompted the development of several theoretical models of stuttering to account for the potential role of suprasegmental properties during speech production in individuals who stutter. Many theorists propose temporal dyssynchrony during speech planning or production due to the delayed retrieval of segmental properties and/or suprasegmental properties. In essence, fluent speech cannot be achieved if one or both properties are delayed prior to production. This entry provides an overview of theoretical models, experimental research, and crosslinguistic data as they relate to the impact of paralinguistic and prosodic factors on stuttering.

Theoretical Models

The *fault-line hypothesis* (FLH) developed by Marcel Wingate describes a stuttered event as a breakdown, or *fault-line*, between the initial sound and the following stress-bearing vowel within the first syllable of a word. This disruption is thought to originate from difficulties in simultaneously processing both the segmental and the prosodic properties of the rhyme (i.e., stressed vowel nucleus) and results in the inability of the motoric system to advance beyond the initial consonant. The FLH generated a number of descriptive studies that generally support the co-occurrence of stuttered speech with stressed syllables during connected speech. However, the unique contribution of syllabic stress is difficult to disambiguate from overlapping factors also thought to increase the likelihood of stuttering (e.g., word-initial position, utterance-initial position, grammatical class, word frequency, word familiarity).

The *neuropsycholinguistic* theory by William Perkins and colleagues provides an elaborate account of both prosodic and paralinguistic factors relative to stuttering. Similar to the FLH, this theory proposes that delayed preparation of prosodic–paralinguistic properties of speech disrupts the integration of segmental and suprasegmental information when abnormal time pressure is present. In their view, the output of suprasegmental processing (i.e., syllabic frames) carries vocal elements of pitch, loudness, and duration, which convey both prosodic information (i.e., acoustic properties related to intelligibility) and paralinguistic information (i.e., speakers' emotional state and communicative intent). Increased or inefficient processing within the more primitive suprasegmental processing system is believed to occur due to internal struggle between dominance or submissiveness experienced by individuals who stutter (similar to Joseph Sheehan's *approach–avoidance hypothesis*). Unlike previous theories, the neuropsycholinguistic theory requires one additional, critical factor to distinguish stuttered speech from typical disfluencies: a perceived *loss of control* by the speaker. The description of a moment of stuttering that is based on the experiences of the speaker, rather than the perception of the listener, is inherently appealing and not without merit. However, as noted by critics of the model, the basic predications of the neuropsycholinguistic theory remain difficult to validate empirically due to limited ability to measure *loss of control* experienced by the speaker during moments of stuttering.

The variability model is described by Ann Packman and colleagues as a departure from previous theories that attempt to identify the underlying cause of stuttering. Instead, the variability model offers an account of how certain motoric properties of prosody, namely duration and syllabic stress, fluctuate when stuttering is alleviated. Across these seemingly disparate tasks (i.e., prolonged speech, choral speech, syllable-timed speech), the recurring factor during fluent speech by individuals who stutter was the reduction of variability in vowel duration (i.e., a more restricted range of long- and short-vowel durations during connected speech). Authors argue that reduced variation in vowel duration is a product of reduced variation in syllabic stress contrasts during connected speech. In turn, the increased motoric demand required to produce contrastive stress during connected speech is considered sufficient to *trigger* moments of stuttered speech.

Experimental Research

In the 1990s Frank Wijnen and colleagues conducted two empirical studies that directly investigated the

FLH predictions of delayed retrieval of the stress-bearing vowel. During an implicit naming paradigm in Dutch-speaking participants, researchers found speech-onset times for trochaic word lists were faster for adults who stutter only when the target words shared both the initial consonant and stress-bearing vowel (e.g., *kogel, kokos, koper, koning, kodak*), rather than just the initial consonant (e.g., *lepel, lila, loeder, larie, luier*), suggesting adults who stutter may have greater difficulty encoding the initial stress-bearing vowel than nonstuttering adults. In their subsequent implicit priming study with a larger number of participants, words with both initial and noninitial stress were included as stimuli. Unfortunately, findings between studies did not converge, suggesting that speech planning and production were not influenced by stress assignment in the manner predicted by the FLH. As noted by Wijnen and colleagues, further investigation into stress-based hypotheses using word sets that are phonemically similar but differ only in stress pattern may account for the potential contribution of lexical processing during response.

In studies conducted in 2006 and 2015, researchers examined the influence of stress during phonological encoding for adults who do and do not stutter in the absence of speech production using a silent phoneme monitoring task. In a 2006 study, adults who do and do not stutter were required to silently identify sounds within compound words (e.g., *BLACK-board*: initial stress) or noun phrases (e.g., *black-BOARD*: noninitial stress) of identical phonemic composition. Findings indicated an overall slowness in response time for adults who stutter, but this slowness did not interact with word type (i.e., stress pattern). Authors noted the potential influence of lexical retrieval during response as a potential confounding factor.

To further isolate the relationship between segmental and suprasegmental encoding in the absence of motoric and lexical processing, a similar silent phoneme monitoring task was conducted in 2015 using bisyllabic nonwords that differed *only* by syllabic stress demarcation. Adults who stutter exhibited delayed encoding when encoding novel words, but only for stimuli with noninitial stress. In addition, adults who stutter exhibited a greater number of phonemic errors and stress assignment errors for stimuli with noninitial stress during posttrial verbal response. In contrast, no differences in monitoring latencies and posttrial accuracy were observed in typically fluent adults, regardless of stress pattern. These data suggest that in addition to the observed articulatory consequences of prosodic stress noted by previous researchers, stress assignment also perturbs during phonological encoding processes in a manner that is unique to adults who stutter, and it is observed more readily during the retention and assembly of new, unfamiliar words prior to production.

Crosslinguistic Data and Future Studies

Despite the use of more refined techniques, experimental and descriptive data to date have not determined a direct link between suprasegmental factors and stuttered speech beyond the frequent co-occurrence during production. At minimum, there is sufficient evidence to suggest that one prosodic factor, namely syllabic stress, may impose greater demand on speech production, as well as speech planning processes, in adults who stutter within stress-based languages. The growing body of research investigating prosodic factors that are phonetically distinct from syllabic stress, such as pitch-accent within mora-timed languages (e.g., pitch-fall in Japanese) and lexical tone within tone-based languages (e.g., high–level, high–rising, falling–rising, high–falling in Mandarin), may provide greater insight into the underlying impact of suprasegmental properties on stuttering across languages. Future research that includes a broader range of prosodic and paralinguistic factors across languages, and in children closer to the onset of speech production, is needed to establish their unique role in relation to the *cause* of stuttering, as well as their contribution to *moments* of stuttered speech, and to further inform our understanding of stuttering across the life span.

Geoffrey A. Coalson

See also Psychological Stress and Speech Disorders; Segmentation of Speech; Suprasegmental Aspects of Speech

Further Readings

Burger, R., & Wijnen, F. (1999). Phonological encoding and word stress in stutter and nonstuttering adults. *Journal of Fluency Disorders, 24,* 91–106.

Chou, F.-C., Zebrowski, P., & Yang, S.-L. (2015). Lexical tone and stuttering loci in Mandarin: Evidence from preschool children who stutter. *Clinical Linguistics and Phonetics, 29,* 115–130.

Coalson, G. A., & Byrd, C. T. (2015). Metrical encoding in adults who do and do not stutter. *Journal of Speech, Language, and Hearing Research, 58,* 601–621.

Matsumoto-Shimamori, S., & Ito, T. (2013). Effect of word accent on the difficulty of transition from core vowels in first syllables to the following segments in Japanese children who stutter. *Clinical Linguistics and Phonetics, 27,* 694–704.

Packman, A., Onslow, M., Richard, F., & van Doorn, J. (1996). Syllabic stress and variability: A model of stuttering. *Clinical Linguistics and Phonetics, 10,* 235–263.

Perkins, W., Kent, R., & Curlee, R. (1991). A theory of neuropsycholinguistic function of stuttering. *Journal of Speech and Hearing Research, 19,* 509–522.

Sasisekaran, J., & de Nil, L. F. (2006). Phoneme monitoring in silent naming and perception in adults who stutter. *Journal of Fluency Disorders, 31,* 284–302.

Wingate, M. E. (1988). *The structure of stuttering: A psycholinguistic analysis.* New York, NY: Springer.

Paraphasia

Paraphasia is the term given to phonemic or word errors found in the expressive language of fluent aphasia. These errors are neither due to motor production deficits found in dysarthria, such as weakness or paralysis of the speech muscles, nor from a motor programming deficit found in apraxia. Paraphasias arise from higher level language errors in the selection of sounds or words. Unlike anomia, the inability to find the word, the speaker knows the word to say, but because of paraphasic errors, the word spoken is a nonword or the wrong word. This entry provides a brief overview of paraphasias, which can be described along a continuum based on types and numbers of errors.

Literal or Phonemic Paraphasia

Literal/phonemic paraphasia involves a single sound error in a word, across adjacent words, or across phrases. These sound selection errors conform to the speech sounds and to the phoneme sequence constraints of the speaker's language. There are several types of phonemic paraphasias based on the sound error made. A substitution error (e.g., "lup" for *cup*) occurs when the substituted sound is unrelated to the target sound (sometimes called a *wild error*). More common substitution errors involve homorganic sound pairs that share the same place of articulation but differ in manner and voicing (e.g., "pop" for *mop*). An anticipatory error occurs when there is a right-to-left movement of the phoneme (e.g., "toto" for *photo*), and a perseveration error happens with a left-to-right movement of the phoneme (e.g., "pork pop" for *pork chop*). A deletion error simplifies a consonant cluster at word initial (e.g., "tuck" for *truck*) or at word final (e.g., "comet" for *comment*).

There is some disagreement as to which type of phonemic paraphasia occurs most frequently. David P. Corina and colleagues found that the more common error is deletion of word final segments or syllables followed by substitution errors, while Sheila Blumstein found that substitutions occurred more frequently than deletions. A confounding variable in these types of studies is the presence of dysarthria and/or apraxia in the speech of people with aphasia. Apraxia/dysarthria arises from damage to the inferior motor strip in the frontal lobe, which causes muscle weakness and/or incoordination that can result in a true distortion of a given phoneme (e.g., *bath* pronounced with an approximate stop for /θ/). This error would not be considered a true phonemic paraphasia.

Neuroanatomically, literal/phonemic paraphasias correlate to damage to both the parietal and temporal areas including the superior and middle temporal gyri and especially the middle superior temporal gyrus.

Verbal or Semantic Paraphasia

Verbal/semantic paraphasia occurs when a real word different from the target word is used. Most instances of a semantic paraphasia involve a word that is semantically related to the target word. Categories of semantic paraphasias are based on the type of semantic relationship that exists between the target word and the spoken word. Corina investigated the frequency of occurrence of semantic paraphasia types and found that coordinate-level errors (e.g., "lion" for *tiger*) accounted for nearly 75% of the errors; part-whole errors (e.g., "finger" for *hand*) occurred in nearly 15% of the errors; and associate-level errors (e.g., "foot" for *shoe*) around 6%. Other types of semantic paraphasias occurred less frequently in their subject population: superordinate errors (e.g., "apple" for *fruit*), visual errors (e.g., "nail" for *knife*), and subordinate errors (e.g., "flower" for *daisy*).

Neuroanatomically, verbal/semantic paraphasias have been linked to damage in a number of cortical structures in the language-dominant hemisphere including the posterior middle temporal gyrus, postcentral gyrus, and the anterior supramarginal gyrus. Corina describes the areas most involved in the production of semantic paraphasias to be the middle posterior central gyrus, the anterior supramarginal gyrus, and the posterior middle temporal gyrus. Cathy Price found that semantic paraphasia errors that were close to the target word (e.g., "dog" instead of *cat*) involved the angular gyrus and the anterior inferior temporal regions. Errors that did not have a semantic relationship to the target (e.g., "dog" for *train*) involved a more global impairment including the supramarginal gyrus, the left angular gyrus, and the posterior superior temporal gyrus extending into the occipital cortex.

Neologism

Neologism (meaning *new word*) is a type of paraphasia that involves more than one sound error in a word so that the spoken word is undecipherable as the target word (e.g., "potch" for *cup*). Neologisms arise from damage to the more posterior areas of the parietal/temporal lobes in the language-dominant hemisphere.

Jargon

Jargon refers to multiword utterances that contain so many errors, both phonemic and semantic, that the message is undecipherable ("kash mon a zomfatatat" for *make me a sandwich*). The listener may be able to grasp the meaning of the jargon utterance only if there is enough context or if the utterance is accompanied by gestures or drawings by the speaker. People with aphasia who have a wider area of damage across the parietal, temporal, and anterior occipital lobes are more likely to produce jargon.

Paraphasias can also occur in written language and are usually the same types of errors heard in verbal utterances. A person with aphasia may use only one type of paraphasia or may use all types. The type of paraphasia can also be diagnostically significant with jargon/neologisms reflecting a more severe impairment than semantic or phonemic paraphasias together or alone.

Carmen Larimore Russell

See also Anomia; Aphasia; Communication Disorders; Jargon and Jargon Aphasia; Neurogenic Communication Disorders; Speech Production, Theories of; Stroke

Further Readings

Blumstein, S. (1973). *A phonological investigation of aphasic speech*. Hague, The Netherlands: Mouton.

Buckingham, H. W. (1986). The scan-copier mechanism and the positional level of language production: Evidence from phonemic paraphasia. *Cognitive Science, 10*, 195–217.

Buckingham, H. W. (1989). Phonological paraphasia. In C. Code (Ed.), *The characteristics of aphasia* (pp. 89–110). New York, NY: Taylor & Francis.

Corina, D. P., Loudermilk, B. C., Detwiler, L., Martin, R. F., Brinkley, J. F., & Ojermann, G. (2010). Analysis of naming errors during cortical stimulation mapping: Implications for models of language representation. *Brain and Language, 115*, 101–112.

Goodglass, H., Kaplan, E., & Barresi, B. (2001). *The assessment of aphasia and related disorders* (3rd ed.). Austin, TX: Pro-Ed.

Price, C. J. (2000). Functional imaging studies in aphasia. In J. C. Mazziotta, A. W. Toga, & R. S. J. Frackowiak (Eds.), *Brain mapping: The disorders* (pp. 181–201). San Diego, CA: Academic Press.

Parkinson's Disease

James Parkinson is credited with writing the first clear medical description of Parkinson's disease (PD) in 1817. In his essay on the "Shaking Palsy,"

Parkinson outlined a clinical syndrome in which he described involuntary tremulous motion with lessened muscular power in parts not in action, even when supported; a propensity to bend the trunk forward, and to pass from a walking to a running pace, with the individuals' senses and intellects remaining uninjured. Building on this historic clinical presentation of PD, researchers have continued to broaden the understanding of the motor and nonmotor characteristics of the disease as well as added pathological definitions. As a result, therapies have been designed that are reliable and effective and can be used as part of the diagnostic criteria. This entry provides an overview of the history of PD and then details its diagnosis, demographics, causes, and treatment.

History of PD

While James Parkinson is credited with providing the first thorough description of PD, evidence of much earlier statements of a clinical syndrome involving rigidity, tremor, slowness, and akinesia has been discovered. The oldest existing Chinese medical text dating back to 500 BCE outlined these symptoms. In addition, Charaka, "the father of Indian medicine," provided a coherent picture of parkinsonisms in 300 BCE.

In Western medicine, Galen (138–201 CE) is credited with the earliest references to symptoms of PD. However, it wasn't until the 1800s that various physicians, patients, and researchers began documenting more thorough descriptors of the disease. Following Parkinson's publication, Jean-Martin Charcot (mid-1800s) expanded the clinical picture, adding the symptoms of masked face, possible contractions in hands and feet, and akathesia (i.e., a feeling of inner restlessness). Charcot also clarified that paralysis was not necessarily part of the syndrome, which, at the time, was often referred to as *paralysis agitans*. In 1876, he suggested the syndrome be referred to as PD from that point forward; the term is used today. Sometimes, *idiopathic PD* is used to describe parkinsonism for which a single cause cannot be identified.

Diagnosis

The diagnosis of PD relies solely on clinical examination, as there are no biomarkers or simple laboratory tests that can confirm a diagnosis, except autopsy. The accuracy of diagnosing using clinical examination as confirmed at autopsy is estimated at between 80% and 90%.

Four major motor clinical symptoms of PD include tremor; bradykinesia (i.e., slowness of movement); rigidity of the arms, legs, or trunk; and postural instability. At least two of the four symptoms must be present before a diagnosis of PD should be considered. The onset of symptoms is insidious and often asymmetric. Because many of these motor symptoms can result from etiologies and conditions unrelated to PD, often imaging is recommended to rule out other causes. Additionally, a thorough review of past and current medications, as well as response to medications that imitate the production of dopamine, can aid in the clinical diagnosis of PD.

Tools have been developed to follow the progression of the disease symptoms. The Unified Parkinson's Disease Rating Scale is the most widely used clinical rating scale for PD. This scale has four parts: Part I (nonmotor experiences of daily living which includes investigations into the patient's cognition, mood, apathy, psychosis, sleep, pain, dysautonomia, and fatigue); Part II (motor experiences of daily living); Part III (motor examination); and Part IV (motor complications). Both patient- and caregiver-derived information is integrated with raters' clinical judgments and observations. The tool is available in English, and it has been translated into various non-English versions including German, Russian, Hungarian, Japanese, Italian, Spanish, French, Chinese, Estonian, and Slovak.

Demographics

PD is the second most common neurodegenerative disorder after Alzheimer's disease. It afflicts more than 4 million people worldwide, and by 2030, it is projected to affect between 8.7 and 9.3 million people. It is unknown whether PD is more common in certain countries because of the limited number of studies conducted to date. While the disease occurs in all races, it seems to be somewhat more prevalent in Caucasians. The incidence of PD increases with age. It is estimated that 4% of individuals with PD are diagnosed before the age of 50 years. The average age of onset is 60 years. PD is diagnosed in men 1.5 more times than in women.

Causes

The cause of most cases of PD is unknown. Both sporadic and familial forms of the disease exist, although familial forms probably make up less than 10% of those diagnosed. While changes in DNA have been reported in a small portion of those with the disease (i.e., 30% of the familial and 3–5% of the sporadic cases), cases rarely are due to genetic change alone. PD likely results from a confluence of inherited and environmental factors. These environmental factors are suspected to influence the expression of the gene(s). Head trauma, toxin and pesticide exposure, and certain occupations and foods are among the higher risk environmental factors. Lower risk factors include cigarette smoking, coffee drinking, and the use of some anti-inflammatory drugs, among others.

Neuropathologically, the symptoms of PD are the result of a progressive and profound loss of neuromelanin containing dopaminergic neurons in the substantia nigra pars compacta with the presence of eosinophilic, intracytoplasmic, proteinaceous inclusions (i.e., Lewy bodies) and dystrophic Lewy neurites in surviving neurons. At mid-stages of the disease, there is often widespread neurodegeneration of the central nervous system.

Treatment

The treatment for PD is symptomatic. As of 2018, there are no options that halt the loss of neurons in PD. Pharmacological management of the classic motor symptoms of PD, as well as of selected non-motor symptoms, is often the first course of treatment. Strong evidence supports the use of levodopa and dopamine agonists for motor symptoms at all stages of PD. Dopamine agonists and drugs that block dopamine metabolism are effective for treating motor fluctuations, and clozapine is effective for treating hallucinations. Cholinesterase inhibitors may improve symptoms of dementia, and antidepressants and pramipexole may improve depression.

Despite the best medical therapy, it is estimated that 40% of patients experience complications such as unpredictable fluctuations of symptoms and dyskinesias as PD advances into the later stages (5 years after initial PD diagnosis). Surgical intervention is an option for some individuals with PD. Deep brain stimulation involves the implantation of electrodes into parts of the brain, often either subthalamic nucleus or globus pallidus. The electrodes are connected to a generator that is implanted into the patient's chest and sends electrical pulses to the brain to improve many motor symptoms of PD. This can reduce the need or amount of levodopa required, which often becomes less effective in the later stages of the disease.

According to Giselle Petzinger, exercise-based behavioral treatments for the motor symptoms of PD may improve function and slow progression of motor symptoms and neural degeneration. Physical, occupational, speech, and dysphagia therapies, among others, are often recommended to improve patient's speech, swallowing, limb function, gait, balance, and activities of daily living. Evidence for the inclusion of exercise therapy in the management of PD has grown, especially short-term benefits.

Individuals with PD have described their communication impairments as embarrassing, often resulting in their withdrawal from social situations and inactivity. Nearly 90% of individuals with PD have speech and voice disorders characterized by reduced loudness, breathy and monotone speech, imprecise articulation, hesitations, and rushes of speech. It is hypothesized that the speech and voice deficits associated with PD are due to inadequate merging of kinesthetic feedback, motor output, and context feedback within basal ganglia necessary to select and reinforce an appropriate gain in the motor command. While deep brain stimulation has positive effects on many of the motor symptoms associated with PD, the effects on speech have been variable and not uniformly positive. However, individuals with PD who participate in behavioral training to increase loudness have had documented success. Data from two randomized controlled trials have demonstrated lasting (24 months after training) increases in vocal sound pressure levels and in frequency variability during speech in speakers with PD who participated in an intensive voice program.

Alana Mantie-Kozlowski

See also Motor Speech Disorders; Neurogenic Communication Disorders; Pharmacological Interventions in Speech and Language Disorders; Voice Disorders; Voice Therapy

Further Readings

Berg, D., Postuma, R. B., Bloem, B., Chan, P., Dubois, B., Gasser, T., . . . Deuschl, G. (2014). Time to redefine PD? Introductory statement of the MDS Task Force on the definition of Parkinson's disease. *Movement Disorders*, 29(4), 454–462.

Connolly, B. S., & Lang, A. E. (2014). Pharmacological treatment of Parkinson disease: A review. *JAMA*, 311, 1670–1683. doi:10.1001/jama.2014.3654

Fox, C., Ebersbach, G., Ramig, L., & Sapir, S. (2012). LSVT LOUD and LSVT BIG: Behavioral treatment programs for speech and body movement in Parkinson Disease. *Parkinson's Disease*, 2012, 391946. Retrieved from http://doi.org/10.1155/2012/391946

Klein, C., & Westenberger, A. (2012). Genetics of Parkinson's disease. *Cold Spring Harbor Perspectives in Medicine*, 2(1), a008888. doi:10.1101/cshperspect.a008888

Martinez-Martin, P., Rodriguez-Blazquez, C., Alvarez-Sanchez, M., Arakaki, T., Bergareche-Yarza, A., Chade, A., . . . Goetz, C. G. (2013). Expanded and independent validation of the Movement Disorder Society-Unified Parkinson's Disease Rating Scale (MDS-UPDRS). *Journal of Neurology*, 260(1), 228–236.

Ovallath, S., & Deepa, P. (2013). The history of Parkinsonism: Descriptions in ancient Indian medical literature. *Movement Disorders*, 28, 566–568. doi:10.1002/mds.25420

Parkinson, J. (1817). *An essay on the shaking palsy. Whittingham and Rowland for Sherwood*. London, UK: Needly and Jones.

Pathophysiology of Stroke

The term *pathophysiology* refers to the study of detrimental changes to normal physiological processes, deriving from infection, disease, or injury. A *cerebrovascular accident* (CVA), or *stroke*, represents a sudden neurovascular event in which blood supply to a portion of the brain is disrupted; when this causes the death of brain cells, it is called a cerebral infarction. CVAs are among the top three causes of death and disability in the United States. They are classified as either ischemic or hemorrhagic. Ischemic CVAs result from a narrowing or blockage in an artery, while hemorrhagic CVAs are caused by rupture of the arterial wall; in either case, blood supply to brain tissue is lost. According to the Centers for Disease Control and Prevention, ischemia accounts for 87% of all strokes and hemorrhage for 13%. This entry provides an overview of the pathophysiology of ischemic and hemorrhagic strokes.

Ischemic CVA

Ischemia is defined as a cessation or significant reduction of blood flow to tissue, due to either obstruction by a free-floating bolus (e.g., a blood clot) or vascular stenosis (e.g., gradual accumulation of atherosclerotic plaque on the arterial wall, narrowing its inner diameter). Atherosclerotic plaque is an agglomeration of lipids, cholesterol, calcium, macrophage foam cells, and other components. Ischemia is called *embolic* when due to bolus obstruction and *thrombotic* when due to stenosis.

During ischemia, cerebral blood flow (CBF) is restricted, immediately depriving cells of oxygen and glucose. The brain, despite accounting for only 2% of the body's weight, requires some 20% of the oxygen and glucose in the bloodstream. Without these molecules, adenosine triphosphate (ATP) cannot be generated. ATP is the energy source that drives many of the metabolic processes in neurons. The brain does not store ATP, so when no new ATP is generated, the extant supply depletes rapidly. To compensate for the loss of CBF, there is an immediate localized autoregulatory response of vasodilation and reallocation of CBF from alternate routes which can provide collateral circulation. If these mechanisms are insufficient and CBF drops below about 30% of the normal flow rate, neuroelectrical and synaptic activity shuts down and the cell goes dormant. If CBF continues to drop below a critical threshold of 15–20% of the normal flow rate, loss of ATP initiates a catastrophic cascade of biochemical processes, culminating in cell necrosis.

In a typical CVA, there is a *core* region of tissue where the CBF has dropped below the critical threshold and the cells die within 1–2 min. Surrounding the core is the *penumbra*; this region may still receive sufficient CBF from intact collateral circulation to survive longer and may eventually recover if there is reperfusion of the tissue within an appropriate time window. The greater the degree of CBF deprivation, the shorter the window of opportunity to reperfuse the area and potentially rescue affected tissue. This may be as brief as minutes (for severe or complete CBF deprivation) to several hours (for mild CBF deprivation). If reperfusion does not occur within this time, then tissue in the penumbra will also become necrotic. It should be noted, however, that reperfusion also carries with it risks (which is discussed later).

The pathophysiology of ischemia involves a number of processes: loss of energy and sodium/potassium homeostasis, loss of calcium homeostasis, excitotoxicity, acidosis, oxidative and nitrative stresses, inflammatory processes, and apoptosis. These processes are interrelated, often forming feedback loops that can cause runaway escalation of the processes leading to cell death. To understand the significance of these processes, a very basic understanding of some of the conditions in an intact nerve cell is helpful. In a normal neuron at rest, there are two gradients across the cell membrane: a chemical gradient and an electrical gradient. The chemical concentration of sodium (Na^+), chloride (Cl^-), and calcium (Ca^{2+}) ions outside the cell is typically far higher than inside the cell at rest, while the chemical gradient for potassium ions (K^+) is in the opposite direction. The separation of these ions by the cell membrane also contributes to the maintenance of the electrical potential gradient across the membrane (approximately 70 mV lower inside the cell when it is at rest). The cell membrane is not perfectly impermeable; normally, the chemical gradients drive some leakage of the ions across the membrane. Countering this, one active ion transport mechanism continually pumps Na^+ out of the cell and K^+ into the cell against their respective gradients, and another active ion transport mechanism pumps Ca^{2+} out of the cell. These active ion transport mechanisms are powered by ATP. The leak currents and the counteracting ATP-driven active ion transport mechanisms together maintain ionic homeostasis in the healthy neuron.

During a stroke, when CBF has dropped below the threshold, ATP is no longer manufactured and the ATP-dependent active ion transport mechanisms in the neuronal membrane stop. The ever-present ion leaks then collapse the ion concentration differentials across the cell membrane, leading to depolarization, and the membrane becomes more permeable to ion species. A by-product of the influx of sodium and chloride into the cell is the creation of osmotic gradients which pull water into the cell and cause cellular edema; this will eventually lead to rupture of the membrane and cell necrosis. Meanwhile, the loss of energy and ion homeostasis sets the stage for further destructive processes.

Next, there is the loss of calcium homeostasis as well as excitotoxicity. The processes described in the preceding paragraph exacerbate the influx of calcium ions into the cell. Under normal circumstances, there is 1/10,000 the amount of calcium inside the cell as outside. This tight regulation of intracellular calcium is necessary to maintain the delicate balance of calcium ion concentration inside the cell, which supplies a variety of processes, including gene expression, synaptic function, and cytoskeletal stability. These processes are disrupted by such large increases in intracellular calcium ions. The elevated intracellular calcium also unleashes destructive enzymes: proteases, phospholipases, protein kinases, and endonucleases. Pathological levels of such enzymes contribute to the destruction of the cytoskeleton, the creation of additional destructive compounds, and other impairments to cell function (which is discussed later). Finally, the sudden influx of calcium ions also causes massive release of the excitatory neurotransmitter glutamate and aspartate to toxic levels, far in excess of the ability of synaptic reuptake mechanisms to clear the extracellular concentration of neurotransmitters. This forms a feedback loop stimulating greater inflow of calcium ions into the cells, thereby exacerbating the processes described previously.

Toxic by-products of the loss of calcium homeostasis (such as nitric oxide synthases and reactive oxygen radicals) are also produced in the affected neurons. Nitric oxide synthases catalyze the production of nitric oxide, which appears to be one of the mechanisms involved in the formation of oxygen free radicals. Additionally, high levels of calcium ions (and sodium ions) induce mitochondria to produce oxygen free radicals. The reactive oxygen species produced in these ways strip electrons from other molecules in the cell (such as proteins, lipids, and nucleic acids) and cause much damage as well as contribute to apoptosis (which is discussed later).

The oxidative and nitrative stresses initiate a complex inflammatory response which takes place in acute, subacute, and chronic phases (from minutes, to hours, to days after onset). It should be noted that the natural process of inflammation may have some benefits, such as increased production of glial cells and vascular supply, facilitating neuroplasticity, and carrying away necrotic debris. It is not clear which, if any, inflammatory responses mitigate or exacerbate the injury and whether treatment of inflammation is warranted—and if so, how that intervention might be phase dependent.

The unfolding inflammatory response over time involves many processes. Resident microglial cells are attracted to the lesion site immediately and express pro-inflammatory molecules. Circulating inflammatory cells (such as neutrophils, macrophages, T cells, monocytes, and other leukocytes) infiltrate the area, contributing to and exacerbating degradation of the cerebral endothelium. Leukocytes, for example, accumulate within about 12 hr and secrete cytotoxic enzymes and generate oxygen free radicals. This in turn undermines the blood–brain barrier and causes microhemorrhage. The cerebral parenchyma becomes susceptible to edema.

Another pathophysiological process that occurs in the anaerobic conditions of CBF loss is the production of lactate (related to lactic acid), which lowers the intracellular pH, causing acidotoxicity in the neuron. This occurs because pH below about 6.5 triggers calcium-permeable acid-sensing ion channels to activate and further permit calcium ions to enter the cell. The acidotoxic processes cause edema and impaired mitochondrial respiration, and they may contribute to the destruction of the blood–brain barrier.

As the previously described processes cause necrosis in the core, spontaneous waves of periinfarct depolarization of neuronal membrane potentials pass through the penumbra region. This appears to be caused by extracellular potassium and glutamate emanating from the core region. These depolarization waves may cause calcium buildup in penumbral cells, leading to tissue necrosis there as well. However, it appears that the majority of penumbral tissue loss is caused by apoptosis rather than necrosis. This is because, given the collateral blood supply in the penumbra, there is some production of ATP so that energy levels do not fall so far as to cause tissue necrosis. Nevertheless, cells may still die through apoptotic mechanisms.

Apoptosis, often referred to as *programmed cell death*, represents a series of processes whereby the cell shuts down and dies in a controlled manner. Indeed, it is a natural and important part of the healthy function of organisms; some 50% of the neurons in the growing human fetus are destroyed through apoptotic processes to facilitate the healthy development of the brain in utero. During ischemia, especially in the penumbra, apoptosis is initiated due to ion imbalances and other processes that lead to the swelling of the neuronal mitochondria and pore formation in its outer membrane. This causes the release of cytochrome c from the outer mitochondrial membrane, which binds with enzymes in the cytosol to form the apoptosome complex. The apoptosome complex and apoptosis-inducing factor (also secreted by the mitochondria) together choreograph a complex set of processes designed to shut down and dismantle the neuron in a controlled manner.

Given the slower process of penumbral necrosis or apoptosis, it is possible to intervene before significant cell death occurs there. Reperfusion must occur within 1–2 min to avoid cell death in the core region and within 3–4 hr to spare the penumbra. During this penumbral window, intravenous administration of a thrombolytic such as recombinant tissue plasminogen activator can re-establish CBF and significantly reduce the likelihood of penumbral necrosis. Thrombolytics, considered the standard of care when indicated, should be administered as soon after the onset of ischemia as possible, ideally within a 60-min *door-to-needle* time frame. Additionally, there are other means of reperfusion, such as intra-arterial thrombolysis (i.e., delivering the thrombolytic directly to the site using a catheter), thrombectomy (i.e., surgical removal of the thrombosis), or balloon angioplasty with or without stent placement (i.e., insertion of a catheter to the site, inflation of a balloon to expand the arterial lumen, and possible placement of a stent to maintain arterial wall integrity). These techniques all carry respective benefits and risk factors which must be weighed by the neurotrauma team.

Unfortunately, reperfusion may have adverse effects. If reperfusion occurs after the penumbral time window, there may be a sudden increase in the production of potent oxygen-derived free radicals. These components exacerbate the degradation of the arterial wall and weakening of the blood–brain barrier which began with the original loss of CBF. Simultaneously, dysautoregulation of capillary blood pressure may cause CBF during reperfusion to exceed normal levels and worsen the cerebral edema. White blood cells accompanying the returning CBF also aggravate this inflammatory response. Collectively, the original loss of CBF and the resulting processes, as well as administration of thrombolytics and reperfusion, may contribute to hemorrhage within the region. This is referred to as *hemorrhagic transformation*; what began as an ischemic CVA may transform into a hemorrhagic CVA.

One final note regarding ischemia is that, apart from the death of neurons, there are also effects on other cell types. However, although astrocytes, oligodendroglial cells, and other tissues in the core and penumbra sustain injury, the pathophysiology of these components is not well understood. Overall, it can be said that loss of CBF affects not only neurons but also glial cells and the cerebral microvasculature. Since 2001, the term *neurovascular unit* has become common, emphasizing that neurons, glial cells, and vascular endothelium are together affected by the ischemic event.

Hemorrhagic CVA

Hemorrhagic CVAs are caused by rupture of the arterial wall, and they may be further subdivided into three types: arterial hemorrhage, ruptured aneurysm, and ruptured arteriovenous malformation (AVM). Arterial hemorrhage, when it occurs epidurally or subdurally, is usually the result of head trauma. Otherwise, arterial hemorrhage can occur intraparenchymally, and these often result from arterial disease affecting the smaller arteries and arterioles of the brain. Aneurysms are a ballooning, or outpouching, of a weakened arterial wall; this may then rupture and hemorrhage. AVMs consist of a tangle of vessels in which arteries are directly connected to veins without intermediary capillaries. Normally, CBF rate is highest in arteries and decreasing as the diameter gets smaller toward arterioles and then capillaries. Blood pressure is also lower in venules and veins. Designed to accommodate lower pressure and flow, the walls of venules and veins are thinner and weaker than those of arteries and arterioles. Thus, in AVMs, when the high-pressure arterial flow is connected directly to veins without the step-down that normally occurs in the capillary beds, the veins receive blood at higher pressure and flow rate and are susceptible to rupture.

Although accounting for only 13% of all CVAs, hemorrhagic strokes tend to be more severe in terms of morbidity, mortality, and long-term clinical outcomes; they comprise some 40–70% of the 1-month mortality rate for strokes. This increased severity is not only due to the fact that there is loss of blood supply (i.e., ischemia) to the tissue that had been served by the hemorrhaging artery but also because there may be a growing hematoma (i.e., pooling volume of blood) at the hemorrhage site. The tissue around the hematoma may also become edematous. If the hemorrhage enters the ventricular system (more common for strokes in and around the thalamus or basal ganglia), then clotting of blood may obstruct the flow of cerebrospinal fluid through the ventricular system, leading to a buildup of cerebrospinal fluid causing potentially catastrophic swelling of the ventricles. All of these mass effects (hematoma, intracerebral edema, and ventricular enlargement) will cause elevated intracranial pressure (ICP).

The mass effects and increased ICP compress tissue near the hematoma site or in the periventricular region if due to ventricular swelling and possibly throughout the brain. Compression of the brain tissue is a serious risk factor, causing additional cell necrosis. Severe ICP elevation may cause herniation of the brainstem through the foramen magnum, possibly causing coma or death. The mass effect may also compress blood vessels, thus causing additional ischemic injury to the areas supplied by the compressed vessels.

Less severe hemorrhagic CVAs stabilize within hours to days. More severe types may worsen progressively over acute, subacute, and chronic phases, before leading to death or ultimately stabilizing. In either case, the process begins with the initial hemorrhage; this causes the first neurological insult: ischemic injury. Thus, hemorrhagic CVAs will also involve the same processes described in the previous section on ischemic CVA. Beyond that, however, the hemorrhaging blood may also form an intracerebral hematoma. Unless the hemorrhage is sealed or coagulated, the hematoma will continue to expand in the acute phase. This may last from days up to 2 weeks (if it stops at all), depending upon the severity of the hemorrhage. In addition to the mass effects, the hematoma may also cause stretching of blood vessels at the periphery of the clot, leading to secondary hemorrhages. An expanding hematoma is the principal cause for progressive worsening of symptoms during the acute phase.

Surrounding the hematoma, edema begins to form and typically peaks several days after onset. This may be due initially to the production of thrombin (i.e., a product of the coagulation process in the early acute phase), which activates enzymes that undermine the blood–brain barrier. Vasogenic edema may be the result of blood clot retraction. During the subacute phase, a second wave of perihematomal edema may evolve due to erythrocyte lysis. Additionally, iron from degraded hemoglobin is cytotoxic and contributes to the edema—indeed, it may be the primary factor. Relatedly, ambient extravascular/extracellular blood degrades into blood breakdown products and may induce vasospasm in intact blood vessels which can cause hemorrhage as well.

While surgical techniques and treatment options have been refined, the essential approaches for hemorrhagic CVA have not changed substantially. One or more of the following comprise the main approach: cessation of any blood thinners the patient may already have been taking prior to the stroke; administration of pharmacological agents to minimize seizures or vasospasm; careful management of blood pressure and ICP; endovascular interventions to coil or clip an aneurysm; surgical removal, or stereotactic radiosurgery, for AVMs; placement of an arterial stent, evacuation of the hematoma and placement of a shunt to manage hydrocephalus; alleviation of ICP via craniectomy; and other techniques.

Pradeep Ramanathan

See also Anatomy of the Human Neurological System; Aphasia; Traumatic Brain Injury; Plasticity of Brain; Regional Cerebral Blood Flow (rCBF); Stroke

Further Readings

Arai, K., Lok, J., Guo, S., Hayakawa, K., Xing, C., & Lo, E. H. (2011). Cellular mechanisms of neurovascular damage and repair after stroke. *Journal of Child Neurology, 26*(9), 1193–1198.

Chen, S., Zeng, L., & Hu, Z. (2014). Progressing hemorrhagic stroke: Categories, causes, mechanisms and managements. *Journal of Neurology, 261*, 2061–2078.

Guo, Y., Li, P., Guo, Q., Shang, K., Yan, D., Du, S., & Lu, Y. (2013). Pathophysiology and biomarkers in acute ischemic stroke—A review. *Tropical Journal of Pharmaceutical Research, 12*(6), 1097–1105.

Jin, R., Yang, G., & Li, G. (2010). Inflammatory mechanisms in ischemic stroke: Role of inflammatory cells. *Journal of Leukocyte Biology, 87*, 779–789.

Kumar, G., Goyal, M. K., Sahota, P. K., & Jain, R. (2010). Penumbra, the basis of neuroimaging in acute stroke treatment: Current evidence. *Journal of the Neurological Sciences, 288*, 13–24.

van Asch, C. J., Luitse, M. J., Rinkel, G. J., van der Tweel, I., Algra, A., & Klijn, C. J. (2010). Incidence, case fatality, and functional outcome of intracerebral haemorrhage over time, according to age, sex, and ethnic origin: A systematic review and meta-analysis. *Lancet Neurology, 9*, 167–176.

Zhang, J., Yang, Y., Sun, H., & Xing, Y. (2014). Hemorrhagic transformation after cerebral infarction: Current concepts and challenges. *Annals of Translational Medicine, 2*(8), 81. doi:10.3978/j.issn.2305-5839.2014.08.08

Pathophysiology of Traumatic Brain Injury

Traumatic brain injuries (TBIs) may be categorized as closed or penetrating. A closed head injury (CHI) occurs when the brain is injured as a result of a blow to the head or a forceful movement resulting in the brain bouncing against the inner skull. A penetrating head injury (PHI) follows the penetration of a projectile through the skull and meninges, the membranes (dura mater, arachnoid, pia mater) that enclose the brain. This topic has become increasingly important because of the relatively high incidence of TBI throughout the world and its association with sports, war, and everyday activities such as driving. Consequently, professionals who evaluate and treat individuals with communication disorders in clinics, schools, and medical settings are encountering persons with TBI on a regular basis. This entry focuses on the communicative consequences of TBI.

Incidence

There are estimated 1.6 million new cases of TBI among civilians each year in the United States. Adolescents and young adults aged 15–24 years have the highest incidence of TBI, typically associated with motor vehicle accidents. Sports-related concussion has also become a common etiologic factor for this age-group, as repeated concussions may result in TBI. In addition, due to advancements in munitions, increased use of improvised explosive devices, and sophisticated body armor, military personnel who have served in Iraq and Afghanistan have a greater risk for brain injury (i.e., blast injury) than those from the Vietnam War (31% vs. 15%). Older adults over the age of 65 years and children under the age of 5 years have the next highest incidence of TBI, most commonly resulting from falls. Males are twice as likely to suffer a TBI as females, and persons with a previous TBI are three times as likely to suffer a second TBI.

Type of Injury

TBI may be classified in general terms as closed or penetrating, based on whether the meninges, the three tissue sacks which enclose the brain, remain intact. A CHI is typically the result of a rapid acceleration and deceleration movement creating a whiplash effect that results in diffuse axonal injury, in which the axons that connect brain cells are stretched, twisted, or torn, while the meninges remain unbroken. This manner of injury is common in motor vehicle accidents. By contrast, in a PHI, some type of missile pierces the skull, the meninges, and the brain. A gunshot wound is an example of this type of injury.

Consequences

The consequences of TBI are many, quite varied, and, in large measure, dependent on the overall severity of injury. Generally speaking, TBI results in physical, cognitive, communicative, and social impairments. Because of the complex sequelae of TBI, once an individual has stabilized medically, the resulting impairments are best managed by an interdisciplinary rehabilitation team that includes physicians, nurses, physical and occupational therapists, psychologists, social workers, and speech–language pathologists. Rehabilitation following TBI is a long multistage process with the ultimate goal of returning the person to his or her previous social role in the community. One of the most important predictors of success toward that objective is communicative proficiency.

Communication Following TBI

Aphasia

Language is disturbed in 75% or more of individuals with TBI. Whether this language disturbance is the result of aphasia is often not clear. Aphasia is an acquired impairment of language processes underlying receptive and expressive modalities caused by damage to brain regions responsible for language function. Incidence of aphasia following TBI has been reported as ranging from 2% to nearly 50%. The discrepancies regarding the incidence of aphasia following TBI are difficult to resolve because of the incomplete descriptions of the TBI patients studied as well as the varied measures of aphasia employed. The most common linguistic deficits observed following TBI are anomia and impaired auditory comprehension. There is overlap in the language deficits between individuals with aphasia and those with TBI, but the qualitative differences in their errors are most useful for distinguishing between aphasic and nonaphasic responses. Another key distinction is that the specific linguistic deficits often confused as aphasia in TBI are often transient, clearing as the patient recovers, which rarely occurs in aphasia secondary to a stroke.

Cognitive–Communication Disorders

The hallmark of TBI consists of the resulting cognitive disturbances often present. The primary deficits nearly always present are difficulties with attention, memory, and executive function. Attentional problems may be mild or severe and are a common long-term sequel of TBI. Numerous definitions of attention appear through the rehabilitation literature, but the most useful have been described with regard to functional dimensions such as focused attention, sustained attention (vigilance), selective attention, alternating attention, and divided attention. This model facilitates a systematic approach to assessing and treating attentional deficits. There are also numerous definitions of memory. Most involve components of attention, encoding (i.e., preparing stimuli for storage), and consolidation (i.e., merging novel information with previously stored information). Although memory deficits may occur in isolation, they are often accompanied by impairments of orientation, attention, and language. Finally, damage to the prefrontal regions of the brain frequently results in executive dysfunction. The prefrontal brain areas are important for coordinating activities involved in cognitive processing. Executive functioning is an amalgam of the abilities necessary for goal-directed behavior, including anticipation, goal selection, planning, plan execution, self-monitoring, and use of feedback. Executive function is absolutely critical for community reentry after TBI.

Communication difficulties that present after TBI have been designated *cognitive–communication disorders* and are characterized by problems with listening, speaking, reading, writing, and social interactions resulting from underlying cognitive impairments such as attention, memory, and executive functions.

Pragmatics

The primary basis of language impairment in the majority of individuals with TBI is the result of difficulty with pragmatics or language use. Pragmatics may be thought of as a system of rules which prescribe the use of language in specific situations and social contexts. It has been observed that persons with aphasia communicate better than they speak, while individuals with TBI speak better than they communicate. It is now well established that individuals with TBI generally present with cognitive–communication disorders, rather than aphasia, and that a key characteristic of the disorder pattern is difficulty with discourse-level language. In casual interactions, individuals with TBI are often perceived as being off-target, disorganized, tangential, and in some cases that they offer little specific information. These deficits are apparent in both monologic (e.g., descriptive, narrative, procedural) and conversational discourse types. There is no evidence to suggest that individuals with TBI may have selective impairments in monologic or conversational discourse. Discourse deficits may range from mild to severe and do not resolve spontaneously. In addition, different mechanisms of injury (i.e., CHI vs. PHI) yield similar problems with discourse. Discourse deficits in individuals with TBI have serious consequences for quality-of-life outcomes such as return to work and the establishment and preservation of social relationships.

Approaches to Assessing Cognitive–Communication Disorders

Clinicians typically initiate evaluations of cognitive–communication deficits by administering an aphasia battery, focused on vocabulary and syntax. Many individuals with TBI do not present with difficulties in these realms, because they are not aphasic. The clinician must then shift to the evaluation of complex language such as discourse as well as cognitive abilities (e.g., attention, memory, executive function). Discourse is defined as a series of related linguistic units that convey a message. The length of the discourse is determined by the purpose of the communication. It has been suggested that discourse is the most natural component of verbal communication. The production and comprehension of discourse entail a complex interaction of linguistic, cognitive, and social abilities, all of which are susceptible to disruption in TBI. As noted previously, individuals with TBI present with a complex array of cognitive–communication deficits. The assessment of these difficulties requires the use of both standardized and nonstandardized instruments.

Standardized Assessments

A primary objective of assessment is to identify strengths, limitations, and directions for intervention that will facilitate the client's maximal participation in his or her community and social role. A variety of standardized assessments have been recommended for use for persons with TBI. It is important to note that not all of these batteries were designed specifically for TBI; consequently, findings should be interpreted cautiously. Although it is appropriate to evaluate discrete cognitive abilities (e.g., attention, memory, executive function), scores will not stipulate how impairments in these abilities compromise communication. There are few language or communication assessments that delve into this realm; therefore, nonstandardized measures must also be included in the evaluation. Such measures are employed for domains (e.g., complex language and pragmatics) that are critical in real-world contexts and for examining the effects of systematic changes in communication and cognitive demands.

Nonstandardized Assessments

There is substantial evidence to support the assessment of communication following TBI beyond what is included in standardized aphasia batteries. These aphasia tests, which evaluate vocabulary and grammatical abilities at the single word and sentence levels, are not sensitive to the subtle nature of discourse impairments. Studying pragmatics at the level of discourse considers both linguistic and cognitive influences and how these components are integrated for successful social interactions. Discourse analyses have demonstrated utility for delineating pragmatic deficits following TBI. For example, in large groups of TBI survivors (i.e., CHI and PHI) regardless of injury type (diffuse or focal), the most typical pattern involves missing and disorganized content.

Discourse analysis begins with the elicitation of a sample of spoken discourse, minimally five sentences in length. Longer samples are preferred, as shorter samples are not sufficiently complex to characterize discourse proficiency. Due to the lack of a standardized instrument for assessing discourse in TBI, there are no widely used protocols. Consequently, a variety of discourse genres may be sampled, for example, descriptive (e.g., describing a picture); procedural (e.g., relating how to make a sandwich); story narrative (e.g., generating or retelling a story); and conversation. The elicited discourse sample is recorded, transcribed verbatim, and segmented into sentence-like elements such as T units (i.e., an independent clause plus any dependent clauses associated with it) prior to analysis.

A variety of discourse analyses may then be applied. Some of the most commonly used have been measures of cohesion (i.e., how meaning is tied across sentences) and grammatical complexity. Other analyses include coherence (i.e., thematic unity of a text), amount and accuracy of content, story grammar, measures of productivity and efficiency, propositional analyses, and lexical selection. There is general agreement that discourse deficits following TBI are often characterized by decreased verbal output and efficiency. Other consistent findings are problems with coherence, content accuracy and organization, and an increased number of irrelevant propositions. Less consistent findings were reported for measures of grammatical complexity and cohesion.

One specific measure, story grammar, is of particular relevance for individuals with TBI. While descriptions of story grammar differ, the episode is central to all models. The components of an episode are statements pertaining to stated goals, attempts at solutions, and outcomes of those attempts. These components, referred to as initiating events, attempts, and direct consequences, are logical and not dependent on content. The formation of episodes is evidence of story grammar knowledge and is considered to be mediated by nonlinguistic cognitive processes that may be disrupted by TBI. This assertion has been supported by studies of two diverse groups of TBI participants. In both studies, one of the primary discriminating factors between the discourse performance of the TBI participants and those participants without brain injury was a story grammar measure. The TBI groups' decreased ability to generate episodes suggested that the interaction between nonlinguistic cognitive abilities and language was difficult for them.

Neural Underpinnings of Discourse

Discourse processing is thought to require a dynamic interplay between the language system and other cognitive mechanisms. For example, personal experiences and accumulated world knowledge are drawn upon in the successful production and comprehension of a story. Current evidence from neuroimaging suggests that this process requires a distributed network of brain regions including classic language areas in the frontal, temporal, and cingulate areas. A frontoparietal network is thought to support the integration of cognitive representations, while the anterior temporal lobe appears to be activated during tasks requiring increased integration. Inferencing is important for the production and comprehension of stories. A narrative is coherent when each sentence relates to the one before and to the story as a whole. The frontomedial prefrontal cortex, posterior cingulate cortex/precuneus, and the orbitofrontal cortex have been shown to be preferentially engaged during comprehension of coherent, connected texts compared to that of unrelated sentences.

Few neuroimaging studies have been performed of narrative production due to the design challenges of studying connected speech including excessive movement of the speech musculature. Positron emission tomography is most often used for imaging of continuous speech production, but it is time-consuming, expensive, and invasive, and it carries technical limitations. The main advantage to positron emission tomography is its invulnerability to the motion artifacts that hamper the use of functional magnetic resonance imaging during imaging of speech production.

Of the studies that have used neuroimaging to examine comprehension and production of discourse, one used an elaborate motion correction procedure after participants retold short, simple stories during functional magnetic resonance imaging. Results suggested that production and comprehension of story narratives appeared to engage both perisylvian and extrasylvian regions, confirming prior neuroimaging evidence that discourse proficiency is not an exclusively language-based ability. Although both comprehension and production engaged similar areas, the right hemisphere seemed to have greater involvement in discourse comprehension, and the left hemisphere was thought to have a greater role in story narrative production. When positron emission tomography has been used to contrast the two discourse processes, a substantial overlap in comprehension and production was observed. It appeared that more bilateral hippocampal function was necessary for comprehension than for production. The overlap in function in the two processes is not surprising as both require integration, maintenance, and manipulation of information.

Findings from lesion symptom mapping studies of participants with TBI and right hemisphere damage suggest that discourse comprehension relies on a frontal–parietal network involving common cognitive abilities within the left hemisphere and language functions mediated by the right hemisphere. These skills include discourse planning/comprehension; understanding humor, sarcasm, metaphors, and indirect requests; and the generation/comprehension of emotional prosody—all of which are critical for social communication. Making use of world knowledge, as discussed previously, further requires incorporation of motor, spatial, verbal, and executive processes. Finally, discourse comprehension does not appear to function autonomously with regard to cognitive and neural underpinnings but rather shares these processes with working memory and social skills. The comprehension and production of stories require an interaction of several brain regions, which integrate language, inferencing, and executive function abilities, all of which determine proficiency in social skills.

Similarly, 15 participants with PHI with lesions in the left dorsolateral prefrontal cortex demonstrated specific difficulties with narrative discourse production. Deficits were observed in narrative coherence and inclusion of critical story components. In terms of discourse performance, those with lesions in the right dorsolateral prefrontal cortex were not significantly different from the group of participants without brain injury. These results would seem to support observations of relatively lesser involvement of the right PFC in more active tasks, in this case the production of a narrative.

Final Thoughts

Successful discourse is an essential human experience. Disruption contributes to the social isolation that often follows TBI. Neuroimaging studies of discourse comprehension and production following TBI will serve as important next steps in delineating the functional network dedicated to this function. These kinds of studies also have the potential to eventually guide clinicians in treatments that will best facilitate neural recovery.

Carl Coelho and Jennifer Mozeiko

See also Cognitive Impairment; Discourse Analysis; Executive Function and Communication; Memory; Neuropragmatics; Pathophysiology of Stroke

Further Readings

Abdul Sabur, N. Y., Xu, Y., Liu, S., Chow, H. M., Baxter, M., Carson, J., & Braun, A. R. (2014). Neural correlates and network connectivity underlying narrative production and comprehension: A combined fMRI and PET study. *Cortex, 57,* 107–127.

Barbey, A. K., Colom, R., & Grafman, J. (2014). Neural mechanisms of discourse comprehension: A human lesion study. *Brain, 137*(Pt 1), 277–287.

Coelho, C., Lê, K., Mozeiko, J., Krueger, F., & Grafman, J. (2012). Discourse production following injury to the dorsolateral prefrontal cortex. *Neuropsychologia, 50*(14), 3564–3572.

Egidi, G., & Caramazza, A. (2013). Cortical systems for local and global integration in discourse comprehension. *Neuroimage, 71,* 59–74.

Ferstl, E. C. (2010). Neuroimaging of text comprehension: Where are we now. *Italian Journal of Linguistics, 22*(1), 61–88.

Ferstl, E. C., Neumann, J., Bogler, C., & Von Cramon, D. Y. (2008). The extended language network: A meta-analysis of neuroimaging studies on text comprehension. *Human Brain Mapping, 29*(5), 581–593.

Mar, R. A. (2004). The neuropsychology of narrative: Story comprehension, story production and their interrelation. *Neuropsychologia, 42*(10), 1414–1434.

Xu, Y., Tong, Y., Liu, S., Chow, H. M., AbdulSabur, N. Y., Mattay, G. S., & Braun, A. R. (2014). Denoising the speaking brain: Toward a robust technique for correcting artifact-contaminated fMRI data under severe motion. *Neuroimage, 103,* 33–47.

Zasler, N., Katz, D., & Zafonte, R. (2013). *Brain injury medicine: Principles and practice* (2nd ed.). New York, NY: Demos Medical.

PEDIATRIC AUDIOLOGICAL ASSESSMENT

The primary goal of an audiological evaluation is to determine whether a child has sufficient hearing (i.e., auditory brain access) to develop speech and language. A complete diagnostic evaluation includes frequency and ear-specific threshold information using both air and bone conduction, immittance testing, otoacoustic emissions (OAEs) testing, and speech perception. Auditory brain response (ABR) and auditory steady-state response are routine for infant evaluations and can provide additional diagnostic information for older children and adults.

Accurate assessment of hearing in infants and children is critical if clinicians are to successfully manage hearing loss (HL). Most infants are now screened at birth so the process of early identification and management can begin very early. Infants will be screened using either ABR or OAE. Infants who do not pass the screen are referred for follow-up using ABR or auditory steady-state response. While ABR, auditory steady-state response, and OAE testing are a critical part of the audiological assessment because they provide important information about the status of the auditory pathways, they are not measures of hearing. No assessment of hearing can be considered complete without behavioral testing, which includes tonal thresholds in each ear and assessment of speech perception. This entry provides an overview audiological test protocols for evaluation of infants and young children.

Auditory Brain Development

For children to have good auditory brain development, it is essential that they have good access to clear speech. To assure access to clear speech, it needs to be determined that children are hearing at normal conversational levels throughout the frequency range and that speech is clear and not muffled. If children do not receive sufficient acoustic access early, they will not have sufficient auditory brain development. Information about critical periods makes it clear that auditory access must happen early and be consistent. Work from Andrej Kral's group has demonstrated the importance of early brain development, and others have clearly demonstrated the importance of fitting technology early for infants with HL.

Behavioral Evaluation of Infants and Young Children

The primary goal of an audiological evaluation is to determine whether a child has sufficient hearing (auditory brain access) to develop speech and language. A complete diagnostic evaluation includes frequency and ear-specific threshold information using both air and bone conduction as well as an assessment of speech perception monaurally and binaurally at normal conversational levels. Immittance testing and OAEs are a routine part of most evaluations.

Behavioral audiological testing is the only direct measure of hearing. If a child is identified with HL, ABR cannot be used to monitor performance with technology, which can only be obtained with behavioral testing. For these reasons, it is critical that accurate threshold information be obtained as clinicians plan for management of HL in children. Behavioral evaluation of thresholds is obtained using behavioral observation audiometry (BOA), visual reinforcement audiometry (VRA), or conditioned play audiometry (CPA), depending on the cognitive age of the child. Infants who are cognitively less than 6 months of age will be tested using BOA, infants 5–36 months of age will be tested using VRA, and children over 30 months of age will be tested using CPA.

An advantage of behavioral testing is that families can observe testing and see the infant's response to sound. This assists in helping them understand HL facilitating their ability and readiness to proceed with management including obtaining and using technology, participating in therapy, and providing good language stimulation.

Determining Cognitive Age

It is critical that the appropriate test protocol be selected in order to obtain accurate test results. To select the appropriate test, audiologists need to be knowledgeable about behavioral developmental milestones. Cognitive age can be determined by observation of the child, interviewing parents and caregivers about developmental milestones, speaking with other clinicians working with an infant, and through direct evaluation. Selecting the wrong test protocol will result in inaccurate test results. For example, asking a 6-month-old to raise his or her hand when he or she hears a sound would result in assuming that the infant is deaf as the infant would not perform the required task.

BOA

BOA uses changes in sucking to observe response to sound. For the best results, infants need to be awake and comfortably seated with torso supported. The importance of having the child well positioned cannot be overstated. It will not be possible to obtain good responses if the infant is fussy and squirming. Responses can be obtained with infant nursing, using a pacifier, or sucking from a bottle. Starting and stopping of sucking are both acceptable responses, and infants may respond to the "on" or "off" of the presentation of the sound. As with all other tests, timing is critical. Responses of changes in sucking should occur within a few seconds of presentation of the stimulus. Stimuli should be presented with more wait time between presentations than would be used when testing older children, as this allows infants to return to sucking comfortably. Stimuli presented too quickly will make it difficult to observe responses. Figure 1 shows thresholds obtained using BOA, VRA, and CPA on one infant, demonstrating the reliability of the test protocol.

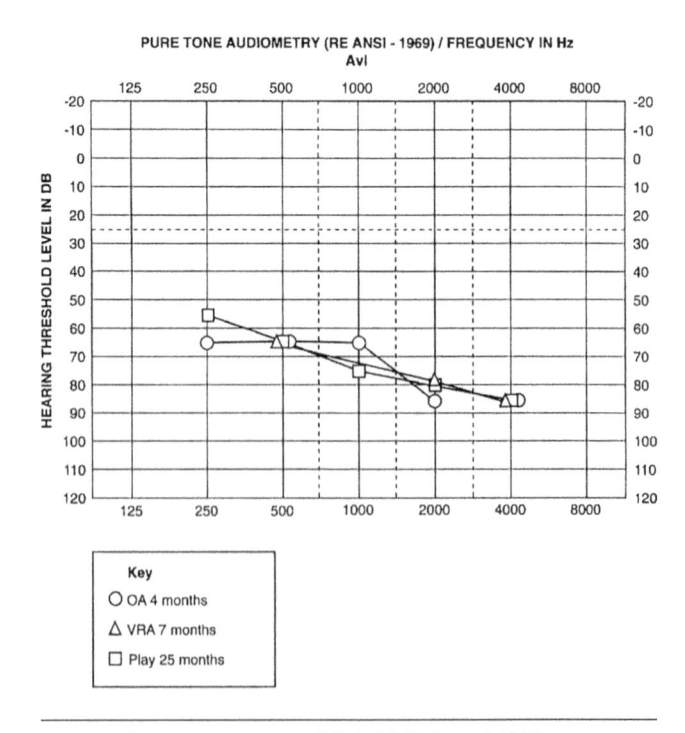

Figure 1 Comparison of BOA, VRA, and CPA thresholds in one infant

Source: Author.

Many audiologists are not comfortable performing BOA on infants. They may build their skills in this area by trying BOA before or after ABR testing, while waiting for an infant to fall asleep. Demonstrations of BOA testing can be found in Madell and Flexer (2014) and Madell, Flexer, Wolfe, and Schafer (2018). As BOA is a technique for infants and children cognitively less than 6 months of age, it can be used with older children with developmental disabilities who are cognitively less than 6 months of age.

VRA

VRA is used to test infants who are cognitively between 5–6 and 30–36 months of age. Testing involves training the infant to make a conditioned head turn in response to the test stimulus. Most infants will turn to a sound source a few times, but to get sufficient information to obtain thresholds throughout the frequency range, the infant will need to be trained to make a conditioned head turn. Shaping head turns using operant conditioning is an easy task. To condition an infant, sound is presented at a level at which the infant is expected to respond. If the infant makes a head turn to seek the sound, the reinforcer is turned on. If the infant does not make a head turn, it may be because he or she did not hear the sound or does not know what to do to respond. If the audiologist is certain that the child has heard the sound, the audiologist can call the child's attention to the VRA toy by pointing to it. After a few attempts, the infant should have learned the task and be making the head turns on her own. Please note, *it is critical that the reinforcer toy not be turned on unless the audiologist is certain that the child hears the stimulus*. Turning on the reinforcer toy when no sound is present will teach the child that the toy goes on at random times and will make accurate testing impossible. Once the child is conditioned to respond, the test assistant should ignore all stimuli and just engage the child with a toy but not to provide any clues to the child that a sound is present. Once the child makes a head turn, the test assistant can applaud and look at the reinforcing toy with the child to provide additional social reinforcement.

Stimuli should be presented when the child is engaged forward watching the test assistant or parent entertaining him or her so that the head turn is clear. For many children, they should not be playing with toys but should be watching others play. The test assistant can be stacking blocks, building with LEGO®, or twirling a pinwheel to keep the child's attention. Toys should be interesting but not too engrossing.

Reinforcers, such as a lighted toy or a bear playing drums, are usually enough of a reinforcer to interest young children. Videos such as cartoons with sound off will not be a good reinforcer for very young children but will work well for older children, keeping their attention for a longer period of time. Reinforcers should ideally be placed at a 90° angle from where the child is facing, but can be placed at a minimum of 45°. Having the toy any closer will make it difficult to be certain the child is really making a head turn to the stimulus.

As with BOA and CPA, positioning is critical. Infants should be seated so that they are comfortable and not wiggling. High chairs work well for any child who can sit. The child can be strapped to keep them in place and well positioned. Children can also be tested sitting on a parent's lap, but parents need to be advised not to respond to the presentation of the sound so as not to clue the child.

CPA

CPA is the appropriate task for children over 30 months of age. While older children may be able to raise a hand or push a button in response to a sound, they may get bored more quickly. Using toys in CPA will help children maintain interest in the task, enabling the audiologist to obtain more information in one test session. CPA can also successfully be used with older children with developmental delays who have difficulty attending to a hand-raising task.

When conditioning a child for CPA, the stimulus needs to be paired with the response. The audiologist or test assistant can teach the "listen and drop" task by holding the toy to his or her ear and putting it into the bucket when the sound is presented. Alternatively, the test assistant can help the child hold the toy to his or her ear and help him or her move the toy into the bucket when the sound is presented. It is essential that the sound used in conditioning be loud enough to be certain that the child can hear the sound. If the child does not hear the sound and sees the test assistant drop the toy into the bucket, the child is being taught to respond randomly.

Only responses that are clear to a stimulus should be accepted. Responses should be demonstrated within a few seconds after the stimulus is presented. If a child puts the toy in the bucket when there is no stimulus, or too long after the stimulus is presented, the test assistant should take the toy out of the bucket and hand it back to the child, which will help the child understand the task. Having a variety of toys will greatly assist keeping a child interested in the task.

Determining Test Protocol

Order of test protocols will be determined by the reason for testing. For most children, the primary goal of testing is to determine whether the child has sufficient hearing to develop speech and language. If that is the case, thresholds at low, middle, and high frequencies need to be obtained. If a child will accept insert earphones, separate ear information can be easily obtained. If the child is uncomfortable with earphones, it may be easiest to begin testing in sound field. Sound field testing will not provide separate ear information but will give information about hearing in the better hearing ear, which will provide enough information to begin management.

A complete audiogram should include thresholds from 250 to 8000 Hz with mid-frequency testing at 3000 and 6000 Hz. However, when testing infants and children, it is not always possible to keep their attention long enough to test every frequency in each ear during one test session. At a minimum, there needs to be a low-, mid-, and high-frequency threshold to plan management.

If concern is primarily about middle ear disease, hearing is likely to be poorer in low frequencies so testing should begin in the high frequencies (e.g., 2000, 3000, or 4000 Hz) which will be easier for the child to hear. Conditioning the child to the test task will be easier at a frequency in which he or she hears better. Once a high-frequency threshold is obtained, testing should proceed to 500 Hz. When middle ear HL is the concern, moving to bone conduction testing is important. Because low-frequency thresholds are likely to be more compromised, bone conduction testing should begin at 500 Hz. If an air–bone gap is present, a conductive HL will be confirmed.

If concern is about sensorineural HL, testing should begin at a low frequency (i.e., 500 Hz) and proceed to a high frequency (i.e., 3000 Hz) as low frequencies are likely to be better. If there is a significant difference in thresholds between low and high frequencies, obtaining thresholds at 1000 and 2000 Hz will be important to get a clear picture of the audiometric contour.

Management can begin with threshold information at one low and one high frequency in each ear, but testing should not be considered complete until thresholds are obtained throughout the frequency range in each ear for air and bone conduction. A complete audiogram will not need to be obtained in one visit. Thresholds at 500 and 2000 Hz may be obtained on Visit 1, 1000 and 4000 on Visit 2, and bone conduction at additional visits. However, with the basic threshold information at one low and one high frequency, there will be enough information to determine whether a child likely has an HL and to begin to set technology.

Speech Audiometry

Speech perception testing is a critical part of the audiological test battery. It provides information about how a child is functioning in a variety of listening situations. Speech perception testing is the only part of the audiology test battery that functionally assesses auditory performance. The information obtained is critical to planning management.

Speech Threshold Testing

Testing is divided into threshold tests and speech recognition tests. When performing threshold tests, the goal is to find the softest level at which a child is able to respond. Testing should be in agreement with pure-tone 3 frequency average. Threshold tests consist of speech awareness threshold (SAT) and speech reception threshold (SRT). When testing SAT, a child is only asked whether he or she can detect the presence of a sound. In SRT testing, the child has to identify the test word by either repeating the word or pointing to a picture or object.

SAT is useful when testing infants and others who are not yet able to participate in more complex testing or when monitoring technology. Testing is often accomplished using conversational speech, but it is important to remember that conversational speech has a very broad frequency range so interpreting test results will be difficult. Frequency-specific SAT testing can be accomplished using Ling Sounds and obtaining thresholds to /ba/, /sh/, and /s/. Thresholds for /ba/ should be in agreement with tonal thresholds at 500 Hz, /sh/ should be in agreement with thresholds at 2000–3000 Hz, and /s/ should be in agreement with thresholds at 4000 Hz.

SRTs

SRTs are obtained using standard spondee words (e.g., *hotdog*, *baseball*, *airplane*). For younger children, or children who have limited language, testing can be accomplished with familiar words (e.g., *eyes*, *nose*, *mouth*) or by asking the child to point to familiar objects (e.g., *car*, *book*, *spoon*).

Speech Recognition Testing

Speech recognition or speech perception testing is accomplished by having a child repeat back or point pictures to determine whether he or she can identify the test stimulus. Testing is accomplished at super threshold levels and is a good measure of how a child is performing in everyday situations. When testing under earphones, tests will be presented at 40 dB sensation level (i.e., 40 dB above the 3 or 4 frequency pure-tone average). To get a better picture of how a child will perform in everyday situations, testing should be accomplished in sound field, at 50 dB HL (i.e., normal conversational level) and at 35 dB HL (i.e., soft conversational level). Testing should also be accomplished in the presence of competing noise to obtain a full picture of how a child hears in typical listening situations. Four-talker babble is an excellent noise source as it is most like the sound that children will find in their daily lives. It is important to select tests that are appropriate to a child's cognitive age. Testing using a picture-pointing task with preschool vocabulary, while excellent for a 4-year-old, is not appropriate for a 9-year-old in third grade.

Scoring Speech Perception Tests

Interpretation of speech recognition tests is critical in planning management. Excellent speech perception is a score of 90–100%, good speech perception is a score of 80–89%, fair speech perception is 70–79%, and poor speech perception is less than 70%. It is important that when reporting scores, appropriate descriptions be used. For example, if a child receives a score of 68% and it is described as "good," parents, teachers, and therapists have no reason to believe that the child needs work to improve performance. If the test results are accurately described as "poor," then everyone knows that work needs to be done to improve the child's performance.

Using Speech Test Information

If children are performing well at normal conversational levels, it is expected that they are able to hear well when the talker is 3–5 feet away from them. If children can hear well at soft conversation, it is expected that children will hear well at 10 feet. If children hear well in competing noise, they will hear well in situations in which noise is present. If children are not doing well in any of the test situations, it will be necessary to determine what needs to be done to improve function. A child who does not hear well at normal or soft speech can be expected to have difficulty hearing in school, which means use of a remote microphone system will be critical, and auditory-based therapy should also be recommended.

Final Thoughts

Careful and complete audiological evaluation covering all aspects of functional hearing will help to select and program technology, plan management, develop school plans, and arrange counsel for both the child experiencing HL and his or her family. The results will likely bring about improvements for children with HL.

Jane Madell

See also Audiology; Auditory Development; Diagnostic Audiological Assessment; Pediatric Audiological Rehabilitation

Further Readings

Cardon, G., Campbell, J., & Sharma, A. (2012). Plasticity in the developing auditory cortex: Evidence from children with sensorineural hearing loss and auditory neuropathy spectrum disorder. *Journal of the American Academy of Audiology, 23*(6), 396–411(16).

Kral, A. (2013). Auditory critical periods: A review from system's perspective. *Neuroscience, 247*, 117–133.

Kral, A., Kronenberger, W. G., Pisoni, D. B., & O'Donoghue, G. M. (2016). Neurocognitive factors in sensory restoration of early deafness: A connectome model. *The Lancet Neurology, 15*(6), 610–621.

Kral, A., & Lenarz, T. (2015). How the brain learns to listen: Deafness and the bionic ear. *E-Neuroforum, 6*(1), 21–28.

Kral, A., & Sharma, A. (2012). Developmental neuroplasticity after cochlear implantation. *Trends in Neurosciences, 35*(2), 111–122.

Madell, J., Batheja, R., Klemp, E., & Hoffman, R. (2011). Evaluating speech perception performance, *Audiology Today, September–October*, 52–56.

Madell, J. R., & Flexer, C. (2014). *Pediatric audiology: Diagnosis, technology and management* (2nd ed.). New York, NY: Thieme Medical.

Madell, J. R., Flexer, C., Wolfe, J., & Schafer, E. (2018). *Pediatric audiology: Diagnosis, technology and management* (3rd ed.). New York, NY: Thieme Medical.

Moon, C., Lagercrantz, H., & Kuhl, P. K. (2013). Language experienced *in utero* affects vowel perception after birth: A two-country study. *Acta Paediatrica, 102*(2), 156–160.

Yoshinaga-Itano, C., Coulter, D., & Thomson, V. (2001). Developmental outcomes of children with hearing loss born in Colorado hospitals with and without universal newborn hearing. *Seminars in Neonatology, 6*(6), 521–529.

PEDIATRIC AUDIOLOGICAL REHABILITATION

The purpose of pediatric audiological rehabilitation is to determine and reduce the impact of permanent hearing loss on a child's development in multiple domains, including auditory function, communication, and social development. Permanent hearing loss in infancy or childhood disrupts the typical development of spoken language and communication. Audiologists, speech–language pathologists, and educators need to be familiar with communication disorders related to hearing loss, as the majority of affected infants and children will require specialized intervention. These professionals need to be familiar with the various approaches to rehabilitation and the relationship between auditory development and communication. They need to understand the core components of intervention, including the role of families in pediatric audiological rehabilitation throughout childhood. This entry provides an overview of audiological rehabilitation for children from early childhood through school age.

Pediatric audiological rehabilitation is viewed as a fundamental service in the sequence of care for children with permanent hearing loss. In most developed countries, universal hearing screening has been widely implemented, leading to early detection and early intervention (rehabilitation) of childhood hearing loss. Consequently, since the 1990s, the population of children receiving early intervention has changed to include children with mild bilateral and unilateral loss in addition to more severe hearing loss. Furthermore, the widespread use of cochlear implants for children with severe and profound hearing loss means that access to "acoustic information" is now available to most children with hearing disorders.

Rehabilitation Approaches

Pediatric audiological rehabilitation is considered essential to achieve spoken language development in the majority of children with hearing loss. Rehabilitation usually implies a program of care that is provided not only to the child but also to the caregivers. Rehabilitation services are provided by various professionals who are specialists in communication disorders and education of the deaf and hard of hearing. Historically, various approaches to audiological rehabilitation have been promoted. Known under various names, these fall into two major categories: (1) oral language development with an auditory-specific emphasis (e.g., auditory–verbal, auditory–oral) and (2) oral language with the addition of visual information, which may include speechreading, cued speech (i.e., systematic system of hand cues added to code the phonemes of speech to facilitate speechreading), and/or sign language. Programs that include sign language support are often known under various terms such as *total communication*, *simultaneous communication*, and *dual communication*. There is no clear evidence to support that one approach is more effective than others in developing spoken language. There is consensus that families should be provided with informed choices when their child is diagnosed with hearing loss. Several characteristics, as described later in this entry, are common to pediatric audiological rehabilitation for children with hearing loss.

Early Auditory and Language Rehabilitation

With early detection and advanced hearing aid and cochlear implant technologies, the majority of children with hearing loss benefit from pediatric audiological rehabilitation with a focus on auditory–oral development. Several key concepts form the foundation of pediatric audiological rehabilitation. Of prime importance is early acoustic accessibility to speech through hearing technology (e.g., hearing aids, cochlear implants, remote microphone systems) and exposure to optimal listening and learning environments. The child's caregivers are seen as essential partners throughout all aspects of the habilitation process.

A core concept underlying early auditory intervention is the notion that optimal auditory development relies heavily on stimulation being provided during the first few years of life, when the auditory system is most receptive to this type of sensory activity. Even when auditory input is flawed compared to that available to the normal hearing system, due to neuroplasticity, the brain is primed to benefit from auditory information, which translates to more typical language acquisition. It is well accepted that developmental synchrony (i.e., development of skills at the time they should occur) permits language acquisition that closely follows natural speech and language trajectories in children with normal hearing. Therefore, due to early identification and good access to audition and speech models, a developmental model with a focus on language learning in natural contexts is widely adopted in rehabilitation. This contrasts with the remedial models that were often more structured but previously required in habilitation programs when late diagnosis was common and children had reduced access to hearing across the full speech spectrum.

Overall, most children can follow typical stages of language development but require specific rehabilitation techniques to enhance spoken language learning. Embellishment of language input is required because despite the best available hearing technologies, children with hearing loss have reduced access to typical speech and language models. This is not only due to the poorer quality and incomplete nature of the speech input they receive but also because they experience considerably more difficulty hearing speech at a distance and in noise, all of which affect overhearing speech patterns and consequently incidental language learning.

Early pediatric rehabilitation is highly dependent on the caregiver's involvement in auditory and language development. Rehabilitation includes supporting and coaching families to use the best available hearing technology, to create optimal listening and learning environments in the home and community, and to implement listening and language facilitation techniques. Caregivers are provided with guidance and practical strategies aimed at achieving hearing device use throughout the child's waking hours. They are taught to provide rich learning environments (e.g., reduce background noise) and to take advantage of integrating language learning opportunities into their child's everyday activities. Caregivers also learn specific skills to encourage and facilitate the development of their child's listening and language skills. For example, a common technique in rehabilitation includes acoustic highlighting, which involves modifying a speech pattern to make it more audible for the child (e.g., elongating vowels, placing emphasis on the last word in a phrase). Another is the selection of verbal input that is acoustically salient in the early stages of intervention, such as words that vary in number of syllables and intensity (e.g., animal sounds, sounds associated with vehicles). These techniques and practices are aimed at developing sound awareness and associating meaning with sound, building a solid auditory function so that children can learn more naturally through hearing. In addition, parents are coached about the usual techniques to facilitate language development such as modeling, expansion, repetition, turn-taking, and questioning. Overall, rehabilitation involves following typical early auditory, speech, and language stages of acquisition while structuring intervention to facilitate learning through audition, because the child with hearing loss is at a disadvantage compared to peers with normal hearing.

Ongoing diagnostic assessment is an integral component of rehabilitation to establish intervention goals, monitor progress, and determine whether communication is aligned with expectations for the child's developmental level. A comprehensive assessment of the child's overall functioning in the areas of listening, communication, and psychosocial development helps to determine whether modifications are required such as introducing other hearing technology (e.g., moving from hearing aids to cochlear implants) and/or other approaches to rehabilitation.

Several factors affect expectations and outcomes of rehabilitation for children with hearing loss. These can be grouped into child, family, and environmental factors. Commonly identified child factors include cognitive/developmental level (e.g., the presence of additional disabilities), severity of hearing loss, and age of diagnosis and intervention. Family factors may include parent engagement, family functioning, and resources. Environmental factors encompass such aspects as access to hearing technology and intervention, type of intervention, and coordinated care.

There is good consensus that the majority of children with greater than a moderate degree of hearing loss require specialized support to develop auditory and spoken language skills, whereas children with mild degrees of hearing loss and unilateral loss may develop language without direct intervention. However, parents of children with any degree of hearing loss require some level of support, especially in the early stages, to understand and mitigate the effects of hearing loss. Most children with typical development can be expected to develop spoken language that is closely aligned with that of their hearing peers. Children who have complex medical and other developmental needs in addition to hearing loss may require special consideration related to expectations for communication development. In particular, those with severe cognitive delay may not be able to develop spoken language at the same rate as typically developing children. Rehabilitation for these children requires ongoing assessment and collaboration with other health and education specialists to adjust expectations for communication, to modify audiological recommendations and intervention approaches, and to appropriately guide parents throughout the process. The overall goal is the provision of intervention services tailored to the child's and family's needs.

Rehabilitation at School Age

Rehabilitation is generally considered a long-term requisite for the majority of children with hearing loss to maintain and/or continue to improve their auditory and language skills. As children enter the school system, various educational options may exist including a special classroom for children with hearing loss, partial integration in general education with typically hearing peers, or full inclusion in general school systems. With increased opportunities for spoken language, there has been a strong shift since the 1990s toward the inclusion of children with hearing loss in general education programs with their hearing peers. However, listening and learning in a mainstream classroom environment present challenges for most children with hearing loss, which can affect not only literacy and academic function but also social development and overall participation in school. Therefore, it is generally accepted that all children require some support services in any school system. Rehabilitation may range from simply monitoring the child's functioning to prevent difficulties or delays to providing intensive direct support. The use of personal remote microphone systems and classroom audio distribution systems is routinely recommended to improve the acoustics to the extent possible in classrooms, which are generally reverberant, noisy, and busy learning environments.

When children with hearing loss reach school age, parent engagement and communication with parents about the child's school functioning continue to be important. However, rehabilitation also shifts to an emphasis on coaching teachers about technology and strategies to maximize learning in the classroom through enhancements such as the use of remote microphone technology, preferential seating, visual material to support teaching, peer support (e.g., note-taking), and communication strategies (e.g., repetition, rephrasing). In addition to an emphasis on continued auditory and language work, there is frequently an integration of literacy and academic material, as well as social skills coaching, into a rehabilitation program. For some children, owing to factors such as late identification, slower progress, or other learning difficulties, some intervention may be more remedial in nature (i.e., focused on filling in language gaps). As previously noted, comprehensive individual assessment of each child's needs is a core component of rehabilitation, and the intensity and type of intervention services are adjusted accordingly.

Final Thoughts

Pediatric audiological rehabilitation involves use of the best available hearing technology coupled with specific therapy techniques and explicit family and school coaching to develop spoken language skills that are aligned with the child's developmental level.

Elizabeth M. Fitzpatrick and Suzanne P. Doucet

See also Cochlear Implant (Re)habilitation; Hearing Aids; Language Acquisition; Language Assessment; Language Therapy and Intervention; Oral Language; Rehabilitation

Further Readings

Cole, E. B., & Flexer, C. (2016). *Children with hearing loss: Developing listening and talking, birth to six* (3rd ed.). San Diego, CA: Plural.

Duncan, J., Rhoades, E. A., & Fitzpatrick, E. M. (2014). *Auditory (re)habilitation for adolescents with hearing loss: Theory and practice*. New York, NY: Oxford University Press.

Estabrooks, W., MacIver-Lux, K., & Rhoades, E. A. (Eds.). (2016). *Auditory-verbal therapy: For young children with hearing loss and their families, and the practitioners who guide them*. San Diego, CA: Plural.

Fitzpatrick, E. M., & Doucet, S. D. (2013). *Pediatric audiological rehabilitation: From infancy to adolescence*. New York, NY: Thieme Medical.

McCreery, R. W., & Walker, E. A. (2017). *Pediatric amplification: Enhancing auditory access*. San Diego, CA: Plural.

Moeller, M. P., Ertmer, D. J., & Stoel-Gammon, C. (Eds.). (2016). *Promoting language and literacy in children who are deaf or hard of hearing*. Baltimore, MA: Paul H. Brookes.

Smaldino, J. J., & Flexer, C. (2012). *Handbook of acoustic accessibility: Best practices for listening, learning, and literacy in the classroom*. New York, NY: Thieme Medical.

Spencer, P. E., & Marschark, M. (Eds.). (2006). *Advances in spoken language development of deaf and hard-of-hearing children*. New York, NY: Oxford University Press.

Perception

Perception refers to any kind of conscious sensory experience whereby external stimuli generate electrical signals in the nervous system of an organism that ultimately allow some kind of interaction with the environment. In human communication, the external stimulus is usually a spoken acoustic signal, and the receiving organism is typically a human listener. The auditory system of the listener transduces this sound into neural impulses in the brain, which are then processed at several stages. The traditional view of speech perception is that the acoustic signal from a speaker is perceived as a sequence of consonants and vowels which are further organized into words and sentences. However, the acoustic waveform contains information about not only basic linguistic elements but also nonlinguistic properties such as the speaker's location in space; the identity of the speaker including size, gender, and place of origin; the speaker's emotional state; and even the acoustic environment in which he or she is speaking, such as the size of the room and the acoustic reflectivity of nearby surfaces. However, communication can also include sign language and lipreading, which rely on both the visual system and the Tadoma method in which an individual who is deafBlind uses tactile information to perceive the movement of the speaker's lips and jaw to understand speech.

In general, perception depends not only on the external stimulus itself but also on the experiences of the receiver as a result of learning, attention, expectation, and the wider context in which the stimulus occurs. Perceptual systems also interact with one another: Speech perception is modulated not only by the sound of the speech arriving at the ear of the listener but also by the image of the speaker's lips moving in synchrony. Similarly, the tactile sensation of a puff of air on the listener's face can even change the perception of a speech sound from /ba/ to /pa/. This entry provides an overview of perception with a particular emphasis on speech perception, including how it works, the similarities between different modalities of perception, and specific phenomena related to contrast effects, learning, and top-down effects.

How Perception Works

Perception begins with a source that generates a stimulus in the form of energy such as light or sound, which is then transmitted to the receiver. These stimuli are transformed into electrical activity in the receiver in a process called *neural transduction*. At the most peripheral levels of neural processing, this electrical activation represents a relatively close correlation to the properties of the external stimulus itself. For example, in hearing, the outer, middle, and inner ear transform pressure variations in the air via mechanical vibrations in the middle ear bones and the flexible basilar membrane of the cochlea. This results in the sequence of neural impulses that encode both frequency and intensity of the incoming stimulus, and the relationship between these physical properties and the neural impulses themselves is monotonic. However, beyond the auditory nerve—or the very first stage of neural processing—this information is transformed into increasingly more complex representations. It is widely believed that, at the highest levels of speech processing, the acoustic waveform corresponding to the speech signal is ultimately represented in the human brain as speech sounds, or phonemes, such as consonants and vowels.

Perception is not just the transduction of external stimuli into a neural code, however. Perception can also be viewed as a process of *receiving* information about the environment that is *acted upon* by the receiver. From this point of view, successful perception means that an organism has sufficient information about external stimuli such that it can function in its environment. Neural representations of stimuli are not necessarily veridical or accurate, however—perception only needs to achieve sufficient agreement with reality to allow the perceiver to attain specific goals.

The fact that perception is not *veridical* results in several phenomena in speech that can be characterized as illusions. For example, in the McGurk effect, when the sound of one speech sound (e.g., /ba/) is played in synchrony with an image of a speaker producing a different speech sound (e.g., /ga/), the combined audiovisual stimulus is perceived as the unrelated syllable /da/. Similarly, in the phonemic restoration effect, the speech sound /w/ of the word *wheel* in the sentence "It was found that the wheel was on the axle" can be completely replaced by the sound of a cough, yet listeners will not be able to report which speech sound is actually missing—although they can clearly hear the cough, they will not be able to say which speech sound was replaced, and the sentence will sound unbroken to the listener.

Perception of one's environment may seem to be a direct representation of the world because perception is remarkably consistent. For example, the McGurk effect and phonemic restoration are highly stable phenomena. Likewise, visual illusions, such as simple Necker cubes (i.e., wireframe representations of blocks), appear to be consistently viewed from either above or below despite being ambiguous. In more realistic situations, one perceives an external object as constant even though the stimuli generated by that object can vary considerably across presentations. For example, if one looks at a chair from different angles, it is still perceived as the same object even though the pattern of light projected onto the eyes can be substantially different depending on the distance from the viewer, the viewing angle, and lighting conditions. Similarly, when one hears a speaker say the word "dog," the actual acoustic waveform will depend largely on the size of the speaker, the pitch of the speaker's voice, the distance between the speaker and the listener, and the acoustic characteristics of the environment in which the word is spoken. Nonetheless, the listener will hear the same word across multiple repetitions and even believe that each token is identical despite potentially large acoustic differences.

Conversely, the critically important acoustic characteristics of a vowel as spoken by a large adult, such as the /ʌ/ sound in "cub," can have similar acoustic properties to the sound /ɑ/ as produced by a small child. It is widely believed that formants (i.e., resonances produced by the vocal tract of the speaker) are the most reliable discriminants of different vowel categories in speech. However, formants are dependent not only on the vowel being produced but also on the size of the speaker. In practice, however, the vowels /ʌ/ and /ɑ/ are never confused; listeners do not perceive these as the same because they usually know the relative size of the speaker which can be inferred from simple visual cues or context (e.g., other speech sounds in the sentence, vocal pitch), and it is known that knowledge of speaker size helps disambiguate these potential confusions.

Because multiple sources can result in the same pattern of perceptual cues, it is often impossible to recover the exact state of the object being perceived. In speech perception, this is referred to as the *inverse problem*—that is, the listener cannot be certain of the sequence of speech events led to the sound being heard, so listeners must rely on other sources of information.

Another important issue in perception is stimulus grouping; multiple stimulus properties are associated with the same external object on the basis of shared characteristics. In vision, different patterns of light are organized into groups that correspond to individual external objects on the basis of similar properties—for example, illumination, converging edges, relative depth, and similar trajectories of motion. In hearing, listeners are typically presented with a multitude of sounds being generated by several different external sources at any given time. However, all of these sounds are combined at the level of the outer ear resulting in a single pattern of pressure variation that is transduced to a neural signal. At the most fundamental level, this pattern is one-dimensional: It is simply the variation in eardrum displacement resulting from pressure fluctuations as a function of time.

The auditory system must process this information and segregate multiple sources of sound into groups that correspond to individual sound-generating objects through a process of *auditory scene analysis*. For example, vowels are largely specified by the frequencies of multiple formants. However, in a given acoustic environment, there may be several talkers or even other sound generators that also produce resonances. In complex acoustic environments, different acoustic elements can be grouped according to the direction of the sound source relative to the listener (i.e., sounds originating from the same location in space are grouped together) or by shared acoustic patterns such as fundamental frequency or onset/offset time (i.e., sounds that have the same acoustic period as well as those that start and stop at the same time are grouped). This ability to segregate/integrate sounds is a critically important perceptual skill, and it is known that hearing impairments often have a detrimental effect on listeners' ability to understand speech in the context of competing noises.

An important aspect of perception is that it must result in action by the receiver, which may include just simple understanding in the case of speech communication. An enduring view of perception has been that organisms form a representation of their environment from their perception, and many researchers have developed the notion that there are *objects* of perception. This is not strictly true. It is more accurate to say that there are *objectives* of perception in that an organism must maintain sufficient agreement with its environment to facilitate adaptive behavior.

For example, in speech perception, it is widely believed that listeners perceive the acoustic waveform in human communication in terms of phonemes or basic speech sounds and that all acoustic events are compared with these references, which are then organized into higher levels of linguistic structure, such as words or sentences. Much of the work in speech perception has been focused on exactly *how* the basic acoustic waveform is categorized with reference to these internal representations—when someone says the vowel /i/, how exactly does the listener know that the vowel is /i/ and not /u/? There is research to show that listeners distill just enough information from the speech stream to facilitate effective communication, while superfluous acoustic properties are discarded or forgotten. Although the example of acoustic information is used here, these concepts apply equally well to other domains such as vision (e.g., lipreading).

Relationship Between Speech Perception and Perception in General

Speech-perception research has often been distinguished from the study of auditory perception in general. However, there are fundamental principles that govern all domains of perception including other modalities, such as vision and touch. For example, successful perception does not generally require perfect recovery of object properties in the real world. Instead, perception describes a relationship between an organism's actions and the world around it. Since perception is imperfect, it is often impossible to recover the exact events that lead to the stimulus itself (e.g., the McGurk effect, phonemic restoration).

Similarly, in vision, one is presented with a two-dimensional projection of a three-dimensional object onto one's eyes. Multiple external objects can give rise to the same patterns, however. In hearing or speech perception, there are a number of events that could give rise to the same auditory representation. For example, the signal from a mobile telephone represents a compromise between the cost of data bandwidth and the minimum acceptable volume of information required for verbal communication. However, this sound bears only a superficial resemblance to the actual acoustic waveform produced by the remote speaker. Speakers and listeners deem this acceptable because one's sensory systems (i.e., ears) make no attempt to perfectly reconstruct one's distal environment but rather process information and respond appropriately.

Information about one's environment can take multiple forms: light, sound, pressure, and so on, and this information is used to understand the world. In general, the physiological mechanisms that humans use to receive this information are severely limited—for example, one can see a very narrow spectrum of light and within that range, most humans decompose waves of light along only three dimensions: red, green, and blue. These limitations mean not only that humans are unable to see wavelengths outside this range, but even within these limits, humans are unable to see complex combinations of color components such that everything is reduced to combinations of just these three colors. Likewise, the human ability to detect fluctuations in pressure that correspond to the propagation of sound through the air is limited by the relative mechanical simplicity of the outer, middle, and inner ear.

The Role of Contrast Effects

For this reason, much of perception relies on *contrast effects* rather than absolute levels of stimulus properties. For example, the perception of color is heavily influenced by hues that are either nearby in space or recent in time. Although one may immediately notice the effects of tinted sunglasses, wearers adapt to this change relatively quickly, and colors quickly appear to be normal if not somewhat impoverished. Likewise, the actual color projected by an object will depend heavily on the illumination of the surrounding scene, and humans rely on contrast between adjacent regions to determine what the natural color of an object is. In hearing, how one hears a sound depends primarily on sounds that occur immediately before, simultaneously, and even after. While this may impact the fidelity of one's perception, these influences effectively increase the dynamic range of one's sensory systems, thereby allowing an individual to discriminate many more levels of a stimulus property than he or she can otherwise identify in isolation. For example, one can identify only a handful of hues when presented alone, yet one can discriminate approximately 1 million different colors when presented as contrasting pairs.

Many researchers believe that contrast effects are critically important in speech perception. For example, the acoustic properties of /k/ differ substantially depending on the following vowel. For this reason, it is impossible to splice together speech sounds to form new words from a collection of acoustic segments in arbitrary ways. However, *relative* changes in the acoustic properties between /k/ and the following vowel sound are quite stable across utterances, and speakers and these relative changes are used in speech perception. Similarly, vowel sounds themselves are rarely static: Individual productions of vowel sounds by human speakers are typically indicated by small changes in acoustic properties that are important in perception. For example, a recording of the word *bib* will sound like *babe* when played backward owing to the fact that formant frequencies for the vowels /ɪ/ and /e/ change in opposite directions over a short period of time. Therefore, it is not the *absolute* properties but rather the *relative* changes within these speech sounds that help in their identification.

The Role of Learning

A very important factor in perception is learning. From the moment humans are exposed to the world around them, their brains attempt to make sense of it, and neural structures are organized to maximize their ability to perceive those stimuli that are important for survival. If an individual is never exposed to a certain type of stimulus, that person may never learn to perceive it. As an extreme example, cats that are never exposed to vertical lines throughout their lives are unable to perceive them, and it has been shown that the visual centers of their brains have been reorganized such that they are physiologically incapable of seeing such lines. Similarly, native speakers of Japanese are unable to perceive the difference between /r/ and /l/ as this contrast does not occur in their language. Unlike the laboratory cats, however, Japanese children do hear /r/ and /l/ as these speech sounds do occur in Japanese speech. However, /r/ and /l/ are functionally equivalent in this language—that is, there are no words in Japanese that differ by these speech sounds alone. The ability to identify this contrast has no bearing on their ability to communicate effectively and therefore serves no purpose in perception—the ability to discriminate them is lost. In general, newborn children have the capacity to identify any speech sound in any language. However, with experience, an individual's perceptual abilities are fine-tuned such that the person becomes much more sensitive to the contrasts that exist in the language that he or she is exposed to.

The Role of Top-Down Effects

Perception is also modulated by attention and expectation. People can be primed to see a particular object or hear a particular word. When presented with an optical illusion or ambiguous figure, a viewer's bias can be shifted by presenting him or her with a similar object or even a written word. Likewise, when listening to an ambiguous utterance, listeners can be primed to hear one word or the other simply by being shown a picture of an object. Perceptual biases can also be tuned by context. For example, when presented with the spoken sentence "The milk was poured in the ___," listeners are more likely to hear the word "cup" spoken than "cub," even if the final word sounds unambiguously like *cub* when presented in isolation.

These phenomena are often referred to as *top-down* effects—individuals' experiences about the world around them have a direct influence on how they perceive it. Such top-down effects can potentially be dangerous, as individuals can have expectations that are completely invalid and cause them to misperceive stimuli regularly. However, top-down effects are essential, as the stimuli individuals receive are often regularly impoverished or ambiguous. If one tries to communicate in a very noisy environment, the speech signal can be so distorted or masked by background noise that top-down effects are essential for any kind of recovery of the intended linguistic message.

Fortunately, most of the stimuli individuals perceive are highly contextualized such that they can recover elements that are absent or difficult to perceive directly. For example, one does not need to see all four legs of a chair to identify it as a platform for sitting. Similarly, one does not need to hear the acoustic waveform corresponding to the last word of the sentence "The groundskeeper mowed the ___" to understand it perfectly. Furthermore, individuals can lead themselves to believe that they heard the last word whether it was actually present (e.g., phonemic restoration).

These context effects are measurable. At the most fundamental level, perception of a stream of unrelated, random speech sounds is quite challenging for the listener, and the magnitude of these top-down effects can potentially be very strong. However, one can determine the influence of context effects on perception. For example, knowledge of vocabulary limits the number of possible words that one expects to hear (e.g., one is more likely to hear the word "dog" than "dob"), and the relative frequency of those words in spoken language also has a strong influence (e.g., one is more likely to hear the word "dog" than "don"). Furthermore, knowledge of sentence structure and word meaning influences perception. For example, one is more likely to hear "Cooks make hot food" than "Cooks make hot flew."

Michael Kiefte

See also Auditory Processing; Auditory Scene Analysis; Speech Perception, Theories of

Further Readings

Goldstein, E. B. (2010). *Sensation and perception.* Belmont, CA: Wadsworth.

Wolfe, J. M., Kluender, K. R., Levi, D. M., Bartoshuk, L. M., Herz, R. S., Klatzky, R. L., ... Merfeld, D. M. (2006). *Sensation and perception.* Sunderland, MA: Sinauer.

PERSON-CENTERED CARE

Person-centered care is a philosophy of care that puts the client (the person) at the center of decision making about treatment approaches and desired outcomes. This means that speech-language pathologists and audiologists—also referred to hereinafter as *communication professionals*—who adopt this approach demonstrate attitudes and behaviors that are respectful of the whole person, including his or her preferences and cultural background. It involves a therapeutic alliance between the communication professional and the person, to maximize treatment outcomes, satisfaction with care, and quality of life. This entry provides an overview of the history and philosophy of person-centered care, then explores examples of person-centered approaches in both pediatric and adult cases. For the purposes of this entry, *person* is inclusive of the individual and his or her family. *Family* will be defined as those whom the person identifies as significant (e.g., caregiver, spouse, parents, friends, designated advocate, and community).

History and Philosophy

The concept of person-centered care was derived from Carl Rogers's (1961) nondirective, humanistic approach to psychotherapy. Rogers's approach was much like that of person-centered care: to be a companion in care and provide a warm and accepting atmosphere in which the person can grow. In the early 21st century, the application of person-centered care has expanded to the treatment of communication disorders across the life span, from pediatric to elderly populations. Person-centered care for children is family-centered, embracing the values and collaboration of the family in setting goals for the child. Person-centered care for adults emphasizes client participation at all stages of intervention, including evaluation, treatment planning, and reporting outcomes.

Contrasting Medical and Person-Centered Models of Care

Health-care services have traditionally followed the medical model. In contrast to person-centered care, the medical model is a hierarchical approach in which care is decided *for* the person *by* the health-care professional. The person's expertise on his or her health condition is seldom considered. The medical model of care addresses only the underlying diagnosis, not the person. Thomas Kitwood (1997) was among the first to propose an alternative to the medical model. He advocated for dementia care that prioritizes the unique qualities of the person and the care environment rather than diagnosis alone. As language is uniquely human and personal, communication professionals practicing within a medical model may be limiting the effectiveness of their care because of lack of patient acceptance or buy-in of clinician-determined therapy goals. To be more person-centered, clinicians developed goal attainment scaling, an interview process to increase the involvement of the person in decisions about their treatment. The clinician and client discuss current levels of functioning and project future levels of change toward a goal, before agreeing upon a treatment plan. Periodic reevaluation of progress toward the goal allows for patient input about the success or weaknesses of the approach as well as potential modifications of the treatment plan.

The following treatment goals illustrate the contrast between person-centered and medical models of care:

1. Mary will use semantic circumlocution during conversation regarding her recent vacation to retrieve words and communicate messages with

90% accuracy, given minimal verbal cues, to increase successful functional communication with family.

2. The patient will use semantic circumlocution to improve word finding to 90% accuracy, given minimal verbal cues, when asked to name common objects.

The first example is a person-centered goal in language and content. The person is referred to by name (Mary), and her specific interests (vacation) and needs (communication with family) are addressed. The second example is an impairment-focused and generic goal. The person is referred to as *the patient*, and the activity is depersonalized.

Multidimensional Model of Care

In their systematic review of the person-centered care literature, Diana White and colleagues (2008) identified a multidimensional model of person-centered care. Dimensions of this model include *personhood*, *knowing the person*, *autonomy and choice*, *nurturing relationship*, and a *supportive environment*. Although this review was focused on studies conducted in long-term care environments for persons with dementia, their findings can be applied to clients across the life span, as illustrated in the subsequent sections.

Personhood

The first dimension, personhood, is acknowledging the person as inherently worthy of value and respect, no matter his or her background or disability. Personhood as applied to care situations emphasizes the person's strengths rather than his or her disability. In dementia care, for example, procedural memory is known to be preserved well into the late stages of the disease. Therefore, procedural tasks, such as reading, cooking, or gardening, can be the context for activities to help the person maintain independent functioning and meaningful connection.

Knowing the Person

The second dimension is knowing the person, which is central to the development of person-centered care. Every person has a unique identity, life history, and significant life experiences. Person-centered care involves learning this information and directly incorporating it into the person's everyday activities. It is important to know the level of functioning a person wants to maintain or enhance; does the person want to continue reading books to a grandchild or serving as a lector at his or her church? Does the child sound intelligible to family, but experiences frustration when communicating with unfamiliar listeners (i.e., same-aged peers), making it difficult to form new friendships? The focus of therapy is therefore not only on with whom the person currently communicates but—from knowing about them—with whom they *want* to communicate. In addition, knowing the person means knowing the activities or interests he or she holds most valuable and incorporating these into treatment. In culturally diverse populations, knowing the person may require multiple sources of information about the person's country of origin, religious practices, and other cultural choices.

Autonomy and Choice

The third dimension is autonomy and choice. Person-centered care seeks to empower the person to make informed decisions about his or her care. This means providing unbiased information on treatment options and realistic outcomes and, when necessary, providing the appropriate communication supports to allow the person to make important decisions. In the case of adult communication disorders, such as aphasia and dementia, providing appropriate visual and picture supports when discussing complex situations is a crucial component to autonomy, choice, and decision making. Speech–language pathologists often provide counseling on alternative methods of feeding if an individual has severe dysphagia (i.e., disordered swallowing), placing him or her at risk of choking or infection. Autonomy and choice in this context would mean providing pros and cons about treatment options (e.g., feeding tube or modified diet) and respecting the family's or person's decision.

Nurturing Relationship

Social connectedness is a fundamental human need and is thus another integral component of person-centered care. The fourth dimension of person-centered care, nurturing relationship, means maximizing the person's ability to feel socially connected and accepted in his or her communication environments. For a person with stroke-induced aphasia, for example, this may mean supporting communication via several modalities (e.g., using a communication book to point to pictures and gesturing) so that the person can once again participate in meaningful activities (e.g., going out to dinner with friends). In addition, social connectedness can be facilitated for children with autism through the use of social stories to teach valuable social skills, such as perspective-taking and initiating interaction.

Supportive Environment

The final dimension is a supportive environment. This means creating an environment that supports the person's remaining abilities and promotes an optimal level of function. In the case of pediatric treatment, this may mean providing treatment in the home or at school with the child's own toys, desired activities, and siblings or friends. A supportive environment for a child with autism, for example, might reduce sensory stimulation that could distract the child (e.g., television or radio). For adults with both communication impairments (e.g., aphasia or dementia) and strengths in reading, a supportive environment would include appropriate text-based cues around the house. If a person with severe dysphagia, who is unsafe for oral feeding, has refused a feeding tube, clinicians could model ways for the family to provide alternative, palliative feedings.

Final Thoughts

Person-centered care is a philosophy of care that places personhood at the center of clinical decision making. It is a therapeutic alliance between the professional and the person and his or her family that allows them to be active participants in the evaluation, treatment, and outcome measuring process. Person-centered care puts professional knowledge secondary to the person's expertise regarding his or her health and communication behaviors. It seeks to emphasize the unique needs of the person, rather than his or her diagnosis, to maximize outcomes, quality of life, and satisfaction with care. It is applicable to both pediatric and adult populations. The five dimensions underlying person-centered approaches (personhood, knowing the person, autonomy and choice, nurturing relationship, and supportive environments) provide the structure to ensure the implementation of this promising model of clinical care.

Vanessa Burshnic and Michelle Bourgeois

See also Aphasia; Autism Spectrum Disorder; Collaboration in Speech–Language Therapy; Dementia; Functional Communication Skills

Further Readings

Camp, C. J., Bourgeois, M. S., & Ekkes, J. (2018). Person-centered care. In G. Smith &Farias, S.T. (Eds.), *APA handbook of dementia.* (pp. 615–629). Washington, DC: American Psychological Association.

Dunst, C.J., Trivette, C.M., Gordon, N.J., & Starnes, A.L. (1993). Family-centered case management practices: characteristics and consequences. In: Singer, G.H. & Powers, L.L. (Eds). Families, disability, and empowerment: active coping skills and strategies for family interventions. (pp 89–118). Baltimore, MD: Brookes.

Kitwood, T. (1997). *Dementia reconsidered: The person comes first.* New York, NY: Open University Press.

Registered Nurses' Association of Ontario. (2015). *Person-and family-centred care.* Toronto, ON: Registered Nurses' Association of Ontario.

Rogers, C. R. (1961). *On becoming a person: A therapist's view of psychotherapy.* Boston, MA: Houghton Mifflin.

Schlosser, R. W. (2004). Goal-attainment scaling as a clinical measurement technique in communication disorders: A critical review. *Journal of Communication Disorders, 37,* 217–239.

Singer, G., & Powers, L. (Eds.). *Families, disability, and empowerment: Active coping skills and strategies for family interventions* (pp. 89–118). Baltimore, MD: Brookes.

White, L. D., Newton-Curtis, L., & Lyons, K. S. (2008). Development and initial testing of a measure of person-directed care. *The Gerontologist, 48,* 114–123.

Woods, J., Wilcox, M. J., Friedman, M., & Murch, T. (2011). Collaborative consultation in natural environments: Strategies to enhance family centered supports and services. *Language, Speech, and Hearing Services in Schools, 42*(3), 379–392. doi:10.1044/0161-1461

Pharmacological Interventions in Hearing Disorders

Numerous pharmacological agents have demonstrated protection and/or rescue from noise-induced hearing loss (NIHL) and/or drug-induced hearing loss (DIHL) in preclinical studies around the world. Some have already progressed to clinical trials. Although none are yet approved for clinical use, it appears likely that in the future one or more of these agents will be available to treat or prevent DIHL or NIHL. Consequently, clinical audiologists and speech–language pathologists need to be aware of the agents being studied and their underlying mechanisms of protection.

NIHL

NIHL is a rapidly growing public health concern. According to Yulia Carrol, evidence of NIHL exists in approximately one in four U.S. adults aged 20–69 years. Hearing loss leads to communication impairments that may have significant social and professional repercussions.

Either intense impulses of noise or prolonged steady-state noise can cause hearing loss. Noise-induced free radical generation leads to both apoptotic and necrotic changes in cochlear outer hair cells (OHCs). Multiple studies report structural changes in cochlear OHCs following noise exposure; these changes include stereocilia damage, cell body swelling, nuclear migration, and OHC death. These structural changes progress up to 5 days after noise cessation, suggesting the primary mode of damage at this time is necrosis. Bo-Hua Hu reported apoptotic changes, karyorrhexis, karyopyknosis, and nuclear swelling in response to noise; he later confirmed apoptosis via caspase-3 activity, an initiator of DNA degradation in apoptotic pathways. W. P. Yang suggested that early pathological changes in cochlear OHCs are secondary to apoptotic pathways, whereas later damage is primarily mediated by both apoptotic and necrotic pathways. Barbara Bohne asserted that a third, unknown, death pathway may be involved in NIHL. In Bohne's study, this third pathway demonstrated characteristics of both necrotic pathways, swollen nuclei and pale staining cells, and apoptotic pathways, pyknosis and shrunken, dark staining cells. Colleen LePrell's review reported that oxidative stress plays a significant role in noise-induced cochlear injury, but vasoconstriction of cochlear capillaries has also been indicated. David Lipscomb demonstrated that cochlear capillary constriction results from the accumulation of reactive oxygen species (ROS) after noise. Josef Miller reported that the specific mechanism involved in posttraumatic vasoconstriction is a direct consequence of 8-isoprostane-$F_{2\beta}$, a vasoactive by-product of ROS. Capillary constriction can lead to reduced blood flow, ischemia, and decreased ROS flushing from the site.

Given the proposed NIHL mechanisms, researchers have investigated multiple antioxidants, vasodilators, and apoptotic pathway inhibitors in the treatment and prevention of NIHL.

DIHL

Cisplatin and aminoglycosides frequently cause DIHL by damaging the basal turn cochlear OHCs, producing predominantly bilateral, high-frequency, sensorineural hearing loss.

Cisplatin

In 1978, Food and Drug Administration approval of cisplatin, a platinum-based chemotherapeutic agent, was a major turning point in the treatment of solid tumors. Cisplatin can cause serious side effects including ototoxicity, nephrotoxicity, neurotoxicity, and myelosuppression. Cisplatin ototoxicity causes bilateral sensorineural hearing loss, primarily of the higher frequencies, that is generally permanent. Cisplatin's primary mechanism of action is to introduce covalent bonds at the N7 position of purine bases in DNA, which leads to DNA damage and apoptosis (see Figure 1).

Cisplatin-induced free radical formation damages cochlear OHCs. ROS, including free radicals such as superoxide (O_2^-) and the hydroxyl radical (OH·), can disrupt cellular structure and function. ROS-induced cellular damage includes initiating DNA strand breaks, fatty acid peroxidation, oxidation of proteins, and disruption of membrane-bound enzymes and carbohydrates. In his review, Leonard Rybak noted three main areas

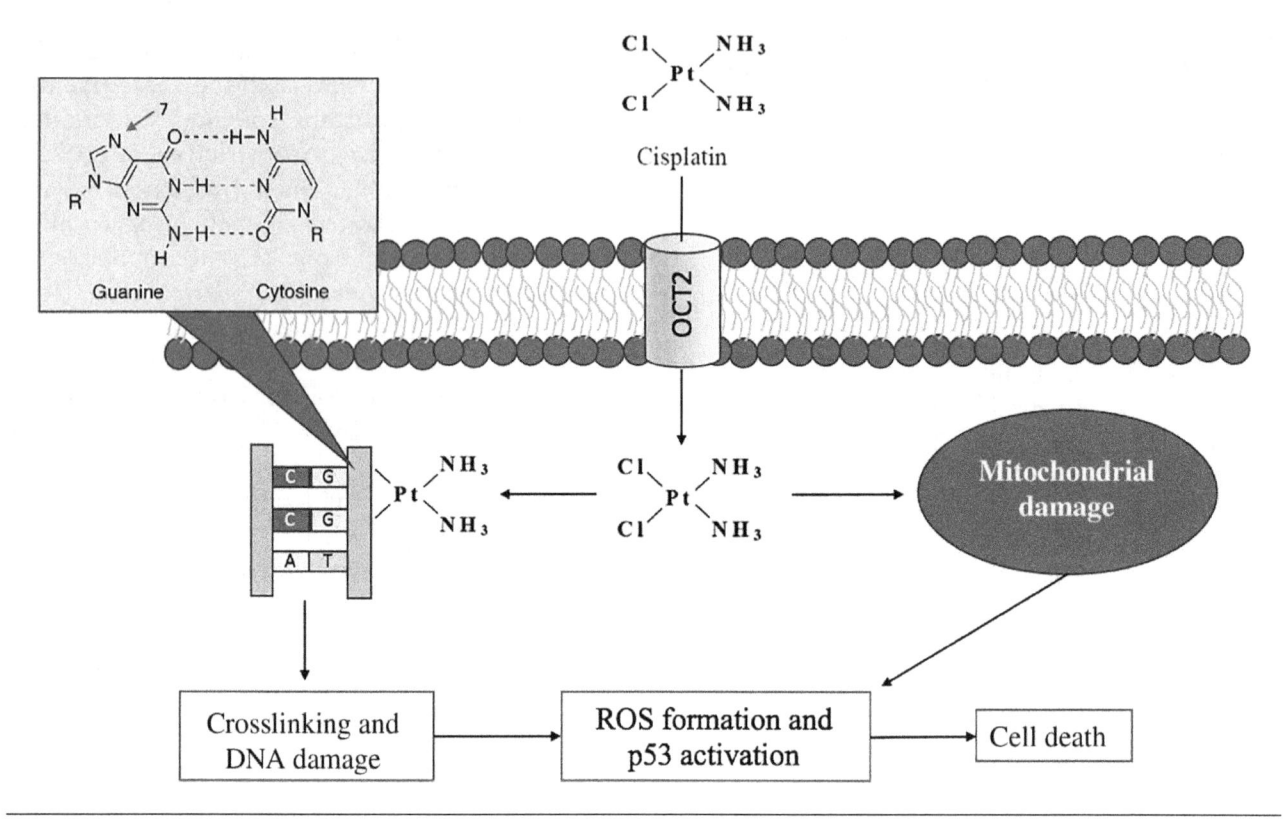

Figure 1 Cisplatin's method of action

of damage: the spiral ganglion cells, OHCs, and the lateral wall tissues (spiral ligament and stria vascularis). Damage to the basal portion of the cochlea is consistent with high-frequency hearing loss. Continued use of cisplatin may progressively damage the cochlea, leading to lower frequency hearing loss. The exact molecular mechanism of cisplatin-induced cochlear damage is not well established. Giuliano Ciarimboli established that cisplatin uptake transporters, CTR1 and OCT2, are expressed in the cochlea; OCT2 is expressed in both the stria vascularis and the hair cells. OCT2 transporters were found to have the highest expression in the basal turn of the cochlea, providing a potential explanation for targeted damage of the OHCs.

Aminoglycosides

Aminoglycosides effectively treat many serious bacterial infections but often produce cochleotoxic and/or vestibulotoxic effects. The manifestation of cochleotoxicity is usually bilateral, permanent, sensorineural hearing loss beginning at high frequencies, whereas vestibulotoxicity can include vertigo, nausea, nystagmus, and/or ataxia. Aminoglycosides bind the 30S subunit of bacterial ribosomes leading to misreading of messenger RNA and faulty protein synthesis. The production of erroneous proteins eventually kills the bacteria. Aminoglycosides differ in their levels of ototoxicity and vestibulotoxicity. Jing Xie reports that gentamycin, kanamycin, amikacin, and tobramycin are ototoxic, but neomycin is regarded as the most highly toxic; conversely, streptomycin and gentamicin are primarily vestibulotoxic and tobramycin is equally cochleo- and vestibulotoxic. Cochleo- and vestibulotoxicity are often dose limiting in the use of aminoglycoside antibiotics.

Aminoglycosides preferentially damage cochlear OHCs via free radicals. Initially, OHCs of the basal turn are affected, leading to high-frequency hearing loss; if aminoglycoside use is continued, damage to the inner hair cells may also occur. Progression leads to lower frequency damage, further impairing speech understanding. Mechanisms of aminoglycoside-induced damage include free radical formation, overactivation of glutamatergic receptors, and disruption of mitochondrial protein synthesis. Free radical oxygen and nitrogen species have been implicated in apoptotic damage caused to OHCs by aminoglycosides. Apoptosis has two major pathways, and both are regulated by caspases. The external pathway is mediated by the activation of death receptors such as Fas and TNFR, whereas in the internal pathway, caspases are activated in response to mitochondrial apoptogenic factor release into the cytoplasm. Daniel Bodmer suggested that OHC apoptosis is primarily mediated by the intrinsic pathway; however, L. Lei found evidence linking Fas protein expression to kanamycin ototoxicity, which suggests that the external pathway may be involved. Although free radical damage is widely accepted as the major mechanism of aminoglycoside ototoxicity, evidence supporting concomitant excitotoxicity is rising. This evidence suggests that aminoglycosides can act as an agonist at the polyamine site on the N-methyl-D-aspartate receptor, leading to increased calcium influx and hair cell degeneration. Aminoglycoside-induced damage may be exacerbated by its increased half-life in cochlear tissues. Tran Ba Huy substantiated that the half-life of aminoglycosides in the inner ear extends past 1 month, and D. Dulon reported that traces may be identified up to 6 months after aminoglycoside cessation.

Otoprotective Agents

Several pharmacological agents reduced and even potentially eliminated NIHL and/or DIHL in preclinical and clinical studies.

Many otoprotective agents can be delivered directly to the cochlea or, in some cases, systemically via injection or oral ingestion.

Antioxidants

D-Methionine

According to studies by Kathleen Campbell, D-Methionine (D-Met) is a promising agent in the treatment of NIHL as well as aminoglycoside- and cisplatin-induced hearing loss. D-Met's primary mechanism of protection appears to be its ability to scavenge free radicals. Cisplatin, aminoglycoside, and NIHL all cause ototoxic damage in part by free radical production. Pathways of ROS production are demonstrated in Figure 2. Preventing ROS-mediated damage could explain D-Met's role in alleviating NIHL and some DIHL. Methionine can be reversibly oxidized to act directly as a free radical scavenger, or it can act indirectly by increasing the intracellular pool of reduced glutathione. The success of D-Met in treating cisplatin-induced hearing loss is also related to its thiol group (–SH). Sulfur has a high affinity for platinum, a major component in cisplatin; sulfur-containing enzymes may be targeted by cisplatin leading to cellular damage. D-Met functions as a decoy for platinum to bind, leaving cellular proteins and enzymes unharmed. Platinum bound to methionine retains most of its antitumor activities, and tumor models demonstrate that D-Met does not inhibit cisplatin tumor kill. Other thiol-containing compounds include N-acetylcysteine (NAC), amifostine, sodium thiosulfate (STS), methylthiobenzoic acid, lipoic acid, tiopronin, and glutathione ester.

D-Met effectively protects against cisplatin ototoxicity when administered directly to the round window membrane of chinchillas, as demonstrated by Kurtis Korver, or when injected intraperitoneally as shown in a rat study by Kathleen Campbell. Although it is more cumbersome, local delivery avoids the risk of systemic side effects and the interruption of cisplatin's tumor-reducing capacity. Kathleen Campbell and Mark Jones also found that systemic delivery of D-Met protects other organ systems from cisplatin toxicities, such as weight loss and nephrotoxicity.

N-Acetylcysteine

NAC, a precursor of glutathione and an ROS scavenger, has been widely studied as an otoprotective agent but has produced mixed results. Richard Kopke verified that significant protection from NIHL was only produced when NAC was combined with high-dose salicylate. Other studies by Kopke show partial protection from NIHL

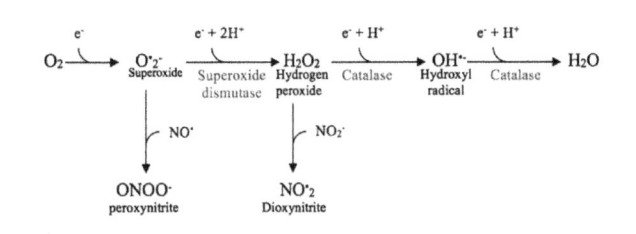

$$O_2 \xrightarrow{e^-} O_2^{\bullet-} \xrightarrow[\text{Superoxide dismutase}]{e^- + 2H^+} H_2O_2 \xrightarrow[\text{Catalase}]{e^- + H^+} OH^{\bullet} \xrightarrow[\text{Catalase}]{e^- + H^+} H_2O$$

Superoxide → NO• → ONOO⁻ peroxynitrite

Hydrogen peroxide → NO₂• → NO•₂ Dioxynitrite

Figure 2 Formation of reactive oxygen species

while using NAC as a single drug therapy, but the Department of Defense did not report significant protection in clinical or preclinical studies.

Ebselen

Ebselen, a seleno-organic compound that mimics glutathione peroxidase, has completed Phase 2 clinical trials for the prevention of NIHL; preclinical studies by Leonard Rybak suggested that ebselen is a promising agent in ameliorating ototoxicity. Although ebselen is not a strong ROS scavenger, it scavenges hydroperoxides. The removal of hydroperoxides is comparable to ROS scavenging in otoprotection. Rybak demonstrated otoprotection from gentamicin and cisplatin by ebselen in several studies. Akram Pourbakht studied ebselen use in guinea pigs and found ebselen also protects against noise-induced OHC damage by preventing $ONOO^-$-mediated cytotoxicity. $ONOO^-$, formed upon the reaction of NO with O_2^-, leads to DNA strand breaks. One study by Tatsuya Yamasoba showed significant decreases in temporary hearing loss, and others by Yamasoba exhibited either partial or complete protection from permanent threshold shifts in hearing when given orally.

Amifostine

Amifostine, a prodrug ROS scavenger, has not exhibited significant results in the treatment and protection from cisplatin-induced hearing loss, according to a meta-analysis by Marc Duval and Sam Daniel. Its use as an otoprotective agent against cisplatin-mediated cochlear damage is refuted by van As, van den Berg, and van Dalen (2014), and amifostine is not recommended for otoprotection by the "American Society of Clinical Oncology 2008 Clinical Practice Guideline Update: Use of Chemotherapy and Radiation Therapy Protectants," as reported by Martee Hensley.

Vitamins ACE With Magnesium

An oral combination of beta-carotene, vitamins C and E, and magnesium (ACE Mg) demonstrated protection against NIHL in a study by Colleen Le Prell. Although Mg and ACE components separately did not confer protection, the combination partially reduced permanent NIHL in guinea pigs. However, this antioxidant combination is contraindicated in smokers; Gilbert Omenn verified that beta-carotene increases the risk of lung cancer in this population. Additionally, Mg is known to cause a laxative effect; therefore, ACE Mg in patients with inflammatory bowel disease should be discouraged.

Acuval, Coenzyme Q10

The combination of a multivitamin, Acuval, with coenzyme Q10 (CoQ10) provides protection from NIHL. Vincenza Cascella demonstrated protection from NIHL when using this formulation of minerals, vitamins, and CoQ10 in rats. Acuval is a supplement containing vitamins A, E, B1, B2, B6, and B12; L-Arginine; *Ginkgo biloba*; and minerals Mg, selenium, and zinc, and it also contains small amounts of CoQ10. The electron transport chain of cells utilizes CoQ10 in the production of energy by the mitochondria, the powerhouse of the cell. Mikael Turunen demonstrated that CoQ10 scavenges free radicals; however, it is much less water soluble. A water-soluble version of CoQ10, Q10 terclatrate, studied by Mora Corvi, has increased efficacy against oxidative injuries, lipid peroxidation, and mitochondrial damage. Rats were divided into four groups: Group A noise exposed, Group B exposed to noise and treated with Acuval, Group C exposed to noise and treated with Acuval plus CoQ10, and Group D only treated with Acuval and CoQ10 with no noise exposure. Groups A and B had significant hearing loss at 4 kHz, but Group C was protected and demonstrated similar hearing profiles to Group D (no noise exposure). This combination protects against hearing loss, but its use is not advised in all populations. *Ginkgo biloba* has been shown to increase bleeding risk in a review by Stephen Bent. Therefore, its use would be contraindicated in surgical candidates, soldiers, and patients with increased risk of bleeding.

Molecular Hydrogen

Hydroxyl radicals are arguably the most cytotoxic of the ROS; molecular hydrogen selectively reduces this radical. Yingni Lin demonstrated molecular hydrogen's protective effects in a study of guinea pigs that either received plain water or hydrogen-rich water for 14 days prior to noise exposure. The animals underwent noise exposure for 3 hr; those in the hydrogen-rich water group had significantly better auditory brainstem responses compared to the plain water group. Members of the hydrogen-rich water group had greater OHC function during recovery. The mechanism relates to hydrogen's ability to facilitate hair cell recovery following noise exposure; this protects and helps OHCs recover after noise induced damage.

Sodium Thiosulfate

STS neutralizes cisplatin, and dosing must be carefully timed to prevent antagonistic effects of cisplatin on tumor treatment. Leslie Muldoon suggested administering STS several hours after cisplatin to prevent tumor protection. Edward Neuwelt investigated the time line of STS and carboplatin administration in guinea pigs in the treatment of blood–brain barrier disrupting brain tumors; to better introduce cisplatin to the brain tumor, he administered mannitol, an osmotic agent that disrupts the blood–brain barrier. He concluded that otoprotection was best achieved with STS administration 8 hr after carboplatin administration, but STS had no effect at 24 hr after carboplatin administration. In a rat model, Edward Neuwelt concluded that STS caused neurotoxic damage when administered immediately after blood–brain barrier disrupting but not when administered 60 min after blood–brain barrier disrupting. Local administration of STS via ear drops is being investigated.

Cochlear Arteriole Vasodilators

Mg produces its otoprotective effects via cochlear arteriole vasodilation leading to increased waste product removal from the cochlea and decreased ischemic damage. Mg may also reduce calcium influx into cells, thus inhibiting apoptotic pathways and ROS damage; however, for greatest protection, Mg should be administered in combination with ACE.

Cochlear Hes1 Suppressors

Corticosteroids, such as dexamethasone, reduce inflammation, inhibit apoptosis, and may promote survival pathways in the organ of Corti through the suppression of Hes. OHCs develop during the embryonic period and don't regenerate postnatally, but when they are provided with the appropriate signals, J. Shou found that supporting cells on the organ of Corti can transdifferentiate into new hair cells, and dexamethasone can promote these transdifferentiation pathways. Math1 and other positive basic helix–loop–helix transcription factors are utilized in inner ear hair cell differentiation. Hes1 (hairy and enhancer of split 1) is a negative basic helix–loop–helix transcription factor that inhibits the differentiation of inner ear hair cells, as discussed by Ryoichiro Kageyama and J. Lisa Zheng in their studies of basic helix–loop–helix factors and inner ear hair cell differentiation, respectively. Bin Wang exposed guinea pigs to loud noise and demonstrated that dexamethasone inhibits Hes1 expression, thus promoting the regeneration of new hair cells and preventing permanent NIHL.

Apoptosis Pathway Inhibitors

Inhibition of apoptosis may be achieved through agents that are inhibitors of caspase, the Jun-N terminal kinase, or calcium and calcineurin. However, inhibition of apoptosis may lead to increased risk of cancer and infection due to its role in immunogenic function. Consequently, local versus systemic use of apoptosis inhibitors should be considered. Loubna Abaamrane investigated apoptotic pathway inhibition by two major mechanisms: inhibiting caspase 3 activation and inhibiting calpains, calcium-activated proteases. Abaamrane's study focused on gunshot-induced hearing loss. This study was performed in guinea pigs and demonstrated that caspase inhibition by z-VAD-FMK after noise exposure reduced OHC loss; unfortunately, calpain inhibition by leupeptin did not yield significant results. This suggests that impulse NIHL relates more closely to caspase activity than calpains. In a human study, Markus Suckfuell administered Jun-N terminal kinase inhibitors intratympanically to subjects within 24 hr of noise exposure and demonstrated significant clinical improvement of acoustic trauma without any severe adverse effects. Calcineurin inhibitors are widely used as immunosuppressants; Isao Uemaetomari demonstrated their efficacy in preventing NIHL of guinea pigs when administered intraperitoneally. Although calcineurin inhibitors are efficacious in preventing NIHL, their propensity to cause calcineurin pain syndrome limits its use in this field.

Final Thoughts

NIHL as well as aminoglycoside- and cisplatin-induced hearing loss are prominent issues in the medical field. Active research in the treatment and prevention of this disorder is ongoing, but several potential treatment options have been identified. Major mechanisms of ototoxic injury include apoptotis, necrosis, ROS formation, and cochlear arteriolar vasoconstriction, as in the case of NIHL. Antioxidants as otoprotective agents have been widely studied and show mixed results. Antioxidants include D-Met, NAC, ebselen, amifostine, ACE Mg, Acuval CoQ10, molecular hydrogen, and STS. D-Met has been shown to effectively protect against noise as well as aminoglycoside- and cisplatin-induced hearing loss. Additionally, ebselen, in clinical trials in 2018, shows promise in the prevention and treatment of NIHL. Whereas NAC has not consistently proved to provide significant protection against acoustic damage, amifostine, tested in cisplatin-induced ototoxicity, is not recommended in the treatment of DIHL. ACE Mg, Acuval CoQ10, and molecular hydrogen have all proved to protect against NIHL, but Mg, a cochlear arteriole vasodilator, as a single agent provides little to no significant protection. Lastly, Hes1 inhibitors and various apoptotic pathway inhibitors have also proved to be useful in the treatment and prevention of NIHL (although systemic and chronic administration of apoptotic pathway inhibitors should be avoided due to adverse reactions that may occur).

Kelly A. Roth and Kathleen C. M. Campbell

See also Hearing Disability and Disorders; Pharmacological Interventions in Speech and Language Disorders; Physiological Basis for Hearing

Further Readings

Anderson, J. M., & Campbell, K. C. M. (2015). Assessment of interventions to prevent drug induced hearing loss. In Miller, J., LePrell, C.G., & Rybak, L. (Eds.) *Free radicals in ENT pathology* (pp. 243–269). New York, NY: Humana Press

Campbell, K. C. M. (2007). *Pharmacology and ototoxicity for audiologists*. Thomson Delmar., Boston, MA

Campbell, K. C. M., Meech, R. P., Klemens, J. J., Gerberi, M. T., Dyrstad, S. S. W., Larsen, D. L. L., . . . Hughes, L. F. (2007). Prevention of noise-and drug-induced hearing loss with D-methionine. *Hearing Research*, 226, 92–103.

Knight, K. R., Kraemer, D. F., Winter, C., & Neuwelt, E. A. (2007). Early changes in auditory function as a result of platinum chemotherapy: Use of extended high-frequency audiometry and functions as a result of platinum chemotherapy. *Journal of Clinical Oncology*, 25(10), 1190–1195.

LePrell, C. G., Yamashita, D., Minami S. B., Yamasoba, T., & Miller, J. M, (2007), Mechanisms of noise-induced hearing loss indicate multiple methods of prevention. *Hearing Research*, 226, 22–43.

Rybak L. P., & Whitworth, C. A. (2005). Ototoxicity: Therapeutic opportunities. *Drug Discovery Today*, 10, 1313–1321.

Schacht, J., Talaska, A. E., & Rybak, L. P. (2012). Cisplatin and aminoglycoside antibiotics: Hearing loss and its prevention. *The Anatomical Record: Advances in Integrative Anatomy and Evolutionary Biology*, 295, 1837–1850.

Tieu, C, & Campbell, KCM (2012). "Current Pharmacologic Otoprotective Agents in or Approaching Clinical Trials: How They Elucidate Mechanisms of Noise-Induced Hearing Loss" Journal of Otolaryngology, 2:4. http://dx.doi.org/10.4172/2161-119X.1000125

van As, J. W., van den Berg, H., & van Dalen, E. C. (2014). Medical interventions for the prevention of platinum-induced hearing loss in children with cancer. *The Cochrane Database of Systematic Reviews*, (7), CD009219. doi:10.1002/14651858. CD009219.pub3

Yorgason, J. G., Fayad, J. N., & Kalinec, F. (2006). Understanding drug ototoxicity: Molecular insights for prevention and clinical management. *Expert Opinion on Drug Safety*, 5(3), 383–399.

Pharmacological Interventions in Speech and Language Disorders

Most psychiatric disorders affect how patients perceive the world around them and/or how the world perceives them via their ability to communicate. Thus, while it could be argued that almost any psychiatric illness has an element of communicative disorder, this entry focuses on such disorders as defined in the *Diagnostic and Statistical Manual of Mental Disorders, Fifth Edition* (*DSM-5*), where disordered communications either are central criteria for their diagnosis or play an outsized role in their clinical manifestation.

Autism Spectrum Disorder

Autism first came to medical attention with Leo Kanner's case reports of children who exhibited extreme aloneness, with notable deficits in social interaction and expressive language abilities. Contemporaneously, Hans Asperger described a group of children with similar levels of decreased functioning in social skill sets, but without notable cognitive or language development delays.

In the intervening period since this original description, a number of reworking and regroupings of the diagnostic definition and subtypes have occurred. The *DSM-5* groups the previously distinct (1) autistic disorder, (2) Asperger's disorder, (3) childhood disintegrative disorder, (4) Rett syndrome, and (5) pervasive developmental disorder not otherwise specified under the umbrella of Autism spectrum disorders (ASDs). This reflects the early 21st-century understanding of the underlying disease process, which recognizes ASD as a group of heterogeneous disorders with a strong inheritable (but not monogenetic) basis that share a common phenotype of impaired social communication several standard deviations below the mean combined with restricted repetitive patterns of behavior, interests, and activities.

Clinically, this may manifest as children who fail to engage in give-and-take conversation, have challenges with nonliteral or imaginative play, or as they grow older, fail to understand that their interests are not universally shared. They may readily become anxious or agitated when their routines are disrupted, and particularly in those individuals with comorbid intellectual disability, there are increased rates of self-injurious and self-stimulating activity.

ASD appears to be more prevalent among males, with an estimated ratio of four males to one female. In the population overall, the rate varies based on study methodology, but estimates of between 1 and 20 per 1,000 appear frequently in the established literature in examination of U.S. and European cohorts. There has been a question of whether the disorders are increasing in prevalence; while there is no definitive answer, the consensus is that the apparent increase more likely reflects changing case definitions and increased awareness.

Treatment for individuals with ASD is an ongoing area of active research, but in general, it is highly individualized to take into account the individual's intellectual functioning, vocabulary and language skills, and other comorbid mental and physical illness, and at its heart, it requires a multidisciplinary approach. Early interventions are thought to produce the best outcomes, with the National Academies of Sciences, Engineering, and Medicine advocating for 12 months a year and 25 hr a week of interventions starting at the first suspicion of the diagnosis; this should be carried out in a mainstream environment where individuals with ASD can interact with children without ASD. Further, National Academies of Sciences, Engineering, and Medicine identified four "priorities of focus": (1) functional spontaneous communication, (2) social instruction delivered throughout the day in various settings, (3) cognitive development and play skills, and (4) proactive approaches to behavior problems.

Social (Pragmatic) Communication Disorder

Social (pragmatic) communication disorder is a new diagnosis that has come about in *DSM-5*. It is essentially the absence of normal social interaction that occurs during communication. While overlapping in part with the clinical picture of ASD, individuals with this illness will not have any history of restricted play or repetitive patterns of behavior, interests, or activities.

One way to distinguish expressive language disorders from ASDs is to identify how much frustration is present in the child. Children with ASD will typically not be frustrated by their disability, but patients with expressive language disorders will not be happy with their condition and typically try their best to improve their condition.

Selective Mutism

Selective mutism is a condition experienced by children with normal language development.

These children will speak in a normal manner in front of their family members and around people with whom they are comfortable. However, situations that are unfamiliar or involve strangers will usually result in the patient staying mute. These patients are socially anxious, and this disorder likely has more of an anxiety component to it. The majority of children outgrow selective mutism as they age.

Mixed Receptive-Expressive Language Disorder

Mixed receptive-expressive language disorder involves an inability to both fully comprehend and fully produce speech. Attention-deficit hyperactivity disorder is present in about 33% of patients with a mixed picture. Mixed receptive-expressive disorder is different from both childhood-onset fluency disorder (stuttering) and speech sound disorder, because in these disorders, patients have no impairments in expression and reception—however, they do have speech incompetence. Some studies indicate that psychotherapy has a role in treating patients with a mixed language disorder who also have significant emotional and behavioral issues. Psychotherapy that involves assessing a patient's self-worth and social skills is essential. More importantly, therapy should include family members in addition to the patient. These family therapy sessions should stress the importance of effective communication methods that diminish arguments and frustration.

Speech Sound Disorder

Speech sound disorder is characterized by difficulty pronouncing sounds. According to *DSM-5*, a patient cannot be diagnosed with speech sound disorder if he or she has a neurological reason for the dysfunction.

Cluttering

Although cluttering is not a formal diagnosis in *DSM-5*, it is a condition worth noting. Cluttering occurs when an individual produces speech patterns that are without any rhythm or symmetry. People who experience cluttering are typically not aware of their deficits; this is in stark contrast to individuals who stutter, who are fully aware of their disability—this is why their rates of anxiety and fear are greater.

Expressive Language Deficits

Expressive language deficits occur when there is an inability to speak but the ability to receive language is preserved. Nonverbal language is also relatively preserved. Psychiatrists and psychologists often utilize the Wechsler Intelligence Scale for Children to help with this diagnosis. They often find that a patient's verbal intelligence is diminished in comparison to the patient's overall intelligence. These patients will most often be verbally much younger than their age. Expressive language deficit children often do not use as many adjectives and often refer to objects without specifically naming them. As a child gets older, the prevalence of expressive language deficits decreases.

Childhood-Onset Fluency Disorder

Childhood-onset fluency disorder (formerly known as *stuttering*) occurs when an individual has a problem with fluency, rhythm, and rate of speech. Eyeblinking, head jerking, involuntary body movements, and facial grimacing are often witnessed during stuttering. Adults with stuttering exhibit higher incidences of social anxiety disorder. In adolescents, social isolation is one of the major negative outcomes of stuttering. Children who stutter have greater rates of being victims of bullying than children who do not. Those who stutter often become fearful and anxious about the possibility of stuttering, especially in social situations or during public speaking. Social anxiety disorders in addition to depression are more prevalent in patients with stuttering compared to the general population.

Psychiatric Comorbidities in Children With Speech and Language Disorder

Language disability can happen through a variety of mechanisms. The most common cause of language disability is congenital. Other less common causes are from trauma, infection, or neurological disorders. Additionally, it can occur in patients who have deafness which is not diagnosed early.

Those children with language disorders have an above average rate of combined psychiatric disorders. Attention-deficit hyperactivity disorder, anxiety disorders, and the combination of oppositional defiant disorder and conduct disorder are most commonly seen in patients with speech and language disorders. School-age children with language deficits face a host of issues related to self-esteem, depression, and bullying.

Pharmacotherapy of Stuttering

As research into the pathophysiological basis of stuttering continues to elucidate the multifactorial nature of this complex and largely unchartered area of neuropsychiatry, so too does the clinician's ability to pharmacologically treat patients who experience stuttering. Originally thought to be the result of anatomical abnormalities of the tongue and larynx, stuttering is now known to be a multifactorial disorder involving a close interplay of genetics, neurophysiology, and the environment.

Although no one brain region has been identified as the source of developmental stuttering, it is evident through positron emission tomography (PET) studies that much of the pathology occurs in brain regions involved in speech or articulation. Studies using PET scans of individuals with stuttering showed abnormal glucose metabolism in speech cortical brain areas and the basal ganglia. In addition, PET studies of individuals with moderate-to-severe developmental stuttering showed significantly higher metabolic uptake in the medial prefrontal cortex, deep orbital cortex, insular cortex, extended amygdala, auditory cortex, and caudate tail.

The Dopamine Hypothesis of Stuttering

Stuttering appears to be related to abnormal elevations of cerebral dopaminergic activity, which is further supported by studies showing increased stuttering symptoms in patients taking stimulant medications or dopamine agonists (e.g., levodopa) known to raise dopamine levels in the brain. As previously mentioned, PET scan studies showing striatal hypometabolism in individuals who stutter may in part be explained by dopamine's general inhibitory properties on striatal metabolism and higher levels of presynaptic dopamine found in individuals with stuttering.

Dopamine's central role in the pathophysiology of stuttering, known as the *dopamine hypothesis*, is well supported by its association with both tic disorders and specific dopaminergic genes found to be related to an increase in susceptibility to stuttering disorder. These revelations have led to clinical trials investigating dopamine antagonists as potential treatment options for patients with stuttering. Dopamine-antagonist medications such as haloperidol, risperidone, olanzapine, asenapine, aripiprazole, and lurasidone have all been shown to significantly improve stuttering.

Also, the selective gamma-aminobutyric acid A (GABA) partial agonist pagoclone has shown benefit for patients with stuttering but more so with respect to the social anxiety than direct effects on fluency of speech. Although it is unclear how this GABAergic medication benefits the fluency, it is likely related to the dopamine-GABA interactions in the basal ganglia and to changes in cortical networks mediated by altered GABAergic regulations. GABA does regulate anxiety so pagoclone's positive effects on patients who stutter with this aspect are quite clear.

Dopamine 2 Antagonists: Typical Antipsychotics

Haloperidol, a widely used and older antipsychotic, is well-known for its dopamine antagonistic properties. Studies as early as the late 1960s showed its efficacy in treating Tourette syndrome and eventually sparked interest in its use as a potential treatment option for stuttering. These early studies on the use of haloperidol in the treatment of stuttering showed clinical improvement in dysfluency, speed of speaking, and a reduction in secondary *struggle* while speaking. However, one of the major drawbacks of haloperidol consists of the multitude of adverse side effects which often reduces compliance in the long term. Dysphoric side effects, sexual dysfunction, extrapyramidal concerns, and risks of tardive dyskinesia are just a few of the adverse effects that create an obstacle for keeping patients in treatment.

Dopamine Antagonists: Atypical Antipsychotics

Risperidone, a second-generation (atypical) antipsychotic, has also been shown to improve stuttering symptoms, but it has a more favorable side effect profile than haloperidol. Significant decreases in percentage of syllables stuttered, time of stuttering, and overall stuttering severity have been reported with risperidone. Although well tolerated overall, risperidone's prolactin-related side effects such as dysphoria, sexual dysfunction, galactorrhea, gynecomastia, and amenorrhea have also hindered long-term compliance.

Olanzapine is an atypical antipsychotic-like risperidone, but it has a different side effect profile with fewer prolactin-related side effects. Olanzapine's long-term usefulness in stuttering treatment is hindered by the compound's relation to weight gain and metabolic disturbances. In a double-blind, placebo-controlled trial, Olanzapine showed significant reduction in stuttering symptoms compared to placebo in patients with developmental stuttering. Of note, all patients in the study opted to enter the open-label phase of the protocol showing improvement in stuttering symptoms over 6 months to over 1 year. These findings suggest an adequate treatment trial of olanzapine to be over a period of months.

Asenapine, a novel atypical antipsychotic, and *Aripiprazole*, a partial dopamine agonist at D_2 and 5-HT_{1A} receptor agonist and 5-HT_{2A} antagonist, have both been shown to improve stuttering symptoms in a small number of case reports. Aripiprazole is an atypical antipsychotic with D_2 partial agonist activity that has been effective in reducing symptom severity in patients with Tourette's disorder. Aripiprazole was identified as a potential therapeutic option for stuttering in two separate case reports on an adult in 2008 and an adolescent in 2016. In the adult study using the Riley Stuttering Severity Instrument 3 following aripiprazole treatment, the patient's stuttering severity decreased. The patient also reported a decrease in social anxiety and reduction in syllables stuttered. In the adolescent case, a 300-word reading sample and a 300-word conversational sample were used to assess stuttering severity, with results showing a decrease in disfluency rate following aripiprazole treatment. In addition to the improvement of stuttering symptoms, the patient reported little akathisia, sedation, or weight gain.

Lurasidone is an atypical antipsychotic D2 receptor antagonist with a favorable side effect profile with little metabolic disturbance and extrapyramidal symptoms. In an open-label study of six patients with stuttering published in 2017, researchers noted improvements in symptoms subjectively using the Clinical Global Impressions scores and the Subjective Screening of Stuttering scale. Patients also reported a decrease in stuttering severity, locus of control, and avoidance.

GABA Receptor Agonists

Pagoclone, a selective $GABA_A$ partial agonist, was actively being developed specifically for the treatment of stuttering. In an 8-week, multicenter, double-blind, placebo-controlled study, pagoclone treatment resulted in significant reductions in percentage of syllables stuttered and was well tolerated with headache being the most common side effect. Additionally, patients in the treatment group reported a greater sense of control over their stuttering and verbal fluency as well as reduced social anxiety. A further study yielded a high placebo response rate on fluency but further development of the compound ceased as funding ended.

Baclofen is a pharmacological compound used as a muscle relaxant but was studied in a 2017 case report of a patient with comorbid alcohol dependence and stuttering. It is pharmacologically similar to Pagoclone by acting as a GABA agonist. This case report observed the cessation of stuttering during treatment with baclofen.

Final Thoughts

Further research and additional clinical trials will be required to further elucidate the properties and mechanisms of each of these compounds in the treatment for stuttering. Physicians should take a multidimensional approach with speech–language pathologists in addition to addressing the patient's social and cognitive needs. The future of stuttering therapy will likely include a comprehensive approach utilizing speech therapy combined with psychotherapy to address comorbid psychiatric symptoms and psychopharmacological treatments to address the stuttering itself and related symptoms.

Spencer Wang, Michael Ingram, Evan Trager, Monish Parmar, and Gerald Maguire

See also Diagnosis of Communication Disorders; *Diagnostic and Statistical Manual of Mental Disorders (DSM)*; Fluency and Fluency Disorders; Psychiatric Disorders With Communication Disorders; Stuttering and Adolescents; Stuttering Treatment

Further Readings

American Psychiatric Association. (2013). *Diagnostic and statistical manual of mental disorders* (5th ed.). Washington, DC.

Charoensook, J., Fernandez, C., Hoang, J., Patel, S., & Maguire, G. (2017). *A case series on the effectiveness of lurasidone in patients with stuttering*. UCR School of Medicine Riverside, CA.

Hoang, J. L., Patel, S., & Maguire, G. A. (2016). Case report of aripiprazole in the treatment of adolescent stuttering. *Ann Clin Psychiatry, 28*(1), 64–65.

Kanner, L. (1968). Autistic disturbances of affective contact. *Acta Paedopsychiatr, 35*(4), 100–136.

Maguire, G. A., Yeh, C. Y., & Ito, B. S. (2012). Overview of the diagnosis and treatment of stuttering. *Journal of Experimental & Clinical Medicine, 4*(2), 92–97.

Sadock, B. J., & Sadock, A. V. (2007). *Kaplan and Sadock's synopsis of psychiatry: Behavioral sciences/clinical psychiatry* (10th ed.). Philadelphia, PA: Lippincott Williams & Wilkins.

Tran, N. L., Maguire, G. A., Franklin, D. L., & Riley, G. D. (2008). Case report of aripiprazole for persistent developmental stuttering. *Journal of Clinical Psychopharmacology, 28*(4), 470–472.

PHENOMENOLOGY

Phenomenology is a branch of philosophy that has spawned methodological innovations in the psychological and social sciences. Phenomenology focuses on the study of human consciousness as experienced from a subjective, first-person viewpoint. This makes it distinctly different from philosophies that posit a strict distinction between subject and object—the person who knows and that which is known—and from research methods that aim at objectifying experience, such as experimental investigations of cognition and perception or survey questionnaires with standardized questions. Consequently, phenomenology has informed qualitative research methods that attempt to describe reality as it is experienced by research participants.

As an example of the kind of problems phenomenology investigates, consider what happens when you bite into an apple. How would you describe this experience to a person who has never tasted apples? You could analyze the taste into its components—say, *fruity*, *sweet*, and *tart*—but those would be true descriptions of the taste of berries, too. Moreover, they would only make sense to someone who has already tasted something fruity, sweet, and tart. In the absence of the experience, any *objective* description—in words or numbers—cannot convey what it is like.

Based on observations like this one, phenomenology argues that conscious experience—thoughts, emotions/feelings, perceptions, and bodily and kinesthetic sensations—cannot be reduced to material processes—brain activity, hormonal fluctuations, flavor compounds hitting taste buds, muscle activation, and so forth—nor can it be investigated by observation of such processes alone. Human experience is always experience *for* someone not simply experience *of* something: It is undergone by a concrete person with a concrete personal or cultural background that shapes his or her interpretation of the experience and his or her motives in interacting with the world. Hence, phenomenology argues that the experience of being human is not adequately addressed by the methods of the natural and experimental sciences and attempts to overcome this problem by devising its own set of investigative techniques.

For the student of communication sciences and disorders, phenomenology has the potential of shedding light on issues that are not commonly addressed by academic research, even though they are obvious to the practicing clinician. Why does my client not wear his hearing aids? Why does this child refuse to participate in the activity that his or her peers engage in with enthusiasm? Why does my client not practice his sounds at home, even though he is clearly bothered by his articulation issues? Why is my swallowing patient rejecting the pureed dish that she ate with enjoyment a week ago? Experimental methods, geared toward objective facts—causal or correlative connections between controlled variables—are ill suited to answering such questions. Investigating people's experience of speech–language and hearing therapy from a phenomenological, first-person standpoint promises fruitful insights into common issues *on the ground*.

History and Development of Phenomenology

Like many strands of Western thought, the roots of phenomenology can be traced to Aristotle (384–322 BCE). In his writings on *Theoretical* and *Practical Knowledge*, Aristotle identified contemplative, subjective experience as one form of theoretical knowledge, and practical knowledge as an intentional, goal-oriented way of being in the world. Phenomenology brings both ideas together, asserting that subjective experience is a form of active knowledge: All conscious experience includes *intentionality*. That is, it is always directed *at* something, and it is always experience *for* someone, shaped by past meanings and intended future uses of its content.

The study of subjective experience fell out of fashion with the emergence of modern science and the philosophies that accompanied it. René Descartes (1596–1650) posited a strict dualism between subject and object—the person who knows and that which is known—and claimed that objective knowledge can be obtained through rational thought. By contrast, David Hume (1711–1776) argued that knowledge is obtained through experience alone. Consequently, he dismissed mental phenomena in favor of experiment and observation. Both Descartes's and Hume's ideas, while in conflict with each other, have informed experimental methods, which combine strict rationality with formalized observation to devise and test hypotheses.

French rationalism and British empiricism were criticized by German and Austrian thinkers. Immanuel Kant (1724–1804) argued that human experience is constrained by the operations of the mind, which always involve space, time, and causality. What lies beyond this *phenomenal* world—the world as accessible to our perception—we cannot know: The *thing-in-itself* cannot be accessed by reasoning or observation. Georg Wilhelm Friedrich Hegel (1770–1831) developed a *phenomenology of the spirit*, a typology of the ways phenomena appear to the mind. Franz Brentano (1838–1917) revisited Aristotle's ideas and formulated *intentionality* as discussed previously. He was the first author to use the term *phenomenology* in the sense of *descriptive psychology*.

Edmund Husserl (1859–1938), a student of Brentano's, became the founder of phenomenology as a philosophical school. In his *Logical Investigations*, published in 1900–1901, Husserl wove together two strands of thought: psychology as formulated by Brentano and by American psychologist William James and philosophical logic and semantics. Building on Brentano's concept of intentionality, Husserl outlined phenomenology as a method to describe and classify the *intentional objects* that constitute people's mental lives.

In Husserl's method, the phenomenological researcher *brackets* her assumptions about the world: Instead of equating an experience of something with the one that is experienced, she abstains from any belief about the latter and turns her attention to the experience itself. For example, instead of asking "What is the taste of an apple?" the phenomenologist might ask "How do I experience the taste of an apple?" or "How do people describe the taste of an apple?" This is a subtle but crucial distinction: The first question asks about a property of an object in the world, whereas the latter two ask about the properties of human consciousness. Thus, they aim at *lived experience*, probing into what it is subjectively like to interact with the world. The world as experienced by a subject constitutes the subject's *lifeworld*, the world as it is *for* the subject.

Husserl's work proved enormously influential in philosophy and the social and psychological sciences. His successors expanded his program of inquiry. Alfred Schütz (1899–1959) devised a phenomenology of the social world, arguing that lived experience always includes meanings and symbols acquired as we grow up into a shared lifeworld. Maurice Merleau-Ponty (1908–1961) focused on *embodiment*, the lived experience of the body. American sociologist Harold Garfinkel (1917–2011) created *ethnomethodology* on phenomenological foundations. This qualitative method of inquiry refrains from theoretical assumptions about social phenomena, describing them in terms of the actors involved. Out of ethnomethodology grew *conversation analysis*, an approach that uses the same principles on talk-in-interaction and that has been deployed in a range of studies in the field of communication sciences and disorders.

The second half of the 20th century saw the rise of a countercurrent to phenomenology. *Philosophical materialism* asserts that conscious experience is identical with corresponding neural states and does not need to be investigated in its own right. This idea gained momentum with the emergence of neuroscience—the study of the brain—and cognitive science—the experimental study of the mind. Both strands of inquiry have since provided important insights into neural and cognitive processes. Their questions, however, are of a different type than those asked by phenomenology, and their methods cannot answer phenomenological questions. The experience of eating an apple is different from the neural activation while eating it or from performance on a task of, say, sorting apples by flavor.

This issue is discussed, in contemporary philosophy and science, as the *qualia problem*. The term *qualia* refers to subjective experiences of material processes. Thomas Nagel famously asked, in a 1974 essay, "What is it like to be a bat?" and argued that subjective experience cannot be captured by observation. We know a lot about the anatomy and physiology of bats, but we cannot know what it is like to be one. Materialist philosopher John Searle subscribes to the idea that intentionality and consciousness are integral aspects of mental states. Thus, phenomenological questions are nowadays debated even in quite different philosophical traditions.

Applications in Communication Sciences and Disorders

Phenomenology has potential to elucidate understudied problems in the field of communication sciences and disorders. Areas that could benefit from phenomenological research include the therapeutic relationship and rapport, client engagement and motivation, fluctuations in client performance, and individual differences in therapy outcomes. However, phenomenology has not been widely used in the field (for notable exceptions see the Further Readings section). Two reasons for this can be identified. First, as is the case for many philosophical and qualitative approaches, phenomenology involves a dazzling array of highly technical terms and concepts not easily accessible to nonphilosophers. Practical guidelines for researchers are available, however, such as those devised by Jonathan Smith and colleagues.

The second and more important reason is that our field is still very much dominated by the medical model and its emphasis on experimental research. This is manifest in the way evidence-based practice (EBP) is conceptualized. The American Speech-Language-Hearing Association identifies three components of EBP: (1) external scientific evidence, (2) clinical expertise and expert opinion, and (3) client/patient/caregiver perspectives. The goal of EBP is to integrate these, and such an integration would indeed provide a well-rounded approach to clinical practice, balancing third-person, objective knowledge (1) with first-person, subjective evidence (2 and 3). However, American Speech-Language-Hearing Association's guidelines to using EBP preclude such a balance. They stipulate that external evidence has primacy over all other types. Clinical expertise is considered the lowest level of evidence; client perspective is not even discussed as a source of evidence. This is unfortunate, for it precludes thoughtful examination of two out of three EBP components.

Ripich and Panagos (1985) provide a stark insight into client perspective. Asked about her view of speech therapy, a child in their study responded, "I'm supposed to make the bad *r* sounds." It can be assumed that this view might affect outcomes. And yet, this type of evidence is not typically considered. Phenomenological research could help close this gap, leading to truly EBP.

Conclusion

Phenomenology is a promising tool for our field, yet underused due to the dominance of experimental methods. It is worth pointing out, in this regard, that phenomenological inquiry is not limited to those who operate under this label. Anyone who examines the contents of the mind—their own or others'—practices phenomenology. Thus, even Hume and Descartes used phenomenology to come to their conclusions. Likewise, anytime clinicians engage in *reflective practice* using *introspection* or *empathy*—examining their own mental states or interpreting those of their clients—they practice a form of phenomenology. In other words, all clinical practice inevitably involves a phenomenological component. This makes phenomenology, arguably, one of the most widespread and at the same time underappreciated forms of inquiry.

Tobias A. Kroll

See also Affect; Conversation Analysis; Emotional Impact of Communication Disorders; Intentionality; Motivation; Qualitative Research

Further Readings

Agar, M. (2013). *The lively science: Remodeling human social research.* Minneapolis, MN: Mill City Press.

Fourie, R., Crowley, N., & Oliviera, A. (2011). A qualitative exploration of therapeutic relationships from the perspective of six children receiving speech-language therapy. *Topics in Language Disorders, 31*, 310–324.

Fourie, R., & Murphy, M. (2011). Alienation and therapeutic connection: A phenomenological account of three patients with communication disorders associated with cancers of the head and neck. *Journal of Interactional Research in Communication Disorders, 2*(1), 1–27.

Hamilton, D. (1994). Traditions, preferences, and postures in applied qualitative research. In N. K. Denzin & Y. S. Lincoln (Eds.), *Handbook of qualitative research* (pp. 60–69). Thousand Oaks, CA: Sage.

Hinckley, J. J. (2005). The piano lesson: An autoethnography about changing clinical paradigms in aphasia practice. *Aphasiology, 19*, 765–779.

Hinckley, J. J. (2014a). A case for the implementation of cognitive-communication screenings in acute stroke. *American Journal of Speech-Language Pathology, 23*, 4–14.

Hinckley, J. J. (2014b). Phenomenology. In M. J. Ball, N. Müller, & R. L. Nelson (Eds.), *Handbook of qualitative research in communication disorders* (pp. 93–111). New York, NY: Psychology Press.

Holstein, J. A., & Gubrium, J. F. (1994). Phenomenology, ethnomethodology, and interpretive practice. In N. K. Denzin & Y. S. Lincoln (Eds.), *Handbook of qualitative research* (pp. 262–272). Thousand Oaks, CA: Sage.

Husserl, E. (2001). *Logical Investigations, Volume 1 (International library of philosophy and scientific method.)* Translated by J. N. Findlay. Edition abridged, reprint, revised. New York, NY: Psychology Press.

Lincoln, Y. S. (2005). Institutional review boards and methodological conservatism: The challenge to and from phenomenological paradigms. In N. K. Denzin & Y. S. Lincoln (Eds.), *Handbook of qualitative research* (3rd ed., pp. 165–181). Thousand Oaks, CA: Sage.

Pascale, C. M. (2011). *Cartographies of knowledge: Exploring qualitative epistemologies.* Thousand Oaks, CA: Sage.

Ripich, D. N., & Panagos, J. M. (1985). Accessing children's knowledge of sociolinguistic rules for speech therapy lessons. *Journal of Speech and Hearing Disorders, 50*, 335–346.

Smith, D. W. (2013). Phenomenology. In E. N. Zalta (Ed.), *The Stanford encyclopedia of philosophy* (Winter 2013 Edition). Retrieved July 8, 2015, from http://plato.stanford.edu/archives/win2013/entries/phenomenology/

Smith, J. A. (1996). Beyond the divide between cognition and discourse: Using interpretative phenomenological analysis in health psychology. *Psychology & Health, 11*, 261–271.

Smith, J. A., Flowers, P., & Larkin, M. (2009). *Interpretative phenomenological analysis: Theory, method and research.* Thousand Oaks, CA: Sage.

PHONATION

See Phonetics; Voice Quality

PHONEME

The term *phoneme* is applied to the minimal unit of speech capable of changing meaning in a given language or language variety. The nature of the phoneme was subject to discussion within linguistics, with some proposing a physical reality, and others a psychological status. Current views tend to support an abstract linguistic status, though many current phonological theories no longer give a central role to the phoneme.

The semantic contrastive nature of the phoneme can be seen, for example, in the use of the English sounds [p] and [k] in the words *pat* and *cat*. These words contrast only through the change in the initial consonants, thus these consonants belong to separate phonemes, shown through the use of slant brackets: /p/, /k/. A *minimal pairs test* is used to separate speech segments (*phones*) into different phonemes. Thus, a pair of words differing in only one segment in the same position in the word is used to demonstrate phonemic contrastivity in the language being studied. In English, *pat* can be contrasted with *cat, bat, sat, mat, pet, pit, put, pack, pan,* and so on.

Phonemes are described as consisting of a set of variants (termed *allophones* and shown in square brackets). These variants may be context dependent. A *complementary distribution test* may be used to demonstrate this. Thus, if two phonetically similar allophones are in complementary distribution, then they are deemed to belong to a single phoneme. So, for English, the clear-l ([lʲ]) is found in syllable initial position in words such as *leaf*, and the dark-l ([lˠ]) in syllable final position in words such as *feel*. These two variants are found in mutually exclusive phonological contexts and cannot be used in English to distinguish the meanings of words, thus they belong to a single /l/ phoneme. Some phones that are in complementary distribution are not considered members of a single phoneme if they are phonetically dissimilar; for example in English, [h] and [ŋ] are in complementary distribution (syllable initial only vs. syllable final only) but are not classed together phonemically.

Some allophones are not context dependent but nevertheless are not capable of changing word meaning. These allophones can be chosen by speakers for stylistic or related reasons. Such allophones are termed as being in *free variation*. An example from English is the choice between aspirated and unreleased variants of /p/ word finally. Thus, *map* can be realized as either [mæpʰ] or [mæp̚] with no change of meaning, and so the two variants are classed as allophones of /p/.

Phoneme inventories differ widely from language to language with totals varying from a low of around a dozen, to a high of over 100.

Phonemic transcription is a record of the abstract phoneme units used by the speaker and not a record of the precise realization of those units. It is always shown in slant brackets. It is rarely useful in the transcription of disordered speech, as these speakers by definition are not using the target phoneme system of the language.

The notion of the phoneme has been extended by some linguists beyond the purely segmental level of phonological analysis, to suprasegmental aspects such as length, pitch, and stress. One proposal to characterize contrastive vowel and consonant length in languages where this is needed, is to add a *chroneme* unit to the phonological system. So, if a language has five long vowels and five equivalent short vowels (all contrastive), rather than positing 10 vowel phonemes, one could include only 5, together with a chroneme. For tone languages, the *toneme* unit can be employed. Here, if a language employs four contrastive tones, then four tonemes are included in the phonological inventory (the allotones representing the context-dependent realizations of specific tones). Finally, a stress unit (the *stroneme*) was also suggested but is rarely encountered in the literature.

Two related problems with phonemic analysis can be mentioned. First is the *biuniqueness* requirement. Phoneme theory requires allophones to belong to one phoneme only. However, examples can be found where this requirement is breached. For example, intervocalic flapping in several varieties of English affects both /t/ and /d/. Thus, *patting* and *padding* may be pronounced with a medial flap [ɾ], and so [ɾ] would be deemed an allophone of both /t/ and /d/. Similar mergers may be found at the phonemic level, characterizing the second problem: *neutralization*. For example, the contrast between fortis and lenis obstruents in Polish occurs at word initial and medial but not at word final position. So, the words *buk* and *bóg* (*beech tree, god*) both have a final /k/, but in their plural forms *buki* has /k/, whereas *bogowie* has /g/. To account for both these problems, archiphonemes have been proposed. These group together two (or sometimes more) phonemes that share most characteristics but one (the one that is neutralized or merged). Thus, transcribing *patting* and *padding* phonemically using an archiphoneme would give /pæDɪŋ/, allowing the transcriber to avoid having to choose between /t/ and /d/. Likewise, with the Polish example, an archiphoneme /K/ could be used.

One early and still commonly found analysis of types of phonological disorder is based on the phoneme principle. This is the SODA system: substitutions, omissions, distortions, and additions. The category of omission refers to deletion of a target phoneme (either from the attempted word or the system altogether). Addition is used to characterize a nontarget sound used in an attempted word (though it is unclear whether this category is to be used only for added phonemes of the language, or any added sound). Substitution is the use of one phoneme of the language in place of the target phoneme, and distortion is the replacement of a target phoneme by a sound that is not another phoneme of the language. This last category is wide and could include incorrect allophones of the language or sounds from outside the phonological system of the target language altogether, including sounds not found in natural language.

Martin J. Ball

See also Clinical Phonology; Phonetic Transcription; Phonetics; Phonology

Further Readings

Ball, M. J., Müller, N., & Rutter, R. (2010). *Phonology for communication disorders.* New York, NY: Psychology Press.
Jones, D. (1950). *The phoneme: Its nature and use.* Cambridge, UK: Heffer.
Lass, R. (1984). *Phonology.* Cambridge, UK: Cambridge University Press.
Twaddell, W. (1935). *On defining the phoneme.* Baltimore, MD: Waverly Press.

Phonetic Transcription

Phonetic transcription in its most general sense is the recording of aspects of pronunciation by any written means. In phonetics, however, it refers to the use of specialized notation systems for representing the phonetic content of speech. Apart from the central role such systems have in the study of phonetics, there are a number of reasons why practitioners of various professions employ phonetic transcription. Foreign language dictionaries and teaching texts need to be able to instruct learners how to pronounce words when sound-spelling correspondences are ambiguous (e.g., <oo> in *book, boot, blood*) or inconsistent (e.g., *cite, site, sight*). Linguists carrying out fieldwork want to be able to write down their consultants' speech with enough precision that other linguists can read it and recover the pronunciations reasonably accurately. Forensic phoneticians often have to compare details of pronunciation in two speech samples to decide how likely it is that they were spoken by the same person and to provide a written record of that comparison as part of legal process. In conversation analysis, it is important to be able to note subtle pronunciation behaviors and correlate them with structural and pragmatic properties of conversational interaction. Speech and language therapists require a quick and convenient means for writing down their records and analyses of clients' (mis)pronunciations. In all these activities, the focus is on details of spoken language which cannot be expressed in ordinary orthography. This entry lists common uses of phonetic transcription, and the relationship of transcription to orthography, before outlining some different kinds of phonetic notation and briefly describing various types of transcription. It then considers how phonetic transcription can be used alongside instrumental analyses of speech.

It is important to appreciate that, although phonetic transcription can be seen to supplement orthographic resources, it would be a mistake to think of it as an alternative way of spelling words. The purpose of spellings is to identify words in the vocabulary of a particular language. For example, the spelling <but> identifies the conjunction *but* (pronounced [bʌt]) in English; however, in French, it identifies the word meaning *goal* (pronounced [by]). One therefore needs to know which language one is dealing with in order to know which lexical item it is; if one is familiar enough with that language, then one will already know how it is pronounced. The transcription [but], however, expresses a phonetic analysis of a pronunciation form, not a lexical item, and is valid for whichever languages have a word, or part of a word, pronounced in that way (e.g., the English word *boot*, the first part of the French word *boutique*, etc).

Phonetic Notation

A phonetic notation system is a set of symbols each of which has assigned to it, by a set of interpretative conventions, a unique phonetic definition in terms of phonetic categories such as places, manners, and aspects of articulation or degrees of pitch height and directions of pitch movement for denoting properties of intonation. By far the most common system in use today is the International Phonetic Alphabet (IPA), supplemented since the 1990s by the Extensions to the IPA and Voice Quality Symbols. Phonetic symbols are enclosed in square brackets. The IPA symbol [b], for example, is defined as the conjunction of the three categories *voiced bilabial plosive*, [s] as *voiceless alveolar fricative*, [ŋ] as *voiced velar nasal*, and so on. From the way symbols are arranged on the IPA chart, it is clear how to interpret them, provided of course that the terms such as *bilabial*, *fricative*, and so on are properly understood. That is to say, an understanding of phonetic theory and terminology is necessary in order to use phonetic notation to its full potential.

Some phonetic notation systems designed their symbols iconically in an attempt to directly represent the organs and actions of the vocal tract. One well-known example is Alexander Melville Bell's *Visible Speech* notation dating from the 1860s. His symbol for [b] was [ᴐ]. It is an *analytic* symbol because each component separately denotes a phonetic category—[ᴐ] = *lips* (the shape represents the mouth facing left), [ı] = *shut* (representing the entrance to the mouth being closed), and [-] = *voice* (representing a closed vibrating glottis). By contrast, most IPA symbols, being derived from alphabetic letters, are *integral* because the whole symbol denotes all the categories at once. There are partial exceptions, however, such as the symbols for retroflex sounds which all have a descending right tail: [ʈ ɖ ʂ ʐ ɳ ɽ ɭ] and glottalic implosives all containing an ascending right hook-top: [ɓ ɗ ʄ ɠ ʛ]. The subset of IPA symbols known as *diacritics* (because they are added to main symbols) contains some iconic members (e.g., the voiceless diacritic [b̥] indicative of an open glottis, here combined with [b] to mean *devoiced bilabial plosive* and [t̪] denoting *dental* with a tooth-shaped diacritic, combined here with [t] for a *voiceless dental plosive*). Symbols for intonation tend toward iconicity in the sense that voice pitch is commonly described as being high or low, and moving up or down, and height and movement are shown by the positions and directions of the

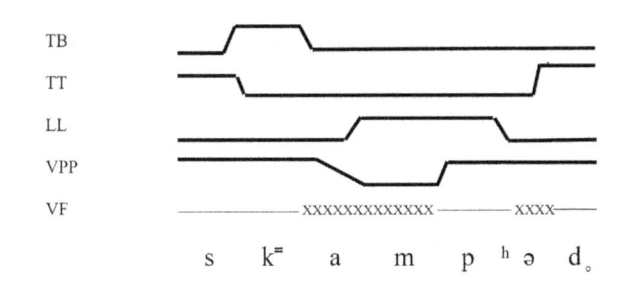

Figure 1 Parametric transcription of *scampered* with an aligned IPA transcription. TB = tongue back; TT = tongue tip; LL = lower lip; VPP = velopharyngeal port; VF = vocal folds; xxx = vibrations

IPA tone marks such as [˧] (mid-tone) and [↘] (global fall).

IPA notation for consonants and vowels relies on the view that speech can be usefully represented as a linear arrangement of discrete symbols, even though it is well-known that, from articulatory and acoustic perspectives, speech is a weave of phonetic properties which overlap and continuously vary through time, not a succession of separate sound segments. Support for IPA notation comes from the argument, perhaps controversial, that what listeners seem to become conscious of in the process of speech perception are discrete identifiable sounds and that therefore analyses of these perceptual objects can legitimately be expressed with IPA symbols.

An alternative type of notation, which does not treat speech as discretely segmental in the time domain, is parametric notation. A tiered array shows the relative timing of articulatory events, with upward and downward movements of the lines representing raising and lowering of speech organs; see Figure 1 for an example of a parametric transcription of a typical nonrhotic pronunciation of *scampered*.

Phonetic Transcription

A symbol in a transcription, in addition to denoting the phonetic categories that define it, represents a piece of real or potential speech data. By bringing the categories and the data together, a transcription expresses an analysis of those data. There are many different types of phonetic transcription depending on the kind of data being transcribed (specific or generic), orientation (to the speaker or listener), level of detail (broad or narrow), method of analysis (perceptual or systematic), and level of linguistic structure (phonemic or allophonic).

Specific and Generic Transcriptions

A specific transcription is a representation of the speech of an individual speaker on a particular occasion, whereas generic transcriptions represent generalizations about how words are typically pronounced by a particular group of speakers. For example, a speech and language therapist might make a specific transcription of a client's utterance and compare it with a generic transcription to draw attention to the atypicalities.

Transcription Orientation

Two specific transcriptions of the same piece of speech may turn out to be different if they are made from different perspectives. One transcriber might be paying attention to the speaker's articulations perhaps with the aid of a video recording or phonetic instrumentation, while the other relies entirely on listening. The former is therefore a speaker-oriented transcription, the latter a listener-oriented one.

Broad and Narrow Transcriptions

The broad–narrow distinction has a long history stretching back to Andrew James Ellis in the mid-19th century, and it has sometimes overlapped with one or other of the two distinctions presented later in this entry. To avoid confusion, it may be helpful to confine the distinction to the level of detail contained in a transcription such that *narrow* means *more detail*. The temptation simply to count symbols and diacritics to assess narrowness has to be resisted in favor of evaluating the richness of the analysis that a transcription expresses. For example, [t̪] contains no more detail than [t], despite the addition of a diacritic.

Perceptual and Systematic Transcriptions

If the analysis expressed in a transcription has been carried out entirely by paying attention to the speaker's utterance, with no, or minimal, reference to knowledge of the phonological system of the language being spoken, then it is a perceptual transcription, also called an *impressionistic transcription*. Among phoneticians, there is some skepticism as to the worth of an impressionistic transcription because of the difficulty of ensuring validity and reliability.

If phonological knowledge does significantly inform a transcription, then the transcription is a systematic one. For example, knowing that /p t k/ in English are typically aspirated means that aspiration need not be transcribed because it is predictable by a phonological rule of English. How /t/ will be realized in a word like *water*, however, is not systematically predictable—it could be [t] or [ʔ]. Free variants can therefore present a problem for systematic transcription.

Transcription and Linguistic Structure

So far, transcription has been discussed largely at the phonetic level of the structure of spoken language. Transcription can, however, express phonological analyses in addition to general phonetic analyses. Phonological analysis groups sounds together as allophones of phonemes, and phonemes can be represented by IPA symbols placed in slant brackets, for example, /t/. The difference between /t/ and [t] is that the former subsumes a set of language-specific allophones, whereas the latter denotes the general phonetic categories *voiceless alveolar plosive*. The phoneme /t/ in English, although usually classified as *voiceless alveolar plosive*, includes the allophones [t tʰ t̪ ɾ s̬ ʔ] not all of which are voiceless, or plosives, or alveolar. Phoneme symbols therefore do not denote general phonetic categories; rather, they denote units of phonological structure. The symbol chosen to represent a phoneme is usually the allophone which occurs as a singleton in syllable onsets, stripped of any phonologically unnecessary diacritics, hence the choice of /t/ rather than /tʰ/ for English.

Transcription and Instrumental Analysis

Transcription is a convenient way to annotate or summarize the phonetic information in spectrograms, palatograms, and other instrumental displays. Figure 2 shows an example of

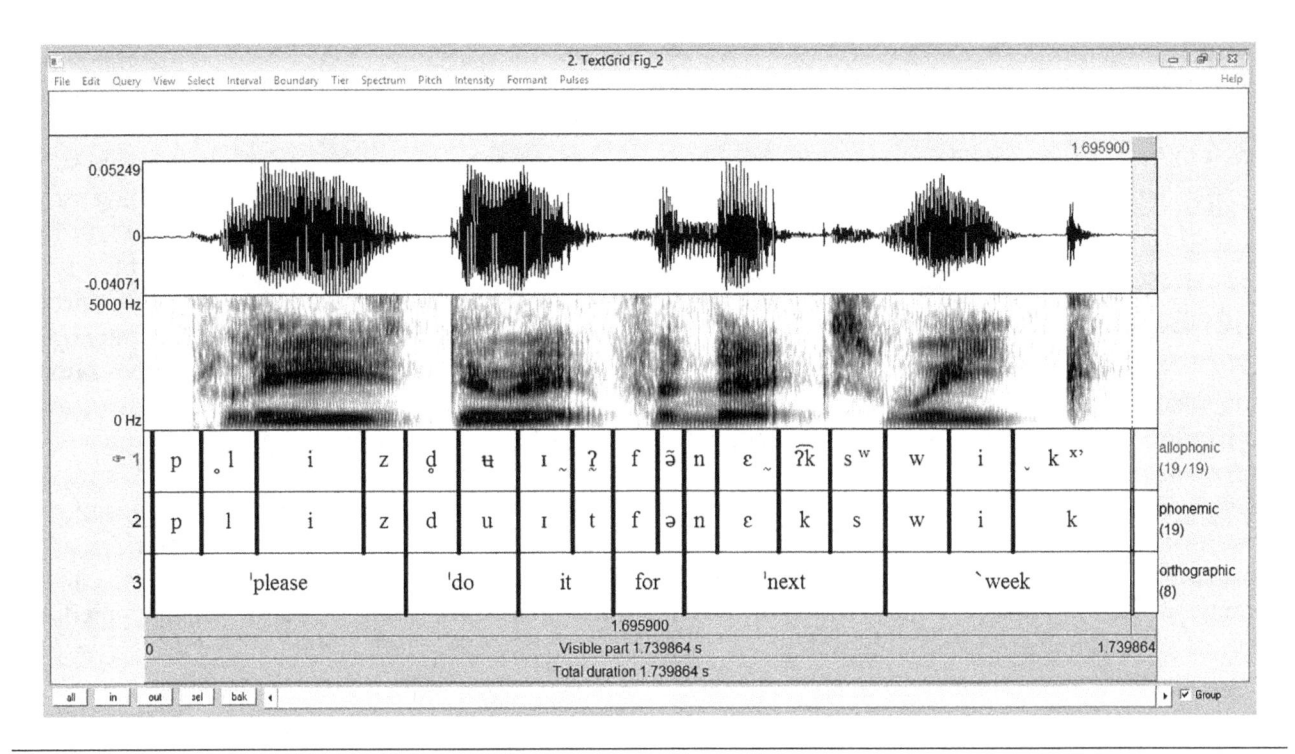

Figure 2 Allophonic, phonemic, and orthographic transcriptions aligned with spectrogram and waveform. Orthographic transcription also marks stress and nuclear tone

orthographic, phonemic, and allophonic transcriptions aligned with a spectrogram and waveform of the utterance, "Please do it for next week." The allophonic transcription enables the reader to identify the acoustic correlates of the allophones, while the phonemic transcription identifies the phonemic structure and the orthographic transcription identifies the lexical items and the sentence, as well as here carrying commonly used marks for rhythmic stress and nuclear tone to express a suprasegmental analysis. Something of the inadequacy of segmental transcription can be seen here. It is not self-evident to which phoneme the voicelessness between the release of /p/ and the voicing of /l/ should be assigned nor whether creaky voice is part of the realization of /ɪ/ and /ɛ/ or of the following consonant, or both, or whether the lip-rounding on the latter part of /s/ anticipates /w/ or is actually part of it.

When perceptual transcriptions are aligned with instrumental records, the instrumental evidence may sometimes be at odds with the perceptual analysis. Some phoneticians regard the instrumental analysis as more accurate because its results are replicable, while others take the view that the two analyses offer complementary perspectives and that trying to explain apparent contradictions can lead to new questions and understandings about the relationship between speech production, transmission, and perception.

Barry Heselwood

See also Articulatory Phonetics; Intonation; Phonetics; Phonology; Segmentation of Speech; Speech Sound Disorders

Further Readings

Abercrombie, D. (1964). *English phonetic texts*. London, UK: Faber and Faber.

Ball, M. J., Rahilly, J., & Tench, P. (1996). *The phonetic transcription of disordered speech*. San Diego, CA: Singular.

Cucchiarini, C. (1996). Assessing transcription agreement. *Clinical Linguistics and Phonetics, 10*, 131–156.

Esling, J. H. (2010). Phonetic notation. In W. J. Hardcastle, J. Laver, & F. E. Gibbon (Eds.), *The handbook of phonetic sciences* (pp. 678–702). Oxford, UK: Wiley-Blackwell.

Heselwood, B. (2013). *Phonetic transcription in theory and practice*. Edinburgh, UK: Edinburgh University Press.

International Phonetic Assocaiation (IPA). (1999). *The handbook of the international phonetic association.* Cambridge, UK: Cambridge University Press.

Müller, N. (Ed.). (2006). *Multilayered transcription.* San Diego, CA: Plural.

PHONETICS

Phonetics is the study of the oral mode of communication. Phoneticians are mostly concerned with spoken language (speech) but may also investigate extralinguistic sounds such as encouragement or annoyance sounds. Phonetics is distinguished from phonology. Whereas phonetics studies the form of speech (e.g., how different types of sounds are produced), phonology studies the function of speech in a particular language or language variety (e.g., the types of syllables and sound combinations allowed). Thus, one can describe both the phonetics of a particular language and the phonology of that language, and one can have general phonetics (i.e., the description of speech in general not restricted to any specific language) and general phonology (i.e., concerned with building theories of phonological representation). This entry provides an overview of the principal strands of phonetics: articulatory, acoustic, and auditory.

Phonetics is often divided into these three broad strands, related to the so-called speech chain. The speech chain envisages the transmission of a message from one person to another through the spoken medium. It commences with the conversion of an idea into linguistic form in the brain of the speaker and the assigning of the phonological makeup of the linguistic units and the subsequent compilation of a motor plan and neural signals to produce the organic changes required to realize the phonological patterns as speech. The result of these steps is the production of an acoustic signal that travels from the speaker to the listener(s). The speech chain then requires the converse with the listener of what was seen with the speaker. The incoming acoustic signal is converted via organic movements into a neural signal that travels to the brain of the speaker, where it is comprehended as a linguistic message. *Articulatory phonetics* is the study of the organic phase of speech production; that is, the movements of the various organs of speech to produce spoken communication. *Acoustic phonetics* is the study of the characteristics of the speech sound wave, and *auditory phonetics* is the study of the reception of the speech sound wave and its onward neural transmission. Aspects of the speech chain not covered here are the psycho- and neurolinguistic aspects and the neurophonetic aspects. While the former lies outside phonetics, the latter has become a focus of interest within the discipline of phonetics and will be returned to below.

Cutting across the three main branches of phonetics just specified is the distinction between *segmental* and *suprasegmental* phonetics. The former is concerned with the individual segments of speech (i.e., the consonants and vowels), and the latter with speech features extending over more than one segment (e.g., syllable stress, intonation). As phoneticians have demonstrated, segments do not have discrete articulatory or acoustic boundaries, so the idea of a single speech segment is a fiction; nevertheless, it is a convenient one.

Articulatory Phonetics

In articulatory phonetics, the production of speech is usually considered as a set of separate systems. *Initiation* is the setting in motion of an airstream in the vocal tract (a requirement for the production of speech). Bellows- or piston-like movements of vocal organs cause an increase or decrease in air pressure in their vicinity (dependent on their action), thus producing an inward (ingressive) or outward (egressive) flow of air. In speech, three initiators are found: the lungs, the glottis, and the tongue dorsum together with the velum. The resultant airstreams are termed *pulmonic*, *glottalic*, and *velaric*. In natural language, four airstreams may be encountered: pulmonic egressive, glottalic egressive, glottalic ingressive, and velaric ingressive (though pulmonic ingressive may be used extralinguistically or found in pathological speech). A pulmonic egressive airstream is used in all languages, and even in those that use one or more of the other types, it is used for most speech sounds, as the other types only provide enough air flow for a single sound at a time. Glottalic egressive sounds are termed *ejectives*, glottalic ingressive sounds are usually mixed with a certain amount of pulmonic egressive airflow, and these mixed sounds are termed *implosives*. Velaric ingressive sounds are termed *clicks*.

Phonation refers to the laryngeal activity imposed on the pulmonic aggressive airstream as it passes through the larynx. The vocal folds can be open (producing *voiceless* sounds) or close together and vibrating (producing *voiced* sounds). Natural languages all exploit these two phonation types. Other phonation types, using different degrees of vocal fold approximation and tenseness, are used linguistically in some languages (e.g., *creaky voice, murmur*). These types are also used extralinguistically, as are *whisper* and *falsetto*. Some phonation types are usually considered pathological, such as *breathy voice* and *ventricular phonation* (i.e., using the false vocal folds).

The resonance system refers to the supraglottal direction of egressive airflow. This can be *oral* only (if the velum is raised), *nasalized* (if the velum is lowered and the oral cavity is not blocked by an articulator), or *nasal* only (if the velum is lowered and the oral cavity is blocked by an articulator). Individual sounds can be classed as oral, nasalized, or nasal, and a speaker's voice quality can also be described in terms of degree of oral or nasal resonance.

Articulation is the production of individual speech sounds by the articulators. For consonants, it is described in terms of manner of articulation and place of articulation. The major manners of articulation are *oral stops* and *nasal stops* (involving a complete closure to oral airflow somewhere in the mouth), *fricatives* (involving a narrow gap left between articulators resulting in turbulent airflow), and *approximants* (involving a wider gap resulting in laminar airflow, at least for voiced approximants). Other types include *affricates* (i.e., an oral stop followed by fricative release), *trills* (i.e., rapid striking of one articulator against another), and *taps* (i.e., a single strike of one articulator against another). Fricatives, affricates, and approximants can have *central* or *lateral* airflow (where the airflow is directed down the side of the tongue). The term *obstruent* is often applied to oral stops, fricatives, affricates, trills, and taps, while *sonorant* is used for nasal stops, approximants, and vowels.

The major places of articulation are *bilabial* (upper and lower lip), *labiodental* (lower lip and upper teeth), *dental* (tongue tip/blade to inside of upper teeth), *alveolar* (tongue tip/blade to alveolar ridge), *palatal* (tongue front to hard palate), *velar* (tongue back to soft palate), *uvular* (tongue back to uvula), *pharyngeal* (tongue back/root to pharynx), and *glottal* (the two vocal folds articulating with each other). Other places such as *postalveolar*, *alveolo-palatal*, and *epiglottal* and simultaneous double articulations such as labial–velar and labial–palatal may also be used in some languages. Finally, it should be noted that a *retroflex* tongue shape is used in some languages whereby the under surface of the tongue blade articulates against the postaleolar or prepalatal area.

Consonants may have secondary articulations as well as their primary ones, and many of these will affect the sound quality of the consonant. Common are *labialization* (secondary approximation of the two lips), *palatalization* (secondary raising of the front of the tongue), *velarization* (secondary raising of the back of the tongue), and *pharyngealization* (secondary retraction of the tongue root).

Vowel articulations are usually described in terms of tongue height, tongue anteriority, lip shape, and state (though the cardinal vowel system is an alternative description system based on perceptual constants). Vowels can thus be described as high, mid-high, mid-low, or low (also close, half-close, half-open, and open); front, mid, or back; and rounded, neutral, or unrounded (also spread). In terms of state, vowels can be *monophthongs* (where the tongue remains static throughout most of its duration), *diphthongs/triphthongs* (where the tongue moves from its start position to a different end position), or *rhotic* (where the tongue adopts a shape to produce a rhotic sound quality simultaneous to the vowel, usually through tongue tip raising). Resonance also plays a part in vowel description, as fully nasalized vowels are found in many languages, and partially nasalized vowels occur as vowel variants before nasal consonants.

Suprasegmental aspects of speech are also a concern of articulatory phonetics. *Tone* (word based) and *intonation* (phrase based) are derived from pitch movements, which in turn are controlled by the speed of vibration and the tension of the vocal folds: The faster the vocal folds vibrate, the higher the perceived pitch. *Stress* is syllable based and may be a combination of loudness, duration, and pitch movement. Duration, termed *length* when used linguistically, is also syllable based though usually expressed in terms of length of consonants or vowels.

Loudness is controlled through the amount of air in the vocal tract and the pressure with which it is moved; while considered a suprasegemental feature, it has only an extralinguistic function. This is true also of *tempo*, the speed of speech. However, both loudness and tempo may be affected in disordered speech. A final suprasegmental feature is *voice quality*. Voice quality is partially derived from phonatory activities, but supraglottal settings also contribute to the long-term perceived voice quality of a speaker. These include resonance settings but also tendencies such as consistent use of palatalization and velarization. Overuse of certain settings may indicate a voice disorder.

Acoustic Phonetics

The concerns of acoustic phonetics are the nature of the sound wave produced through speech articulation. Acoustic analysis via sound spectrography allows the phonetician to access information on acoustic characteristics such as *duration, frequency, amplitude, intensity,* and *resonance* and how they relate to specific segmental and suprasegmental aspects of speech.

Duration in acoustic analysis is measured in milliseconds, and differences of a few tens of milliseconds can be detected by listeners and thus play a contrastive role. An example from English is the difference between the so-called voiced and voiceless oral stops (also termed *plosives*). The air pressure that builds up behind the total obstruction with oral stops is released as *plosion* when the articulators move apart. Voiced plosives (also termed *lenis* plosives) are followed by an almost immediate onset of vocal fold vibration for the next voiced sound (indeed the vocal folds may have been continually vibrating through the closed stage of the stop if in intervocalic position). On the other hand, voiceless (or *fortis*) plosives (especially in stressed word-initial position) are followed by a brief period of voiceless turbulent airflow (termed *aspiration*) before the voicing commences for the next sound. This voice onset time lasts between 50 and 80 ms for English fortis plosives and is one of the main cues listeners use to distinguish fortis sounds from the lenis. Voice onset time values differ among languages, however, and many languages do not have aspiration following voiceless oral stops.

Duration is also an important characteristic of vowels in English. English has some vowels that are basically short in duration and some that are long. For example, the vowel in *seed* is longer than that in *Sid* (e.g., one measurement gives the former as 290 ms and the latter as 174 ms). However, with both the long and short vowels, vowel duration is clipped if the following consonant is voiced: *seat* being 168 ms and *sit* 143 ms.

Frequency is measured in Hz, that is, cycles per second. Frequency measures derive from the repetition patterns found in periodic sound waves (i.e., sound waves that repeat a pattern). Aperiodic sound waves are not amenable to frequency analysis. Aperiodic sound waves are found in speech in the turbulent airflow associated with fricatives, affricates, and plosive aspiration; (complex) periodic waves are found in voiced sonorants. Sounds such as voiced fricatives will have periodic waves in the voicing component and aperiodic in the frication component. An important measure of frequency in speech is the fundamental frequency (F_0) of the speaker's voice. A pitch analysis, for example, involves tracking the changes in frequency of a speaker's voice from time to time within a phrase. So, a question such as "Are you leaving today," spoken with a rising pitch at the end, will see a typical male speaker's F_0 change from a beginning point of around 2000 Hz to an end point of about 4800 Hz (ignoring various intermediate changes).

Intensity is a measure derived from a combination of the frequency of a sound wave and its amplitude (i.e., the extent of the wave's displacement). It is related proportionately to these components: to the square of the frequency and the square of the amplitude. In speech, intensity is normally considered via its perceptual equivalent of loudness, and loudness is measured using the logarithmic dB scale. Intensity is one difference between stressed and unstressed syllables. For example, in *import*, when the stress is on the first syllable, the intensity measures for one speaker were 88 dB versus 83 dB for first and second syllables respectively; where *import* was stressed on the second syllable, the measures were 76 dB versus 80 dB for the first and second syllables.

Resonance is the term given in acoustics to instances where one, driven, system is set in motion through the forced vibrations of another, driving, system. The natural frequency of the driven system (i.e., the frequency it would vibrate at if it were subject to free rather than forced vibration) will be boosted at the expense of other frequencies in the driving system. In other words, resonance acts like a filter, where certain frequencies are boosted and others absorbed. In speech, the vocal fold vibrations can be considered the basic system that drives other resonators in the pharynx and oral and nasal cavities. Because these cavities are adjustable (or in the case of the nasal cavity, can be excluded), this means speakers alter the filtering characteristics from moment to moment as they speak. Sound spectrography allows an examination of the sound spectra of speech: that is, a measure of what frequencies are found in any particular sound and what the relative intensity of these frequencies is.

Sound spectra analysis reveals that bands of frequency at high intensity levels can be identified for periodic sounds, and these bands are termed *formants*. The first three formants are normally listed in acoustic analysis of speech and can be used to classify vowels, for example. In English, the vowel in *seat* for a typical male speaker would have $F1$ 270 Hz, $F2$ 2290 Hz, and $F3$ 3010 Hz; the vowel in *spa* would have $F1$ 730 Hz, $F2$ 1090 Hz, and $F3$ 2440 Hz. At the boundaries between sounds, there are formant transitions, and listeners may use these transitions as important cues to the place of articulation of consonants.

Auditory Phonetics

The organic phase of auditory phonetics covers the conversion of the incoming sound waves to neural impulses via the tympanum (i.e., eardrum), which transmits vibrations into the middle ear; these vibrations are then forwarded via the auditory ossicles to the inner ear. The cochlea in the inner ear converts the incoming vibrations into movements of the hair cells in the organ of Corti, and nerve fibers from the auditory nerve located near the hair cells take these movements as electrochemical impulses to the auditory center of the brain.

Of greater interest to phoneticians perhaps is the study of speech perception. Psychoacoustic experimentation has been used extensively to investigate speech perception. Using either synthetic speech or edited real speech, researchers have investigated a range of speech features. Various acoustic cues have been manipulated (such as duration, formant frequencies, and noise components) to ascertain which cues are used by listeners to distinguish and categorize speech sounds. One result of this research is the notion of categorical perception, that is, that listeners tend to place speech sounds into discrete categories and if a sound is manipulated such that over a series of steps it becomes more like another sound, listeners will still assign each step to one or another category, switching over at a particular point in the progression.

Auditory phonetics has also described perceptual units of speech. These include the syllable, the mora, and the phoneme. Syllable shapes (i.e., the arrangement of consonants and vowels) have also been the focus of research, and sonority theory attempts to account for commonly occurring syllable shapes by positing that syllable nuclei will be filled by highly sonorous sounds and syllable peripheries by less sonorous ones (where sonority refers to relative loudness of speech segments). It should be noted that there are problems with this analysis, and not all phoneticians accept sonority theory.

Finally, auditory phonetics makes use of a series of perceptually based scales to describe pitch and loudness. The mel scale and the bark scale measure pitch perceptually, expressing how much higher or lower one frequency is perceived to be compared to another. In loudness measurements, the phon scale measures loudness independently from differences of frequency, whereas the sone scale allows a sound to be measured in relation to another, so a sound of two sones is perceived as twice as loud as a sound of one sone. Working with these scales also allows auditory phoneticians to ascertain just noticeable differences in pitch and loudness. So, for example, a tone of 1000 Hz at 5 dB must be doubled to 10 dB before a difference is noted.

Other Aspects

Instrumental phonetics can apply to all three main areas. Speech production can be investigated via a range of instrumentation including aerometry (initiation), glottography/laryngography (phonation), nasometry (resonance), electropalatography, and ultrasound (articulation). Other instrumental techniques require access to more extensive imaging methods and include electromagnetic articulography, magnetic resonance imaging, and radiography. Speech acoustics is investigated via speech spectrography, with freely available software on personal computers. Auditory phonetics makes use of psychoacoustic experimentation referred to previously and techniques such as dichotic listening (to test hemispheric dominance) and delayed auditory feedback (to investigate auditory feedback). Both these last techniques also have clinical applications.

Neurophonetics is a comparatively recent area of the discipline, and it aims to elucidate the neural mechanisms that underlie speech. Disordered speech from speakers with acquired speech disorders has informed work in this area along with developments in functional imaging of the brain.

Martin J. Ball

See also Acoustic Phonetics; Articulatory Phonetics; Auditory Phonetics; Electropalatography (EPG); Phonetic Transcription; Psychoacoustics; Sound Spectrography; Speech Perception, Theories of; Ultrasonography; Vowels

Further Readings

Hardcastle, W., Laver, J., & Gibbon, F. (Eds.) (2010). *The handbook of phonetics sciences*. (2nd ed.). Chichester, UK: John Wiley.

Johnson, K. (2011). *Acoustic and auditory phonetics* (3rd ed.). Chichester, UK: John Wiley.

Lass, N. (1996). *Principles of experimental phonetics*. St. Louis, MO: Mosby.

Laver, J. (1994). *Principles of phonetics*. Cambridge, UK: Cambridge University Press.

Pisoni, D., & Remez, R. (Eds.) (2007). *The handbook of speech perception*. Chichester, UK: John Wiley.

Stevens, K. (1998). *Acoustic phonetics*. Cambridge: MIT Press.

Phonological and Phonemic Awareness

Phonological awareness (PA) is the ability to attend, identify, and manipulate a variety of sounds within the speech stream. It implies conscious knowledge, at any age, of the sound structure of spoken words, from syllables to phonemes. *Phonemic awareness* (or *phoneme awareness*) is one aspect of PA, related to consciousness of the smallest speech units: the consonant and vowel *phonemes*, displayed here in slashes (//). Other aspects of PA are the skills of detecting rhymes and alliteration; recognizing that words within the speech stream can be broken down into smaller chunks such as syllables and phonemes; using metalanguage to talk about, reflect upon, and manipulate phonemes; and understanding, explicitly, the relationship between spoken and written language.

As a subtype of PA, phonemic awareness relates to an individual's cognizance of the phonemes in a given word. The skills it covers include identification of word onsets (e.g., knowing *batty* begins with /b/); phoneme isolation and segmentation (knowing that *batty* can be broken down into the sequence of phonemes identified as /b/, /æ/, /t/, and /i/); and phoneme manipulation (e.g., knowing /b/ /æ/ /t/ /i/ is *batty* and /t/ /æ/ /b/ /i/ is *tabby*; that adding /ɹ/ after /b/ in batty results in *bratty* and that removing /t/ from *tabby* makes *abbey*).

This entry provides an overview of the development of PA/phonemic awareness and its relationship to literacy and speech as well as the assessment and treatment of low PA in at-risk children. Children's ages are expressed in years; months; for example, 5; 0 indicates 5 years; 0 months and 3; 11 indicates 3 years; 11 months.

Development of PA

PA acquisition is a gradual, incremental process, forming the bedrock of learning to read. Many 4-year-olds have syllable awareness (e.g., they can be successfully instructed to tap once if they hear *bat* and twice for *batty* or tell you *bat* has one beat, and *batty* two), and the majority achieve rhyme awareness by age 6. With appropriate instruction, prereaders with strong PA advance quite easily to becoming competent readers or *decoders*, while children who have difficulty with PA are expected to face challenges in becoming so.

Development of Phonemic Awareness

Most children have limited phoneme awareness before they start to read, with around half showing some sensitivity to single onset consonants by 5 years. Micah, 5; 0, knows that his name, and several other words, start with /m/, but, as is typical, his proficiency varies according to the nature of the phonemic awareness task presented. Few 5-year-olds can deconstruct consonant clusters (e.g., tell you that *pram* starts with /p/ then /ɹ/), or delete (*pram-ram*, *pram-Pam*), add (*ram-ramp*), or move (*Pam-map*) consonants in words.

Related Terms

Three related terms, important in understanding the role of PA in early literacy, are *phonological representations* (PRs), *phonics*, and the *alphabetic principle*.

PRs

Knowledge of the phonological form of words an individual knows is *stored* mentally as PRs also called *underlying representations* and *phonemic representations*. Jan, a first grade teacher, can observe an object (e.g., a hook) and, even without saying its name aloud or picturing its spelling, will know what sound its name begins with (in this example, /h/). That information has come from Jan's PR of the word, and she can use metalanguage to explain what she knows.

Development of PRs

The status of young children's PRs is difficult to determine because their metalinguistic skills (i.e., their ability to use language to talk about language) are still taking shape, so that they cannot explain to adults what they know about words. Nonetheless, it has been proposed that while very young children are acquiring their first words, their PRs are holistic, fuzzy, underspecified units, with features omitted. Claudia, 1; 4, with typical language development, pronounces *finished* as [pɪntʃt] and *pinched* as [pɪntʃt], and it is probable that her PR for both words is /pɪntʃt/. As Claudia's expressive vocabulary expands, she will need her words to be distinctive in order to convey meaning unambiguously (*finished* and *pinched* must not be homonyms: *Doggie finished my dinner* and *Doggie pinched my dinner* must sound different from each other). Most likely her PRs will become more detailed; her representation for *pinched* will remain the same, and her PR for *finished* will resemble the adult form, /fɪnɪʃt/, reflecting Claudia's increasingly accurate production. A surge in specification will likely happen, when she has a typical vocabulary spurt (word spurt) at 18 months, followed by a gradual segmentation of her PRs into smaller and smaller units.

In typically developing children, this process of refinement continues through the first 2 or 3 years of formal schooling. School itself promotes headway, as teachers—particularly if they use a *phonics*-based approach—nurture and encourage a child's increasing awareness of letter-sound correspondences, or the alphabetic principle.

The word productions of school-age children do not directly reflect the child's PR for that word. When asked to make judgments of their own word mispronunciations, children with typical language development accurately recognize most of their own errors, and even children with developmental language disorder (also called *specific language impairment*) spot around half of their own production errors.

Phonics and the Alphabetic Principle

Phonics is a method of teaching children to read and spell that has strong scientific support. It is often contrasted with the *whole language* approach, which has many supporters in the context of a scant evidence base. The various phonics approaches (i.e., *phonics*, the *analytic phonics* of the 1960s, *synthetic phonics*, *linguistic phonics*, and *embedded phonics*), and the commercially available programs used to implement them, are overlapping reading and spelling instruction methodologies based on teaching children the relationship between the letters of written language and the sounds (phonemes) of spoken language. Letters are organized into *graphemes* that represent phonemes. A grapheme may consist of several letters (e.g., *igh* for /aɪ/, *th* for /θ/ and /ð/, *ng* for /ŋ/, and *sh* for /ʃ/). Phonics instruction focuses on one-to-one correspondences between graphemes and sounds or the alphabetic principle: the understanding that words are made up of letters and letters represent sounds. Phonics knowledge involves understanding that some words (e.g., *mitt*, *mat*) can be decoded with simple sounding-out strategies; some reflect more complex position-sensitive grapheme patterns (e.g., the patterns underlying the grapheme choices for the instances of /k/ in *kick* and *cook* and /s/ in *circus* and *sissy*); some words obey common spelling rules, such as the "magic e" in *mate* and *mite*, and many grapheme choices reflect crosslinguistic influences, such as *kh* in *khaki* from Hindustani (Urdu).

If they are well grounded in phonics, typical students learn to decode and become fluent readers. They practice by reading aloud to a parent, teacher, or other helper, beginning with simple books or *readers* from a reading scheme such as *Jolly Phonics*, *Keyword*, *Letterland*, the *Oxford Readers*, and the *Usborne Reading Programme*, graduating to longer, more complex texts. Once students attain fluency, usually by the end of their third year of schooling, with decoding that is rapid, accurate, and automatic, they can focus almost entirely on meaning (i.e., comprehension) and enjoyment of what they read, and further phonics instruction is unnecessary. PA, interwoven with orthographic (i.e., spelling) awareness and vocabulary growth, continues its important role in the fourth year of schooling and beyond.

Low-Progress Readers and Children With Speech Sound Disorders (SSDs)

PA and PRs have an intimate, reciprocal, and probably obvious relationship with early literacy development, and difficulties with them are often implicated in low-progress readers. Less obviously, PRs are significant in *word learning* and *speech production*. We have to extricate whole words from the speech stream, so we need PRs that are sufficiently flexible to allow their recognition in different forms (e.g., across varieties of English), while being established and precise enough to drive consistent, intelligible output. Limitations in forming and accessing PRs may underpin the difficulties many children with SSDs exhibit in both PA and early literacy. It must be noted, however, that although phoneme level PA (i.e., phonemic awareness) is important in the early phase of literacy acquisition, explicit PA is not a prerequisite for typical speech development. Furthermore, little is known about the levels of PA needed to elicit change in children with SSD.

Children with SSD at risk of literacy difficulties include those with percentages of consonants correct below 50% when formal reading instruction starts, those who are unintelligible at 5; 6, those who also have semantic and syntactic difficulties, and those who have persistent, mild SSD beyond 6; 9.

Assessing PA and PRs

Examiners choose standardized PA assessments carefully, ensuring they reflect reading instruction practices, exposure to literacy, and school-starting age in the child's milieu, as these vary between and within countries and cultures, leading to different rates of PA development from 4 to 6 years of age.

Assessing PA in At-Risk and Low-Progress Readers

Since PA is a dependable indicator of later reading prowess, efficient and reliable PA assessment tools are central to identifying children at risk of literacy difficulties; for gauging the response to intervention of children having help with reading; and, as a diagnostic tool, to tease out the level or levels of difficulty a child has. PA assessment is most useful when it coincides with three crossroads in PA development. First, when children start school and their basic PA forms the foundation of understanding the alphabetic code. Second, in the second or third year of school when their PA is normally quite refined and their PRs clearly specified. Third, PA assessment is pertinent in the fourth year of school, when it is anticipated that PA and orthographic awareness will be integrated.

To be comprehensive for school starters, including at-risk children, assessment taps understanding of the word *sound*, rhyming, syllabification, identification of onset phonemes, and alphabet knowledge. For children who are faltering with reading in the second or third year, PA assessment covers the crucial skills of blending and segmenting sounds in words and consonant clusters, and isolating rimes from onsets, using onset deletion tasks (e.g., "Say *meeting* without the /m/"). PA assessment for low-progress readers in the fourth year of school concentrates on phoneme manipulation, orthographic awareness, and nonword reading.

Assessing PA and PRs in Children At Risk of and With SSDs

Children at risk for SSD include those who have: failure to babble or late onset of canonical babbling, episodic otitis media with effusion between 12 and 18 months, atypical phonological patterns, small phonetic inventories, prevalent final consonant deletion beyond 34–39 months, and vowel production errors that persist beyond 35 months.

It is necessary to assess both PA and PRs in children with SSD because some children with SSD have age-appropriate PA abilities and PRs. Children with SSD and good PA tend to respond better to speech intervention, and their early literacy performance matches that of age peers who do not have SSD. Assessment tasks should not require spoken responses because speech errors may prevent appropriate interpretation of the child's output. Anne Hesketh, a UK expert in the field, says that as there is wide variation in PA abilities in typical development it can be hard to know really whether there is a problem. She notes that because speech intervention of whatever kind inherently involves PA and can trigger further PA development, appropriately qualified professionals can be more confident in diagnosing a significant PA problem based on the assessment of a 5-year-old child at the end of therapy than in a 4-year-old child prior to intervention. PRs in older children can be assessed with explicit, *silent* PA tasks, such as silent deletion of phonemes, and from age 3; 9, mispronunciation detection, or judgment of correctness, tasks can be used.

PA and PR Intervention

Robust evidence is available to support working on PA in low-progress readers to improve their PA, reading, and spelling. The evidence is less clear-cut for low-progress readers with speech–language impairment (SSD and/or DLD). Untreated, or unsuccessfully treated, PA deficits in children with speech–language impairment may persist into adolescence. Simply improving intelligibility will not necessarily result in improvements in phonemic awareness, reading, or spelling. Rather, children with speech–language impairment need specific instruction in phoneme awareness.

For children with SSD, there are no absolute guidelines for when, how, and whether to target PA, so treatment decisions rest on clinical judgment and individual, ongoing assessment. There is evidence that working on PA changes PA itself, but the findings on whether improved PA leads to speech improvement are mixed. In a New Zealand study by Gail T. Gillon and colleagues, children aged 5; 6 to 7; 4 with speech and language impairment showed improvement in speech and early reading when they received an integrated PA intervention aimed at simultaneous facilitation of speech production, PA, and letter-sound knowledge (phonics). In an associated study, preschoolers, aged 3; 0 to 3; 11 at the outset, showed similar gains. There have been few investigations into intervention that directly targets children's PRs, and this is an area of research need. There is logic, however, in integrating PR-type activities as well as PA, relevant to a child's current speech targets, into his or her therapy sessions.

Caroline Bowen

See also Metalinguistics; Phoneme; Reading and Reading Disorders; Speech Sound Disorders; Vocabulary

Further Readings

Gillon, G. T. (2012). *Phonological awareness: From research to practice* (3rd ed.). New York, NY: Guilford Press.

Hesketh, A. (2015). Phoneme awareness intervention for children with speech disorder: Who, when and how? In C. Bowen (Ed.), *Children's speech sound disorders* (2nd ed., pp. 210–214). Oxford, UK: Wiley-Blackwell.

Neilson, R. (2009). Assessment of phonological awareness in low-progress readers. *Australian Journal of Learning Difficulties, 14*(1), 53–66.

Websites

Five from Five: Retrieved from http://www.fivefromfive.org.au/

Phonological awareness and other resources provided by Gail T. Gillon. Retrieved from http://www.education.canterbury.ac.nz/people/gillon/resources.shtml

Phonological Development

Phonological development entails the acquisition of knowledge about the sound system of the ambient language for the purpose of comprehending that language and producing it intelligibly. The process of phonological development is long and complex because the sound system of any language is organized in a hierarchical fashion across many interacting tiers so that the child must acquire many types of knowledge. If a child's acquisition of even a simple word such as *doggies* (in English) is considered, it is clear that several tiers of phonological structure are invoked: There are two syllables produced with a strong–weak stress pattern; the syllables are composed of segments, specifically consonants (C) and vowels (V), slotted into onset (/d/, /g/), nucleus (/ɑ/, /i/), and coda (/g/, /z/) positions within the syllables; and each of these C and V segments are characterized by bundles of distinctive features that differentiate, for example, the obstruents (/d/, /g/, /s/) from sonorants (/ɑ/, /i/), stops (/g/, /d/) from the fricative (/s/), voiced (/d/, /g/) from voiceless (/s/), and coronal (/d/, /s/) from dorsal (/g/) consonants. Furthermore, knowledge of these tiers of the phonological hierarchy must be acquired at multiple levels of phonological representation. Knowledge of acoustic-phonetic features permits perception of speech and supports production learning by providing an acoustic target for production practice. Articulatory-phonetic knowledge includes the specific articulatory gestures associated with individual speech sounds as well as the ability to produce varying sequences of speech sounds smoothly. Phonological knowledge involves learning to manipulate phonological units at multiple tiers of the phonological hierarchy so as to contrast meaning, using rules that are specific to the ambient language. For example, in English, /d/ and /g/ are separate phonemes that can occur in the same syllable positions to contrast meaning across word pairs such as /dɪg/ and /dɪd/ or /dɔg/ and /gɔd/. This kind of phonemic knowledge is required to ensure that [d] and [g] are produced distinctly and in the correct order to produce the word *doggies*.

Incomplete phonological knowledge, leading to substitutions or omissions at any of the tiers of the phonological hierarchy, would change the intended meaning of an utterance. Therefore, even at a young age, a child must master a fair degree of precision in the acoustic-phonetic, articulatory-phonetic, and phonological domains to produce intelligible speech. To produce lengthy complex utterances at the rate and precision typical of an adult speaker requires so much practice that phonological development is not complete until the late teenage years. Developmentally, phonetic knowledge emerges before phonemic knowledge. Therefore, a 6-month-old infant may be capable of producing utterances that contain the [h], [m], [æ], and [t] sounds without knowing the meaning of a single word. An adult, aware that the words *hat* and *mat* have different meanings, perceives the acoustic differences between the phones [h] and [m] and comprehends the functional contrast between the phonemes /h/-/m/. Phonological knowledge as defined here is concerned with the comprehension and production of meaningful utterances and requires the integration of acoustic-phonetic, articulatory-phonetic, and phonological knowledge at multiple tiers of the phonological hierarchy. For this reason, the earliest stages of speech perception and speech production development are referred to as *prelinguistic*, even though much language-specific perceptual knowledge emerges and the onset of babbling occurs during the first year of life. This entry explores the stages of phonological development, from early word learning to increased segmental accuracy and, eventually, to mastery of speech accuracy. This account of phonological development begins during the second year of life when the infant begins to understand and produce meaningful words.

Early Word Learning: Perception and Comprehension

An important aspect of word learning is the ability to recognize an acoustic-phonetic form, even when produced variably (as when produced by different talkers) or in variable contexts (as in different sentences, "Look! Doggie!" or "See the doggie over there"). The word segmentation and recognition abilities involved are present as early as 8 months of age but are not considered to be fully linguistic until the infant shows evidence of clearly associating the acoustic-phonetic form with its referent, and more particularly with an abstract representation of the referent as evidenced by comprehending that the word *doggie* applies to beagles and poodles and labradors and the stuffed version of a pug on one's bed.

Several laboratory tasks have been devised to assess infant acquisition of referential word knowledge. These studies reveal that infants learn to associate novel word forms with new referents between approximately 12 and 14 months of age, but only when the word forms are dissimilar from each other (i.e., dissimilar word shapes, [bos]–[os], or similar shapes with distinct phonetic content, [lɪf]–[nim]). Later in the second year, between 17 and 20 months of age, infants are able to associate similar sounding word forms with new referents (i.e., [bɪ]–[dɪ]), within the same laboratory experiment. Throughout this period, it is clear that the infant is capable of processing and remembering fine phonetic details since minimal pairs can be discriminated at birth; furthermore, discrimination ability is retained into the second year and beyond for language-specific contrasts as long as the task is purely perceptual in nature. Laboratory studies have also shown that toddlers can differentiate correctly pronounced versions of familiar words (i.e., *apple*) from slightly mispronounced versions of the same words (i.e., *opple*). However, perceived variations in acoustic-phonetic details at prosodic, segmental, and suprasegmental levels continue to interfere with infant word learning late into the second year, while the infant sorts out which details have functional significance. Considerable experience with speech input is required before the toddler's phonological representations for words stabilize. An important feature of the toddler's phonological representations in the second year is that they are word based—in other words, unanalyzed wholes rather than strings of discrete segments. Laboratory studies of infant speech perception performance and modeling studies of phonological development have examined the relationship between lexical and phonological learning. These studies suggest that word learning occurs in parallel with the acquisition of phonological units (specifically phonemic category learning) but with interactions between learning in these domains.

Early Word Learning: Production

At approximately 12 months of age, most infants produce their first word and then demonstrate a slow, gradual increase in productive output over the next 6 months, after which time the rate of word acquisition increases markedly. Crosslinguistically, early words are extremely variable in form and composed of a restricted range of consonant and vowel segments. Segmental preferences for [p,b,t,d,m,n,i,a,o] in early words suggest continuity with babble from the prelinguistic stage, presumably as a function of articulatory constraints. Some of these characteristics are apparent in Table 1, showing a speech sample recorded from an 18-month-old English-learning toddler.

During the early word learning period, toddlers use several strategies to produce speech that can be understood by communication partners, despite the challenges of within-word variability and a restricted phonetic repertoire. One strategy is to aim for lexical contrast as can be seen in some of the productions shown in Table 1: Most words are produced variably with bare approximation to the adult target; however, there is less overlap in phonetic form between words than one might expect. Another common strategy is selection of words from the input language that can be produced according to a repertoire of preferred templates, with each template conforming to a global word shape with gross constraints on segment production within the template. An associated strategy is to avoid words that are not consistent with preferred templates. For example, Table 1 shows that the child attempted almost exclusively single syllable words (e.g., *bee*, *pig*) and avoided more complex words that slightly older children attempted (e.g., *chicken*, *tractor*) when playing with the same set of toys. Alternatively, words may be adapted to a preferred template even if the result bears little resemblance to the input form, a strategy that can be observed in Table 1, with respect to the modification of CVg input forms to fit a gV template (e.g., *pig* pronounced as [go]).

Table 1 Word Forms Produced by 18-Month-Old English-Learning Child

Target	Child Form	Target	Child Form
eye	[aj]	duck	[kʌ]² [bæp] [dʌ]
oink	[oj]²	dog	[gɑ]² [aigə]
under	[hʌjə]	one	[ʌ] [ʌm]
Ernie	[gɚni]	want	[wɑ] [wæn] [wɪn]
head	[hɛ]	what	[wʌ]
yeah	[ʌ] [jæ] [jɛ]	moo	[muː] [hu]
yellow	[ja.ʊ]	woof	[wʌ]³ [wʊ]³ [wʊf]³ [wʊfə]
right	[dai]² [ai] [tʰai] [tʰɛi]	ball	[bɑ]⁸ [bɑw]³ [bɑːəl] [bɑl] [bo]
no	[no]² [dõ] [do]	bee	[ji]
two	[ju]	book	[bʌ]
there	[dɛ]⁸ [tʰɛ]² [wɛ] [ɛ] [ɛjo]	pig	[go]
this	[dɪʃ]	frog	[kʰɑ]

Note: Superscripts indicate the number of tokens where more than one occurrence of a given token occurred. These data were recorded from Participant ME-306 in the context of the study reported in MacLeod, A. N., Laukys, K., & Rvachew, S. (2011). Impact of bilingual language learning on whole-word complexity and segmental accuracy among preschoolers. *International Journal of Speech-Language Pathology, 13*(6), 490–499.

As a consequence of production practice, maturation of speech motor control, and increased vocabulary size, rapid change occurs in the nature of the toddler's productive phonology toward the end of the second year. The emergence of new phones and word shapes permits a reduction in homonymy (i.e., words with different meanings having the same phonetic form). The earliest consonant inventory is likely to contain an approximant, a stop, and a nasal representing at least one place of articulation. Expansion will establish one or two additional places of articulation within these manner classes when permitted within the ambient language (e.g., labial as in [m, b, p], and/or coronal as in [n, d, t] and/or dorsal as in [g, k]). Expansion of the consonant inventory to include new manner classes also occurs with the addition of at least one liquid (e.g., [ɹ] as in *row*) or fricative (e.g., [s] as in *sun*) or affricate (e.g., [ts] as in *catsup*). There are crosslinguistic differences in the consonants that are likely to be added to the inventory at this stage: Affricates are common early consonants in Cantonese, whereas /ɹ/ can emerge early in English, but the lateral /l/ emerges early in Spanish, Arabic, and Icelandic (relative to English, Swedish, and Dutch), for example. When the ambient language has a small consonant inventory, early emergence of a consonant is predicted by high input frequency; however, when the ambient language has a large consonant inventory, early emergence of a consonant is predicted by high functional load (i.e., the consonant is part of many contrastive word pairs in the language). Syllable shapes also become elaborated during this time to include structures such as coda consonants (e.g., syllable final consonants as in *cup* or *naptime*) and consonant sequences (e.g., clusters such as *stop* or *pants*), in accordance with the possibilities presented by the input language. In fact, the development of word shape and prosody is strongly impacted by the input language from an early age, perhaps even prelinguistically, so that most words produced by Finnish toddlers contain two or more syllables whereas English-learning toddlers tend not to produce words longer than two syllables even when extraordinary efforts are made to elicit them.

Increasing Segment Accuracy During the Preschool Period

The third year of life is marked by the emergence of phoneme contrasts along with more stable and segmentalized underlying representations for words, supporting increased consistency and accuracy of speech overall. However, some regressions in production accuracy may also occur. Returning to Table 1, the child might stabilize the pattern of substituting a glide for the liquid /l/ and generalize this pattern to the liquid /ɹ/, resulting in consistent productions such as "ball"→[bɑw], "there"→[dɛw], and "right"→[waɪt]. The formerly correct "ball"→[bɑl] would be referred to as a progressive idiom, which disappears in conformity with a phonological pattern that emerges as the child transitions from word-based to phoneme-based underlying representations.

Phonological patterns, such as replacing all the liquids with a glide, are usually called *natural phonological processes*—natural because they are expected to be common in child speech crosslinguistically and because they may also occur in adult speech, especially when speaking casually or quickly. Segmental processes involve substitution of one phoneme for another, whereas syllable structure processes usually involve deletion of segments so that the word shape is altered. Examples of some commonly occurring phonological processes, as observed in English and French child samples, are shown in Table 2. The examples are shown one word at a time, but a process cannot be identified as such unless the error pattern is consistently applied across a natural class of phonemes. Therefore, the replacement of liquids with glides would not be identified as the process "gliding of liquids" unless it occurred with a considerable degree of consistency, within and across words, and across /l/ and /ɹ/ targets. Furthermore, distortions of speech sounds do not result in a phonological process when there is no collapse of a phonological contrast.

Despite clear regularity in children's error patterns between 2 and 5 years of age, there is more inconsistency than would be expected, especially across syllable positions because many phonological error patterns are context dependent. For example, velar fronting is much more likely in the coda than the onset of a syllable. Furthermore, there are language-specific patterns so that a process that may be expected in one language is atypical when it appears in the speech of children learning another

Table 2 Examples of Phonological Processes Observed in the Speech of English- and French-Learning Preschoolers

	English		French	
Phonological Process	*Target*	*Child Form*	*Target*	*Child Form*
Syllable deletion	tɛləfoʊn spəgɛɾi	[tɛfoʊn] [gɛɾi]	akwaʁjɔm elikɔptɛʁ	[kwaʁjɔm] [likɔptɛʁ]
Consonant cluster reduction	spʌn tɹeɪn	[pʌn] [teɪn]	avjɔ̃ fʁɑ̃bwaz	[navɔ̃] [fɑ̃bwaz]
Final consonant deletion	dɑlfɪn gɪtɑɹ	[dɑlfɪ] [gɪtɑ]	ʒiʁaf joguʁ	[ʒiʁa] [jogu]
Stopping	naɪf ʃu	[naɪp] [tu]	velo ʃapo	[belo] [tapo]
Fronting	gɑɹdɛn fɪʃɪŋ	[dɑdɛn] [fɪsɪŋ]	kamjɔ̃ ʃato	[tamjɔ̃] [sato]
Gliding	lɛmɪn ɹæbɪt	[wɛmɪn] [wæbɪt]	lynɛt tʁɛno	[wynɛt] [twɛno]

Source: Provided with permission from Francoise Brosseau-Lapre

language. Deletion of onset consonants is highly unusual in English-learning children for example but occurs relatively frequently in Finnish, a difference that reflects differences in the phonetic repertoire and the prosody of the two languages; specifically perceptual attention is preferentially attracted to onset consonants in English and to word medial geminates (i.e., double-length consonants) in Finnish. As another example, fronting is common in English (e.g., as in /ʃ/→[s]), whereas backing in common in Japanese (e.g., as in /s/→[ʃ]), another crosslinguistic difference that is grounded in perceptual factors. Despite individual differences in the number and type of error patterns that occur, steady improvements in accuracy occur throughout the preschool period, resulting in speech that is intelligible to familiar and unfamiliar listeners. By the age of 4 or 5 years, learners of most, if not all, languages will have acquired a complete set of phonological contrasts so that the phonological processes described in Table 2 have largely been resolved. Vowels and tone contrasts (i.e., manipulation of pitch to distinguish words) are mastered early in the preschool period, whereas the consonant contrasts show a longer course of acquisition. By the time they are 5 years old, most children will produce most consonants correctly more often than not.

Mastery of Speech Production Accuracy

The final stage of phonological development involves ongoing refinements in accuracy of speech sound production, manifested as the elimination of distortion errors, mastery of difficult word shapes, and full integration of all levels of the phonological system (i.e., contrastive use of prosodic structure, tone, and distinctive features, as well as appropriate manipulation of suprasegmental aspects at the word and phrase levels). With respect to mastery of the late developing consonants, it has been shown that articulatory difficulty of specific speech sounds explains age of mastery crosslinguistically; specifically, the late developing phonemes require fine force control and involve relatively complex tongue gestures. In English, /s/, /z/, and /ɹ/ are the latest phonemes to be mastered, sometimes not until 9 years of age. In general, one or more of the sibilants /s, z, ʃ, ʒ/ are relatively late developing in many languages including Cantonese, Dutch, German, Icelandic, Finnish, and Swedish.

Difficult sound sequences within complex syllables or longer words are also subject to a longer course of phonological development. For example, in French, the individual segments are mastered at a relatively early age but consistent and accurate inclusion of all segments in the characteristically long words in this language is often not mastered even at the age of 7 years: For example, "escalier" /ɛskalje/→[ɛstalje], "bibliothèque" /bibliɔtɛk/ →[blibliɔtɛk], and "hélicoptère" /elikɔptɛʁ/ →[ekɔktɛʁ], produced by children who correctly pronounced all of the misarticulated phonemes in less complex words. Similarly, in English, the production of words that have word internal codas and word internal clusters such as *ambulance, computer,* and *octopus* is vulnerable to deletions by school-aged children, an age when deletions of consonants from monosyllabic words do not occur. As with the late emerging phonemes, late resolution of these syllable structure errors is often attributed to articulatory factors given that these consonant sequences are assumed to present a coarticulatory challenge. However, it has also been shown that these errors often occur in contexts that present a perceptual challenge due to the low prominence of unstressed syllables. Finally, phonological factors are involved given the low frequency of some of the phonotactic sequences. When the words themselves have low input frequency and low neighborhood density, there is even less phonological pressure for the child to correct errors that do not result in homonyms that will create lexical uncertainty. Indeed, throughout the first 9 years of life, it is the interplay of perceptual, articulatory, phonological, and lexical factors that supports the gradual accumulation of knowledge and skill that results ultimately in adultlike speech accuracy.

Susan Rvachew and Françoise Brosseau-Lapré

See also Delayed Phonological Development; Motor Speech Disorders

Further Readings

Ball, M. J. (2016). *Principles of clinical phonology: Theoretical approaches.* London, UK: Routledge.

Curtin, S., & Zamuner, T. S. (2014). Understanding the developing sound system: Interactions between sounds and words. *Wiley Interdisciplinary Reviews: Cognitive Science, 5*(5), 589–602. doi:10.1002/wcs.1307

Dodd, B., Holm, A., Hua, Z., & Crosbie, S. (2003). Phonological development: A normative study of British English-speaking children. *Clinical Linguistics & Phonetics, 17*(8), 617–643.

Másdóttir, T., & Stokes, S. S. (2016). Influence of consonant frequency on Icelandic-speaking children's speech acquisition. *Journal of Speech-Language Pathology, 18,* 111–121.

McLeod, S. (Ed). (2007). *The international guide to speech acquisition.* Clifton Park, NY: Thomson Delmar Learning.

Rvachew, S., & Brosseau-Lapré, F. (2018). *Developmental phonological disorders: Foundations of clinical practice* (2nd ed.). San Diego, CA: Plural.

Smit, A. B., Hand, L., Freilinger, J. J., Bernthal, J. E., & Bird, A. (1990). The Iowa articulation norms project and its Nebraska replication. *Journal of Speech and Hearing Disorders, 55,* 779–798.

Stokes, S. F., & Suredran, D. (2005). Articulatory complexity, ambient frequency, and functional load as predictors of consonant development in children. *Journal of Speech, Language, and Hearing Research, 48,* 577–591.

Vihman, M. (2016). Learning words and learning sounds: Advances in language development. *British Journal of Psychology, 108,* 1–27.

Phonological Disorders

Phonological disorders involve difficulties in the perception, production, representation, processing, and/or acquisition of the speech sounds and sequences of words of a language. Phonological disorders may affect speakers of any age, but the term is used most often in reference to childhood disorders. It is estimated that 10% of all preschoolers present with some form of phonological disorder; indeed, phonological disorders are one of the most common language disorders of childhood. The majority of children with phonological disorders require clinical intervention. The American Speech-Language-Hearing Association reports that children with phonological disorders constitute the single largest population on the caseload of practicing clinicians in U.S. public schools. The disorder also carries potential risks for related developmental, speech, academic, and other difficulties with possible lifelong consequences. Thus, children with phonological disorders are a population of significant concern for developmental, health, clinical, and educational reasons. This entry provides an overview of the structure of phonology in the context of acquisition and then explores the causes, incidence, risk, diagnosis, and common error patterns of phonological disorders as well as treatment methods and efficacy.

Phonological Structure and Acquisition

To better understand the complexity of a phonological disorder, an overview of the structure of the phonology in the context of acquisition is in order as this delineates the full scope and impact of the disability. All languages, whether spoken or signed, have a phonological system with distinct structure. There are four elements that all phonologies share: (1) phonetic inventory, (2) phonemic inventory, (3) distribution, and (4) phonological rules. The phonetic inventory is the full listing of sounds articulated by a speaker of a given language. The phonetic inventory reflects articulation, whereas the phonemic inventory is an abstraction from the physical to the mental representation of sounds in words of the lexicon. The phonemic inventory is the subset of sounds used specifically to denote meaning through the occurrence of minimal pairs. A minimal pair is two words that differ by one sound. The word *pit*, for example, is minimally distinct from *bit*, *fit*, and *sit*, among others; thus, /p/, /b/, /f/, and /s/ are phonemes. Distribution refers to the allowable context of occurrence of sounds in words. In the word *pit*, /p/ assumes the initial position, but English also allows its occurrence intervocalically (e.g., *tipping*) and finally (e.g., *sip*). Distribution also reveals constraints on the phonology; for example, in English, the sound "ng" (e.g., *ring*) is never permitted word-initially. Phonological rules are systematic changes in production of sounds that are predictable by phonetic context. The English plural is a good example because it is implemented in three different ways: [s] following a voiceless sound (e.g., *pits*), [z] following a voiced sound (e.g., *pigs*), and [əz] following a sibilant (e.g., *buses*). Because the different productions of the plural are systematically predicted by context, they can be derived by rule. This eliminates the need to store each plural variant as a separate entry in the mental lexicon and aids economy of storage and processing. Together, the four elements of phonological structure underlie the perception, production, and processing of words.

In the course of language acquisition, the child must learn each of the aforementioned elements. A long-standing hypothesis is that the seeds of phonology are planted during word learning. When the child learns a new word, there is an initial mapping of the sounds and sound patterns of that word in the mental lexicon. According to this hypothesis, the initial phonological form of the word is incomplete or *fuzzy* such that only the grossest canonical (consonant–vowel) structure is encoded. As the lexicon grows in size, the representation of sounds in words becomes more elaborate and refined to facilitate word recognition and production. This takes place over time with experience, use, and attention to the predictable patterns of word and sounds in the input. Eventually, the representation of the word becomes segmentally specified and adultlike.

If the child presents with a phonological disorder, difficulties may occur in any of the aforementioned aspects of phonological structure and/or acquisition. Articulation may be affected, impacting the range of sounds produced or resulting in residual errors. The child may not differentiate meaning among words perceptually or productively, affecting the size and/or composition of the phonemic inventory. The distribution of sounds may be limited, such that production is restricted to a single word position. Rules of the target language may not be learned, and still others may be invented and applied when they should not. Word learning too may contribute, such that the child may fail to elaborate the phonological content of words and thus the representation remains non-adultlike. In all, a phonological disorder may impact all aspects of the phonology—perception, production, recognition, processing, and/or acquisition.

Other more restrictive terminology, such as articulation disorder or speech sound disorder, has been used to describe this population. However, it can be seen that the term *phonological disorder* takes into account language performance, competence, and acquisition from the dual view of linguistics and psycholinguistics. This disciplinary grounding is relevant because it offers a foundation of testable theoretical models for insight into the mechanisms, causes, prognosis, and treatment of the disorder.

Causes, Incidence, and Risks

Phonological disorders are largely functional in nature, having no organic and no known cause. While the phonology is impaired, other skills tend to be unaffected. This notwithstanding, it has been observed that the occurrence of a phonological disorder is correlated with recurrent otitis media. Phonological disorders are also known to co-occur with other speech and language disorders of childhood, including stuttering and specific language impairment, respectively. Children with phonological disorders may have difficulties learning words, processing auditory information, or retaining phonological information in working memory. Reading, writing, and spelling may be subsequently affected because these skills require recoding sounds heard in the auditory domain to orthographic letters seen in the visual domain. Other symbolic skills may be compromised, including the ability to learn math. Generally, 50–70% of children with phonological disorders require remedial services, with academic difficulties often extending through grade 12.

It is well established that phonological disorders affect boys on the order of 3 to 1 relative to girls. In some cases, phonological disorders run in families, with grandparents, parents, and siblings affected in similar linguistic ways. New research is exploring possible genetic bases of phonological disorders, but the phenotypic patterns are complex.

The impact of a phonological disorder may persist across the life span. Retrospective studies of adults, who as children presented with a phonological disorder, report a perseveration of language difficulties. General comprehension, retrieval, and manipulation of linguistic information are slowed, and more errors are made relative to other adults with no prior history of the disorder. Effects are not limited to language. Adults with a prior history of the disorder reportedly achieve fewer years of formal education and occupational attainment is likewise impacted. Such life challenges are not likely caused by a phonological disorder; rather, the disorder may be one of many interrelated factors that shape the goals, perspectives, and achievements of the individual.

Diagnosis

Children with phonological disorders are typically identified during the transition from toddlerhood to the early preschool years. Often, the family, pediatrician, or other invested party notices that the child produces words in error, experiences lags or plateaus in language or word learning, or is unintelligible relative to peers. A speech–language pathologist makes the differential diagnosis, often in conjunction with a team of related professionals. A case history is requested from the parent to establish developmental milestones, family background, and behavioral, social, motor, or emotional patterns and concerns. A battery of diagnostic tests is administered to assess hearing acuity, articulation, and oral-motor structure and function. Stimulability may be established; this refers to the child's ability to produce an erred sound correctly when provided with instructional models or visual and physical cues. Receptive and expressive vocabulary and language, intelligence, and phonological working memory are some of the other complementary skills that may be evaluated through testing.

The collective diagnostic information helps to determine whether the child has a phonological disorder as distinct from or co-occurring with other speech, hearing, or language deficits. Once this is in place, detailed speech samples are usually obtained. These may include connected speech elicited in play or conversation as well as structured probes to measure the accuracy of each sound of the language in each relevant word position as sampled in multiple words. These data are used to establish severity of the disorder and to characterize the child's errors and error patterns so as to inform the course of treatment.

Historically, the most basic characterization relies on age-referenced developmental norms of speech sound mastery. Normative scales provide a tentative index of the age at which children are likely to produce sounds of the language correctly. When norms are consulted, the characterization that results is a listing of sounds in error and corresponding ages of mastery for use in planning an ordered set of goals for treatment. While potentially useful, normative scales are based on three inherent assumptions: Normative scales portray learning as a fixed and ordered sequence, first acquired skills are assumed to be easy, and first acquired skills are presumed prerequisites for later skills. For phonological learning, these assumptions do not hold. Individual variability in phonological learning is well-documented. Children do not acquire sounds in a fixed sequence within or even across languages. Sounds deemed late acquired may be learned before others noted as early acquired. A further clinical concern is that developmental norms do not recognize phonology as an integrated linguistic system, where sets of sounds pattern together based on their characteristics and function in the language. This is relevant to phonological treatment because the overarching goal is to promote system-wide improvement in the phonology for the greatest impact.

Contemporary methods of phonological description dating to 1979 remedy the limitations of norms through use of complementary relational and independent analyses of children's phonologies. Relational analyses establish patterns of error by comparing one-to-one the child's outputs to the adult target and then grouping commonalities in production. One relational analysis is the place–voice–manner analysis, where the child's errors are coded as representing a change in phonetic place, voice, or manner of articulation relative to the intended target. For example, the child's production of [t] for target /s/ represents a change in manner, such that a stop is substituted for a target fricative. If that same child also substituted [p] for target /f/ and [d] for target /z/, then errors may be grouped to form a broader and consistent pattern of production that impacts manner of articulation. For treatment, the relevance is that manner may be targeted as an overarching goal. Another relational analysis codes error patterns using phonological processes, which are descriptive linguistic labels. The identification of patterns is much the same as in the place–voice–manner method, but here, substitutions are coded as processes. Returning to the previous example, the child's substitution of stops for fricatives would be coded as *stopping*. Likewise, treatment would aim to eradicate the broader pattern. The place–voice–manner analysis and phonological process analysis yield much the same characterization of the child's sound system and, for the most part, are notational variants.

An independent analysis views the child's phonology as a unique grammar without reference to the adult. Accuracy of production is not pertinent; rather, an independent analysis relies on conventional analytic techniques used by linguists to describe the phonology of any natural language. An independent analysis identifies the child's phonetic and phonemic inventories, contextual distribution of sounds in the inventories, and phonological rules, in accord with the four elements of phonological structure that are common to all languages.

The phonetic inventory has been operationalized as a two-time occurrence of a sound regardless of its accuracy or position in words. The resulting inventory may then be coded for complexity using a universal typology that applies crosslinguistically. Complexity of the phonetic inventory is not associated with the size of the phonetic inventory or the chronological age of the child.

The phonemic inventory has been operationalized as a conjunction of minimal pairs and accuracy. A sound is included in the phonemic inventory if the two unique sets of minimal pairs are identified and also if that sound is produced with some (>6%) accuracy. Minimal pairs are based on the child's contrastive use of sounds in minimal pairs, not the adult's. To illustrate, a child produces [mɪ] "milk" and [sɪ] "sit" and also [mu] "boo" and [su] "shoe." These outputs meet the criteria of two unique sets of minimal pairs because /m s/ signal a difference in meaning for the child. Yet, notice that *milk* and *sit* are not a minimal pair of adult English because the words differ by more than one segment. Notice too that *boo* and *shoe* are a minimal pair of adult English, but the adult contrast is between /b ʃ/, whereas the child contrasts /m s/. Lastly, notice that the child does not produce any of the target words correctly, yet sounds used contrastively are identified as phonemes of the grammar. This example hints of the various ways that the child's minimal pairs might stand apart from the adult's to derive a unique phonemic inventory.

The distribution is determined by noting the contextual occurrence of sounds in words for each sound in the phonetic inventory and separately, each sound in the phonemic inventory. Gaps in the distribution identify the phonological rules of the grammar. There are two types of rules, static and dynamic. Static rules are called *phonotactic constraints* and reflect absolute exclusions. There are three types of phonotactic constraints. Inventory constraints ban the occurrence of a sound entirely (e.g., no /s/). Positional constraints restrict sound occurrence by context (e.g., /s/ but only word-finally). Sequence constraints limit the occurrence of contiguous sequences (e.g., /sk-/ but never /ks-/ in word-initial position). Phonotactic constraints are identified directly from the phonemic inventory and its distribution. By comparison, dynamic rules capture predictable sound changes by context and are either neutralizing or allophonic. Dynamic rules are identified by evidence of free variation, where a given word is produced in multiple ways, and by morphophonemic alternations. The latter occurs when a base word is produced in a given way and that same base, when suffixed (or prefixed), is produced in another way. An example often cited in the literature is the child's production of "dog" as [dɔ] but "doggie" as [dɔgi]. The relevant question for clinical treatment is, how does the child represent the word *dog* in the mental lexicon, with or without /g/? Morphophonemic alternations reveal the answer to inform a phonological rule. In the example, the child lexically represents *dog* with /g/, but that segment is deleted systematically and predictably in final position. A phonological rule of final consonant deletion is motivated if this pattern were observed consistently in the grammar, affecting sounds other than /g/.

When the results of relational and independent analyses are integrated, they reveal what the child knows about the phonology and what remains to be learned through treatment. This combination provides the most comprehensive characterization of the phonology and is recommended as the diagnostic standard.

Common Error Patterns

At the most general level, children with phonological disorders typically present with a reduced phonetic and phonemic inventory, which renders them unintelligible. They tend to produce nasals, stops, and glides to the exclusion of other manner classes. They also tend to simplify syllables, such that consonant clusters are lacking. Children with phonological disorders may have vowel errors as well, but these must be differentiated from dialectal differences.

More specifically, children with phonological disorders tend to produce unmarked sounds and sequences in lieu of marked patterns. *Markedness* is a linguistic term used to describe universal co-occurrence relationships among sounds and sound sequences in language. Markedness relationships are implicational, such that the occurrence of X in a grammar implies the occurrence of Y, but not vice versa. The implying property X is more complex and termed marked structure; the implied property Y is less complex, termed unmarked structure. Implicational relationships thus predict that complex structure predicts simpler structure. Some common markedness relationships are as follows. (Note that the complex property is shown on the left and predictive of the simpler property shown on the right. The simpler property tends to be the default output for children with phonological disorders.)

- Voiced obstruents (stops, fricatives, or affricates) imply voiceless obstruents.
- Fricatives imply stops.
- Affricates imply fricatives.
- Consonant clusters imply affricates.
- Liquids imply nasals.

The lawful nature of markedness relationships is advantageous to phonological treatment. Studies have shown that when treatment focuses on the complex marked property, the simpler unmarked property is acquired for *free* without direct instruction. Examples of other unmarked patterns of production include final consonant deletion, velar fronting, liquid gliding, and cluster reduction.

Children with phonological disorders may also evidence patterns of production that involve interactions between segments. Coalescence describes one such error in production of clusters. In coalescence, the manner or place of contiguous segments fuses. For example, when *spoon* is produced as [fun], the fricative manner of articulation of /s/ is fused with the labial place of articulation of /p/, resulting in the output [f]. Assimilation is another interacting pattern where segments become alike, but the interaction takes place at a distance in the word. An initial consonant may harmonize with a final consonant as in *boom* produced as [mum], or vice versa as in *take* produced as [tet].

Another observation is that children with phonological disorders may produce nonambient sounds that do not occur in the target language but do occur in other fully developed systems. Use of bilabial or velar fricatives is commonly cited in the literature. The intrigue is how the child might have learned nonambient sounds, which are never heard or modeled in the target language. Another puzzling pattern is the chain shift. A chain shift occurs when a sound is produced incorrectly, but that very sound is produced accurately as a substitute. A common chain shift in children with phonological disorders involves the accurate [f] production for target /f/, the substitution of [f] for target /θ/, but the substitution of [θ] for target /s/. The question is why target /θ/ is incorrect when the child is clearly capable of producing [θ] as the substitute for /s/.

Perhaps the most striking finding is that the characteristic error patterns of phonological disorders are not so very different from those reported in typical phonological development. Moreover, the same patterns are also seen in fully developed languages. This finding is of theoretical interest because it suggests the universality of phonological systems. If errors are to be made, they will not be haphazard or random but will follow from the basic structures shared more generally by all languages. There may be degrees of freedom in productive outputs within and across languages, but these are constrained and well-defined. Such observations bear on long-standing debates about the innateness of language.

Treatment Methods

There are two families of treatment, each with methodological variants. The traditional approach, put forth by Charles Van Riper, is based on the view that phonological disorders are maturational and have a perceptual-motor basis. The assumption is that the child's errors result from developmental lags associated with faulty perception and/or poor articulatory skills. As such, treatment is designed to teach sounds in the developmental order of emergence, with each sound a separate goal; this is called a *vertical goal attack strategy*.

Treatment involves sequential activities to first improve perception and then productive skills. In perception, activities may include auditory bombardment, where the child receives massed auditory exposure to the treated sound with emphasis on listening. Additional perceptual activities are identification and discrimination of the treated sound relative to other erred renditions of that same sound. In production, treatment begins with production of the treated sound in isolation with gradual advances to syllables, words, phrases, sentences, and running connected speech. The contextual occurrence of the treated sound varies, starting with production in initial, then final, and lastly, intervocalic position. Production activities take advantage of the contexts that facilitate production accuracy.

Two novel variations of traditional treatment are of mention. One method is cycles approach, which employs a sequence of auditory bombardment, followed by production practice, then again auditory bombardment in each treatment session. Cycles approach is distinct from traditional treatment in that error patterns are the focus of treatment such that a range of treated sounds is taught in illustration of the pattern; this is called a *horizontal goal strategy*. Another method, Speech Assessment and Interactive Learning System, employs a series of computerized perceptual identification training modules. The modules target a subset of sounds that are often found to be in error by children with phonological disorders. All modules are to be completed, regardless of the child's particular errors. In administration of Speech Assessment and Interactive Learning System, the child listens to natural tokens of a given sound in words that are spoken by a variety of speakers. In some trials, the words that are spoken are correct productions, and in other trials, the words are misarticulated. The child is to judge the perceived production by pointing to a corresponding picture or to reject the production by pointing to an X. As in traditional treatment, Speech Assessment and Interactive Learning System incorporates perceptual modules with conventional production practice.

The second family of phonological treatment adopts a cognitive–linguistic approach, where the child's phonology is viewed as being systematic, structured, and similar to other natural languages.

The goal of treatment is to interrupt broader patterns of error by teaching one or more sounds that exemplify the pattern, much the same as in cycles approach. In doing so, change in other affected sounds is expected vis-à-vis the cognitive process of generalization. Generalization is the transfer of learning from treatment to other untreated aspects of the phonology. When generalization occurs, improvements are expected in the treated sound and other untreated sounds and word positions for system-wide gains in the phonology. The cognitive–linguistic approach is primarily defined by the minimal pair method of treatment. Recall that a minimal pair is two words that differ by one sound relevant to the differentiation of meaning; for example, *tip–sip* is a minimal pair, with meaning denoted by the contrast between /t s/. In treatment, the child is presented with sets of minimal pairs specific to his or her error pattern and is taught that a collapse of contrast leads to homonymy and miscommunication. This is achieved by feigned miscommunication on the part of the clinician and/or explicit production of the contrast by the child.

There are several riffs on minimal pair treatment that vary the target–substitute relationship, number of treated sounds, and number and type of contrastive differences among sounds. Conventional minimal pair treatment couples the target sound with the child's corresponding substitute; for example, if /s/ is produced as [t], then these sounds are paired as in *sip–tip*. Maximal opposition treatment couples the target sound with a known sound produced accurately by the child; for example, if /s/ is erred, it may be paired with the child's accurate use of [m] in *sat–mat*. Another variant involves coupling two target sounds with each other; for example, if /s/ and /r/ are both erred, then *sat–rat* is a relevant pair. Multiple opposition treatment is still another variant that couples those target sounds that share a common substitute; for example, if [t] is substituted for targets /d s l/, then *toe–doe*, *tie–sigh*, and *tip–lip* are relevant contrasts.

Metaphon is another cognitive–linguistic method that uses minimal pairs, but it appeals to real-world contrasts to illustrate linguistic contrasts. Conceptual and production activities are employed, with a child first learning a real-world contrast, for example, front–back. The real-world contrast is then extended to a similar distinction in phonology, for example, /t/, an anterior sound contrasts with /k/, a posterior sound. The thought is that real-world contrasts provide the child with a conceptual frame for understanding and communicating about phonological distinctions.

Many other methods of phonological treatment are available including, for example, whole language, core vocabulary, or stimulability training. Treatment may also be administered in individual sessions or in groups, using a pull-out or push-in model in the schools, with or without the involvement of parents as instructors.

Treatment Efficacy

The efficacy of phonological treatment has been established in descriptive, experimental, and clinical studies that address three related questions: Does treatment work? Is one treatment method better than another? And, what are the learning gains that accrue from phonological treatment? These questions define the study of effectiveness, efficiency, and effects, respectively.

In terms of effectiveness, a general finding is that treatment is better than no treatment for children with phonological disorders. This result is important in light of the known critical period for speech sound normalization. Normalization refers to the alignment of the child's productions with the intended target, such that erred outputs are accurate as expected. The optimal time frame for normalization occurs between the ages of 4 and 6, with rapid learning again between the ages of 7 and 8. Normalization plateaus around age 8 years, 5 months; thus, early intervention is encouraged.

With respect to efficiency, few studies have attempted to differentiate among methods. Moreover, the available work tends to stray from the recommended format of a given method by modifying its implementation. A possible reason for this is that phonological treatment methods differ widely in goals, programmatic steps, activities, stimuli, feedback, and child response. This then results in apples-to-oranges comparisons. Indeed, surveys report that speech–language pathologists rely primarily on an eclectic approach to treatment, piecing together elements of several different methods to address the unique phonological needs of each child.

In terms of treatment effects, the majority of studies on phonological treatment have focused on isolating the teaching conditions that lead to optimal learning as defined by system-wide generalization with broad improvements in production of treated and untreated sounds in new words and new contexts. There have been two strands of study, one that identifies the optimal sounds for treatment and another that identifies the optimal words.

Numerous studies have demonstrated that treatment of sounds that are more complex leads to cascading generalization, which fans across the phonology. Sound complexity has been defined in terms of markedness, such that more marked properties lead to greater learning. This includes treatment of voiced obstruents, fricatives, affricates, clusters, and liquids. Complexity has also been defined by normative sequence of sound mastery. Treatment of either a developmentally early acquired sound or a later acquired sound has similar effects, with improved production of treated and untreated sounds from the same manner class. However, only developmentally later acquired sounds lead to improved accuracy of sounds from untreated manner classes for system-wide generalization. The cascading effects associated with complexity are of interest because similar findings have been noted in other instructional domains and for other clinical populations. One suggestion is that complexity represents a general cognitive preference that defines the circumstances under which human learning excels.

Related studies of treated words have found that greater phonological learning takes place when later as opposed to early acquired words are used as stimuli. Likewise, frequent words promote greater generalization than infrequent words. Treated words that are composed of commonly occurring sounds, and those with many rhyming counterparts also lead to system-wide improvements in the phonology. When taken together, the findings associated with treatment effects begin to define the ideal conditions for phonological learning, which may be assembled to maximize the benefits of treatment.

While much progress has been made on the treatment front, outstanding questions remain. Most notably, meta-analyses of phonological treatment are largely lacking. Meta-analyses are considered the benchmark for establishing principles of evidence-based clinical practice. One reason meta-analyses are lacking is because phonological treatment research has primarily employed single-subject experimental design. While well suited to clinical applications, single-subject design precludes the cross-comparison of studies in meta-analyses. To correct the situation, recent innovations in single-subject design are beginning to recommend effect size as a uniform statistic for establishing the magnitude of gain in learning associated with treatment. The application of a constant scale-free statistic such as effect size has the potential to pave the way for meta-analyses of phonological treatment. This will represent a significant advance in establishing evidence-based procedures for treatment of phonological disorders.

Judith A. Gierut

See also Clinical Phonetics; Clinical Phonology; Delayed Phonological Development; Phonological Treatment; Phonology; Speech Sound Disorders

Further Readings

Baker, E., & McLeod, S. (2011). Evidence-based practice for children with speech sound disorders: Part 1 narrative review. *Language, Speech and Hearing Services in Schools, 42,* 102–139.

Barlow, J. A., & Gierut, J. A. (2002). Minimal pair approaches to phonological remediation. *Seminars in Speech and Language, 23,* 57–68.

Felsenfeld, S., Broen, P. A., & McGue, M. (1992). A 28-year follow-up of adults with a history of moderate phonological disorder, linguistic and personality results. *Journal of Speech and Hearing Research, 35,* 1114–1125.

Felsenfeld, S., Broen, P. A., & McGue, M. (1994). A 28-year follow-up of adults with a history of moderate phonological disorder, educational and occupational results. *Journal of Speech and Hearing Research, 37,* 1341–1353.

Fey, M. E. (1992). Articulation and phonology: Inextricable constructs in speech pathology. *Language, Speech and Hearing Services in Schools, 23,* 225–232.

Gierut, J. A. (2007). Phonological complexity and language learnability. *American Journal of Speech-Language Pathology, 16,* 6–17.

Gierut, J. A., Morrisette, M. L., Hughes, M. T., & Rowland, S. (1996). Phonological treatment efficacy and developmental norms. *Language, Speech and Hearing Services in Schools, 27,* 215–230.

Ingram, D. (1989). *Phonological disability in children* (2nd ed.). London, UK: Cole and Whurr.

Law, J., Garrett, Z., & Nye, C. (2004). The efficacy of treatment for children with developmental speech and language delay/disorder: A meta-analysis. *Journal of Speech, Language, and Hearing Research, 47,* 924–943.

Shriberg, L. D., Gruber, F. A., & Kwiatkowski, J. (1994). Developmental phonological disorders III: Long-term speech-sound normalization. *Journal of Speech and Hearing Research, 37,* 1151–1177.

Shriberg, L. D., Kwiatkowski, J., & Gruber, F. A. (1994). Developmental phonological disorders II, Short-term speech-sound normalization. *Journal of Speech and Hearing Research, 37,* 1127–1150.

Smit, A. B., Hand, L., Freilinger, J. J., Bernthal, J. E., & Bird, A. (1990). The Iowa Articulation Norms Project and its Nebraska replication. *Journal of Speech and Hearing Disorders, 55,* 779–798.

Storkel, H. L., & Morrisette, M. L. (2002). The lexicon and phonology: Interactions in language acquisition. *Language, Speech and Hearing Services in Schools, 33,* 24–37.

PHONOLOGICAL PROCESSES

Phonological processes describe speech sound errors in terms of patterns. Grounded in David Stampe's Natural Phonology, these descriptors define how the child's production differs from the adult form. Natural phonological processes are presumed to be innate and motivated by human physiological limitations on the production of speech. Hence, it is presumed that these processes are common across languages. While phonological processes can be used as a synonym for phonological rules, the latter specifically refers to linguistic principles associated with a particular language. These rules describe relationships among phonological elements at different levels of phonology (i.e., surface vs. deep levels) and are written using formulas to describe changes in the basic features underlying unique phonemes (i.e., distinctive features).

Phonological processes then simplify the information provided by phonological rules. They describe speech production patterns in terms of sound changes and can be used to explain differences between the target and actual productions in casual speech, dialects, and speech sound development and disorders. This entry provides an overview of phonological processes, which can be broadly defined as syllable structure, substitution, and assimilation processes, as well as how these processes relate to the assessment and treatment of speech sound disorders.

Syllable Structure Processes

These processes describe ways in which a child's speech productions can be altered by syllable and/or phoneme deletions and insertions. Frequently occurring phonological processes include:

Weak syllable deletion—an unstressed syllable in a multisyllabic word is omitted:/pədʒæməz/→[dʒæməz].

Cluster reduction—a consonant cluster is reduced by phoneme omission(s): /swɛtɚ/→[wɛtɚ] or /strit/→[tit].

Final consonant deletion—the final consonant in a word is deleted: /swɪmɪŋ/→[swɪmɪ].

Reduplication—a stressed syllable in a mulitsyllabic word is repeated either identically or partially. This is most common in young children:/kændi/→[kækæ].

Migration—a sound moves to another position within the word: /stɪks/→[kɪts].

Metathesis—the transposition of sounds: /mæsk/→[mæks].

Epenthesis—a segment is inserted within a word or at the end of a word: /swɛdɚ/→[səwɛdɚ].

There are a few other syllable structure processes that occur during casual speech and also might occur in children with speech sound disorders. These include:

Prothesis—a vowel is added at the beginning of a word, especially when a cluster is present. This might be most noticeable in children who are second language learners: /skul/→[əskul].

Diphthongization—stressed vowels are broken up and become two vowels: /fæst/→[fæɪst].

Diphthong reduction—a diphthong is reduced to one vowel: /paɪ/→[pa:].

Syncope—a syllable is omitted in a colloquial production of a word: /ɪntɚɛst/→[ɪntrɛst].

Substitution Processes

These phonological processes are used to simplify phoneme productions, resulting in place and manner substitutions. The first group of substitution processes affects consonant place.

Fronting—Target phonemes are substituted with phones produced more forward in the mouth. While this process can be used too generally in referring to any phoneme produced more anteriorally, many clinicians use more specific terms. Examples include:

Fronting of velars—a velar phoneme is replaced with an alveolar phoneme: /gʌm/→[dʌm].

Palatal fronting (Depalatalization)—a palatal phoneme is replaced with an alveolar phoneme: /ʃu/→[su].

Backing—This is not a natural phonological process, but frequently manifests itself as backing of alveolars in severe speech sound disorders: /doɚ/→[goɚ].

Another group of processes simplifies consonant manner:

Stopping—a fricative or affricate is replaced with a plosive: /zɪpɚ/→[dɪpɚ] or /tʃu/→[tu].

Deaffrication—an affricate is replaced with a homorganic fricative: /wɑtʃɪs/→[wɑʃɪs].

Liquid (and Nasal) Simplification—sonorant phonemes are simplified to glides or plosives.

Gliding of liquids—/rɑk/→[wɑ].

Vowelization (also known as *Vocalization*)—/tʃɛɚ/→[tʃɛə] or /tebəl/→[tebo].

Denasalization—/mek/→[bek].

Glottal replacement—a medial or final consonant is replaced by a glottal stop: /ʧɪkɪn/→[ʧɪʔɪn] or /tʌb/→[tʌʔ]. While considered to be an atypical process in speech sound development, this process is a normal substitution for /t, d/ in some dialects.

Assimilation Processes

This group of phonological processes is characterized by having one sound become more similar to another sound in the word.

Alveolar assimilation—/kʌt/→[tʌt].

Velar assimilation—/foɚk/→[koɚk].

Labial assimilation—/pedʒ/→[pef].

Nasal assimilation—/spun/→[mun].

The last group of assimilation processes describe context-dependent phoneme voicing, that is, the voicing of the target phoneme becomes like the voicing of the segment that follows.

Prevocalic voicing—/ʃu/→[ʒu].

Final consonant devoicing—/aɪs kjubz/→[aɪs kjus].

Typically, phonological patterns change one aspect of sound production, either place, manner, or voice. As such, it is possible that multiple processes are needed to explain a single phoneme substitution. For example, if the child produces [dop] for /sop/, the /s/ is stopped to a [t] and then it is voiced to a [d]. It is also possible to have multiple processes operating within a single word, like [bu] for /spun/, where the cluster /sp/ is reduced to [p], then voiced to [b], and the final phoneme /n/ is omitted. In this case, one could also argue that the processes were applied in a particular order: Consonant cluster reduction occurred before the prevocalic voicing. The final consonant deletion could occur at any time.

Developmental Sequencing of Processes

As young children learn to speak, they often adapt the adult target to fit their physiological capabilities and/or understanding of the target phonology. There is considerable agreement as to when these developmental processes are suppressed (i.e., no longer used). Processes like final consonant deletion, reduplication, and assimilation processes occur less frequently after the age of 3 years, while processes like gliding and stopping of /θ/ and /ð/ may persist past the age of 5 years. The most common phonological processes used by children ages 3–3.5 years are cluster reduction, weak syllable deletion, glottal replacement, labial assimilation, and gliding of liquids, with weak syllable deletion and cluster reduction continuing in many children until ages 4.5–5 years. Other researchers have found that cluster reduction and gliding of liquids persist in some children until the age of 8 years.

Use of Phonological Processes in the Assessment of Speech Sound Disorder

The patterned suppression of developmental phonological processes has made them attractive for use in the clinical assessment of speech sound disorders. Clinicians evaluate articulation test data or conversational speech samples to determine phonological delay/deviance and to identify patterns affecting entire classes of sounds, thereby clarifying the path to increased speech intelligibility. In other words, instead of listing out sound substitutions and omissions, the clinician now has a list of phonological processes that affect entire classes of sounds (i.e., fricatives or glides) or sound segments (i.e., consonant sequences).

Numerous assessment devices have been developed to assist clinicians in identifying phonological process use. Many of these tests elicit single word productions that are crafted to elicit specific consonant and consonant sequences representing common phonological processes. Examples include the *Hodson Assessment of Phonological Patterns 3*, *Bernthal-Bankson Test of Phonology*, and the *Diagnostic Evaluation of Articulation and Phonology*, to name a few. Others describe methods that identify phonological processes from standard articulation tests (*Khan-Lewis Phonological Analysis-3*) or from an analysis of conversational speech (*Systemic Phonological Analysis of Child Speech*). The goal of all of these assessment techniques is to provide a structured approach to the identification of phonological processes.

The primary difference between these approaches is the nature and number of phonological processes that are identified. For instance, the *Khan-Lewis Phonological Analysis-3* focuses on the identification of 12 core phonological processes and adds a supplementary analysis of 12 less frequently occurring processes. On the other hand, the Hodson Assessment of Phonological Patterns 3 groups errors by syllable type, word position, and distinctive feature to arrive at a severity score and then allows the clinician to identify specific phonological processes in a separate analysis. Most phonological process tests are criterion referenced in that they generate scores that reflect the frequency of process use and compare these frequencies to developmental expectations.

Treatment Approaches Using Phonological Processes

The identification of phonological processes has led to new thoughts about treatment targets and generalization patterns. As such, treatment focus has shifted from the remediation of speech sounds that are early developing and stimulable to the suppression of a phonological pattern that leads to increased intelligibility. Since phonological processes describe the systematicity of phoneme simplifications, treatment emphasis is on expanding the child's phonetic and phonemic inventories to match the complexity evident in the adult system. This results in an ability to treat an entire class of sounds instead of a single phoneme. Hence, phonological processes have not changed the way that clinicians view the therapeutic process, only the process of treatment target selection.

Phonological processes are most useful in treating children who are severely unintelligible, as the primary goal would be to improve speech intelligibility as quickly as possible. This goal is accomplished by selecting representative sounds within a phonemic category with the possibility of influencing the production of all phonemes within that group. For instance, if the child lacks knowledge of a phoneme class, like fricatives, or a syllable shape, such as consonant clusters, the clinician could select an exemplar from the target class (e.g., /s/ or an /s/ cluster, like /sp/ or /ts/) and hope to affect the production of all fricatives or clusters by demonstrating the existence of a pattern previously unused by the child.

There are several ways in which treatment can be conducted. One could use *minimal pairs*, which relies on meaning to strengthen the contrast between the error and target. The phonemic contrasts here can go beyond single distinctive features to include multiple feature contrasts, as in the *maximal oppositions* approach espoused by Judith Gierut. In contrast, Barbara Hodson and Elaine Paden describe a *cycles approach* whereby phonological processes are treated individually within a time period that accounts for how many processes are in error. The goal of this technique is to provide exposure and phonetic practice for targets within a phonological process for which the child is ready to learn (i.e., has shown the ability to produce correctly). This treatment approach does not focus on mastery of the target but instead emphasizes impact on the entire phonological system. Finally, a newer procedure, *multiple oppositions*, treats several phonemes produced as a single phone, known as a *phonemic collapse* (e.g., /s/, /tʃ/, /st/ and /ʃ/ are all produced as [t]), with minimal pairs representing multiple phonological processes (in this case, stopping, cluster reduction, and deaffrication). This approach is designed to treat the entire rule set instead of targeting individual contrasts sequentially.

The goal of treatment using phonological processes is to alter the child's speech sound productions, moving them toward an adultlike system. All three of the phonological approaches described previously can be successful if one considers the severity of the speech sound disorder and the child's preferred learning style. Treatment effectiveness also depends on the child's sensorimotor abilities, attention/memory, and treatment frequency.

Ruth Huntley Bahr and Toby Macrae

See also Articulation (Phonetic) Assessment; Phonological Disorders; Phonological Treatment; Relational Analyses; Speech Sound Disorders

Further Readings

Ball, M. J. (2016). *Principles of clinical phonology: Theoretical approaches.* New York, NY: Routledge.

Gierut, J. A. (1989). Maximal opposition approach to phonological treatment. *Journal of Speech and Hearing Disorders, 54,* 9–19.

Haelsig, P. C., & Madison, C. L. (1986). A study of phonological processes exhibited by 3-, 4-, and 5-year-old children. *Language, Speech, and Hearing Services in Schools, 17,* 107–114.

Hodson, B. W., & Paden, E. P. (1991). *Targeting intelligible speech: A phonological approach to remediation* (2nd ed.). Austin, TX: Pro-Ed.

Kamhi, A. G., & Pollock, K. E. (2005). *Phonological disorders in children: Clinical decision making in assessment and intervention.* Baltimore, MD: Brookes.

Roberts, J. E., Burchinal, M., & Footo, M. M. (1990). Phonological process decline from 2 1/2 to 8 years. *Journal of Communication Disorders, 23,* 205–217.

Velleman, S. L. (2016). *Speech sound disorders.* Philadelphia, PA: Wolters Kluwer.

Williams, A. L. (2000). Multiple oppositions: Case studies of variables in phonological intervention. *American Journal of Speech-Language Pathology, 9,* 289–299.

Phonological Treatment

Phonological treatment is often recommended for preschool and school-age children diagnosed with a phonological disorder. Phonological disorders result in reduced consonantal inventories that impact a child's speech intelligibility. A majority of these children have a disorder severe enough to require phonological treatment to improve sound productions and promote more intelligible speech. Treatment usually introduces a treatment target(s) in a specific context (i.e., word position) in words in a range of perception and production activities. The goal is to establish accurate productions in the treatment stimuli as a means of promoting a transfer of learning to other untreated words, contexts, and untreated target sounds that are also produced in error. This transfer of learning is referred to as *generalization*. Three types of generalization are of interest and have been documented as a result of phonological treatment: treated sound generalization, within-class generalization, and across-class generalization. *Treated sound generalization* involves a transfer of learning of the treated sound to untreated words and contexts. For example, if a child is taught the target sound /s/ in word-initial context, treated sound generalization is illustrated by the production of /s/ in untreated words not only in the word-initial context but also in the intervocalic and word-final contexts as well. *Within-class generalization* refers to a transfer of learning to untreated sounds from the same class of sounds as the treated sound. For example, treatment of the fricative /s/ may promote within-class generalization to other untreated fricatives that the child also produced in error. *Across-class generalization* is a transfer of learning to untreated sounds from other sound classes unrelated to the treated sound. For example, when treating a fricative, it is important to measure for across-class generalization to other untreated stops, affricates, or liquids that were also produced in error. The type and magnitude of generalization learning has been shown to be influenced by the treatment sound(s) selected and the treatment words selected for phonological treatment. The method of instruction is also an important consideration for phonological treatment. This entry provides an overview of these three considerations: sound selection, treatment word selection, and method of instruction.

Treatment Sound Selection

Historically, three factors that have been considered in target selection for phonological treatment include consistency of errors, stimulability, and the recommended age of sound acquisition. *Consistency of errors* refers to how often a target sound is produced in error. Sounds that are inconsistently in error are produced with some accuracy, whereas sounds that are consistently in error are produced with 0% accuracy in all contexts. *Stimulability* refers to a child's ability to imitate a target sound following a clinician's model. A child is stimulable for sounds that are correctly articulated following a model, whereas nonstimulable sounds continue to be produced in error despite visual and auditory cues provided by a model. *Recommended age of sound acquisition* is based on normative scales documenting the order and age of sound emergence in development. Sounds that are acquired at a younger age are considered relatively early acquired, whereas sounds that are acquired at older ages are considered relatively late acquired. Conventionally, a developmental approach to sound selection has focused on sounds that were inconsistently in error, stimulable, and developmentally early acquired. Sound selection following a developmental approach has been documented to result in treated sound generalization and within-class generalization. Experimental evidence has challenged this approach by selecting more complex treatment targets that are consistently in error, nonstimulable, and late acquired. Learning data demonstrates that a complexity approach to sound selection results in not only treated sound generalization and within-class generalization but also broader system-wide gains that emerge through across-class generalization.

A complexity approach to target sound selection has been further demonstrated as efficacious in the selection of target onset clusters for treatment of children with phonological disorders. Onset clusters have been traditionally grouped as target /l-/ clusters, /r-/ clusters, or /s-/ clusters, for example. An alternative approach, adopting linguistic methods of analysis, has suggested examining clusters on the basis of sonority difference. *Sonority* refers to the degree of constriction of the vocal tract. A *sonority scale* can then be applied to assign a numerical value to the target sounds that constitute a cluster, with least sonorous sounds assigned a higher value. Permissible onset clusters in a language are composed of a less sonorous consonant followed by a more sonorous consonant. For example, voiceless stops are the least sonorous segments and assigned a value of 7, followed by voiced stops (6), then voiceless fricatives (5), voiced fricatives (4), nasals (3), liquids (2), and glides (1). Using the sonority scale, it is then possible to determine the *sonority distance*, or difference in sonority values, between those sounds that constitute a target cluster. For example, the target onset cluster /sl-/ is composed of a voiceless fricative (5) followed by a liquid (2). Thus, the sonority difference for the onset cluster /sl-/ is 5−2 = 3. Research findings suggest that treatment of more complex clusters with smaller sonority differences (e.g., /sl-/ with a sonority difference of 3) results in greater generalization learning for children with phonological disorders than less complex clusters with greater sonority differences (e.g., /pl-/ with a sonority difference of 5). The smallest sonority difference, or *minimal distance*, for permissible onset clusters in English is 2 and corresponds to the target onset clusters /sm- sn-/. While treatment of smaller sonority differences has been shown more efficacious, the selection of target /sm- sn-/ requires further analysis of children's productions to determine whether these are appropriate targets, depending on other sounds in the child's phonemic repertoire. It should also be noted that treatment of the onset clusters /sp- st- sk-/ is not supported by research findings because they were shown to result in negligible generalization.

Treatment Word Selection

Embedding treatment targets in word-level stimuli is a common practice in phonological treatment. While some approaches initiate treatment in isolation or at a syllable level, generalization to conversational speech has been documented following phonological treatment with as few as three to five stimulus words. Contributions from psycholinguistic research have led to an emerging body of literature focused on the types of words that are used to elicit the treated sounds. Findings have shown that the characteristics of the words selected result in differences in the type and magnitude of phonological generalization. Three word-level characteristics have been examined: word frequency, neighborhood density, and age of word acquisition. *Word frequency* is determined by how often a word occurs in the language, with a distinction between relatively frequent as opposed to infrequent words. *Neighborhood density* refers to the number of words that are phonologically similar to a given word, based on the substitution, deletion, or addition of a single phoneme. For example, the word *sat* is phonologically similar to words like *cat, sit, sad, at,* and *scat*. These phonologically similar words are called *neighbors of sat*. Words like *sat* that have a lot of neighbors are said to reside in dense lexical neighborhoods, whereas words like *sofa* that don't have many neighbors are said to reside in sparse lexical neighborhoods.

Age of word acquisition is based on adults' ratings of when they learned a word. Words rated as residing in the lexicon the longest are considered relatively early acquired, whereas words that have not been in the lexicon as long are considered late acquired. For word frequency and neighborhood density, research has pointed to frequent words from dense neighborhoods as beneficial for promoting children's generalization of treated and untreated sounds. For age of word acquisition, findings suggest that teaching target sounds in late acquired words (as opposed to early) promotes greater generalization learning to treated and untreated sounds.

One further consideration related to treatment word selection is the use of nonwords in phonological treatment. *Nonwords* are crafted as permissible sound sequences that do not hold lexical status in a child's vocabulary. Nonwords have historically been used as stimuli in phonological treatment dating back to the days of Charles Van Riper. Van Riper recommended presenting a target sound first in a nonword syllable context before advancing to syllables that were *real* words in the language. Experimental findings have further demonstrated the clinical utility of treating target sounds in nonwords. Comparisons of nonwords and real words suggest that training target sound production in nonwords resulted in greater generalization to treated and untreated sounds. Training sounds in nonwords was also shown to boost phonological generalization more rapidly in treatment when compared to real words.

Methods of Instruction

A wide range of methods have been utilized in phonological treatment in research and clinical settings. Two key components that are common to phonological treatment include perception training and production training.

Perception Training

Perception training may include auditory bombardment (i.e., ear training) and/or identification and discrimination activities. *In Auditory Bombardment children are not required to respond, only listen*. The purpose is to ready the listener for production training by exposing the child to a set of stimuli that are related to the treatment sound. Conventionally, the related stimuli would contain the treatment sound in the same context selected for production practice. For example, if a child were taught the treatment target /s/ in the initial position of words like *sat*, auditory bombardment would expose the child to related /s/ initial words like *sun*, *seal*, and *same* in a list format or a story context before moving to production practice. Auditory bombardment does not require a response from the children only that they listen. Experimental findings have demonstrated a more efficacious method of auditory bombardment. When children with phonological disorders were exposed to related stimuli that were the phonologically similar neighbors of the treatment words, greater generalization resulted. For example, if /s/ were taught in a treatment word, like *sat*, auditory bombardment would expose the child to the neighbors: *cat*, *hat*, and *rat*. Moreover, this line of research also discovered that auditory bombardment was most beneficial to children's generalization learning when it was presented at the start of a treatment session, before production practice began.

Identification and discrimination activities have also been incorporated in some approaches to treatment. The goal is to promote children's accurate judgments of the treatment target relative to their own production error (or sound substitute) as a way of focusing their attention and promoting self-correction and monitoring skills. *Identification* involves the child detecting correct and/or error sound productions relative to a standard (i.e., the treatment target). For example, if a child substitutes [t] for the treatment target /s/, a list of words, such as "sew," "two," and "say," is read and the child may be asked to raise his or her hand when the treatment sound /s/ is heard. *Discrimination* involves the child making same or different judgments of the treatment target and the error sound. For example, the child listens to word pairs, such as "sew"-"toe," "sew"-"sew," "sue"-"two," and is asked to judge each pair as the same or different. The benefit of these tasks in promoting generalization has been debated in the literature.

Production Training

Production training typically involves two modes of responding from the child: *imitation* and *spontaneous* productions. Phonological treatment begins production practice by having a child produce the target sound in the treatment stimuli in imitation of the clinician's model. Production practice in imitation continues until a child has reached a time- or performance-based criterion. The next step is to have the child practice production of the target sound in the treatment stimuli spontaneously without the clinician's model. For both imitation and spontaneous productions, the treatment stimuli are generally elicited in turn, one after the other in a random order, and feedback is provided. Feedback serves as a mechanism to shape the child's production closer and closer to the adult target. If the child produces the target sound in error in a given stimulus form, the clinician attempts to correct the child's production by providing feedback and modeling the production of the stimulus form a second time, eliciting another production from the child. If the child continues to produce the target sound in error on the second try, the clinician gives feedback about the production but then moves on to the next stimulus form. If accuracy in production is achieved on a stimulus form, the clinician continues to the next form and so on. There is broad consensus that production training promotes generalization for children with phonological disorders.

The perception and production training activities described here are used to varying degrees in different approaches to phonological treatment. To date, there are over two dozen documented phonological treatment approaches. Some of the more common and long-standing approaches follow. However, it has been noted in the literature that many clinicians employ an eclectic, or hybrid, approach to phonological treatment by adopting and combining methods from a range of different approaches.

Traditional Approach

The *traditional approach* has an articulatory or motor-skill focus and includes both perception and production training. Treatment begins with auditory bombardment and may also include identification and discrimination activities. Production training introduces a target sound first in isolation, then progresses gradually to more complex linguistic units including syllables, words, phrases, utterances, and conversational speech. For each linguistic unit, children are exposed to each permissible context and progress from imitation to spontaneous productions. The goal is to teach the target sound to a level of mastery with performance-based criterion established for advancement. The target sound remains the focus of treatment until generalization is demonstrated to a conversational level.

Cycles Approach

The *cycles approach* focuses on error patterns in children's productions as opposed to an individual target sound(s). For example, a child that substitutes stops for target fricatives demonstrates an error pattern (or phonological process) of stopping. The cycles approach would target the error pattern of stopping as a cycle of treatment. The cycles approach includes both perception and production training. Within a given session, treatment starts with auditory bombardment and then shifts to production training. While a cycle represents an error pattern, there are usually two to three sounds affected by that error pattern that are targeted within a cycle. Each sound is then taught for a specific time period (e.g., 60 min) before progressing to the next sound. Once a cycle is completed, focus shifts to the next error pattern, and patterns may then be recycled until generalization occurs.

Minimal Pair Approaches

Minimal pair approaches expose a child to sound contrasts in word pairs. The goal is to eliminate instances of homonymy. *Homonymy* occurs when two or more words are produced the same. For example, a child may produce the words *fan* and *pan* both as "pan." Perception training may be included in the form of discrimination of the word pairs or to demonstrate miscommunication when homonymy occurs. Production training is also a key component of minimal pair treatment. Conventionally, minimal pair treatment selects a target sound and contrasts it with the child's substitute for that sound. For example, if a child substitutes [p] for target /f/ in initial position, then minimal pair stimulus words would be selected to highlight this contrast in the language (e.g., "fan"-"pan"). In this example, the target sound would be unknown to the child, whereas the substituted sound is known and used in the child's phonology. This example also illustrates that the sound contrasts are minimally different in that they share a common place of articulation (i.e., both are labial) and voicing (i.e., both are voiceless) and differ only in manner of articulation (i.e., one is a fricative and one a stop). Research findings have demonstrated that a more efficacious approach is to contrast two maximally opposed sounds that are both excluded from a child's sound system. This approach then selects two unknown sounds that differ in place, voice, and manner of articulation. For example, if both /f/ and /r/ are excluded from a child's sound system, these would represent a maximal opposition contrast. That is, the target sounds differ in place (labial vs. coronal), voice (voiceless vs. voiced), and manner (obstruent vs. sonorant).

Measuring for Generalization

Throughout and following phonological treatment, it is important to measure for children's generalization learning. Measuring for generalization allows a clinician to evaluate a child's progress and attribute changes to the treatment administered. Additionally, it is critical for a clinician to be able to document the type and extent of generalization to inform treatment decisions and the need for continued treatment. This is generally accomplished through probe measures.

Probes are used to elicit word productions from a child and are typically administered as a spontaneous picture-naming task. Probes are designed to measure for transfer of the treatment sound to untreated words and contexts. Moreover, probes are used to monitor other sounds produced in error prior to the start of treatment. This allows for an evaluation of within-class and across-class generalizations. Probe words are kept distinct from treatment word stimuli and allow an opportunity to sample a child's productions in multiple word forms for each context. Probes administered prior to the start of treatment allow a measure of baseline performance and may be used to establish stability in productions. Baseline performance provides a necessary point of comparison to establish learning (or the lack thereof). Stability in productions (typically with low accuracy) also allows a clinician to attribute a child's improvements to the treatment provided (as opposed to other external or spurious variables). Probes are then readministered periodically throughout treatment and at the end of treatment with performance evaluated relative to the baseline. This allows a clinician to document the type and extent of generalization that results from phonological treatment.

Future Directions

Research related to phonological treatment has focused largely on treatment sound selection and treatment word selection, with less emphasis on the methods of instruction. While treatment methods and approaches have been shown to improve children's perceptual and productive skills, many questions remain. For example, clinicians lack clear guidelines to determine which approach is most efficacious for an individual child or diagnostic profile. There are also limited data available as to whether one treatment approach is better than another in promoting gains. Moreover, with more eclectic approaches being implemented in clinical practice, there is a need to understand the influence of different treatment methods and how it is best to combine methods to facilitate children's generalization learning. It will be important for future research to empirically evaluate these questions through controlled experimental clinical studies.

Michele Morrisette

See also Phonological Disorders; Phonology; Speech Sound Disorders; Speech–Language Pathology; Treatment Research

Further Readings

Fey, M. E. (1992). Articulation and phonology: Inextricable constructs in speech pathology. *Language, Speech, and Hearing Services in Schools, 23,* 225–232.

Gierut, J. A. (2001). Complexity in phonological treatment: Clinical factors. *Language, Speech and Hearing Services in Schools, 32,* 229–241.

Gierut, J. A., & Morrisette, M. L. (2012a). Age-of-word-acquisition effects in treatment of children with phonological delays. *Applied Psycholinguistics, 33,* 121–144.

Gierut, J. A., & Morrisette, M. L. (2012b). Density, frequency and the expressive phonology of children with phonological delay. *Journal of Child Language, 39,* 804–834.

Morrisette, M. L., Farris, A. W., & Gierut, J. A. (2006). Applications of learnability theory to clinical phonology. *Advances in Speech-Language Pathology, 8,* 207–219.

Phonology

One of the central components of a language's grammar is its phonology. The phonology of a language is a highly structured, intricate linguistic system that governs pronunciation. It interfaces most directly with the lexicon and word-formation processes. The phonological component of grammar is responsible for regulating (a) the speech sounds that can and cannot occur in a particular language (i.e., the phonetic inventory); (b) the function of sounds in distinguishing the meaning of words (i.e., the phonemic inventory); (c) the distribution of sounds, sound sequences, and stress within words (i.e., phonotactics); and (d) the behavior of sounds in different phonetic contexts (i.e., phonological processes). This entry highlights some basic accounts of these facts as they derive from contemporary generative theories of phonology.

The accounts appeal to an interplay of language-specific and universal grammatical principles and abstract constructs and structures. Two abstract levels of representation are assumed. The phonetic level of representation is closer to the surface and parses the continuous speech signal into segment-size units that are themselves analyzable as a complex of distinctive features. The phonetic level also includes prosodic structures, which group sequences of sounds into hierarchically organized syllables and, in turn, syllables into higher order feet. The underlying level of representation is more abstract and reflects the speaker's internalized mental representation of words in the lexicon. While there is controversy about the extent to which underlying representations can differ from phonetic representations, it is nevertheless assumed that phonological processes (i.e., rules and/or ranked constraints) connect the two levels of representation. The phonological phenomena exemplified here are drawn from fully developed languages, but all of the same points hold as well for the developing phonologies of young children (typical or atypical) and second-language learners.

Phonetic Inventories and Distinctive Features

The International Phonetic Alphabet provides a conventional means for describing and transcribing the set of sounds that can occur in languages. The International Phonetic Alphabet symbols for speech sounds are, however, merely an abbreviation for a bundled complex of distinctive features. The features that are associated with a sound, when taken together, describe that sound, and individual features distinguish one sound from another. For example, the binary feature [+consonantal] is a property of all consonants and distinguishes the class of consonants from vowels and glides. Other features associated with consonants include, but are not limited to, those that relate to laryngeal activity (e.g., [voice], [spread glottis]); consonantal place of articulation (e.g., [labial], [coronal], [dorsal]); and the manner of articulation (e.g., [continuant], [sonorant], [nasal]). Distinctive features associated with vowels include, among others, those that relate to the tongue-body position (e.g., [high], [low], [back]); the configuration of the lips ([round]); and the state of the velum (i.e., lowered for nasal vowels [+nasal] and raised for oral vowels [−nasal]). Distinctive features also serve to identify natural classes of sounds, that is, sounds that share one or more features and are the focal point of a phonological law or generalization. One such generalization that typifies the phonology of Spanish is that all vowels (i.e., all segments that share the feature [−consonantal]) in that language are oral (i.e., [−nasal]). This statement represents a severe restriction on the vowel inventory of Spanish and contributes to the characterization of that language as distinct from other languages such as French, which allows both oral and nasal vowels.

Language-specific considerations largely determine the sounds that are permitted to occur in a particular language. However, phonetic inventories are also further constrained by implicational universals (also known as *markedness relations*). These implicational universals are based on extensive empirical investigations of the world's languages and describe observed typological asymmetries. For example, while some languages might disallow nasal vowels, and other languages allow both oral and nasal vowels, no language permits nasal vowels to occur without also allowing oral vowels to occur in that same language. This means that the occurrence of nasal vowels in a language implies necessarily the occurrence of oral vowels in that language, but not vice versa. Nasal vowels are, thus, considered marked relative to oral vowels, which are unmarked. Marked sounds imply unmarked sounds. Some examples of other similar asymmetries include the following: The occurrence of fricatives in a language implies necessarily the occurrence of stops in that language. The occurrence of voiced obstruents (e.g., stops, fricatives, affricates) implies the occurrence of voiceless obstruents. Voiceless sonorants (e.g., vowels, nasals, liquids) imply the occurrence of voiced sonorants. Aspirated consonants imply unaspirated consonants. Mid-vowels imply high vowels.

Function of Sounds and the Phonemic Inventory

The correspondence between the sounds within words and their associated meanings is arbitrary. Out of all of the sounds that might occur in a language, some of those sounds have the special function of distinguishing the meaning of words. Consider, for example, the two English words *bus* [bʌs] and *buzz* [bʌz]. These words are phonetically identical, except for their final consonants. The meaning difference is signaled solely by the final consonant of these two words. Words such as these constitute a minimal pair and reveal an important unpredictable property of pronunciation in English, namely that the difference between [s] and [z] is contrastive or phonemic, with each sound being a realization of a separate phoneme, namely /s/ and /z/, respectively. English, of course, includes many other sounds that are phonemic, and this can be established by identifying minimal pairs. The phonemic inventory is, however, different from the phonetic inventory. This is because English and other languages include many sounds that do not function to distinguish meaning. That is, some phonemes can have several different phonetic variants that are governed by context.

While phonemes are abstract phonological constructs, they can be reliably inferred from minimal pairs. Also, speakers' perceptual judgments about sounds are more properly judgments about phonemes, rather than the sound itself. Contrastive properties of pronunciation must be learned and, as such, are incorporated segmentally in the underlying (i.e., mental) representation of words in the lexicon on a word-by-word basis.

Distribution of Sounds and Stress: The Special Role of Syllable Structure and Sonority

As noted previously, the function of sounds largely depends on the context in which those sounds occur within words. The consequence is that the same sounds in different languages might function differently, depending on their distributional properties. Compare, for example, the function and distribution of [s] and [z] in English versus Spanish. While these sounds occur in both languages, they exhibit different distributional traits and thus function differently. Recall for English that [s] and [z] can occur in the same position within a word, signaling a difference in meaning (i.e., a minimal pair). However, in Spanish, these two sounds never occur in the same contexts within different words and thus never contrast. In fact, [s] and [z] are in complementary distribution in Spanish, with [z] occurring exclusively before voiced consonants (e.g., before [m], [l], and so on), while [s] occurs elsewhere. This is a typical distributional fact that follows from a characteristic set of phonological processes, that is, an allophonic process. When phonetically similar sounds, such as [s] and [z] in Spanish, occur in complementary distribution, they are judged to be different phonetic realizations (allophones) of one and the same single phoneme. The phonemic inventory of Spanish would, thus, include the phoneme /s/ but not a separate phoneme /z/. Naive native speakers of a language are generally not aware of the phonetic differences between allophones of a single phoneme; yet, they produce the differences systematically in the appropriate context without fail in a lawlike fashion. Allophonic processes are so entrenched in speakers' phonologies that they pose a special problem for second-language learners, who find it especially difficult to suppress those processes when speaking another language.

Many of the generalizations about the distributional restrictions on sounds and rhythmic stress are best captured by appeal to abstract prosodic structures such as syllables and their subconstituents. A syllable is a sequence of hierarchically organized sounds that conforms to a general template that is itself controlled by both language-specific and universal principles. The core syllable of all languages is constituted by an onset consonant followed by a vowel nucleus (e.g., English *boo* [bu]). Consonants can also serve as the nucleus of a syllable in some languages (e.g., English *bottom* [baɾm̩], *shovel* [ʃʌvl̩]). Languages differ in the permissible degrees of complexity associated with the subconstituents of syllables. For example, many West African languages disallow syllable-final coda consonants. Additionally, some languages require that all syllables begin with an onset consonant (e.g., Arabic), but no language requires that all syllables begin with a vowel. Onset-less syllables are thus marked relative to syllables with an onset. Languages also differ by whether they allow consonant clusters in onsets and/or codas. For example, Spanish allows onset clusters but disallows coda clusters. English, on the other hand, allows clusters in both onsets and codas. If a language allows a cluster in the onset or the coda, it will also allow a singleton consonant in that same syllable subconstituent. Clusters are thus marked relative to singleton consonants.

The role of subsyllabic structure is aptly illustrated by Malayalam in the distribution of its allophones for the phoneme /r/. That is, /r/ is palatalized in the onset, syllabic in the nucleus, and a tap in the coda. Syllable edges can also be relevant to the distribution of sounds. For example, in English, voiceless stops are aspirated in syllable-initial position and are unaspirated elsewhere.

While German voiced and voiceless obstruents contrast in syllable onsets, they fail to contrast syllable finally and are uniformly voiceless in that context. The overall shape of syllables can also be relevant to the distribution of sounds. For example, in Mohawk, stressed vowels are always long in open (i.e., Consonant-Vowel, CV) syllables. In some dialects of Spanish, closed (i.e., CVC) syllables cause mid-vowels to be realized as lax, while they are tense elsewhere.

Syllables and their internal structure also play a significant role in predicting the location of primary and secondary word stress in many languages. For example, heavy syllables (i.e., closed syllables or syllables with a long vowel) tend to attract stress (e.g., Sierra Miwok, English). Conversely, stressed vowels in open syllables tend to lengthen, making the syllable heavy (e.g., Mohawk). In some languages, stress is distributed to multiple syllables within a word in an alternating pattern, for example, stressed–unstressed–stressed–unstressed. Such patterns reveal higher order prosodic structure whereby syllables are grouped into one or more binary feet that are either iambic (unstressed–stressed) or trochaic (stressed–unstressed).

The internal composition of syllables is further restricted by sonority considerations. To demonstrate this, consider the widely held universal scale, which rank orders speech sounds in terms of relative sonority, with vowels being most sonorous and obstruents being least sonorous. Between these extremes, glides are less sonorous than vowels but more sonorous than liquid consonants, which are in turn more sonorous than nasal consonants. In the physical realm, this rank ordering associates high sonority with low intraoral air pressure and high acoustic energy as would occur with a vocal tract configuration that allows for continuous, relatively unrestricted airflow and spontaneous vocal cord vibration. Conversely, low sonority correlates with high intraoral air pressure and low acoustic energy. Taking advantage of this scale, the nucleus of a syllable will be the most sonorous element, and the onset and coda (if present) will be less sonorous. Sonority further constrains the sequential order of the onset by favoring a sequence of consonants that rises in sonority as it approaches the nucleus. On the other hand, a cluster of consonants in the coda tends to fall in sonority going away from the nucleus.

Languages can impose further restrictions on the sonority profile of onset clusters that go beyond the requirement that they must rise in sonority, and those restrictions have implications for the range of permissible clusters in that language. For example, some languages (e.g., Mono, Panobo) require that the first and second segments of the onset must differ in sonority as much as possible. This means that an onset cluster consisting of an obstruent followed by a glide (e.g., [kw]) would be permissible, but all other onset clusters with smaller sonority differences (e.g., *[kl], *[kn], *[nw], *[lw]) would be prohibited. Other languages (e.g., Greek) allow clusters consisting of segments that differ minimally in sonority (e.g., [pn]) along with those that involve larger sonority differences. English is somewhere between these two extremes, allowing onset clusters that differ by at least two or more steps on the sonority scale (e.g., [kl], [kw], [mj] as permissible but not *[kn], *[nl]). The implicational universal that captures these patterns states that the occurrence of an onset cluster with a small sonority difference in a given language entails the occurrence of clusters with a larger sonority difference in that same language, but not vice versa. Onset clusters with large sonority differences are thus less marked (and acquired earlier) than clusters with smaller sonority differences.

The sonority scale also reflects a series of implicational universals regarding the range of permissible singleton segments in syllable onsets and syllable codas. Languages prefer less sonorous sounds in onsets, with the scale reversed for codas, preferring more sonorous sounds in codas. The implicational relationship for onsets is such that, if a language allows an onset with some high degree of sonority, it will also allow onsets with lesser degrees of sonority. For codas, the implicational relationships are just the reverse. That is, the occurrence of low sonority codas in a language implies the occurrence of more sonorous codas in that language.

Finally, it is generally assumed that syllable boundaries are entirely predictable. Given a CVCV sequence in any language, that sequence will be parsed as two open syllables (i.e., CV.CV) and not as a closed syllable followed by an onset-less open syllable (i.e., *CVC.V). The fact is that no language distinguishes the meaning of words by syllabification alone.

Behavior of Sounds and Associated Phonological Processes

The underlying internalized representation of a sound is often forced to change in its phonetic realization, depending on the context in which it occurs. The relevant contexts tend to include immediately adjacent sounds or syllables or are restricted by the sound's position within the word or syllable. These changes are attributed to phonological processes (i.e., rules or ranked constraints, depending on theoretical framework). Segmental phonological processes are either allophonic (i.e., accounting for the complementary distribution of sounds) or neutralizing (i.e., accounting for the merger or loss of a contrast in a limited, well-defined context). Many times, the change involves the sound taking on properties of the adjacent sound, resulting in either regressive or progressive assimilation. Some common regressive assimilation processes include the following: Nasal consonants often adopt the place of articulation of a following consonant (e.g., nasal assimilation in Spanish and Japanese). Vowels nasalize before nasal consonants (e.g., English). Obstruents take on the voicing of the following obstruent (e.g., Catalan). Other feature-changing processes can be nonassimilatory, and those processes are often restricted by the position within a word or syllable, for example, syllable-final obstruent devoicing in Dutch, syllable-initial aspiration in English, word-final syllable stress in French, and word-initial syllable stress in Finnish.

Certain other types of changes are brought about by insertion and/or deletion processes. For example, many speakers of English will, in casual speech, delete the unstressed vowel schwa [ə] between consonants, yielding clusters such as [kr], [vl], [pr], and [ml]. For example, the parenthesized vowel in the following spoken English words is unstressed and can be deleted: "c(o)rrect," "env(e)lope," "sep(a)rate," and "fam(i)ly." This deletion process, however, is further constrained by sonority considerations: Deletion is possible if and only if the resultant consonant cluster rises in sonority. To illustrate, consider the following English words where the capitalized vowel is unstressed, but it cannot be deleted because the process would yield a cluster with falling sonority: "pirAting" (*[rt]), "monItor" (*[nt]), and "melOdy" (*[ld]).

The most compelling evidence that a sound has undergone a change due to an active phonological process comes from observed alternations in the realization of a morpheme (i.e., the smallest meaningful unit of a word). When morphemes at the underlying level of representation are strung together to form a word, novel contexts are often created for the sounds at the edges of those adjacent morphemes. The resultant combinations of sounds in those contexts may be phonetically impermissible in the language and will require a change. Phonological processes can intervene to convert the abstract-internalized underlying sequence into something pronounceable for that language. Consider, for example, the three different phonetic realizations (i.e., allomorphs) of the English plural morpheme in the following representative words: "dogs" [dɔgz], "cats" [kʰæts], and "buses" [bʌsəz]. Assuming for the moment that the underlying internalized representation for the plural morpheme is /-z/, at least one issue arises immediately and is common to the impermissible sequences in /kæt-z/ and /bʌs-z/, namely that the word-final /z/ is preceded by a voiceless consonant. This is a universally impermissible sequence for a syllable coda. More specifically, once vocal fold vibration ceases following the nucleus, voicing cannot resume within the same syllable. There are several logically possible remedies for this, but English adopts a relatively simple and efficient strategy. A process of progressive devoicing is invoked that spreads the voicelessness of the preceding /t/ to the final /z/ of /kæt-z/ to yield a final [s] in the output [kʰæts]. This process does not apply to /bʌs-z/ because it would not result in an improvement inasmuch as English does not allow geminates syllable internally. Instead, English invokes a process of schwa insertion to break up the geminate cluster yielding the output [bʌsəz]. The insertion process in this instance allows the [voice] feature of the plural morpheme to be retained, being realized phonetically in the same way it is represented underlyingly.

Returning to the rationale behind the assumption about the plural morpheme's underlying representation, the discovery of the substance of any morpheme's underlying representation is aided by looking for its realization in a context where no phonological processes are operative, namely a context that reveals the contrastive unpredictable properties of pronunciation. Recall that voiced and voiceless obstruents contrast word finally in English when preceded by a vowel. Since no processes are operative in that context, evidence about the underlying representation of the plural morpheme would, therefore, be provided by the plural of a noun ending in a vowel, for example, "peas" [pʰijz] (cf., contrasting form "piece" [pʰijs]).

The variation associated with the plural morpheme of English is not an isolated phenomenon nor is it morphologically restricted. Instead, the variation is a consequence of an empirically motivated assumption about the morpheme's underlying representation and two independently motivated phonological processes that convert that underlying representation into its various allomorphs. Those same processes and same considerations for establishing the substance of underlying representations hold for the variation associated with certain other morphemes in English. For example, the realization of the past tense morpheme for verbs can be assumed to be represented underlyingly as /-d/, for example, "bagged" [bægd], "walked" [wɔkt], and "fitted" [fɪrəd]. Also, in English, the third-person singular morpheme for verbs and the possessive morpheme for nouns exhibit exactly the same variation as the plural morpheme and are likewise represented underlyingly as /-z/.

Contemporary Theoretical Models

As a final note, phonological research has been guided by rapidly evolving theories of grammar, especially since the 1960s with the Chomskyan revolution and the move away from behaviorism and taxonomic phonemics. The vast majority of the available descriptive studies of the world's languages have been conducted within the rule-based linear and nonlinear frameworks of Generative Phonology and have served to evaluate and refine the theory. Despite the many significant advances that emerged from those theoretical innovations, new questions arose that eluded explanation. Some perplexing questions were related to why many of the same phonological processes occur in genetically unrelated languages, why young children in the early stages of acquisition often exhibit phonological processes that have no basis in the language they are acquiring, how markedness considerations can be incorporated into phonological processes, and what mechanism is available to capture the functional unity of different phonological processes. Answers to these and other questions began to come to light in the mid-1990s with the advent of the revolutionary constraint-based framework known as *Optimality Theory*. The architecture of Optimality Theory does away with phonological rules and appeals instead to universal, violable constraints that are rank ordered on the basis of language-specific evidence. As findings continue to unfold, other new questions are certain to arise and lead to further refinements of phonological theory.

Daniel A. Dinnsen

See also Markedness; Optimality Theory; Phoneme; Phonological Processes; Sonority; Syllable

Further Readings

Anderson, S. R. (1981). Why phonology isn't "Natural." *Linguistic Inquiry, 12*, 493–539.

Barlow, J. A. (2016). Sonority in acquisition: A review. In M. J. Ball (Ed.), *Challenging sonority: Cross-linguistic evidence from normal and disordered language* (pp. 295–336). London, UK: Equinox.

Dinnsen, D. A., & Gierut, J. A. (2008). *Optimality theory, phonological acquisition and disorders. Advances in optimality theory*. London, UK: Equinox.

Goldsmith, J., Riggle, J., & Yu, A. (2011). *Handbook of phonological theory* (2nd ed.). Hoboken, NJ: Wiley-Blackwell.

Kager, R. (1999). *Optimality theory*. Cambridge, UK: Cambridge University Press.

Kenstowicz, M. (1994). *Phonology in generative grammar*. Hoboken, NJ: Wiley-Blackwell.

Physiological Basis of Hearing

An understanding of the normal physiology of hearing allows an understanding of hearing loss and its differential diagnosis, and of the normal and abnormal perception of speech and music. This entry explores the normal physiology of hearing with an overview of the acoustic roles of the outer ear (pinna and ear canal), the middle ear (three bones, two muscles, tendons, and ligaments), and the spiraling cochlea of the inner ear, as well as a brief description of the neural circuitry of the brainstem and higher auditory centers (Figure 1).

The Role of the Outer Ear

Each external ear (*pinna*) collects sound and funnels it into the ear canal (the *external auditory meatus*), amplifying sound about 3-fold (i.e.,

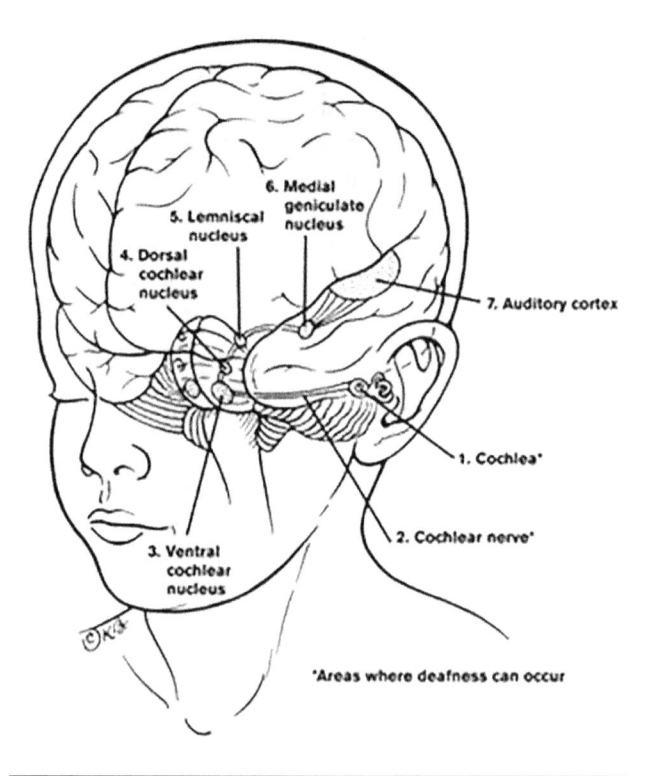

Figure 1 Sound is partly amplified and processed by the frequency- and direction-dependent reflections within the external pinnae, before further amplification and filtering through the ear canal and middle ear. Even more amplification and processing within the cochlea is due to the place-dependent active mechanical resonances along the cochlear partition. The highly tuned vibration of the organ of Corti is detected by inner and outer hair cells (IHC and OHC), with OHCs canceling friction and IHCs detecting the vibration and transmitting it to the central nervous system via the release of glutamate onto the primary afferent dendrites. Action potentials (APs) travel along the auditory nerve to the brainstem and higher centers, where the information is processed by many neural networks working in parallel and specialized to analyze different aspects of the incoming sound

10 decibel [dB] at 6 kilohertz [kHz] depending on direction), with the acoustic funneling of the ear canal amplifying a further 3-fold (i.e., 10 dB). This amplification of the outer ear adds to the amplifications of the middle ear (about 30 dB near 1 kHz) and organ of Corti (about 60 dB). The outer ears and their placement on the side of the head also serve a role in directional hearing. When listening to sound in *free-field* (rather than *dichotic* listening through headphones), the lateral (i.e., left–right) direction of the sound is conveyed partly by the difference in the arrival time of sound at the two ears (the *interaural time difference* at high and low frequencies is about 750ms from the side), and partly by the *interaural intensity difference* (IID or ILD; at most 15 dB from the side). The IID is only present for high frequencies where the head produces an acoustic shadow. At low frequencies, sound diffracts around the head, no acoustic shadow is produced, and sound level is the same on both sides (so some stereos have a single bass speaker). Above 6 kHz, there are also monaural directional cues for the front–back (azimuth) and up–down (elevation) sound location, available at each ear independently, due to the complex reflections within the folds of each pinna. These reflections produce narrowband notch filtering that changes with direction (the *head-related transfer function*, simulated in computer gaming to produce 3-D hearing). This is important in aging and hearing aids because (a) a hearing loss can remove the high-frequency cues, producing *the cocktail party effect*; (b) some aids do not transmit very high frequencies or occlude the pinna's folds with their ear mold, and/or (c) some aids introduce intensity and timing changes (e.g., software latencies). The pinnae in some nonhuman mammals are also highly mobile and can act as steerable reflectors. While the human pinnae are not highly mobile, the *post-auricular muscles* attached to them do respond to even soft sounds, and this reflex response can be measured electrically and used as an assay of hearing sensitivity (the *post-auricular muscle reflex*).

The Role of the Middle Ear

Normal hearing requires that sound produces normal vibration in the cochlea, and this can occur inefficiently through vibration of the whole skull (*bone conduction*, which contains no directional cues), or 200-fold (+46 dB) more efficiently by vibration of the tympanum and middle ear ossicles (*air conduction*). This explains how an audiometric comparison of bone conduction and air conduction sensitivities helps diagnose middle ear conditions or cochlear and retrocochlear issues by exclusion. Total immobility of the middle ear bones with infection or ossification produces at most a 45-dB *conductive hearing loss*, but a larger loss of 55 dB occurs, when the connection between the tympanum and stapes is broken completely by bone dislocation (e.g., head trauma) or bone erosion (e.g., bacterial infection). Importantly, inefficient bone conduction still stimulates an otherwise normal cochlea, providing normal analysis and perception.

The middle ear also serves other roles, including partial protection of the cochlea from trauma, infection, acoustic overload, and slow but large environmental pressure changes. Its main role, however, is to match the acoustic properties of sound in air (i.e., small forces against a low impedance producing large movement) to those in the more dense water within the cochlea (i.e., higher forces against higher impedances producing smaller movements). Without this transformer action, significant reflection of sound would occur at a direct air-water interface, reducing the efficiency of hearing. This acoustic matching uses four different mechanisms: acoustic funneling of the ear canal; coupling of in-and-out drum movement to torsion of the malleus; a difference in the areas of the tympanum and stapes footplate; and different lever ratios of the malleus, incus, and stapes. The middle ear also contains two muscles that attenuate low-frequency sound when they contract: The stapedius muscle stiffens the stapes and is controlled by the facial nerve, and tensor tympani muscle stiffens the tympanum and is controlled by the medial pterygoid branch of the trigeminal nerve. Contrary to popular belief, both muscles are not very effective in protecting against either prolonged sounds (adapting within minutes) or transient sounds or impulses (sound passes before either muscle contracts). Moreover, the two muscles serve different roles: the stapedius contraction is a simple reflex response to high-intensity (low-frequency) sound, while tensor tympani either contracts before self-vocalization, or with startle or stress, so there is not one middle ear reflex but two. This is important because prior stressful exposure to sound can produce overactivity in tensor tympani, and its hyperresponsiveness to sound (and other stimuli) can sometimes produce ear pain, leading to more stress, and a vicious cycle known as *tonic tensor tympani syndrome* or *acoustic shock*.

The middle ear also helps reject very slow pressure changes that could overwhelm the cochlea's detection processes. Overall, five mechanisms reject these slow fluctuations: (1) a functional Eustachian tube from the nose to the middle ear keeps middle ear air pressure near surrounding air pressure, so that the tympanum responds to only sound; (2) the slip joint between malleus and incus in humans prevents large and slow movements of the drum from overdriving the stapes; (3) the *helicotrema* shunts slow fluid pressure fluctuations; (4) IHCs are insensitive to slow movements because their hair bundles are viscously coupled to the overlying tectorial membrane; and (5) other mechanisms like OHC motility allow the cochlea to adapt to slow changes. Too large a slow movement of the stapes can tear the annular ligament that supports it, producing a leak of cochlear fluid (i.e., *perilymphatic fistula*, as in barotrauma from diving, pressure blasts, or head trauma), which produces a sensorineural hearing loss due to cochlear disruption, and a conductive loss due to flooding of the middle ear.

The Role of the Cochlea and Its Organ of Corti

The cochlea is a 35 mm spiraling bony shell, mostly filled with the sodium-rich fluid perilymph, and divided along almost its complete length by the cochlear partition (filled with potassium-rich endolymph). Researchers saw the cochlear spiral as three parallel staircases (from the Latin *scalae*), ascending from the cochlear base to its apex: One staircase ascended from the entry hall or vestibule behind the oval window (scala vestibuli), one ascended from behind the round window looking out at the ear drum (scala tympani), and a third sat in the middle of the first two (scala media). The middle structure surrounding scala media is called the cochlear partition. There is a gap called the *helicotrema* (Greek for "coil hole") at the apex of the cochlear spiral, just after the partition comes to a blind end. The helicotrema joins the two perilymph-filled chambers of scala vestibuli and scala tympani and shunts very low-frequency pressures. The cochlear partition itself has a triangular cross section, bounded by its three main walls: the flimsy Reissner's membrane separating scala vestibuli and scala media, the cochlear bony wall covered by the vascular ion pumping epithelium of stria vascularis, and the vibrating basilar membrane, with the organ of Corti perched upon it. The organ of Corti includes stretch-sensitive hair cells, named for the stiff microvilli-like protrusions from their apical surface called *stereocilia*. The two types of cochlear hair cell (i.e., IHCs and OHCs) are named due to their radial position relative to the central neural core of the cochlea, the modiolus. The stereocilia are surrounded by the K+-rich endolymph in scala media which is at an unusual +95 millivolts (mV). Both the fluid and the voltage (the endocochlear potential) are created by stria vascularis.

There are about 20 primary auditory neurones (Type I afferents) coupling each IHC to the auditory brainstem, with a total of about 10,000 auditory nerve fiber per ear with one fiber per *secure* synapse. A secure synapse is one where each quantum of glutamate transmitter released produces a single excitatory postsynaptic potential, which initiates a single AP. This means that the spontaneous firing rate of afferent neurones is normally determined by the spontaneous release of vesicles of glutamate, itself determined by intracellular Ca^{2+} levels, determined by the hair cell membrane potential. The stochastic nature of the vesicular release means that AP firing is also stochastic or randomized (and private to each synapse), unless a periodicity is forced onto the release by incoming sound. This randomization of neural firing helps higher neurones to average across the population of primary afferent neurones, lowering the noise floor of the system, and also avoids a regular neural firing due to membrane properties being interpreted as the pitch of a sound.

The fast parallel processing of the many auditory brainstem circuits allows humans to respond in a reflexive way to auditory cues (within tens of milliseconds), without any delay introduced by thought (the analysis by higher neural centers at the auditory cortex and beyond that takes a fraction of a second). Although the OHCs are also connected to the brainstem through only 5% of the afferents (Type II afferents), these are unmyelinated fibers, probably serving a homeostatic role.

In any case, in a normal ear, sound vibrates the ear drum and middle ear bones, causing vibration of the stapes footplate, pressure fluctuations in the cochlear fluids, and vibration of the *basilar membrane*. Longitudinal sound waves in free fluid travel at 1500 m/s and distribute within the cochlea in microseconds, so their wavelengths are far longer than any cochlear structures, including its coiling. Importantly, the sound vibration detected by the stretch-sensitive hair cells is *not* the longitudinal waves in the fluid, but the transverse *interface wave* subsequently produced along the cochlear partition (Georg von *Békésy's* traveling waves). Just like longitudinal pressure waves in the bulk water of a pond travel near 1500 m/s, while the transverse surface ripples travel more slowly, the transverse cochlear waves mostly travel slowly away from the stapes toward the cochlear apex. The travel away from the stapes is not because vibration is introduced at the stapes (vibrations through the cochlear wall do the same). It occurs because the cochlear partition is resonant at higher frequencies in the base and responds with less delay than in the apex. If the apex were stiffer than the base, the direction of travel would be reversed. For a *pure-tone* stimulus of a particular frequency, the wave's amplitude grows as it travels from base to apex, before reaching a maximum at its resonant *characteristic place*. Beyond that it collapses abruptly so that no vibration exists beyond its *cutoff region*. This characteristic place is positioned along the cochlear length according to a species-specific, logarithmic, *place-frequency or tonotopic map* (higher frequencies toward the cochlear base and lower frequencies closer to the cochlear apex). The map has a slope of about 1.5 mm/octave in gerbils, 2.5 mm/octave in guinea pigs, and about 4.8 mm/octave in humans, which is relevant to cochlear implants. The mapping is largely determined by the grading in stiffness of the cochlear partition, which has evolved to avoid reflections that would be confusing and limit timing resolution (interaural time difference) and directional hearing.

One important clinical aspect of vibration is that a normal cochlea produces very slight reflections from small imperfections along its length. Originally known as Kemp echoes, they are now called transient evoked otoacoustic emissions, are idiosyncratic of any individual, are delayed according to their cochlear site of origin and therefore frequency, and are measured in the ear canal by a sensitive but quiet microphone as a rapid screening test for normal OHCs and vibration. As an aside, there is little direct coupling between adjacent segments along the cochlear partition, so the traveling waves should *not* be thought of as a rug being shaken near the stapes, producing waves that travel apically through the rug itself. A better analogy is a series of boats moored side by side, with vibration transferred through the water supporting them. If a section of a rug were immobilized, the vibration could travel no further, but if a single boat were immobilized, the wave would simply bypass it and continue downstream. This difference is important clinically because immobilizing the cochlear partition in the base (e.g., with scar tissue) produces a high-frequency hearing loss in the base but not a low-frequency hearing loss more apically.

It is useful to consider two ways of representing this vibration pattern (Figure 2A): a *panoramic view* where one imagines looking through the cochlear wall at the entire traveling wave produced by a pure tone of a fixed frequency, or a *local view* where one imagines looking through a keyhole in the cochlear wall at the response at one location along the cochlear length. The response at a single observation site can be the vibration amplitude in nanometer, the hair cell response in millivolt (mV), or the neural firing rate in AP/s. Whichever, the local view can be plotted as a *frequency tuning curve* or *frequency threshold curve* (FTC) in two ways: as the response amplitude for a fixed sound level at different frequencies (iso-input) or the sound level required for a fixed response (iso-output). For very low frequencies (the *low-frequency tail*), the traveling wave races past one's observation site at high speed but low amplitude (like a tsunami out at sea), so high sound levels are needed to reach a fixed amplitude (Point A of Figure 2B). Conversely, for very high-frequency tones, the traveling wave collapses before it reaches one's observation site, and so no amount of sound produces vibration (Point C of Figure 2B). Finally, near the Characteristic frequency (CF) of one's observation site, the

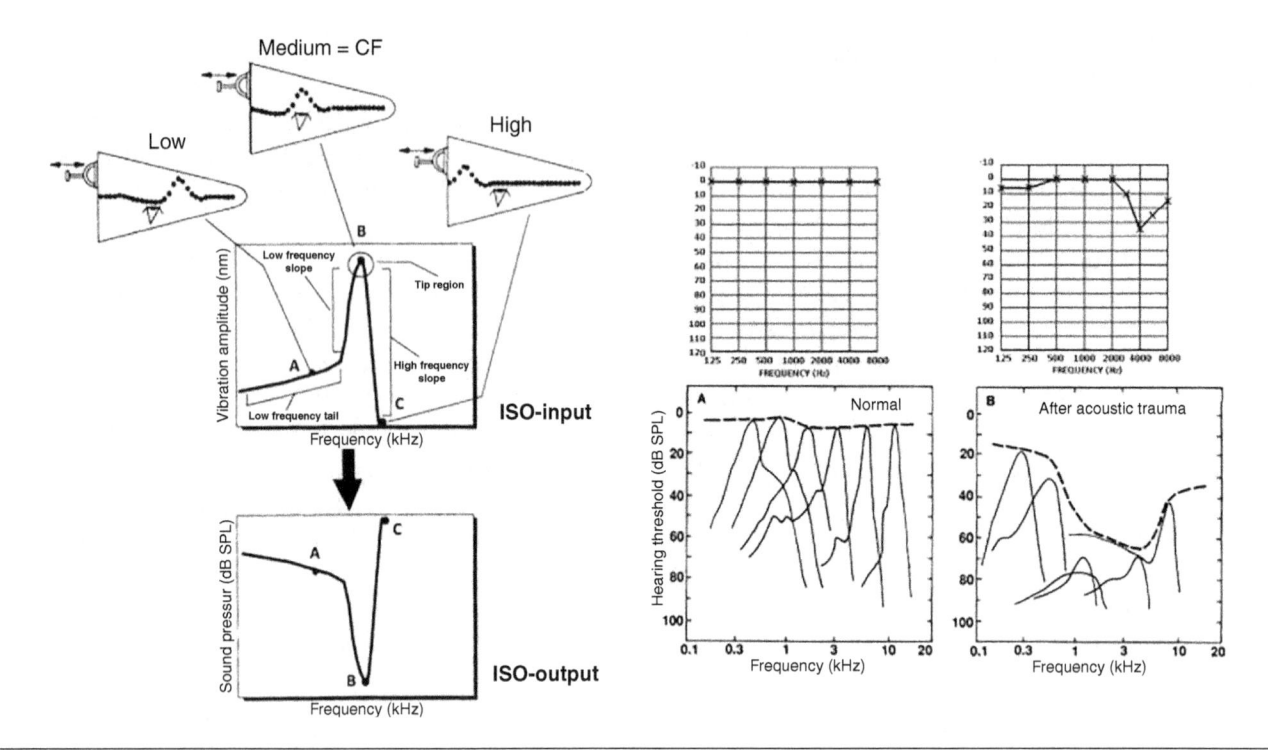

Figure 2 (A) The resonant or tuned vibration of the organ of Corti can be summarized as a panoramic view of the entire length of the basilar membrane in response to sound of different frequencies (upper icons) or as a local view of the vibration of a particular location along the cochlea as a function stimulus frequency (lower curves). This local view can itself be presented as the vibration amplitude for sound at a fixed level (middle iso-input frequency tuning curve or FTC) or as the sound required to produce a fixed vibration amplitude (lowest iso-output FTC). (B) All of the individual iso-output FTCs for the afferent neurones representing neural threshold can be plotted (upside down compared to the lowest FTC in A), and the sensitive tips of the complete set of FTCs determine a person's full clinical audiogram (upper panel). (C) If OHCs are disrupted, vibration and neural FTCs are less sensitive and blunted, and the clinical audiogram is lowered in that region (upper panel illustrating an industrial noise notch)

vibration is resonant and large, and very little sound is required (the so-called tip of the FTC; Point B of Figure 2B). The neural FTC can be thought of as the *audiogram* of a single auditory neurone, with the full clinical audiogram skimming over the tips of the complete set of neural FTCs (Figure 2C).

The Dual Role of Hair Cells

Detecting the vibration of the cochlear partition is the task of the two types of vibration-sensitive hair cells: the IHCs that lie in a single row along the cochlear length and synapse with about 95% of the primary afferent neurones (Type I afferents) and the OHCs that lie in three or four parallel rows, outnumber the IHCs almost 3–1, and synapse with only 5% of the afferent neurones (Type II afferents). The transverse (up–down) vibration of the Organ of Corti (OC) (Point 1 of Figure 3) produces a radial shearing between its tectorial membrane and reticular lamina, and ultimately a deflection of the hair bundles at the hair cell apex, leading to the opening and closing of *mechanoelectrical transduction* (MET) *channels* near the tip of each stereocilium (about 300 channels per cell). This modulates the electrical resistance of the hair cell apex (Points 2 and 2' of Figure 3), and because there is a voltage across the apical membrane of the hair cells which drives K⁺ ions into the cells from endolymph, there is a fluctuation in the K⁺ current through the hair cells known as their *receptor current*. The driving voltage (110 mV for IHCs and 170 mV for OHCs) is made up of two components: the +95 mV Electric Potential (EP) in scala media, and each hair cell's

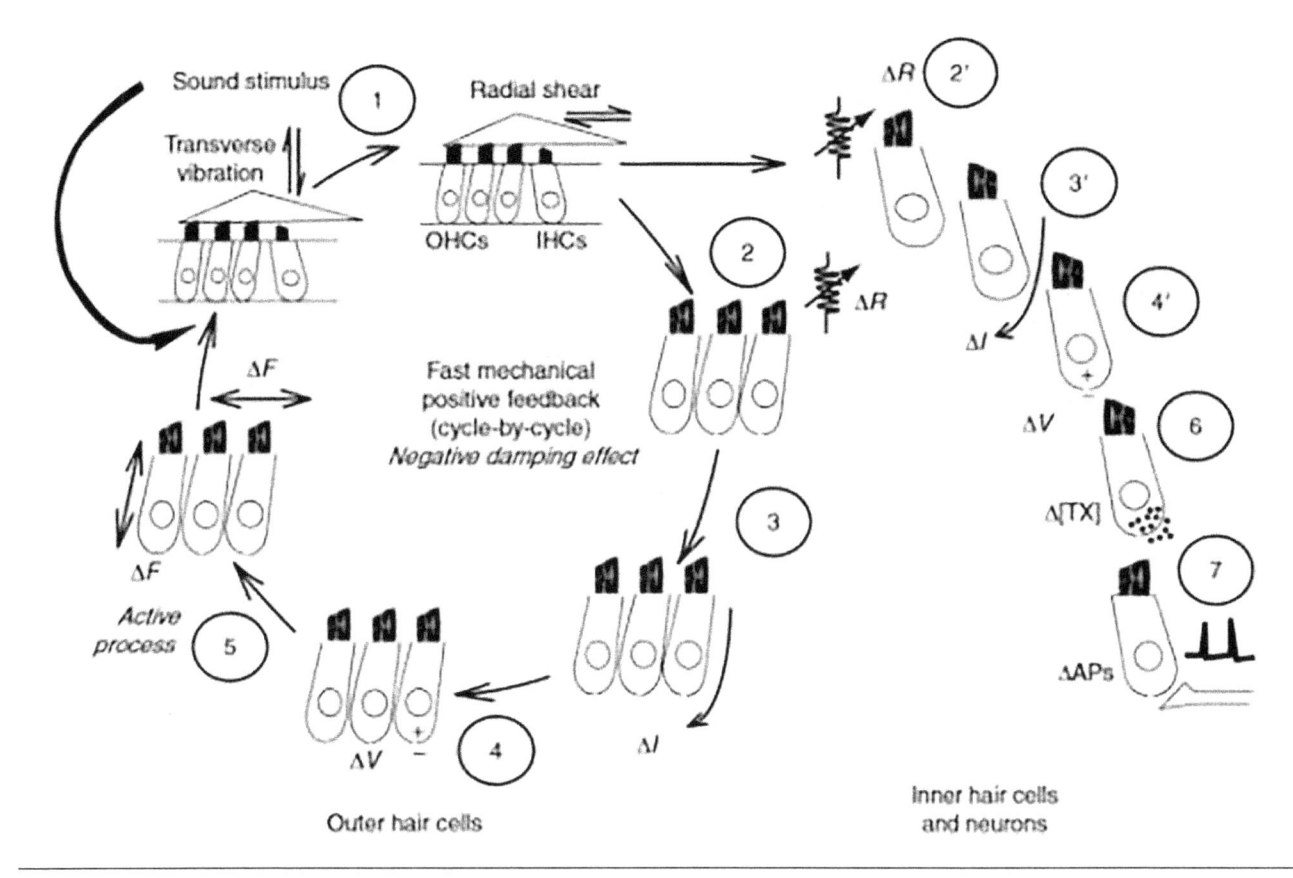

Figure 3 The stages of transduction of the cochlea. (1) Transverse OC vibration transformed to radial shear between tectorial membrane and reticular lamina which deflects hair bundles; (2) bending of hair bundles modulates resistance of the apical membrane of hair cells (mechanoelectrical transduction or MET); (3) modulation of hair cell apical resistance modulates the K+ receptor current through the cells; (4) fluctuating receptor current produces a fluctuating receptor potential within the hair cells, which (5) in OHCs produces cell length changes and hair bundle movement, and (6) neurotransmitter release from inner hair cells and (7) neural firing. The OHC processes can be called *motor processes*, while the inner hair cell and neural processes can be called *sensory processes*

membrane potential (about −40 mV in IHCs and −70 mV in OHCs). Because the hair cell membrane potential is maintained by each cells' own metabolic resources, even complete failure of stria vascularis (e.g., with a stroke) does not necessarily produce profound deafness. Importantly, the rise and fall of receptor current during a cycle of a tone is governed by the highly nonlinear *MET channel transfer function* (current vs. hair bundle displacement; see icons in Figure 3). This MET transfer curve is highly asymmetric for all IHCs and apical turn OHCs but symmetric for basal turn OHCs. This means that for all but basal turn OHCs, a sustained tone produces not only a cyclic fluctuation in receptor current (the *AC* receptor), but a net increase in receptor current during a tone (the *DC* receptor). The near-symmetry of the MET transfer curve of basal turn OHCs, however, means that they produce very little DC receptor current, which has implications for both high-frequency hearing and electrodiagnosis. The receptor currents (Points 3 and 3' of Figure 3) produce *receptor potentials* within hair cells that depend on the electrical properties of each cell's basolateral wall (Points 4 and 4' of Figure 3), which contain an assortment of K^+ channels (some act to stabilize membrane potential, while others are controlled by efferent neurones from the brainstem's medial olivocochlear system). The AC and DC components of the receptor potentials open voltage-sensitive Ca^{2+} channels that control the flow of Ca^{+2} into the hair cells, which then control the quantal release of the main hair cell neurotransmitter (glutamate) at the primary auditory synapses. This opens glutamate-sensitive postsynaptic receptors, allowing the transient flow of Na⁺ into the auditory dendrites, producing excitatory postsynaptic potentials within the dendrites which trigger APs that propagate through the *internal auditory meatus* and *dura mater* to the *cochlear nuclei* of the *auditory brainstem*. A set of efferent neurones from the brainstem's lateral olivocochlear system also synapses on the dendrites, possibly stabilizing dendritic membrane potential and initiation of APs. The hair cell receptor currents, the dendritic currents, and the currents producing APs all produce extracellular potentials measured at or near the round window during *electrocochleography*.

Active Enhancement of Vibration of the Organ of Corti

While the receptor potentials within IHCs and OHCs control neurotransmitters (Point 6 of Figure 3) and spiking in afferent neurones (Point 7 of Figure 3), OHC receptor potentials also flex a set of *motor proteins* (*prestin*) arranged on the inside surface of the OHC basolateral wall. Only 0.5 mV depolarization of IHCs is enough to increase glutamate release and AP firing so a sound is heard. There is so much prestin that the receptor potential changes the OHC length (*electromotility*; although similar forces arise from the hair bundles themselves; Point 5 of Figure 3). Because the opening of MET channels is synchronous with the sound vibration, the receptor current and receptor potential also increase and decrease through a cycle of a tone, so that neurotransmitter release, neural firing, and OHC length do too. This cycle-by-cycle fluctuation of cell length is crucial to normal vibration. Just as a child on a swing moves his or her legs back and forth at the swing's natural frequency to increase the oscillation by canceling friction in the hinge, the OHCs act to cancel friction and increase vibration of the OC. In a normal cochlea, the vibration is increased about 1,000-fold (60 dB) relative to the vibration without OHC help. This cancelation of friction is called *negative damping*, and the combination of

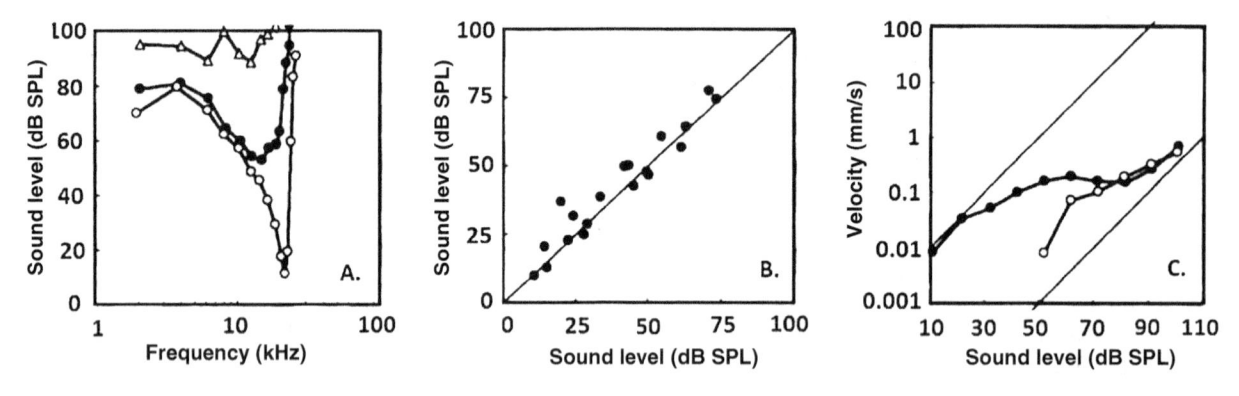

Figure 4 (A) Vibration of the organ of Corti (here at the 18 kHz location in a guinea pig) is normally highly sensitive and sharply tuned (open circles), but it is also labile, becoming less sensitive and more broadly tuned if OHCs are disrupted (black circles). Loss of sensitivity is most pronounced near the FTC tip because that is where OHCs are most effective. With more trauma IHCs and neurones are also disrupted, and the entire FTC is elevated (open triangles). (B) A drop in the sensitivity of neurons is often explained by a drop in mechanical sensitivity (sound level for just detectable neural response on vertical axis; sound level for just detectable vibration response [0.35 nm] on horizontal axis). (C) Because the modulation of the apical resistance of OHCs is not proportional to hair bundle deflection, the generation of OHC receptor current and OHC length changes are limited at higher sound levels. This produces a nonlinear growth of OC vibration with increase in sound level at each cochlear location at that locations resonance frequency (growth rate near 0.2 dB/dB). After trauma and disruption of OHCs, vibration is passive, less sensitive, and more proportional (open circles; 1 dB/dB). This produces an abnormally rapid growth in loudness perception called *recruitment*

the *forward transduction* (i.e., vibration to receptor potential) and *reverse transduction* (i.e., receptor potential to force) is called the *active process*. Because the sensitivity of any resonant movement is inversely proportional to the net friction, the sensitivity of the enhanced vibration at CF depends crucially on the active process and its negative damping: the 1,000-fold enhancement observed requires that friction is almost entirely cancelled (0.1% remaining), and this also means that normal hearing is highly sensitive to OHC disruption (producing a *sensorineural hearing loss*; see Figure 4). A small 20% drop in the receptor current through OHCs can reduce the vibration sensitivity 10-fold (i.e., a 20-dB hearing loss), and a 50% drop can produce a 100-fold drop in hearing sensitivity (i.e., a 40-dB hearing loss). This also means that slight nonlinear aspects of OHC transduction (i.e., distortion) produce disproportional growth of vibration amplitude with sound level (Figure 4C), and dramatic interactions between two sounds presented simultaneously. Vibration is about 0.3 nm at threshold, and above 100 nm hearing loss occurs: Human hearing is a miracle of sensitivity, not of robustness.

The Cochlea's Coding of Timing, Intensity, and Frequency

The quantal release of the glutamate neurotransmitter from hair cells onto afferent dendrites occurs stochastically in silence (due to the standing Ca^{2+} inflow near each synapse), and this Ca^{2+} inflow and transmitter release is modulated by sound. With low-frequency sound (<2 kHz) in all cochlear regions, the hair cell receptor potential and stochastic neural firing can rise and fall through a cycle of a tone, and this is called *phase-locking* or *volleying*. In the high-frequency regions, however, any high-frequency sound (>2 kHz) produces a receptor potential with a prominent DC component but only a small AC component because of the low-pass electrical filtering of the receptor potential by the sluggish charge/discharge of the hair cell's basolateral wall. This means that for high frequencies the stochastic release rate increases progressively with sound intensity to a maximum near 400/s, with minimal cycle-by-cycle fluctuation. This means that human perception of pitch occurs by two different mechanisms. For high frequencies, the steady neural firing during a tone makes it impossible for the central nervous system to decode frequency based on the timing of a cyclic rise and fall of firing rate, and pitch perception relies entirely on which neurones are stimulated. This is called the *place principle* of pitch detection. The decoding of which neurones are firing requires neural networks to compare the firing across the whole neural population. For low frequencies, however, there is not only information conveyed by the place of neural firing, but the firing rate of each neurone rises and falls cyclically during the tone (called *volleying*), and the interval between the peaks and dips of firing allows the detection of pitch by neural networks in the brainstem (known as *periodicity pitch*). At intermediate frequencies, both place and periodicity information are available, and both are used.

The synapse between IHCs and afferent dendrites also plays a role in improving the analysis of sound. For a high-frequency tone burst that turns on and off abruptly, the DC receptor potential in IHCs rises rapidly to its steady-state level over about 1 ms (due to the hair cell's electrical properties) and remains there during the tone (i.e., the receptor potential does not adapt). However, the release of neurotransmitter does adapt, due to the transmitter storage and release mechanisms within hair cells: Initially, there is a burst of transmitter at the onset of the sound that adapts within milliseconds to a lower steady-state release rate during the tone. At the end of the tone, the transmitter release falls to a very low level (zero at some synapses) before recovering to the synapse's normal spontaneous rate. These synaptic properties enhance the transients in the incoming sound (helping timing circuits in the brainstem) and also compress the range of sustained neural firing rates, helping other brainstem circuits that analyze intensity and frequency content.

Nonlinear Growth of Vibration Amplitude With Sound Intensity

The clipping of OHC receptor current and feedback forces at high sound levels (i.e., *saturation feedback*) not only allows the cochlea to compress a 1,000,000:1 range of sound level into a 100:1 range of vibration, but it creates two-tone interactions: *low-frequency intermodulation* (i.e., sensitivity fluctuates through a cycle of low-frequency tones), *two-tone suppression* at higher frequencies (i.e., vibration due to one tone is reduced by the presence of another), and *distortion product generation* (i.e., two tones produce other tones). Two simultaneous tones at frequencies f1 and f2 produce distortion product otoacoustic emissions (DPOAEs) at f2–f1 (the quadratic distortion tone) and 2 f1–f2 (the cubic distortion tone). Normal DPOAEs measured in the ear canal indicate normal OHCs and vibration and explain musical harmony: For only some musical ratios of f1/f2 are the DPOAEs part of a stable chord. Because the DPOAEs are disrupted by any pathology that disrupts OHC function (the motor processes), they can also be used for objective hearing screening like the transient evoked otoacoustic emissions, especially in infants. As for which elements in the cochlea cause the nonlinear phenomena (i.e., *nonlinear compression, rectification, low-frequency intermodulation*, two-tone suppression, and *distortion tone generation*), there are potentially five: nonlinear hair bundle gating stiffness, nonlinear MET at the apex of hair cells, further distortion of receptor potentials by nonlinear conductances at the OHC basolateral wall, nonlinear electromechanical transduction from OHC membrane potential to prestin forces, and hair bundle adaptation at the apex of the hair cells. In some cases, it is clearly the forward transduction of the MET channels that determines the clipping and distortion, but in others it is not so clear.

Coding and Decoding of Neural Firing in the Auditory System

All of the acoustic processing of the auditory periphery can be considered as preprocessing of the sound, so frequency, intensity, timing, and direction information are presented to the brainstem as predigested firing of the primary afferent neurones. The randomized (stochastic) neural firing also has the advantage that averaging across a population of neurones by summing dendritic signals (excitatory postsynaptic potentials Inhibitory Post-synaptic Potential (IPSP) and at subsequent auditory nuclei improves the signal-to-noise ratio for signal detection. The periphery ensures that the sound has been amplified, but interfering signals like slow pressures and biological noise have been rejected, and the whole process is robust and compact. The acoustic stimulus has been modified by the periphery to indicate source direction, separated into its frequency components, and crushed into a very small range of neural firing rate (from spontaneous rate to an instantaneous driven rate less than 1,000 APs/s). The adaptation of transmitter release has emphasized the onset and offset of transient sounds, and it has also contributed to the dynamic compression of sustained neural firing. Even so, the enormous wealth of information encoded in the final neural firing needs to be decoded, and no one neural circuit can do it all, and no single ear is sufficient. As a result, the auditory brainstem has the role of decoding the many aspects of the coded neural firing with many different neural circuits operating in parallel. The frequency content of the incoming sound is maintained in all of these parallel circuits as a tonotopic map or maps in each brainstem nucleus, but the different brainstem nuclei are optimized to decode different aspects of the primary afferent firing, and higher levels of the auditory system extract information preprocessed by the lower levels. It should be mentioned here that while most of the neural circuits function to analyze the incoming sound, some must be for simply keeping the periphery and central circuits stable and robust.

A summary of the neurones analyzing the firing of the primary afferent neurones is shown in Figure 5. The first layer of auditory postprocessing occurs in the cochlear nuclei of the brainstem. Unfortunately, things can be confusing because these nuclei and the cells they contain are named on the basis of their location and appearance, and not on their function. Having said that, some things are clear. Any neural circuit concerned with timing (notably the anteroventral cochlear nucleus) needs to maintain and even enhance the onset and offset aspects of neural firing, with neurones that fire abruptly at the onset of a sound (*primary like* neurones, and *bushy cells* in particular). These neurones play an important role in the detection of the prosodic aspects of speech, and in the calculation of the lateral direction of a sound source, based on a comparison of the time of firing of neurones from the left and right anteroventral cochlear nucleus in the higher medial superior olive. Similar circuits are combined with neural

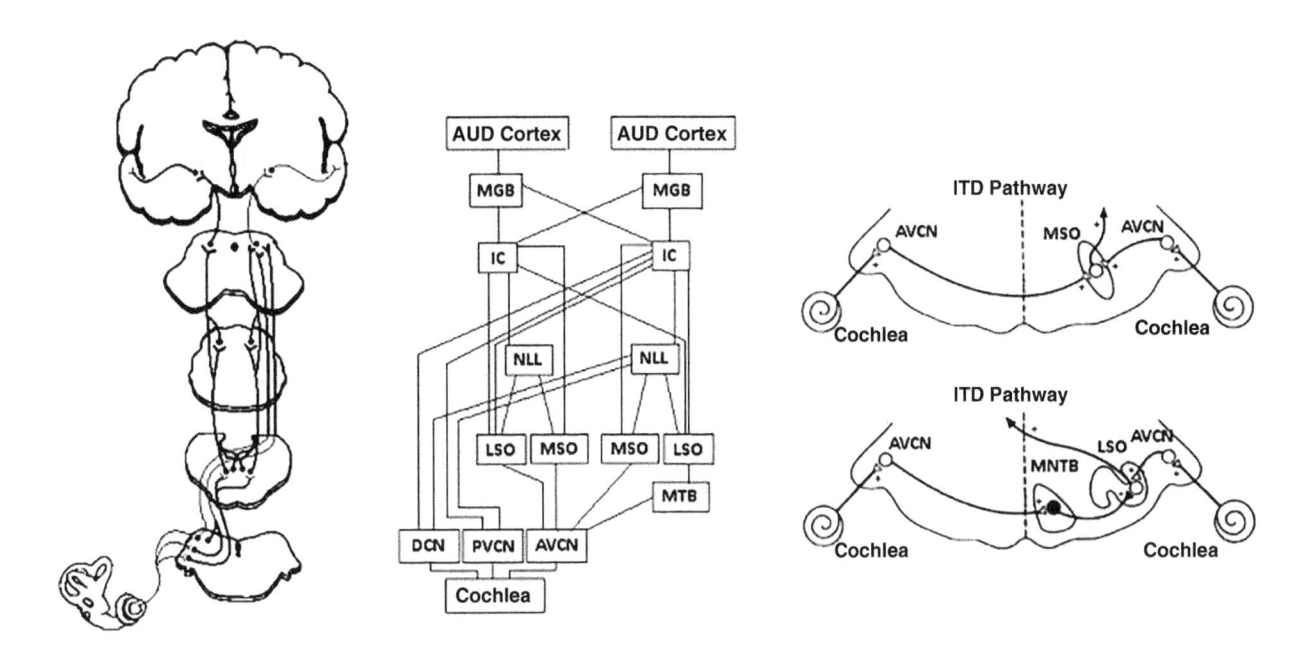

Figure 5 (A) About 10,000 primary afferent fibers feed information to the auditory brainstem from each. The information is processed through many specialized neural networks working in parallel. Higher centers of within the auditory pathway analyze the partially processed information from lower centers, comparing left and right inputs to extract even more information, such as position of the sound source. (B) Much is known of the auditory circuitry, and the neural wiring (dorsal cochlear nucleus, DCN; anteroventral cochlear nucleus, AVCN; posteroventral cochlear nucleus, PVCN; medial nucleus of the trapezoid body, MNTB; lateral superior olive, LSO; medial superior olive, MSO; nucleus of the lateral lemniscus, NLL; inferior colliculus, IC; medial geniculate body, MGB). (C) The detailed wiring and neural processing in many auditory circuits is now well understood. The examples here are for the processing of interaural timing differences, and interaural intensity differences (ILD), which provide information about the location of the sound source

delay to calculate firing intervals, allowing the detection of periodicity pitch. Similarly, the estimation of lateral source direction from IIDs is based on a comparison of left and right ongoing firing rates, accomplished by combining excitatory firing from one side with inhibitory firing from the other, in the lateral superior olive. The conversion from excitation to inhibition occurs in the medial nucleus of the trapezoid body. Analysis of the monaural spectral cues providing up–down and front–back source location occurs in the dorsal cochlear nucleus, containing cells that analyze the ongoing firing of many neurones along the cochlear length with different CFs, comparing the pattern of incoming firing with stored templates that represent different direction of sound (both IIDs and pinna cues). Even higher auditory nuclei (the inferior colliculi) use this directional information to steer human responses to sounds in 3-D, and in nonhuman mammals to also steer the pinna to sound targets.

While all of this auditory information is analyzed in real time by the auditory brainstem, it is not always passed on to the higher auditory cortex (which may be inactive during sleep) because the medial geniculate body acts as a gate or switch, isolating the auditory brainstem from the higher auditory cortex. This is important clinically because a person who is asleep or unconscious does not produce cortical responses, but still produces auditory brainstem responses, which means it is possible to test subjects who are asleep, unconscious, or undeveloped (i.e., neonatal). The role of the nucleus of the lateral lemniscus is not yet fully understood, but it has both timing and intensity information and is important in generating an acoustic startle reflex.

Robert B. Patuzzi

See also Acoustic Reflex; Acoustics; Air and Bone Conduction; Anatomy of the Hearing Mechanism and Central Audiology Nervous System; Decibel; Electrocochleography (ECochG); Frequency Resolution; Loudness; Masking; Otoacoustic Emissions (OAE); Ototoxicity; Pitch; Psychoacoustics; Sound Localization

Further Readings

Møller, A. R. (2006). *Hearing: Anatomy, physiology, and disorders of the auditory system* (2nd ed.). Academic Press Cambridge, MA.

Moore, B. C. J. (2012). *An introduction to the psychology of hearing* (6th ed.). West Yorkshire, UK: Emerald.

Musiek, F. E., & Baran, J. A. (2007). *The auditory system: Anatomy, physiology and clinical correlates.* Pearson Boston, MA.

Pickles, J. O. (2013). *An introduction to the physiology of hearing* (4th ed.). Leiden, The Netherlands: Brill.

Stanley A. G. (2010). *Hearing: An introduction to psychological and physiological acoustics* (5th ed.). Informa Healthcare London, UK.

Physiological Basis of Swallowing

Human swallowing is a complex phenomenon that is essential to human existence on many levels. The *pathway* for human swallowing begins in the mouth and ends in the stomach. Between these two *levels*, a highly complex interaction occurs between sensory and motor function to accommodate ingesting a variety of foods and liquids. As swallowing is due to the complex and coordinated effort, it is susceptible to impairment from a multitude of diseases and health status changes. Any disruption or impairment in the swallowing process may be defined as dysphagia. Dysphagia contributes to a variety of negative health status changes, most notably, increased risk of malnutrition and pneumonia. At its extreme severity, dysphagia can contribute to declining health status and even mortality. However, impairments in human swallowing are responsive to active rehabilitation efforts. Given the essential nature of swallowing, knowledge of typical physiology of this complex group of behaviors is paramount. This entry focuses on the basis for typical swallow function, examining each of the structures and stages involved in swallowing from *teeth to tummy* and the impact of different types of food and liquid on normal swallowing. This entry then briefly describes how swallowing physiology is affected by age and various disease processes.

Stages of Human Swallowing

The preparation and movement of a food or liquid bolus through the swallowing mechanism can be theoretically thought of as a series of valves that need to open and close in a coordinated manner for effective and efficient flow. The movement of the bolus creates zones of high pressure around the bolus and zones of low or negative pressure below the bolus. The combination of this mismatch in pressure with gravity aids the bolus in moving through the swallowing mechanism.

Human swallowing is typically discussed in four stages: (1) the oral preparatory stage, where the food is typically masticated in preparation for transfer through the mouth; (2) the oral stage, where the food or liquid bolus is transferred through the mouth; (3) the pharyngeal stage, where the bolus travels away from the oropharynx into the upper esophagus; and (4) the esophageal stage, where the material travels through the esophagus in to the stomach. Each of these stages is discussed individually; however, it must be noted that although the discussion of the stages of swallowing has theoretical appeal, in reality, the stages are closely linked and flow seamlessly from one to the next.

Oral Preparatory Stage

The primary functions of the oral component of swallowing are to process foods to support adequate swallowing and to transit oral contents to the pharynx. Evidence from swallowing impairment research suggests that humans have voluntary control over this stage of swallowing with input from the cerebral cortex in the brain.

In the oral preparatory stage, complex oral processing of the food or liquid bolus occurs. This oral processing is highly dependent on sensory input. A food or liquid bolus in the mouth stimulates sensory receptors, including taste, pressure (touch), and temperature. For taste, receptors are located on the tongue, palate, pharynx, and above the larynx. Taste receptors are further activated by saliva, which is produced by the salivary glands. Salivary glands are stimulated by tongue and jaw movements in the process of chewing foods or by the inherent taste of a food or liquid. Additionally, appreciation of taste also depends on smell perception. Smell sensations are directly from the food and also perceived when they travel to the back of the nose when food is chewed. Information on taste and smell is then sent via nerves to the brainstem and then the cortex.

The tongue plays a primary role in containing and moving liquids and solid foods within the mouth to facilitate mastication (chewing) and to mix drier foods with saliva for lubrication. The tongue and jaw move the bolus laterally to the molars, where it gets chewed. Further, the tongue also pushes the bolus against the hard palate (roof of the mouth) to aid in breaking it down. The tongue ultimately manipulates, shapes, holds, and then transfers the bolus to the pharynx to trigger the next stage of swallowing.

Oral Stage

In the oral preparatory stage, the bolus is prepared to get it *ready* to swallow. Once the bolus is manipulated adequately (depending on the size, texture, and type of bolus), the tip of the tongue elevates to the anterior portion of the roof of the mouth and the sides of the tongue curve up. Both these actions help in containing the bolus against the hard palate. The posterior portion of the tongue then transports the bolus toward the pharynx. As the bolus is being transported posteriorly, muscles in the soft palate move posteriorly to help seal off the nasal cavity from the oral cavity, preventing the food or liquid bolus from regurgitating via the nose. Almost simultaneously, while this transfer is occurring, respiration ceases (swallow apnea), the larynx (voice box) elevates, and the vocal folds close to protect the airway from food or liquid material entering it. As the larynx is elevating, a cartilaginous structure called the *epiglottis* drops down over the airway adding another layer to protect the airway from food or liquid and directing the food toward the esophagus (food pipe). Laryngeal movement is part of several inbuilt protective mechanisms to prevent food or liquid from entering the airway, crucial to swallow safety. Reparation and swallowing are closely linked in that the same anatomic structures are used for both these functions, and the control for both these functions comes from the brainstem. This is further underscored by the fact that respiration ceases during the process of swallowing, in what is known as *swallow apnea*. The duration of this apnea in typical individuals ranges from 0.75 to 1.25 s depending on the age of the individual and the size of the bolus. The larger the bolus, the longer the duration of apnea.

Pharyngeal Stage

The pharyngeal stage begins when the bolus arrives in the pharynx and ends when the bolus has entered the esophagus. This stage is involuntary (unlike the ability to have voluntary control over the oral stage) and is arguably the most critical stage of the swallow. During this phase, the larynx continues to move up, and several mechanisms are in place to protect the airway from food or liquid material entering it. These include (a) swallow apnea, (b) true and false vocal cords closing, (c) closure of the laryngeal aditus (i.e., the opening that connects the pharynx and the larynx), and (d) division of the bolus through the valleculae that directs the bolus to go around the superior aspect of the airway. These processes are occurring in this stage simultaneously as the muscles in the pharynx constrict sequentially from superior to inferior, creating a peristaltic type motion to direct the bolus to the esophagus. The movement of these muscles also aids in *pulling open* the upper esophageal sphincter (UES), which is the opening to the esophagus. Simultaneously, messages are also received from the brainstem to relax these muscles to aid in the opening. The opening of the UES is also influenced by the type and size of the bolus. Larger, heavier boluses result in a larger opening. Once the bolus passes through the UES, the UES closes, the larynx descends, and the airway reopens. These activities signal the end of the pharyngeal stage of swallowing.

Esophageal Stage

The esophagus is closed at rest and *opens* only as the bolus is moving through the pharynx toward the UES. The proximal one third of the esophagus is made up of striated muscle, similar to the pharynx, and the distal two thirds of the esophagus is made up of smooth muscle, similar to the stomach. Bolus movement through the zones of the esophagus is characterized by orderly, ringlike, progressive contractions termed *peristalsis*. This occurs throughout the esophagus until the bolus reaches the lower esophageal sphincter (LES) on its way to the stomach. This motor activity in the esophagus is rapid at the cervical end of the esophagus and gradually slows as the bolus enters the mid and distal esophagus. The LES starts to relax as the bolus approaches the distal esophagus and contracts to close after the bolus passes through the stomach. The LES remains closed without the signal from an incoming bolus, as this prevents the stomach contents from refluxing into the esophagus. Transient relaxations of the LES that are unrelated to a particular swallowing task result in the experience of gastroesophageal reflux, characterized by heartburn.

Accommodations to Food and Liquid Type

Typical human swallowing is also able to adjust to alterations in volume, texture, taste, and delivery of different solid and liquid boluses. This is termed *bolus accommodation*. With this in mind, diet modifications are often used in the treatment of individuals with dysphagia as a means to compensate for deficits. These prescribed modifications are based on research evidence of the impact of changes in texture, viscosity, and volume of swallowed material on swallow biomechanics.

When considering bolus size, evidence has suggested that in the oral cavity, the tongue changes contour to contain larger boluses. In the pharyngeal stage, some studies have documented greater upward displacement of the hyoid bone (which is part of the larynx) but no evidence of a change in the speed of pharyngeal transit. However, there does appear to be a direct relationship between volume of the bolus and the length of time the UES stays open. This suggests a possible relationship between sensory aspects of the oral stage of swallowing, such as bolus volume, and the mechanics in the pharyngeal stage of UES opening. This further underscores the interdependence of one stage of swallowing with the next.

When considering bolus viscosity, researchers agree that changes in swallow biomechanics, especially pressures generated in the swallowing mechanism, are more sensitive to changes in viscosity than to changes in volume of the bolus. Thicker boluses require greater tongue pressure and force to transport the bolus through the oral cavity.

Bolus taste has also been shown to influence biomechanics. Sweet, sour, and salty boluses have been shown to increase muscle activation and swallowing pressures by varying degrees compared to water boluses. Similarly, carbonation has been shown to result in increased swallow-related pressures in the swallowing mechanism compared to water.

Any number of these modifications are often used individually or in combination as a treatment strategy in individuals with dysphagia in order to trigger faster activation, greater pressures, or increased movement.

Neurologic Control of Swallowing

Given the diverse aspects and control required for human swallowing, neurologic infrastructure is widespread and complex. Significant overlap exists between control for swallowing and non-swallowing movements in the upper aerodigestive tract. The literature refers to a *central pattern generator* in the rostral brainstem that receives sensory information from the oral cavity, pharynx, and esophagus and then provides output for this complex motor activity. Bolus accommodation discussed previously is evidence for an automatic brainstem control in swallowing. In adults, this permits humans to ingest a wide variety of foods and liquids without conscious or voluntary participation in eating and drinking. The brainstem swallowing center not only controls and modulates oropharyngeal aspects of swallowing, but it also coordinates swallowing activity with respiration. The brainstem swallowing controls include two-way communication between the peripheral neuromuscular system, sending output to the muscles for swallowing, and the cerebral hemispheres in the brain. The brainstem basically serves as a *junction box* between hemispheric neural control and peripheral sensorimotor aspects of swallowing.

In the cortex, swallowing control is thought to be bilaterally represented and diffuse. Brain imaging techniques such as transcranial magnetic stimulation, functional magnetic imaging, and functional near-infrared spectroscopy have been used to suggest that swallowing function is not only diffusely represented in the cortex but is not related to control for speech or handedness. It is suggested that this diffuse representation for swallowing function exists as a degree of neuroplasticity, whereby a region in the other hemisphere can take over swallowing function if neurological damage occurs. Despite the diffuse nature of cortical activation for swallowing, imaging studies indicate that swallowing has a distinct pattern of control. Interestingly, however, swallowing different materials (e.g., liquids, puddings, hard solids) has been shown to result in different patterns of activation in the cortex. Furthermore, hemisphere swallowing controls seem to adjust with increasing age. This is presumed to be in response to age-related changes in sensorimotor processing.

More detailed knowledge on the nature of hemispheric control for swallowing is emerging. The current understanding is that there exists a neural network that is flexible to the changing motoric demands required to swallow various materials; it adjusts to sensorimotor changes that occur with aging; and it is plastic in that if neurologic damage occurs, the other hemisphere can take over control of swallowing function.

Swallow Physiology in Typical Aging

A discussion of swallowing physiology would be incomplete without an understanding of how the mechanism changes over the human life span. Swallow physiology changes with advancing age, sometimes beginning as early as 45 years of age. These age-related changes can impact negatively the safe, effective, and efficient flow of food and liquid material through the swallowing mechanism. Age-related changes may also interact with each other to decompensate swallowing further.

In general, a subtle slowing in the process of swallowing (as with other motor functions) occurs with advancing age. This slowing can be related to loss of muscle strength (force) and mass, speed of muscle movement, and extent of muscle movement. Over time, cumulative effects can occur from these subtle changes, resulting in swallowed material entering the airway (commonly referred to as *going down the wrong pipe*) or remaining as residue in the pharynx. Current evidence also suggests that in aging individuals, typical swallow biomechanics may change under stress, which is likely to occur as a result of disease and hospitalization. Additionally, beyond these subtle motor changes with swallowing, aging is associated with decrements in oral moisture (saliva), taste perception, and smell acuity. These changes may also contribute to reduced swallowing performance or a voluntary alteration in dietary intake in the elderly. Clinically, it is imperative to separate the effects of typical aging on swallowing from swallow changes that occur as a result of disease processes.

Impact of Disease

Swallow is movement. Physiologic changes often lead to either of the hallmark characteristics of dysphagia: (a) delay in the transport of the bolus as it travels from the mouth to the stomach or (b) misdirection of the bolus toward the airway or lungs. It is important to note that the degree of change in physiology often determines the diagnosis of dysphagia. For example, as discussed previously, physiologic changes occur in the swallowing mechanism in healthy aging. These changes may impact the propulsion of the bolus by delaying its progress due to a reduction in strength or extent of muscle movement. However, only when these changes result in a significant change in eating habits (e.g., avoidance of foods) or in medical complications (e.g., undernutrition or aspiration pneumonia), then the person can truly be characterized as having a dysphagia. On the other hand, it is also possible that swallowing musculature is normal, but the person may not be alert or have the cognitive capacity to use the musculature appropriately. In such cases, the person may be identified as being at risk of dysphagia because of his or her compromised medical condition. When physiology of swallowing is affected, swallowing rehabilitation, especially that which effects motoric improvement in swallowing performance, can provide tremendous functional benefit for patients with dysphagia.

Final Thoughts

Human swallowing is a complex sensorimotor task that requires a network of neural connections from the cerebral cortex to peripheral neuromuscular systems. Some aspects of swallowing such as oral control of different boluses and initiation of material-specific swallow responses are under voluntary control, appearing to be governed by a flexible, diffuse cortical network. Other aspects of swallowing such as pharyngeal swallowing and coordination with respiration are under more automatic brainstem control. Aging and a variety of health conditions can affect typical physiology and lead to dysphagia. Therefore, it is essential to have an understanding of these interdependent voluntary and involuntary behaviors to accurately evaluate or rehabilitate the swallowing mechanism.

Aarthi Madhavan

See also Anatomy of the Human Articulators; Anatomy of the Human Larynx; Aspiration: Swallowing; Fiberoptic Endoscopic Evaluation of Swallowing (FEES); Swallowing Assessment; Swallowing Disorders; Swallowing Intervention

Further Readings

Groher, M. E., & Crary, M. A. (2016). *Dysphagia: Clinical management in adults and children* (2nd ed.). St. Louis, MO: Mosby Elsevier.

Jean, A. (2001). Brainstem control of swallowing: Neuronal network and cellular mechanisms. *Physiological Reviews, 81,* 929–969.

Madhavan, A., Haak, N. J., Carnaby, G. D., & Crary, M. A. (2015). Neural control of swallowing and treatment of motor impairments in dysphagia. In R. E. Bahr & E. R. Siliman (Eds.), *Routledge handbook of communication disorders* (pp. 78–89). Abingdon, UK: Routledge.

Michou, E., & Hamdy, S. (2009). Cortical input in control of swallowing. *Current Opinion in Otolaryngology Head and Neck Surgery, 17,* 166–171.

Steele, C. M., & Miller, A. J. (2010). Sensory input pathways and mechanisms in swallowing: A review. *Dysphagia, 25,* 323–333.

Physiological Basis for Voice

Phonation refers to the process of using the vocal folds for the purpose of voicing speech. Many nonhuman animals use the vocal folds (also called *vocal cords*) to produce sound, but humans have taken this process to a much higher level. This entry examines the complex physiological basis for voice, focusing on the interaction between the airway and the vocal folds.

The vocal mechanism consists of the larynx, which sits atop the trachea. The larynx is actually a valve that closes off the airway to protect the lungs from foreign objects. The larynx provides a mechanism for completely closing off the airway through muscular effort, which can occur either through reflexive (e.g., coughing) or voluntary action. Voluntary closing of the larynx occurs in voicing for speech. In contrast with coughing, phonation is highly controllable and can be initiated and terminated at will.

The most critical element of phonation is the vocal folds. The vocal folds are made of muscle and connective tissue and course between the arytenoid cartilages in the posterior aspect of the larynx and the anterior thyroid cartilage. The muscle and connective tissue create a mass with elastic characteristics that make the vocal folds capable of vibration under the right circumstances. The vocal folds are moveable, in that they can be adducted (i.e., brought together toward the midline) or abducted (i.e., pulled apart away from midline). When the vocal folds are fully abducted, they leave the airway unimpeded for the strong respiratory effort of exercise, and when they are fully and tightly adducted, they prohibit not only airflow but also entry by foreign objects. Use of the vocal folds for speech falls somewhere in between these two extremes of function. Vocal fold vibration requires discussion of the Bernoulli effect.

Bernoulli Effect in Phonation

The Bernoulli effect (or Bernoulli principle) describes the effects of constriction placed in a flow of liquid or air, stating that *given a laminar flow through a tube, placing a constriction in that flow will significantly alter the characteristics of flow at the constriction.* Bernoulli found that when an obstruction is placed on the wall of a tube through which liquid flows, there will be a drop in pressure perpendicular to the constriction as well as an increase in the rate of flow at the constriction. Because the overall rate of flow is constant, placing a constriction in the flow requires the fluid or air to move faster to get around the constriction at the same rate as the overall flow. Pressure is reduced at the constriction because there are fewer molecules of air at the constriction and subsequently less molecular force exerted on the wall at that point. Pressure is equal to force over unit area ($P = F/A$), and reducing force causes a drop in pressure.

Vibration of the Vocal Folds and Myoelastic Aerodynamic Theory

The vocal folds are essentially masses of tissue placed in the airflow of the respiratory passageway. Recall that the vocal mechanism of the larynx consists of a complex set of muscles capable of adducting and abducting the vocal folds. When the vocal folds are abducted, there is minimal constriction in the airway, so the Bernoulli principle need not be invoked. When the vocal folds are moved toward the midline and are made to make contact (to approximate), there is a significant constriction in the airway, with a drop in pressure at the constriction. When pressure drops between the folds, the vocal folds are sucked together by the force of the negative pressure generated between them. When the folds are pulled together, airflow stops instantaneously, so that the Bernoulli effect is no longer applicable. At that instant, the vocal folds are blown apart by the air pressure below the folds (i.e., subglottal pressure), and airflow between the folds invokes the Bernoulli principle once again, pulling the vocal folds back to midline and closure. This *blowing open* and *sucking closed* occurs repeatedly as long as there is airflow, and this produces phonation.

There is also an elastic component to vocal fold vibration, provided by the *lamina propria* of the vocal folds. Elasticity is the quality of a material that causes it to return to its original condition after being deformed, and when the vocal folds are blown apart, they tend to return to their original position once the forces that blew them apart are no longer in play. When the pressure between the folds goes negative due to airflow across the constriction, the force driving the folds apart is replaced by the aerodynamic force pulling them together, which is supplemented by elasticity of the vocal folds. Taken together, these components make up the heart of the myoelastic aerodynamic theory of phonation. Ingo Titze's expanded model (the mucoviscoaerodynamic theory of phonation) treats the vocal folds as a group of linked masses and accounts for the rich harmonics of voice.

Table 1 Muscles Involved With Laryngeal Adjustments

Function	Muscle(s)
Adduction of vocal folds; medial compression	Lateral cricoarytenoid; oblique arytenoids; transverse arytenoids
Abduction of vocal folds	Posterior cricoarytenoid
Tensing of vocal folds	Thyrovocalis
Relaxing of vocal folds	Thyromuscularis
Elongating and tensing of vocal folds for F0 increase	Cricothyroid, pars recta
Shortening of vocal folds for F0 decrease	Sternothyroid; sternohyoid (indirectly)

Source: Seikel et al. (2016).

The vocal folds adduct and abduct as a result of muscular activity (see Table 1). Adduction of the vocal folds causes the arytenoid cartilages to rock in toward the midline for phonation. The force of adduction is referred to as medial compression. Abduction of the vocal folds rocks the arytenoids laterally, opening the airway and terminating phonation. The arytenoid cartilages can also glide in an anterior–posterior orientation, which occurs during modulation of fundamental frequency (F0).

Frequency of Vocal Fold Vibration

Frequency of phonation refers to how often a cycle of vibration occurs (cycles per second or hertz [Hz]). The average frequency of vibration of the vocal folds (i.e., F0) is about 120 Hz for adult males and 220 Hz for adult females. The F0 arises from the tissue characteristics of the vocal folds. Tissue elasticity causes the vocal folds to return to their original form after being distended, while stiffness of the vocal folds defines the force with which they will return to their original position. More massive vocal folds vibrate at a lower F0 than do less massive folds, defining the essential difference seen between male and female vocal folds. The interplay of mass, tension, and elasticity governs the specific frequency of vibration of the vocal folds, which are manipulated to change the F0 for speech.

Quality of voice is directly related to the symmetry of the vocal folds, tissue elasticity and stiffness, and muscular support involved in controlling the folds. The primary mechanism for changing F0 is to tense the vocal folds. When the vocal folds are elongated, they are tensed, increasing the frequency of vibration. Elongation is performed by the cricothyroid muscle, which rocks the cricoid and thyroid cartilages together in the anterior aspect of the larynx and stretches the vocal folds. In addition, the thyrovocalis muscles contract to fine-tune the tension. Relaxing the vocal folds requires moving the cricoid and thyroid cartilages apart in front, which can be accomplished by the thyrohyoid muscle. For speech or singing, fine adjustments are critical in order to maintain the desired vocal quality, and these are accomplished by the delicate action of the thyrovocalis and thyromuscularis.

Vocal Intensity

Vocal intensity refers to the sound pressure level of speech. Increase in vocal intensity arises from increased medial compression, which causes increased resistance to airflow. When medial compression increases, subglottal air pressure must increase to overcome the added resistance. The vocal folds are blown apart more vigorously and return to the closed phase of vibration much more vigorously, with the result being increased vocal intensity due to increased energy being used in the phonatory process.

One more change occurs in phonation coincident with increased vocal intensity. During a modal vibratory cycle of conversational speech, the vocal folds will spend approximately 50% of the time opening, 37% closing, and 13% closed. As medial compression increases, the forces toward the midline cause the cycle to shift so that the vocal folds spend markedly more time in the closed phase (approximately 30% at higher intensities), which reduces the opening and closing phase proportions. The vocal folds thus are held together more tightly, blown apart with greater subglottal pressure, and remain closed longer during a phonatory cycle, all resulting in greater vocal intensity.

Vocal Attack

The vocal folds are adducted in conjunction with the flow of air through the respiratory passageway. It is very important to realize that the vocal folds are vibrating without repetitive muscular contractions: The folds are adducted toward the midline to initiate phonation and abducted away from midline to terminate phonation. The timing of adduction and respiratory flow has been characterized as being one of three types of attack: glottal, breathy, or simultaneous. In all three types of attack, the vocal folds are being moved toward the midline position (adducted) to initiate phonation, but the difference is how that movement integrates with the onset of airflow.

Glottal attack refers to the condition in which the adduction of the vocal folds precedes the onset of airflow (e.g., vowels). *Breathy attack* occurs when airflow begins before the adduction (e.g., voiceless fricatives). *Simultaneous attack* occurs when the airflow and adduction occur at the same time (e.g., voiced continuants). Termination of phonation occurs when the vocal folds are abducted sufficiently to cause vibration to cease. These processes require great precision in speech because they happen rapidly.

Vocal Register

The pattern of activity of the vocal folds during sustained phonation is termed the *mode of vibration*. Voice science has identified a number of perceptual changes in voice called *vocal registers*, and these relate to physical changes that occur in the vibrating vocal folds. *Modal register* refers to the manner of vibration in everyday speech. In a cycle of modal phonation, the vocal folds open from inferior to superior and close from inferior to superior, in an undulating phonatory pattern. In the anterior–posterior dimension, the vocal folds tend to open posterior to anterior and to close anterior to posterior.

Glottal fry is the phonatory characteristic attributed to the *pulse register*, resulting in extremely low F0 (i.e., 30–90 Hz) and very low subglottal pressure (i.e., around 2-cm H_2O), reduced vocal fold tension, and strong medial compression. The vibrating margins of the vocal folds are flaccid and thick, resulting in a syncopated vibratory pattern in which there is a secondary beat for every cycle of F0.

Falsetto is the third mode of vibration, resulting in extremely high F0. In falsetto, the vocal folds are elongated and tensed so that only the free margins vibrate. The posterior vocal folds are compressed together with increased force, shortening the vibratory portion of the folds and further increasing the F0. The undulating pattern is replaced with vocal folds that vibrate in a reed-like pattern as a unit, along the free margins. Falsetto results in an F0 in the 300- to 600-Hz range.

Pressed phonation results from greatly increased medial compression, resulting in increased stridency or harshness in voice quality and the perception of strain. *Whistle register* is a fifth phonatory mode. In this mode, the vocal folds do not vibrate at all, but rather turbulence at the edges of the tensed vocal folds causes a whistlelike tone with frequencies as high as 2500 Hz. *Breathy phonation* results from vocal folds being inadequately approximated. In this mode of vibration, the vibrating margins allow airflow between them when in the closed phase, resulting in the perception of breathiness. *Whispering* is not a phonatory mode since no voicing occurs. In whispering, the vocal folds are partially adducted and tensed to develop turbulence at the margins. The turbulence is used to excite the vocal tract for nonvoiced speech. Since there is no vibration of the vocal folds, there is no frequency of vibration.

Characteristic Frequencies of Vibration

Pitch is the perceptual correlate of frequency, and as frequency increases, pitch increases. Several phonatory characteristics have been labeled as they relate to the perceptual element (i.e., pitch), but they actually refer to the physical parameter of frequency.

Optimal pitch refers to the frequency of vocal fold vibration that is optimal or most appropriate for an individual, as determined by the physical characteristics of the vocal folds during modal phonation. *Habitual pitch* refers to the frequency of vibration that is used by an individual during typical speech, governed by the personal adjustments of the vocal mechanism to meet physical or psychological needs. *Average F0* refers to the long-term average of F0 for a given task (e.g., reading). As an individual's larynx grows during childhood, the F0 changes as well. At about 5 years of age, males and females have an F0 of between 250 and 300 Hz, but at puberty the F0 of the typical male drops, settling to an adult value of about 135 Hz by 20 years of age. The typical female F0 has a less severe decline to about 220 Hz by 20 years of age. This mean F0 is stable throughout life until about 65 years of age when the male F0 starts to rise again, most likely reflecting atrophy of the vocal folds. The typical female F0 holds fairly constant throughout adult life.

A final concept of vocal fold physiology relates to *vocal jitter*, also referred to as *perturbation*. Vocal jitter is a measure of the periodicity of the vibration of the vocal folds, which, in turn, is seen as an indication of the health of the vocal mechanism. Vocal jitter is defined as the average deviation of the period of each cycle from the long-term average of the period. The period of a cycle of vibration is the time it takes for a cycle to repeat. Greater deviation can indicate vocal folds that lack muscle tone or have asymmetrical mass.

Final Thoughts

The vocal folds can be adducted or abducted to initiate or terminate phonation, and the degree of medially placed force exerted by the focal folds (i.e., medial compression) can be precisely controlled to support increased vocal intensity. The Bernoulli effect states that given a constriction in a laminar flow of air or liquid, there will be a pressure drop and velocity increase at the constriction, and vibration of the vocal folds arises from this effect, combined with tissue elasticity and the forces of subglottal pressure. The myoelastic aerodynamic theory of vocal fold function accurately models the basic vibratory pattern, and the mucoviscoaerodynamic theory elaborates on the cause of the complex acoustic signal produced by that vibration. Frequency refers to how often an event occurs for a unit of time and is measured in cycles per second or Hz, and the average F0 of vibration of vocal folds is about 120 Hz for the typical adult male and 220 Hz for the typical adult female. The primary mechanism for increasing F0 is by tensing the vocal folds.

Increased vocal intensity arises from increasing subglottal air pressure and increasing medial compression, resulting in more vigorous phonation with altered vibratory cycle. Glottal attack is one in which the vocal folds adduct before respiration begins, while breathy attack is the mode in which vocal folds adduct after respiration has begun. Simultaneous attack is that in which adduction and respiration begin at the same time.

There are different modes of vibration, characterized as vocal registers. In modal phonation, vocal folds open from inferior to superior and close from inferior to superior and simultaneously open from posterior to anterior and to close anterior to posterior. Glottal fry is characterized by extremely low F0, arising from very low subglottal pressure and reduced vocal fold tension with strong medial compression. Falsetto uses elongated and tensed vocal folds that vibrate along the edge, producing extremely high F0.

Pressed phonation results from greatly increased medial compression, producing increased stridency or harshness in voice quality. In whistle register, the vocal folds do not vibrate at all, but turbulence along the vocal fold margins causes a whistlelike tone. Breathy phonation results from vocal folds being inadequately approximated. In whispering, the vocal folds are partially adducted and tensed to develop turbulence at the margins.

Optimal *pitch* refers to the frequency of vocal fold vibration that is optimal for an individual vocal mechanism, while habitual pitch refers to the frequency of vibration that is used by an individual during typical speech. Average F0 refers to the long-term average of F0 for a given speaker, and this changes as an individual ages.

Tony Seikel

See also Anatomy of the Human Larynx; Bernoulli Effect; Electroglottography (EGG)/Electrolaryngography (ELG); Jitter and Shimmer; Prosody

Further Readings

Alipour-Haghighi, F., & Titze, I. R. (1991). Elastic models of vocal fold tissues. *The Journal of the Acoustical Society of America, 90*(3), 1326–1331.

Behrman, A. (2007). *Speech and voice science.* San Diego, CA: Plural.

Bless, D. M., & Abbs, J. H. (1995). *Vocal fold physiology* (2nd ed.). San Diego, CA: Singular.

Chhetri, D. K., Neurbauer, J., & Berry, D. A. (2012). Neuromuscular control of fundamental frequency at phonation onset. *Journal of the Acoustical Society of America, 131*(2), 1401–1412.

Kent, R. D., Kent, J. F., & Rosenbek, J. C. (1987). Maximum performance tests of speech production. *Journal of Speech and Hearing Disorders, 52,* 367–387.

McHanwell, S. (2008). Larynx. In S. Standring (Ed.), *Gray's anatomy: The anatomical and clinical basis of practice* (40th ed., pp. 577–594). London, UK: Churchill Livingstone.

Plant, R. L., & Younger, R. M. (2000). The interrelationship of subglottal pressure, fundamental frequency, and vocal intensity during speech. *Journal of voice, 14*(2), 170–177.

Seikel, J. A., Drumright, D. G., & King, D. W. (2016). *Anatomy and physiology for speech, language and hearing* (5th ed.). Clifton Park, NY: Cengage Learning.

Storck, C., Juergens, P., Fischer, C., Wolfensberger, M., Honegger, F., Sorantin, E., . . . Gugatschka, M. (2012). Biomechanics of the cricoarytenoid joint: Three-dimensional imaging and vector analysis. *Journal of Voice, 25*(4), 406–410.

Titze, I. (1973). The human vocal cords: A mathematical model, Part I. *Phonetica, 28,* 129–170.

van den Berg, J. W. (1958). Myoelastic-aerodynamic theory of voice production. *Journal of Speech and Hearing Research, 1,* 227–244.

Pidgin and Creole Languages

Linguists use the terms *pidgin* and *creole* (P/C) to refer to languages that arose in bilingual or multilingual contact settings with no shared language. Pidgins serve as lingua franca for limited purposes while creoles are full-fledged languages that serve all the communicative needs of a community. The differences are fuzzy because the terms developed from lay terminology in specific sociocultural contexts. The term *pidgin* developed from English *business* and was first applied to Chinese Pidgin English. Creole derives from Spanish *criollo*; originally used to refer to persons of European Spanish origin born in the Americas, it was later extended to *things*, including language, that are unique to that context. Naming conventions are not always indicative of their status. Languages that include pidgin in their name such as Solomon Pijin or West African Pidgin English are linguistically similar to creoles and those without such an identifier are prototypical pidgins (e.g., Russenorsk) or creoles (e.g., Matawai). Some researchers also reject the inclusion of the lexifier (e.g., English) in the name, as it wrongly asserts a close link to their lexifier. Research on P/Cs has a long tradition starting with missionary and colonial writings from as early as the 17th century. However, the Mona, Jamaica conferences (1959 and 1961) and the resulting edited volume (*Pidginization and Creolization of Languages*) are considered to be the cradle of P/C studies. Since P/Cs challenge historical linguistic notions about language development, their formation continues to attract the greatest amount of discussion. Besides historical and structural linguistic research, there is also research on types of P/Cs, sociolinguistic and applied matters. The following sections discuss each in turn.

Emergence and Development of P/Cs

P/Cs are typically linked to European expansion starting in the 15th century. However, there is now an increased focus on Arabic, African and American contexts that are not (directly) related to this context. Creoles were believed to develop from pidgins, but a solid case has only been made for Pacific varieties (e.g., Tok Pisin, Bislama). In the Americas, pidgins served as inputs to their formation, but a pidgin phase is not attested. Prototypical pidgins such as Russenorsk and Chinook Pidgin emerged in trade contexts, such as between Pacific Islanders and Europeans engaged in trade, between different first nations in the Americas, or between the latter and Europeans. Other contexts were multilingual crews and domestic service encounters. Labor migration from African and Asian countries is currently giving rise to Arabic Pidgins in the Gulf States, for instance. These contexts typically involved low interactional intensity and limited purposes.

Creoles have their origin in the European plantation contexts in the Caribbean, North America, Indian Ocean, Australia, and the Pacific. For example, enslaved Africans from two or more regions in Africa were transported to Caribbean islands, such as Barbados, and to the American continent to work on sugarcane plantations where, in the absence of a common language, they had to develop ways of communicating with fellow Africans and to a lesser extent with American Indians, European indentured laborers, and plantation owners. African African communications were interactionally rich and involved a wide range of purposes, quickly giving rise to rich means of communication that developed into community languages.

Pidgin formation (or pidginization) is conceptualized as linguistic reduction, whereas creole formation (or creolization) involves expansion. Both consist of several interlinking processes. The former involves not only simplification but also retention and innovation, while the latter is characterized by retention and innovation. Creators of pidgins simplified the input languages, retaining small lexicons drawn from one or all of the contributing languages that include few functional elements. Pidgins involve mostly analytical structures, a small number of syntactic and morphological patterns, word orders, and have low derivational depth. Creole formation closely resembles second-language acquisition except that its agents were not aiming to learn the socially dominant language. Creators of creoles identified (seemingly) similar lexical items in varieties of the dominant language with those in their language repertoire and thereby projected the properties of the latter onto the former, thus generating mixed lexical items and structural patterns that resemble those of the input languages in various ways. Both processes were subject to cognitive processing constraints. Subsequent to their emergence, P/C grammars were subject to internally and externally motivated processes of change.

Types of P/Cs

P/Cs are traditionally classified according to their lexical input (e.g., Portuguese-based Creole).

Researchers currently focus on sociohistorical, usage-based, and linguistic criteria. P/Cs make up a continuum consisting of prototypical pidgins (Delaware Pidgin) that are limited-purpose lingua francas with reduced structures on one end and full-fledged community languages that developed with limited influence from the lexifier, in other words radical creoles (e.g., Suriname), on the other. In-between are pidgincreoles that started out as pidgins and subsequently expanded structurally and functionally such as Tok Pisin and intermediate creoles (Bajan) that emerged in contexts with fairly intense contact with varieties of the socially dominant language.

It is difficult to make general statements about the linguistic nature of P/Cs because they emerged from contact between different sets of languages.

Derek Bickerton made the most explicit claims about structural characteristics, claiming that prototypical creoles can be identified on the basis of 12 structural features. This view was successfully refuted on the basis of structural and historical linguistic research. More recent attempts included fewer features but were also not successful in delimiting P/Cs from other languages.

Sociolinguistics

Sociolinguistic research has focused on determining patterns of language use in P/C communities and the relationship between P/Cs and other languages in these contexts. There is a close connection between research on P/Cs and sociolinguistics because sociolinguistic approaches and methods have played an important role in the research on P/Cs, and models developed for P/Cs have been applied to other contexts. The *post-creole continuum* notion strongly influenced early understandings of English-official communities in the Caribbean. It posits that variation between a creole and (local) Standard English is seamless: After emancipation, with greater access to English, creole speakers gradually adapted the *deep* creole or basilect in the direction of English, or the acrolect. This process, called *decreolization*, produced intermediate lects or mesolects. This model has been successfully challenged on sociohistorical, sociolinguistic, and linguistic grounds but continues to persist, particularly outside of P/C research circles. It is nowadays widely acknowledged that P/C communities resemble other bilingual or multilingual communities, where two or more socially and linguistically distinct languages coexist. While each is iconically linked to particular social contexts, groups of people and types of interactions, language use is dynamic and involves hybrid practices (e.g., code switching, contact-induced language change) that function to assert social and interactional identities and categories.

The *acts of identity* framework also developed from research on P/Cs. It argues that linguistic practices are dynamic and that linguistic variation performs important social functions in that individuals design their linguistic practices to create alignment with or dissociation from identifiable social groups through the process of linguistic focusing. This model has, however, not been widely applied because it requires training in anthropology and linguistics and detailed knowledge of the language situation.

While early sociolinguistic research was quantitative and focused mostly on linguistic aspects, more recent research has paid greater attention to the social meanings and functions of variation and applied both qualitative and quantitative analytical approaches. It has also broadened its database, investigating not just vernacular speech obtained through the sociolinguistic interview but also literary texts, popular music, computer-mediated and media speech, including both formal and informal linguistic practices. Finally, there is also growing interest in language ideologies and the pragmatics of language use both in the traditional communities and in diaspora communities.

Applied Linguistic Research

Given the circumstances of their emergence and the fact that P/Cs are traditionally considered low-prestige languages, applied linguistic research has primarily focused on improving views about them, identifying obstacles hindering their acceptance, and advocating for their inclusions into social domains from which they were (and in many cases still are) barred in order to facilitate creole-dominant populations. While a fair amount of progress has been made over the last few decades not least because of the rise of new forms of communication, change takes place at different speeds in different societies and in different social domains.

The area of primary and secondary education has probably received the most attention. From very early on, Caribbean scholars have argued that P/C-speaking children should be taught through the P/C to maximally support their learning. In contexts where this is currently not possible, P/Cs should nevertheless be actively embraced by the education system. Teachers should actively and in a positive manner raise awareness of the structural differences between P/Cs and their lexifiers/the socially dominant language using structured, communication-based, and culturally adapted activities. This might involve measures such as contrastive grammar exercises, creative writing and performance, and translation activities. Research on their implementation has shown that they significantly enhance participation by P/C-speaking children and improve educational attainments. While some educational programs only focus on raising the profile of P/Cs and/or facilitating the acquisition of the dominant language, others go a step further and integrate P/Cs as subjects or, less typically, as (main) means of instruction into the curriculum. Such projects were set up with varying degrees of success in Nicaragua, Jamaica, French overseas territories, Curaçao, and the Seychelles. While it has not always been easy to set up such projects, they have produced positive educational outcomes and have significantly helped to improve views about P/Cs and the relationship between local populations and the educational system.

The other area that has figured prominently is language development research focusing on codifying P/Cs for developing them as a written medium, a crucial prerequisite for making them educational media. Research has focused on identifying a target variety for linguistic codification which initially proved challenging due to lack of research on variation and a lack of consensus on whether or not it would be beneficial to emphasize P/Cs distinctiveness from their lexifier. The development of writing systems initially also proved contentious for similar reasons. However, the advent of mobile and computer-mediated communication, which has led to an increase in written productions in P/Cs, is set to make a positive contribution toward resolving these issues in a democratic matter. It does not always lead to the wholesale adoption of the homogenized systems advocated by scholars nor does it remove variation because, as in spoken communication, it plays an important role in people's identity management. Over the years, grammars and dictionaries have been produced for many P/Cs to both enhance their standing and facilitate their integration into the education system. However, we still lack research on them and their use, and there is still a dearth of written productions—novels, dramas, textbooks, and so on—in these languages.

There is also some research on other institutional contexts such as the broad area of law enforcement and health. In relation to the former, it was shown that making P/Cs official languages contributes to their greater acceptance but does not ensure that they will be actively used by police, courtroom, and other personnel to facilitate interactions with creole-speaking populations. It requires training and targeted activities that will also entail corpus-planning activities, besides research on language practices in situated institutional interactions.

Conclusion

Research on P/Cs was initially slow because they were considered to be low-status languages not worthy of academic attention. Over the last few decades, it has developed into a vibrant area of research, which has made important contributions to various subfields of linguistics.

Bettina Migge

See also African American English; Applied Linguistics; Bilingualism; Jargon and Jargon Aphasia; Language Acquisition; Multilingualism; Second-Language Acquisition; Sociolinguistics; Universal Grammar

Further Readings

Hymes, D. (1971). *Pidginization and creolization of languages*. Cambridge, UK: Cambridge University Press.

Keesing, R. (1988). *Melanesian Pidgin English and the Oceanic substrate*. Stanford, CA: Stanford University Press.

Kouwenberg, S., & Singler, J. V. (Eds.). (2008). *The handbook of pidgin and creole studies*. Malden, MA: Blackwell.

Michaelis, S. M., Maurer, P., Haspelmath, M., & Huber, M. (Eds.). (2013). *The atlas of pidgin and creole language structures (APiCS)*. Oxford, UK: Oxford University Press.

Winford, D. (2003). *An introduction of contact linguistics*. Malden, MA: Blackwell.

Websites

Creole Language Library. Retrieved from https://benjamins.com/#catalog/books/cll.52/main

Journal of Pidgin and Creole Languages. Retrieved from https://benjamins.com/#catalog/journals/jpcl/main

Pitch

Pitch is a perceptual feature of speech. It is the ear's response to frequency. Pitch changes, it becomes higher or lower, when the frequency of the voice changes. The human voice is a complex sound composed of many frequencies. A listener's perception of a speaker's pitch depends mostly on the lowest frequency or fundamental frequency (F0) of voice, which is the frequency of vibration of the vocal folds. Pitch is also a suprasegmental feature of speech; "segments" are the sounds of speech, and the suprasegmentals are properties that are "overlaid" on those segments. Pitch is not a property of a single sound but extends over words and utterances. It carries important linguistic and extralinguistic functions. It can change the meaning of words and utterances and it can convey our attitudes and emotions.

Pitch is the perceptual correlate of the fundamental frequency of voice. Frequency is a physical phenomenon. It can be objectively measured by instruments. Pitch, on the other hand, is a psychological phenomenon. It is the perceptual interpretation of frequency and can be measured only by asking listeners to judge the frequency of a speaker's voice. In general, when frequency is increased this results in a rise in pitch and when it is decreased the pitch is perceived as lower. However, the relationship between frequency and pitch is not strictly linear. The human ear cannot perceive very small frequency changes, and a change in the perception of pitch typically requires a larger change in frequency, especially in higher frequencies.

The fundamental frequency of voice and, hence, pitch varies as a function of sex and age. Males have an average F0 of about 100–125 Hz (i.e., vocal folds vibrate about 100–125 per second), whereas females have an average F0 of about 200 Hz. This difference in fundamental frequency and pitch is mostly the result of the anatomical differences between males' and females' vocal folds. On average, men have longer and more massive vocal folds than women. The greater the length and mass of the vocal folds, the lower the fundamental frequency. At rest, vocal folds are about 15–20 mm long in adult males and about 9–13 mm in adult females. The F0 of human voice also varies over the lifespan. Before puberty, both males' and females' fundamental frequencies are very similar, around 250–300 Hz. From the onset of puberty until their 20s, F0 drops to around 100–125 Hz in males and to around 200–225 Hz in females. In males, F0 continues to decrease until about the age of 60, when it begins to rise again, whereas in females F0 is generally more stable and decreases gradually over the lifespan.

Although pitch and F0 are typically described using average values, in reality, when speaking, pitch and fundamental frequency do not remain invariant but they constantly change. The mechanism for changing pitch is complex. The easiest thing to modify appears to be the tension of the vocal folds. Tensing the vocal folds increases pitch because it decreases the mass of the vocal folds and increases their elasticity. This results in a higher frequency of vibration and thus a higher F0 and higher pitch. Conversely, an increase of the mass of the vocal folds lowers pitch. Each speaker varies the fundamental frequency of his or her speech within a given pitch range, bound by the anatomical characteristics of that individual's vocal folds. It is generally believed that within that range of frequencies there is an optimal speaking pitch level at which the vocal mechanism works most effectively.

These variations of fundamental frequency during speech can affect the meaning of an utterance. Intonation is the linguistic use of pitch patterns over a phrase or a sentence that signals syntactic and semantic information. A very common use of intonation in English is a rising intonation at the end of a question. For example, the phrase "Ben went to the movies" can be produced with either a declarative or an interrogative sentence pattern depending on whether pitch falls or rises at the end of the utterance. Intonation can also be used to highlight new over given information in a sentence. For instance, in the phrase "Ben went to the movies" we can emphasize any part of the utterance by employing pitch changes on the relevant word. If the phrase was a response to the question "Who went to the movies?" it would be probably produced with a large fall of pitch on "Ben."

Although all languages have intonation systems, in some languages the variation of fundamental frequency does not only alter the meaning of phrases but can also alter the meaning of words. The linguistic use of pitch at the word level is referred to as tone. In tonal languages, such as Mandarin Chinese, sets of words that have exactly the same strings of sounds can have different meaning if produced with different pitch patterns. In English, on the other hand, producing the same word with a different pitch does not change its meaning.

Pitch modifications can also have extralinguistic functions. They can be used to express the attitudes and emotions of a speaker. It is possible for an utterance to be produced in a way that overrides the literal meaning of the words being spoken. Depending on the pitch pattern used, the phrase "Good job" can convey genuine approval or irony. Emotions can also be partly conveyed through the pitch of our voice. Typically, a high average F0, a rising pitch pattern, and a wider pitch range are used to express happy emotions. On the other hand, sad emotions tend to be associated with lower than normal fundamental frequency, a falling pitch pattern, and a narrower pitch range.

In the field of speech and language pathology, there are several examples of voice disorders that affect vocal pitch. For instance, patients with neurological speech disorders, that is, dysarthria, are often described as having abnormal pitch (consistently high or low for age and sex), pitch breaks (sudden and uncontrolled variations of F0), or monopitch (minimal F0 variations). These problems can limit the patient's communicative effectiveness because they can result in inefficient intonation patterns, or, at the very least, they can render speech unnatural and evoke negative listener perceptions. Another example of pitch-related disorder is puberphonia, the persistence of unusually high pitch beyond puberty in the absence of an organic cause. It is a psychogenic voice disorder that usually affects males and is caused by increased tension and contraction of the laryngeal muscles. Given that pitch is an important cue of gender identity, it is also relevant when working with transgender clients. Speech and language pathologist can employ a variety of behavioral strategies that aim to help the client acquire a male- or a female-sounding voice.

Ioannis Papakyritsis

See also Intonation; Suprasegmental Aspects of Speech; Vocal Production: Physics; Voice Disorders; Voice Therapy

Further Readings

Baken, R. J., & Orlikoff, R. F. (2000). *Clinical measurement of speech and voice*. San Diego, CA: Singular Publishing.

Kent, R. D. (2001). *Acoustic analysis of speech*. San Diego, CA: Singular Publishing.

Raphael, L. J., Borden, G. J., & Harris, K. S. (2011). *Speech science primer* (6th ed.). Philadelphia, PA: Lippincott Williams & Wilkins.

Placebo Effect

Placebo refers to a procedure, agent, or treatment that, on the surface, should have an inert or no therapeutic impact. The *placebo effect* is the response an individual has to the introduction of a placebo. The word *placebo* comes from a Latin verb connoting "I shall please." Medical history contains numerous accounts of the use of placebo to address and treat the troubles and desires of patients throughout the recorded history of the world. From the current use of pharmaceuticals to the historic use of drugs derived from minerals, vegetables, and other animal origins extending all the way to seemingly strange practices involving animal and human excrement, humanity has turned to an astonishing array of treatments for its varied ills. To achieve potency from the substances, these various remedies have been dispensed in equally diverse ways, from pills to plasters, from injections to incantations, all prescribed in ritualized manner by individuals believed to hold expertise in the dispersal of the intervening agent.

Throughout ancient and modern history, the placebo effect has been recorded in some form or another, but it is only in this and the previous centuries that the phenomenon has come under specific investigation. The placebo effect has impacted all disciplines and fields of study associated with understanding and treating the human condition. Disciplines associated with communication disorders have been influenced, often unknowingly, by these phenomena and yet many clinicians are unaware of the significance the placebo effect holds for both their practice and the progress (or lack of progress) their clients experience.

Defining Placebo Effect

Prior to the 20th century, placebo primarily referred to an inert substance or action deliberately given by healers to placate the needs of patients when other solutions were not available to benefit them. In the 18th century, medical texts referred to placebo as a commonplace method or medicine and was widely perceived as a viable treatment for many maladies. With medical and biological advancements of the 20th century, the meaning of placebo has expanded and evolved. While the type of placebo and nature of the study vary, it is not uncommon for the placebo effect to account for 50% or more of the change observed in treatment studies. Nevertheless, medical and clinical professionals often derisively view gains attributed to the placebo effect, not knowing whether to embrace or discard it. Placebo effects typically are interpreted in three responses. First, positive responses include favorable changes or reactions within the person or interaction. Second, negative responses, sometimes referred to as the *nocebo*, include those unfavorable changes that result in an aggravation of symptoms or negative effect in the group or individual. The third effect of placebo is the absent response where no observable effect occurs.

Identifying Placebo Effects

Placebo effect may arise from any therapeutic procedure or element of a procedure that is not objectively and specifically active for the prescribed phenomena or condition. Research has found that the placebo can arise from treatments deliberately prescribed but can also arise unknowingly as a consequence of treatment not intended to address the specific condition. From a research perspective, placebo is also often referred to as an acceptable control in experimental studies of interventions. This view of placebo arose in the early 20th century, with the introduction of the scientific method in behavioral research. The perception of placebo as an inert agent used as an experimental control emerged and substantially shaped attitudes and practices of the evaluation of treatments. Combined with statistical analysis, placebos were given in randomized control trials, first as a single-blind control, and later under double-blind conditions in order to more adequately differentiate between active and inactive treatments. The use of placebo as a double-blind control hinges on a belief that placebos are inert.

However, for the last 40 years, researchers of the placebo effect have questioned the assumption of placebos as inert versus active agents. At issue is the medical belief that an inactive substance does not exist. Rather, the dosage of any substance determines whether its function is inert or active. In areas of psychotherapy and fields such as communication disorders, conceptualizations of inert verses active therapy become quite challenging and contribute to difficulties associated with understanding placebo effect in behavioral and social intervention research. For example, one might ask: What would constitute an inert psychotherapy or an inert intervention provided by a speech–language pathologist? The complexity of this question may account for why inquiries into the placebo effect with treatments of communication disorders are often overlooked. When efforts are made to adequately consider the effect, researchers do so through the use of a controlled study comparison. However, the development of placebo controls in studies of communication disorders present a major problem associated with what constitutes credible interventions capable of serving as a therapeutic control. To determine the placebo effect, the control used must be identical to the therapy under investigation with the exception of the specific technique or theoretical principle to be evaluated. This would mean that a credible placebo intervention must contain the same level of therapist investment and client motivation, in addition to duration and number of intervention sessions and other variables of validity and reliability. To illustrate this challenge with one variable, consider the notion that double-blinded random control intervention studies in communication disorders require that the clinician be blinded to the intervention treatment the client is receiving. Without the clinician blinding to the intervention method, therapist investment in the placebo condition would function as a potential biasing effect. A circumstance where clinicians do not know the intervention they were providing is tough to conceptualize and more arduous to implement. Extensions of similar related and conflicting issues are not hard to envision.

Placebo effects reported in the literature related to communication disorders are limited. Random controlled studies using double-blinded methodologies most routinely involve a pharmacological agent and persons with diagnosed what is believed to be a neurogenic-based disorder (e.g., autism, aphasia, traumatic brain injury, dementia, attention deficit hyperactivity disorder). When behavioral interventions have been studied, rarely has the methodology included randomization and most studies meeting this requirement are single-blinded with the clinician being aware of the specific treatment contention implemented. Therefore, narrowly controlled single-subject designs and treatment comparisons studies are more often used to account for therapeutic effects in communication disorders.

While the practicality of double-blinded experimentation is limited in this field, efforts to control for placebo effect through other means have been attempted even if this purpose was not overtly stated in the methodology. To address challenges of creating placebo-controlled studies, researchers may turn to single-subject designs where the client functions as their own control. Other methods attempt to contrast one therapy with another. The assumption is that by using clinicians experienced in the specific practices being contrasted, influencing variables can be adequately controlled and therefore gains in one intervention over that of others would be representative of change not attributable to placebo effects. However, failure to observe differentiated gains between treatments would not rule out placebo effect. If a number of such interventions, along with inquiries into the accompanying elements, are studied and one or more treatment consistently yields superior results, the assumption would suggest the responses are not due to placebo effect. While these methodological innovations are valuable in understanding efficacy of intervention, experienced researchers appreciate how difficult it is to focus on authentic communicative phenomena while controlling the associated and influencing variables.

How Do Placebo Effects Work?

Truthfully, researchers and clinicians are not certain how exactly placebo effects emerge. Yet much has been learned about factors and mechanisms involved in the response. In medicine and other disciplines, culture and method of treatment dispersal (e.g., injections vs. pills vs. topical solutions) as well as age, location, social status, religiosity, and a host of other variables have been found to contribute to placebo effects. However, for the purposes of this entry relevant to communication disorders, client and clinician attributes will be expanded upon briefly. Client attributes and expectancies are known to contribute to the placebo effect. Personal openness to suggestibility and an individual belief of treatment efficacy has been found to influence outcomes. Placebo effect has been observed in clients who talked to themselves with an active voice, demonstrated a sense of information seeking, and exhibited a sense of internal locus of control. Participation in interventions may raise clients' awareness of communication issues and cause them to change their behaviors in ways that modify and improve behaviors and perspective of those behaviors. This may be true whether clients involved in research studies are in the treatment group or the placebo group and may account for some of the observed placebo effect. Extending beyond the client, it is plausible that family members, caregivers, or significant others who are looking for possible responses to an intervention may engage their loved one in activities more intensively in a way that influences how they respond to therapy. Nevertheless, there is ample evidence that attributes associated with those receiving therapy influence the placebo effect.

Clinician attributes are known to influence responses to placebos. Clinicians who showed confidence, warm feelings for their clients, and enthusiasm for treatments are thought to be more likely to contribute to placebo effects. For example, clinicians who see their clients more frequently may be more likely to convey attributes more conducive to placebo effects than those who see their patients infrequently or vice versa. Clinicians' practices are guided by theories. Whether or not they overtly acknowledge it, practices are shaped by belief systems. This provokes in the clinician a kind of intensity or purpose to engage in the effort of helping the client make changes. With this belief comes a certain affective charge that has been found to affect the performance of clients in a variety of talk and rehabilitative therapies. Clinicians create particular interpersonal contexts that contribute to the delivery of interventions and the clients' perceived confidence in expected outcomes. These attributes of clinicians may not be directly related to the prescribed intervention, though they can and often are purposeful, and yet they surely contribute intervention gains that may be attributed to the placebo effect.

The Meaning Effect

For the past 20 years, some researchers have suggested that placebo effects should be approached and conceptualized in dramatically different ways if we hope to better understand how clients improve. Daniel Moerman proposes that positive responses and negative responses (nocebos) to placebos be viewed as meaning responses. What is often important in interventions is that clients, significant others, clinicians, and all those involved are in some way convinced that techniques are powerful and effective and that undeniable evidence of effectiveness exists. This conviction provokes or contributes to a meaning response resulting in the therapeutic change. Such power can come from places of personal experience, cultural beliefs and practices, religious belief, medical beliefs, personal experiences, scientific assertions, or any other host of sources. The significance is that somewhere or somehow, the treatment is meaningful to those involved. In communication disorders, it may be more reasonable to conceptualize therapy as evoking meaning responses in clients that allows individuals and groups of individuals to marshal resources in ways not directly observable and yet meaningful to the client in ways that result in behavioral change.

Ryan Nelson

See also Evidence-Based Practice; Experimental Research; Locus of Control; Meaning; Validity

Further Readings

Bensing, J. M., & Verheul, W. (2010). The silent healer: The role of communication in placebo effects. *Patient Education and Counseling, 80*(3), 293–299. https://doi.org/10.1016/j.pec.2010.05.033

Gruber, F. A., Lowery, S. D., Seung, H., & Deal, R. E. (2003). Approaches to speech-language intervention and the true believer. *Journal of Medical Speech-Language Pathology, 11*(2), 95–104.

Moerman, D. (2002). *Meaning, medicine and the "placebo effect."* Cambridge, UK: University Press.

Sandler, A. (2005). Placebo effects in developmental disabilities: Implications for research and practice. *Mental Retardation & Developmental Disabilities Research Reviews, 11*(2), 164–170. https://doi.org/10.1002/mrdd.20065

Shapiro, A., & Shapiro, E. (1997). *The powerful placebo: From ancient priest to modern physician.* Baltimore, MD: Johns Hopkins University Press.

PLASTICITY OF THE BRAIN

Understanding how the brain changes and learns is fundamental to understanding rehabilitation and the mechanisms that underlie all behavioral interventions. This entry provides a broad overview of neuroplasticity and how it relates to normal learning and learning after brain injury.

What Is Neuroplasticity?

The human adult cerebral neural system was once thought to be unyielding and incapable of regeneration and large-scale change. In the last 15–20 years, the extraordinary potential for neuronal plasticity in the human central nervous system has been recognized. The term *neuroplasticity* has gathered increased attention in the literature as scientists use new technologies to measure a natural phenomenon that has been happening since the evolution of humankind. Neuroplasticity is simply the brain's ability to learn and adapt, to wire and rewire neuronal connections to more efficiently perform every task we do as humans. However, much of what is known about neuroplasticity derives from animal models and motor recovery in humans, and caution must be exercised when extrapolating from these models to higher-order functions including cognition and language.

Neuroplasticity underpins automatic functions such as sitting upright through to complex tasks such as using language to debate a topic, playing tennis, learn a new language, cooking a new recipe, or learning to play a musical instrument. Neuroplasticity is an umbrella term that describes the structural and functional adaptation of the connectivity of brain cells (neurons) that form neural synapses and pathways. Neuroplasticity is based on our interactions with the environment, our experiences, learning, thinking, and our emotions. It is an accumulation of the fundamental cellular mechanisms that underpin every learned function that people perform. Neuroplasticity is use-dependent, reliant on memory and not limited to humans. Laying down neural pathways in infantile development uses very similar neurobiological processes as it does when that behavior or task has to be relearned following brain injury. Repetition is the major component of new learning, but it takes more than repetition to be efficient and effective at a skill. Skill development and mastery require (a) repetition in high doses, or massed practice; (b) task specificity, or "train as you play"; and (c) task saliency, or "meaningful practice." In short, to learn a task, an adult human needs to complete over 3,000 task-specific repetitions, in an environment that emulates the real world, to achieve skill competency. At a cellular level, such high-dose, task-specific, and meaningful practice results in neuronal long-term potentiation (LTP), which is the rapidly induced and sustained efficiency of neural transmission at a synapse that results in learning and memory. Increased efficiency of the synaptic transmission, stronger cellular growth, and improved system reorganization have been shown in early brain recovery when highly repetitious trained tasks are used as part of rehabilitation. One proposed mechanism for this finding is the ongoing GABAergic transmission and associated efficiency of this transmission in learned behaviors (LTP).

Cellular- and Systems-Level Plasticity

Neuroplasticity occurs at a cellular level (secondary to learning) and at a systems level. Cellular-level plasticity involves single neurons changing their structure, for example, increasing axons and developing more synapses with other adjoining neurons. Systems-level neuroplasticity results in cortical remapping or adaptation of the cortical representation of a learned behavior.

Neuroplasticity encompasses synaptic and nonsynaptic plasticity. *Synaptic plasticity* refers to the capacity of a neural synapse (minute space between neurons in which impulses communicated via neurotransmitters) to strengthen or weaken in response to the activity of the synapse. That is, a synapse will increase in efficiency and strength if the behavior that requires the impulse to be transmitted is increased (commonly known as the "use it" principle). Similarly, a synapse will weaken and can disappear if an impulse is not regularly fired. This most frequently happens when the behavior driving the precise synaptic response is not carried out (referred to as the "lose it" principle). This complex process requires many concomitant mechanisms to work in conjunction with one another to produce an effective system. Synaptic plasticity is affected by the amount and type of neurotransmitters involved in the transmission of the impulse, the efficiency of the uptake of the neurotransmitter, and the behavior/task being undertaken at the time the impulse is being transmitted. Synaptic plasticity is the collective term for the neurochemical mechanisms referred to in the Hebbian theory and underpins many rehabilitative theories including "use it or lose it" and "neurons that fire together—wire together."

Nonsynaptic plasticity involves changes in the electrical function (ion balance and channels) of the axons, dendrites, and cell body of a neuron. Nonsynaptic plasticity results in particular intrinsic cellular changes as a result the excitatory and inhibitory potentials of the cell itself. Nonsynaptic plasticity plays a major role in neuroplasticity and is responsible for the cellular exchanges that allow for learning and memory. This complex phenomenon is not within the scope of this entry, and further reading to better understand the physiological mechanisms underlying neuronal functioning and what affects this process is suggested below.

What Happens After Brain Injury?

Neuronal death begins to occur within 2 minutes when normal metabolic substrates (oxygen and glucose) are not delivered in sufficient quantities. Primary cellular changes occur causing neuronal death. Neuronal cell death can be caused by hypoxia, trauma, hemorrhage, or ischemia. Subsequent brain tissue changes ensue. These primary cellular changes occur to all cells deprived of oxygen and glucose and collectively result in an area of infarcted tissue. This area of infarction is surrounded by an area known as the penumbra, which experiences secondary edema. The penumbra experiences resultant decreased electrical activity due to a disruption of metabolic function. This leads to a process of diaschisis, which is the loss of electrical activity in areas related by function, but not necessarily local to the area of cell death. Therefore, not only is the function of the area of infarction and the penumbra affected but so are distant areas of function by virtue of the loss of electrical activity to interconnected areas. Diaschisis has specific relevance in the human communication system as this system involves an enormously complex neuronal network that is dynamically engaged in language processing.

The area immediately surrounding the penumbra is termed the perilesional area. Both the penumbra and perilesional areas have hypoperfused blood supply resulting in reduced levels of tissue oxygenation. Hypoperfusion does not cause cellular death, but it renders the cells in these areas incapable of normal function. During the time frame of the cellular changes, despite the experienced hypoperfusion in the perilesional area, the electrophysiological function remains relatively normal. This is important because the penumbra and perilesional areas are thought to be recruited to take over function of the infarcted tissue in the process of neurorecovery. The rapid and early functional recovery that is reflected during the period immediately following the infarction is often referred to as spontaneous recovery.

Secondary changes to the neuronal tissue occur as a direct consequence of the brain insult and occur in a temporal sequence. Collectively, these processes underlie neurorecovery and allow the brain to regain function after injury. They are as follows: transneuronal degeneration, denervation supersensitivity (also termed denervation hypersensitivity), resolution of diaschisis, upregulation, collateral sprouting, and synaptogenesis. *Transneuronal degeneration* is the degeneration of tissue that loses its usual connections to the infarcted area. *Denervation supersensitivity* applies to the penumbra where the cells that have lost function become supersensitive to any residual electrical input. *Resolution of diaschisis* is the process of regaining the electrical activity that has previously been lost to areas distant to the infarcted tissue. *Unmasking* or *upregulation* refers to the recruitment of previously present but inactive tissue connections, and *collateral sprouting* involves the regeneration of axonal and dendritic branches. Last, *synaptogenesis* is the formation of new synapses.

A Temporal Model of Neurorecovery

The previously described neuroplastic processes and how they are believed to relate to the timing of clinical recovery are important to consider. Although in practical terms, mapping the correlation of neuroplastic mechanisms to timing of cellular recovery is not possible, there is a body of literature that proposes temporal models for brain recovery. The bulk of this evidence relates to motor function, and it is important to keep this in mind when reviewing this information. In general terms, there are five phases relating to motor neurorecovery after stroke: the hyperacute, acute, subacute, consolidation, and chronic phases.

The hyperacute phase is the time frame defined from the onset of stroke to 9 hours poststroke when the direct consequences of ischemia are most prominent. **The acute phase** covers the time frame from 9 hours to 4 days poststroke, when secondary changes reach a peak. It is during the hyperacute and acute phases that the primary and secondary changes described above occur.

The subacute phase commences at 48 hours (therefore overlapping with the acute phase) and continues for up to 4 weeks poststroke. It corresponds to the time where the events in the hyperacute and acute phases have subsided and the area of cell death is stable. This involves the resolution of secondary changes and continuation of neuroplasticity, which occurs to its greatest extent in this phase. During this phase, the perilesional network is exceedingly active in adapting to internal mechanisms of deafferentation and externally to mechanisms that compensate for the areas producing functional deficit.

The consolidation phase is defined in various models as a time onward of 4 weeks, lasting up to several months, coinciding with the chronic phase, which is from 6 months onward. During the consolidation phase there is a leveling of metabolic change. Cortical excitability is thought to continue well into this phase and could reflect a stabilization of the imbalance of the network activation and inhibition in the perilesional and contralesional areas.

Behavioral Interventions and Neuroplasticity: Principles Underlying Experience-Dependent Brain Change

There are 10 general principles proffered in the literature to underpin experience-dependent learning (rehabilitation) following brain injury. Variations in these principles are noted based on the foci of the research being presented; however, these principles are the foundation of all rehabilitation after brain injury. These principles are the following:

1. Use it or lose it: This refers to functional degradation if the function is not frequently used.

2. Use it and improve it: This refers to strengthening and improving functional activity that is frequently performed.

3. Task specificity: The nature of the activity dictates the nature of the plasticity; this can be likened to "match fitness," that is, the task needs to be practiced the way that it will be performed in real life.

4. Repetition: Neural change requires repetition of the task/activity.

5. Intensity: Neural change requires sufficient intensity to permanently establish pathways.

6. Time postonset: Neural plasticity occurs at different times and rates post-brain injury; early rehabilitation is thought to take advantage of natural recovery processes.

7. Salience: Tasks and activities should be meaningful (this assists with task specificity, repetition, and intensity).

8. Age: Younger brains are more receptive to new learning and neural change.

9. Transference: New training is likely to enhance similar but not necessarily trained tasks or behaviors.

10. Interference: Acquisition of new behaviors can be interfered with by other experiences.

Yet to this point rehabilitation efficacy standards have not been set to a level that induces neuronal plasticity in all people with brain injury. The knowledge base of neuroplasticity is developing rapidly; however, there are many limitations to applying this knowledge in clinical settings. Many of these limitations are "system perpetuated"; others require "discovery scientists" (in all areas, not basic science alone) to develop new and improved ways of looking at the problem. The system-perpetuated limitations see a siloed approach whereby basic scientists work in labs that are distinct from the service providers. Similarly, service providers work in distinct disciplines (medical, allied health, nursing) and in distinct health care institutions, which in turn work in either acute care, rehabilitation, or community facilities. This approach never really facilitates cross-pollination of ideas or seamless service delivery.

Clinicians must ensure that they understand and translate theoretical, anatomical, and behavioral perspectives into each and every session of intervention provided. With an ever-stretched health service, clinicians need to be providing the right therapy to the right people at the right time.

They can only do this with self-reflection and ongoing development of their science and service delivery.

Erin Godecke

See also Anatomy of the Human Neurological System; Aphasia; Brain Imaging; Neurogenic Disorders

Further Readings

Jones, T. A., & Schallert, T. (1994). Use-dependent growth of pyramidal neurons after neocortical damage. *Journal of Neuroscience, 14*(4), 2140–2152. https://doi.org/10.1523/JNEUROSCI.14-04-02140.1994

Kleim, J. A., & Jones, T. A. (2008). Principles of experience-dependent neural plasticity: Implications for rehabilitation after brain injury. *Journal of Speech, Language, and Hearing Research, 51*(1), S225–S239. https://doi.org/10.1044/1092-4388(2008/018)

Kreisel, S. H., Bäzner, H., & Hennerici, M. G. (2006). Pathophysiology of stroke rehabilitation: Temporal aspects of neurofunctional recovery. *Cerebrovascular Diseases, 21*, 6–17. https://doi.org/10.1159/000089588

Kwakkel, G., Kollen, B., & Lindeman, E. (2004). Understanding the pattern of functional recovery after stroke: Facts and theories. *Restorative Neurology and Neurosciences, 22*, 281–299.

Marsh, E. B., & Hillis, A. E. (2005). Recovery from aphasia following brain injury: The role of reorganization. *Progress in Brain Research, 157*, 143–156.

Saur, D., Lange, R., Baumgaertner, A., Schraknepper, V., Willmes, K., Rijntjes, M., & Weiller, C. (2006). Dynamics of language reorganization after stroke. *Brain, 129*, 1371–1384. https://doi.org/10.1093/brain/awl090

Speelman, C., & Maybery, M. (1998). *Automaticity and skill acquisition*. In K. Kirsner, C. Speelman, M. Maybery, A. O'Brien-Malone, M. Anderson, & C. MacLeod (Eds.), *Implicit and explicit mental processes* (pp. 79–98). Mahwah, NJ: Erlbaum.

Play

Play can be defined as an activity that is self-chosen, motivated by means rather than ends, has mental rules, and includes a strong aspect of imagination. Everyone has experienced and observed play: play with friends, organized sports, board games, and watching children on the playground. Few people are familiar with how play is related to early human development and what happens as an infant grows to use mental symbols. When a child picks up a plastic stacking cup and puts it to his or her lips to pretend to drink a little milk, the stacking cup is a symbol for a real cup. Likewise, when a child pretends a banana is a telephone (old technology) or a domino is a smartphone (new technology), that object is a symbol in the child's mind for the object pictured in the mind. When a child says his or her first word, *dada*, the spoken word is the symbol for the father. The ability to manipulate symbols, both in play and in language, represents a significant cognitive milestone in the development of the growing child. Researchers have wondered if play precedes language or if language dominates play. Likewise, they have wondered if there is, or is not, a relationship between the two cognitive abilities. This entry provides an overview of play and its stages, the relationship between play and cognitive development from the perspectives of domain-specific and domain-general theories, and the importance of symbolic play in communication development.

Play Skills and the Domain General View of Cognitive Development

An early cognitive achievement of the infant is the ability to use representational thought. Jean Piaget in 1970 documented a consistent developmental sequence in symbolic skills beginning when a child is in his or her pre-operational period (i.e., 18 months to 5–7 years of age). Language and pretend play both necessitate that the child mentally represent reality, though language is more difficult than play. Research by Carol Westby and colleagues in the early 1980s investigated the relationship between play and language development. They hypothesized that words do not represent reality in any clear way and play sequences are more loosely connected than the rule-governed structure of grammar in spoken language. Westby based her understanding of the relationship between play skills and language on her understanding of Piaget's work. Early symbolic play skills were understood to be prerequisites for the development of early language and were thought to progress in a stagelike fashion:

Stage 1 (9–12 months of age): Children no longer simply mouth objects but have developed the ability to find a toy hidden under a small blanket (object permanence) and can pull a string to get a toy on the end of the string (means-end). Children vocalize to request or command.

Stage 2 (13–17 months of age): Children can quickly discover how to operate a toy by pressing a button or pulling on a lever. If children fail to operate the toy, they will hand the toy to an adult to find how to operate it. Some children may use a single word at this stage, but it is often dependent on the context and may not be used in other situations. Children do use utterances and gestures for many more communication functions: greet, protest, request, label, and indicate "Look at me!"

Stage 3 (17–19 months of age): Children direct symbolic actions on themselves (e.g., self-pretending to sleep or drink from a cup). Verbal language begins and children use words for a variety of functions. Children talk about the here and now, not absent subjects. This signifies the beginning of representational thought.

Stage 4 (19–22 months of age): Children begin to extend symbolic play actions away to other actors (e.g., giving a bottle to a doll, or brushing mother's hair with a toy brush). Children can speak with word combinations (e.g., *mommy sock*) and talk about things not present. Possessive function is seen when children talk about *my car* while in a small group of children.

Stage 5 (24 months of age): Children pretend the activities of other children. Children pretend real events from life (e.g., pretending to be the mommy or the daddy). Pretend objects are more lifelike rather than miniature. Block play is stacking and knocking down. Blocks are not incorporated into play by being made into buildings. Sand and water play is filling and dumping from containers. Children are speaking in short sentences and the "–ing" begins to appear on verbs. Sometimes plurals are also marked by adding "-s."

Stage 6 (2½ years of age): Children pretend other life events. Doctor-sick child is one example. The events are short, and often children switch roles quickly. Realistic toys are still used. Parallel play (i.e., play in which two children will sit side by side, playing with the same toys and not interact with each other) dominates. Linguistically, children begin to answer *wh*-questions, although responses to *why* questions are usually wrong.

Stage 7 (3 years of age): Children can now sequence play events (e.g., the child is hurt, mom calls the doctor, and the ambulance takes the child to the hospital). These events are not planned but evolve as the children play. Realistic toys are still used. Children do not yet use full cooperative play but begin to play together in what is termed *associative play*. Children can talk about things that happened in the past or will happen in the future.

Stage 8 (3–3½ years of age): Children move away from realistic toys and begin to use miniature barns and villages. Real objects become play props. Chairs in a row can be seats on an airplane. There is a marked growth in descriptive vocabulary. As children begin to pretend with less real objects, they also begin to take another person's perspective. This allows children to create dialogue between the characters (e.g., "The doctor will tell the lady she needs a shot").

Stage 9 (4 years of age): Children are able to problem solve about events that have not been experienced. They can also make predictions about future events. Children are able to reject items as *too big* or *too flimsy* without using trial and error. Play structures become more elaborate. Children are beginning to be able to use modals such as *might* or *could*. Doll and puppet play become more elaborate as children act out scenes based on "What would happen if?"

Stage 10 (5 years of age): Children are required to use language to organize the play. Full cooperative play with others is now possible. Plans are made and many different play scenes and events can be managed. Children are no longer dependent on realistic toys and can use their imagination. Time relational terms such as *first*, *then*, and *when* are used.

Westby and colleagues suggested that this play stage progression could be used to determine what language might need to be taught to a child. She theorized that unless the child has the cognitive play skill ability, the child may not be able to learn a targeted language skill.

Other Views of Cognitive Development

Since 2010, researchers have questioned whether symbolic play is a prerequisite for language development as Westby and others suggested. As has been seen, her work follows Piaget whose argument in the mid-1950s that cognitive processes operate across different areas of knowledge in similar ways at similar rates has become representative of the *domain-general* view of cognitive development. A major principle of Piaget's theory is that cognition development precedes and is the basis for language development. Domain-general theories suggest positive relationships between play and language through development over time. Contrasted with domain-general theories is the view that symbolic cognitive development is *domain-specific*. Investigations have hypothesized that each form of symbolic use develops in different areas of the brain and unrelated to one another. Particularly, language theorists Steven Pinker and Noam Chomsky believe language is domain specific and viewed as developing independently of any other cognitive systems. Domain-specific theories suggest symbolic play and language develop independently.

Lev Vygotsky in the late 1970s brought another view to this relationship. Like Piaget, Vygotsky viewed symbolic functioning as emerging toward the end of the second year of life. However, to Vygotsky, the representational function does not emerge entirely from cognition but from early speech and nonverbal systems. After integration, language enhances cognition through internalization to become private speech when children are around 4–5 years of age. Vygotsky believed symbolic function allowed domain-general change in the child's cognitive abilities and yet language has a fundamental role not dependent on the change. Of all symbolic activities, Vygotsky viewed language as the most important symbol system. Similar to Vygotsky, Michael Tomasello in the late 1990s put an emphasis on language. Language was viewed as developing from and acquired as a joint attentional activity to share and direct attention with others. Language emerged from a succession of increasing complex attentional behaviors progressing from simple gaze, to gaze-following, to imitation, and then to pointing and declarative gestures. Theories from Piaget, Vygotsky, and Tomasello both propose language and symbolic play develop in a fixed sequence, while Vygotsky and Tomasello suggest that language emerges first and predicts play abilities over time. Indeed, 2013 research by Julie Kirkham and colleagues revealed that domain-general symbolic development in a child's 4th year, with play and language and graphic symbolic skills all interrelated and developing in parallel (supporting the domain-general pattern), was found in a longitudinal portion of the study to reveal only that language measures in year 4 predicted play and graphic symbol use in year 5. This confirmed the theories of Vygotsky and Tomasello.

The Importance of Symbolic Play

Of interest to clinicians, the importance of symbolic play has been recognized as a diagnostic marker for children with autistic spectrum disorders. Amy Wetherby and Barry Prizant in the early 2000s developed the first normed edition of Communication and Symbolic Behavior Scale (CSBS) for use with very young children (aged 8 months to 2 years) who might be at risk of developing communication impairment. The CSBS procedure uses action-based toys, books for young children, and play objects to assess how a child uses and plays with the toys symbolically. In addition, *communication temptations*, such as a few Cheerios in a jar with the lid tightly screwed on, invite the child to communicate. The CSBS measured clusters of child behaviors to score a child's: (1) communication functions, (2) gestural communicative means, (3) vocal communicative means, (4) verbal communicative means, (5) reciprocity, (6) social–affective signaling, and (7) symbolic behavior (play). Wetherby and Prizant recognized the complicated interweaving of early language, early communication, and early play could provide a diagnostic tool for very young children. A screening tool from the CSBS included the CSBS Infant Toddle Checklist and was later validated in an investigation of its use by Wetherby and colleagues. The CSBS Developmental Profile (DP) functions as a screening tool, a norm-referenced test, or for progress reports. Unlike many standardized tests, items from the CSBS DP can be taken as goals for the child's therapy.

Play, as a form of symbolic behavior, provides a window into the very young child's mind as he or she begins to understand and use symbols. From the simple mouthing of, or batting at, a toy; through symbolic acts directed at first, the self, accompanied by single words and later, to another; to the combinations of play sequences that typically accompany the child's ability to combine words, it can be seen that play and language develop in tandem in a child's mind until language becomes dominant as the child prepares to enter school.

Pam Britton Reese

See also Autism Spectrum Disorder; Delayed Language Development; Joint Attention; Language Acquisition

Further Readings

Chomsky, N. (1957). *Syntactic structures.* The Hague, The Netherlands: Mouton.

Piaget, J. (1952). *The origins of intelligence in children.* New York, NY: Norton.

Piaget, J. (1970). *The psychology of intelligence.* New York, NY: Orion Press.

Pinker, S. (1997). *How the mind works.* New York, NY: Norton.

Tomasello, M. (1999). *The cultural origins of human cognition.* Cambridge, MA: Harvard University Press.

Vygotsky, L. (1978). *Mind in society: The development of higher psychological processes.* Cambridge, MA: Harvard University Press.

Westby, C. (1980). Language abilities through play. *Language, Speech and Hearing services in the Schools, XI,* 154–168.

Wetherby, A. M., & Prizant, B. (2002). *Communication and symbolic behavior scales developmental profile–first normed edition.* Baltimore, MD: Brookes.

PLAY THERAPY

Play has been described as an activity that has the following five characteristics, according to Peter Gray: (1) it is self-chosen and self-directed; (2) intrinsically motivated; (3) guided by mental rules; (4) imaginative; and (5) conducted in an active, alert, but relatively nonstressed frame of mind. Play has been used as the context, and the impetus for many interventions aimed at improving the mental and physical welfare of both children and adults. In the early 1900s, mental health concerns for children and the pioneering efforts of a handful of psychoanalysts gave rise to the intervention known as *play therapy.* This entry provides an overview of play therapy, focusing on child-centered play therapy (CCPT) and its use as well as the role of play therapy in treating children with autism spectrum disorder (ASD) and children with communication disorders.

Overview

Play therapy is a recognized intervention based on theoretical assumptions whose goal is to reduce problematic behaviors, assist with coping, and decrease the effects of trauma. Adults often are able to work through problems using words; however, play is the context through which children can explore and express their feelings. Toys, manipulatives, and other props are used to help the recipient of play therapy to express emotions and communicate thoughts in a culturally and developmentally appropriate manner. Play therapy has been reported as an efficacious approach for significantly improving social adjustment, behavior, and personality issues across different providers and different settings, with evidence of large effect sizes (.80) in meta-analyses. Length of play therapy and the amount of parent involvement have been found to moderate the success of play therapy.

CCPT

Over the past 100 years, several types of play therapy motivated by different theoretical views have been developed that fall largely into one of two domains: directive and nondirective. One of the first nondirective types of play therapy was developed by Carl Rogers, in 1951. He extended an existing therapy approach, Relationship Therapy, which focused on the relationship between the therapist and child as the therapeutic element of the intervention, and established client-centered therapy or person-centered therapy. Roger's student, Virginia Mae Axline, extended this work to become what is known as *CCPT.* In CCPT, the child guides the therapy process. The therapist's relationship with the child is friendly, accepting, and respectful. The therapist mirrors feelings and emotions back to the child for reflection and problem solving. It is the child's responsibility to make decisions and to make changes as a result of the guidance from the therapist. Innate resiliency and self-growth combined with the guidance of a skilled play therapist leads to self-healing and self-realization, which are deemed to be within the capabilities of the child. CCPT is unlike other play interventions in that it takes into account the child's feelings as well as the child's behaviors. Importantly, it is the therapist who follows the child's lead.

In the 1940s, CCPT studies were conducted to better understand the effectiveness of play therapy on intelligence as well as on reading abilities and language development. CCPT has been found to be effective for reducing disruptive behaviors in preschoolers and elementary school-age children. Since the mid-1960s, CCPT has been utilized with children who are at risk for academic failure, children with expressive and receptive language disorders, children with articulation disorders, children with fluency disorders, children with attention deficit disorders, children with selective mutism, and children with behavioral and/or social–emotional disorders individually and in small groups. The use of CCPT with children at risk for academic failure resulted in improvements in spoken language skills, reading and writing abilities, math skills, and overall early achievement. Children with expressive and receptive language disorders also have shown language outcome benefits from CCPT.

Play Therapy and Children With ASD

Children with ASD have been the recipients of play therapy that has taken different forms depending on the professional providing the intervention. For example, Axline's classic description of CCPT was documented with a case study, Dibs. It is believed that in the 21st century, Dibs would have been diagnosed as having ASD. Other researchers have reported positive outcomes of using adapted play therapy with children with ASD. One play therapy program called *Learn to Play* was introduced by Karen Stagnitti and her colleagues, in 2012. This program was a method for teaching 5- and 6-year-olds with intellectual disabilities and ASD and/or developmental delays how to engage in pretend play. It was based on the earlier work of Lorraine McCune-Nicolich who posited three play/language relationships: (1) the onset of pretend play and emergence of vocabulary; (2) symbolic play combinations and word combinations; and (3) hierarchical play combinations and emergence of rule-governed language. Teachers, speech–language pathologists, and occupational therapists implemented the *Learn to Play* program over 6 months. The program focused on increasing the children's play skills, and as part of the process, they were encouraged to discuss their emotions and to become emotionally involved during play. Stagnitti and her colleagues found that children in the treatment group made gains in both pretend play and social interaction skills, and that these skills were highly correlated.

Play Therapy and Children With Communication Disorders

The importance of play for a child's expression, along with child-centered guidance by the therapist, is reflected in early intervention approaches in speech–language pathology. The child-centered nature of early intervention in communication disorders follows the theoretical basis of the social interactionist view of language development as well as the cognitive/social view of language development. Jerome Bruner proposed that play is the natural context in which language is developed, with caregivers providing scaffolding through joint reference and attention and linguistic stimulation. The speech–language pathologist has historically used play in two respects, one as a natural context for improving speech, language, and social interaction abilities and the other as a targeted skill that is linked to language skills. Whether a session takes place one-on-one in a therapy room, in the home, in a small group, or in the preschool classroom, play is typically the context in which all activities aimed at improving a child's speech, language, and interaction skills takes place. The speech–language pathologist follows the child's lead during play and uses the natural setting of play to provide linguistic models, prompts, and feedback to the child, which are tailored to individual communicative goals. In playgroups, children may participate in role-playing or dramatic play activities, which allow the child access to new vocabulary, social games/rules, and syntactic or morphological targets. In other cases, particularly when children are experiencing difficulty with social interactions, but also in the case of language delay, play skills are assessed and as a result, the speech–language pathologist may help children to develop play skills such as object play, functional play, symbolic play, and/or peer play.

Final Thoughts

The definition of play is largely the same across professions that use it as an integral element of their interventions. However, play therapy has its own unique meaning in different disciplines and uses different tools to accomplish its goals. In therapy, the goal is to improve the mental health of the child. Allowing the child to express himself or herself through play with the guidance of the counselor or psychologist is a key element of play therapy. In contrast, in speech–language pathology, the goal is to improve the communication skills of the child. The child is taught play skills in a nondirective play environment that provides the opportunity for linguistic models that are contingent on the child's play and verbal or nonverbal communication. Although different professions use play and play therapy for specific goals consistent with their own profession, the end result of play therapy or CCPT is typically the same. That is, it leads to the increased wellness of the child. That wellness may be observed through improved mental health functioning and/or communication skills.

Diane Frome Loeb and Eric S. Davis

See also Autism Spectrum Disorder; Language Therapy and Intervention; Late Talkers; Mediation in Therapy; Play; Preschool Language Intervention; Usage-Based Approach to Language Acquisition

Further Readings

Axline, V. M. (1964). *Dibs: In search of self: Personality development in play therapy*. Boston, MA: Houghton Mifflin.

Blaco, P. J., Ray, D. C., & Holliman, R. (2012). Long-term child centered play therapy and academic achievement of children: A follow-up study. *International Journal of Play Therapy, 21*(1), 1–13.

Bratton, S. C., Ray, D., Rhine, T., & Jones, L. (2005). The efficacy of play therapy with children: A meta-analytic review of treatment outcomes. *Professional Psychology: Research and Practice, 36*(4), 376–390.

Bruner, J. S. (1975). The ontogenesis of speech acts. *Journal of Child Language, 2*, 1–19.

Casby, M. W. (2003). The development of play in infants, toddlers, and young children. *Communication Disorders Quarterly, 24*(4), 163–174.

Danger, S., & Landreth, G. L. (2005). Child-centered group play therapy with children with speech difficulties. *International Journal of Play Therapy, 14*, 81–102.

Gray, P. (2013). Definitions of play. *Scholarpedia, 8*(7), 30578. doi:10.4249/scholarpedia.30578

Landreth, G. L. (2012). *Play therapy: The art of the relationship* (3rd ed.). New York, NY: Routledge.

McCune-Nicolich, L. (1981). Toward symbolic functioning: Structure of early pretend games and potential parallels with language. *Child Development, 52*, 785–797.

Rogers, C. (1951). *Client-centered therapy: Its current practice*. Boston, MA: Houghton Mifflin.

Staginatti, K., O'Connor, C., & Sheppard, L. (2012). Impact of the learn to play program on play, social competence and language for children age 5-8 years who attend a specialist school. *Australian Occupational Therapy Journal, 59*, 302–311.

POSITIVE PSYCHOLOGY AND WELLNESS

Positive psychology as a phrase first appeared in the literature in the work of Abraham Maslow in the 1950s with his description of self-actualization and creativity as an aspect of humanistic psychology. However, as a distinct and formalized branch of psychology, it did not appear until Martin Seligman pushed the initiative in his role as president of the American Psychological Association in 1998. Positive psychology is a close relative of humanistic psychology with perhaps a greater appreciation for the scientific method and empirical methods of inquiry. Additionally, more so than humanistic thought, positive psychology holds an acceptance of the bad as well as the good in humanity as being genuine and worthy of study, without the assumption that people are inherently good. Wellness and the tenets that make up positive psychology hold a long history of research and interest in a number of disciplines, but it is only since the late 1990s that these ideas have entered mainstream awareness and, to some extent, gained acceptance. This entry provides an overview of the history of positive psychology and wellness, examining its history, definition, and its rise and expansion since the late 1990s.

History

The field of human communication disorders has been shaped in part by the various movements in psychology. From narrow applications of behaviorism to understandings of constructivist thought, psychology's various movements have, for better or worse, influenced theories of prevention, assessments, and interventions for persons with communicative disorders. Most pervasively, a medical model focused on deficits has driven advancements since the field emerged as a specific discipline. The medical, disease-oriented model of human functioning has maintained a preoccupation with localizing deficits and repairing disorders found within individuals.

Two of the more influential pioneering advocates of positive psychology, namely Martin Seligman and Christopher Peterson, have traced the movement, in general, as a shift in the field, responding to a solitary focus established immediately following World War II. Prior to World War II, psychology focused on three main missions: curing mental illness, improving the productivity of all people, and improving and enhancing human performance. Following World War II, the missions of psychology narrowed solely to that of addressing mental illness. In the decades that followed, there were important and impactful branches of psychology that offered reconceptualizations and new looks at the human condition, but much of the overall field of psychology remained focused on studying the deficits and frailties of humanity. Much of the research and clinical thought that formed the foundation of related disciplines, such as communicative disorders, adopted the rehabilitative focus that arose from such a deficit-based perspective. Without a doubt, the medical model positively informed understanding and remediation of maladies and contexts affecting the lives of individuals. However, the disease model developed into a pervasive assumption guiding most efforts to improve lives, which translates into individuals being diagnosed with exclusively intrinsic challenges often at the expense of acknowledging external influences on performance and functioning. Limited attention is placed on individual strengths and institutions in life that are valuable and functioning productively. Positive psychology overtly sought to overcome this imbalance by focusing on strengths and the construction of the best things in life. Attention was placed upon understanding the lives of healthy people and making their lives better.

Positive psychology, while new as an official branch of psychology, draws from a long history of thought, writings, and research. Focused on understanding what equates to a good life and what it means to be happy or satisfied, contemporary positive psychology recruits ideas from philosophy, religious figures, and theologians of the past several centuries. The field emphasizes a life of meaning regardless of where it is found (e.g., secular or spiritual pursuits) and turns to society and culture as well as to the individual for understanding.

Defining Positive Psychology

A basic premise of positive psychology and wellness approaches is that human goodness and the aspects and institutions of life that are going well are as important as personal flaws and impairments. Additionally, such underlying assumption posits that by tapping into these beliefs, improvements addressing impairments can be more successfully attained.

Some critics of positive psychology simply dismissed the field as "happy-ology" or a more rigorous assertion of trite commonsense adages of what culture might define as "the good life." However, what constitutes a good life and the path to achieving it is an empirical matter and at the heart of research within the framework of positive psychology and wellness. Three main topics make up the general focus of the field. First is the identification and understanding of positive individual traits. Traits within this focus consist of individual interests, talents, personal values, and strengths of character including optimism and resilience. A second general focus is the description and interpretation of positive subjective experiences. The issue in this focus is the study of happiness, pleasure, life fulfillment, gratification, and intrinsic motivations. The third topic of focus in positive psychology centers on understanding and developing positive institutions such as families, schools, communities, businesses, and other such socially created structures which contribute to the good life of humanity.

To illustrate, within many industrialized nations such as the United States, many may hold the belief that happiness is found through health and financial security. This may be viewed as a commonsense truism of the good life. However, positive psychology's research into happiness reveals far greater complexity. While health and money may contribute to happiness, resilience, optimism, relationships, and social connectedness, the feeling of belonging to something bigger than oneself combined with a sense of control over important aspects of life play significant, if not greater, roles in overall happiness. Furthermore, how these and a multitude of other variables unfold within the specific individual's view of a good life holds additional complexities. For disciplines serving those with communication disorders, such research may shift focus from solely addressing rehabilitation of health toward the construction and maintenance of relationships and greater appreciation for the control and agency of clients in therapeutic decision-making. Further applications to communicative disorders include understanding and developing the institutions that will foster wellness through use of the individual's personal character strengths and a transaction with the organizations and social networks associated with wellness. For example, cooperative learning groups consisting of participants at different levels of proficiency can be provided with opportunities to work on projects and activities where the individual's strengths are allowed to be displayed and valued in the successful completion of the group activity. Institutionally, in case management settings, clients and caregivers can be allowed to take more of a directive role in the determination of treatment goals and the implementation of actions to meet those goals. Additionally, clinicians can push for therapeutic outcomes that begin to focus on enhancement of what is currently functioning effectively rather than strictly on the remediation of deficits.

Wellness has been defined objectively through mortality rates, medical health records, and variables associated with poverty. It has also been conceptualized in terms of personal beliefs and reports of the presence or absence of psychological distress and the reporting of affective states. The wellness perspective arising from positive psychology holds that positive characteristics and experiences and the institutions that enable their development should be studied and utilized in efforts to enhance the lives of all people, including those with communicative disorders.

The Rise of Positive Psychology and Positive Emotions, Engagement, Relationships, Meaning, and Accomplishment

Since the late 1990s, positive psychology has been recognized as a legitimate field of study, with many universities offering related graduate degrees, while disciplines such as speech–language pathology, social work, and education have begun to embrace the original tenets and adapt practices to consider wellness and clinical outcomes more effectively. The properties guiding these extensions and applications can be summarized from Seligman's work since 2009, which is captured in the acronym of PERMA (Positive Emotions, Engagement, Relationships, Meaning, and Accomplishment).

- *Positive Emotion:* Wellness is enhanced when individuals have an ongoing positive affect. This may take the form of remembrances or reminders of good things they have experienced. It includes the ability to savor those experiences and draw satisfaction from them. Furthermore, the ability to draw from experiences while developing or remaining optimistic about the future is guided by positive emotions. A wellness mind-set capitalizes on one's resilience going forward and employs that toward realizing the good life.
- *Engagement:* Wellness is developed and enhanced when an individual is able to lose

him- or herself in ongoing activities that hold personal value and satisfaction. This absorption in ongoing activities is the capacity to be truly present in an activity or interaction. Frequent participation in these absorbing and immersive moments is unique to the individual and the contextualized moment; nevertheless, they are key to virtually all empirically demonstrated descriptions of wellness and the good life.

- *Relationships:* Positive psychology has assisted in underscoring the importance relationships play in wellness and life satisfaction. Many persons with both acquired and developmental communication disorders have connected happiness and the good life with social group connectivity. There is power in both being able and having opportunities to choose to share life's experiences with others and to experience the kindnesses associated with relationships.
- *Meaning:* Wellness and life satisfaction also require a connection to something that matters beyond oneself. The meaningful life allows one to use character strengths in some way that is authentically valued. These connections need not be large in scale, but they must include connection through some personal contribution to a greater good. Again, the articulation of what that greater good may be is determined through the personal lens of life.
- *Accomplishment:* Positive psychology research has furthered understandings of the importance of the accomplishment of goals that matter to the good life of the individual. Determination of what matters is as strictly individualized as are interpretations of what constitutes the good life. That is, the ability to pursue and achieve goals that matter to the day-to-day functioning of the individual has been found to significantly contribute to wellness and pursuit of the good life.

Audrey L. Holland and Ryan L. Nelson have explicitly extended positive psychology, including PERMA, and concepts of wellness to the field of communication disorders in their work on counseling. They, and others, have shown how clinicians can augment where appropriate and reconceptualize where necessary methods to develop happiness personally and to foster it in the clients they serve. The shift in valuing engagement, relationships, and accomplishments of clients with communication disorders is a fertile field for research, growth, and understanding. To the extent that such a shift is accomplished, increased positive social flourishing is possible.

Ryan Nelson

See also Adaptation Theory; Competence and Performance; Resilience; Self-Advocacy

Further Readings

Holland, A. L., & Nelson, R. (2018). *Counseling in communication disorders: A wellness perspective* (3rd ed.). San Diego, CA: Plural.

Lyons, R., & Roulstone, S. (2018). Well-being and resilience in children with speech and language disorders. *Journal of Speech, Language and Hearing Research, 61,* 324–344.

Peterson, C. (2006). *A primer in positive psychology.* New York, NY: Oxford University Press.

Seligman, M. E. P. (2011). *Flourish: A visionary new understanding of happiness and well-being.* New York, NY: Free Press.

Post-Polio Syndrome (PPS)

Post-polio syndrome (PPS) has been described as a slowly progressive neuromuscular disease, which while rarely fatal, may place those individuals with symptoms of respiratory dysfunction and/or dysphagia at a poor prognosis/increased risk level. The syndrome is represented by a cluster of signs and symptoms that become evident years after the initial onset of polio (as many as 30–40 years later). Early descriptions of epidemics caused by the poliomyelitis virus first appeared in medical literature in the early 19th century, but this virus is believed to have existed for thousands of years. A successful polio vaccine was developed in the 1950s, and as a result, new cases are now rare. However, a population of individuals who contracted the poliovirus survived and at least partially recovered function still exists. Some of the survivors have developed post-poliomyelitis syndrome, which represents a cluster of common signs and symptoms that can be disabling. Such symptoms may include progressive muscle and joint weakness and pain, muscle atrophy, and general fatigue and exhaustion following limited activity. Additional symptoms have been reported to include breathing or swallowing problems, sleep-related issues (e.g., apnea), and reduced tolerance of cold temperatures. Specific criteria established for PPS can be found in the Steering Committee Report from the 2001 March of Dimes International Conference on Post-Polio Syndrome. This entry provides an overview of PPS, its diagnosis, symptoms, background information, and treatment goals.

Diagnosis

The diagnosis of PPS is based on the exclusion of other possible conditions that could cause similar signs and/or symptoms, medical history, and physical examination. While electromyography, muscle biopsy, imaging, and blood test data may help rule out alternate diagnoses, there is no single diagnostic test for PPS. Three indicators generally stand out in the person's medical history: (1) previous history of poliomyelitis infection, (2) a long interval between the recovery from initial diagnosis of polio, and (3) gradual manifestation of PPS signs and symptoms.

Symptoms

Among the symptoms reported by people with PPS, new weakness may occur in muscles that had been previously weakened by the illness or in muscles that were not previously clinically involved. This new muscle weakness may resolve, but in some cases, it remains chronic. Other less frequently occurring, but notable, difficulties may include, but are not limited to, reduced respiratory function, dysarthria (a motor speech disorder), and dysphagia (a swallowing disorder).

In a 1995 study, Brian Driscoll and colleagues detailed the laryngeal function of nine patients with PPS who had complained of swallowing difficulties. All the nine participants had some degree of phonatory or laryngeal deficit. Those with dysphagia demonstrated vocal fold paralysis, which lead to the conclusion that PPS patients who complain of swallowing difficulties are at risk for laryngeal pathology.

In 1992, researchers used cinefluorography to evaluate 20 people with a remote history of polio and recent onset of PPS symptoms, specifically progressive swallowing problems. Pharyngeal abnormalities were identified in 19 of the individuals. Such pharyngeal findings included atrophy of prevertebral soft tissues, unilateral or bilateral weakness of tongue or soft palate, paresis or paralysis of the pharyngeal constrictor muscle, incomplete or absence of epiglottis tilt, poor laryngeal elevation, poor laryngeal closure with laryngeal penetration, aspiration (often silent), and luminal narrowing at the cricopharyngeal level. It was concluded that dysphagia can occur as a late complication of poliomyelitis and should be included as part of the spectrum of symptoms in PPS. Researchers felt careful examination of PPS patients with dysphagia requires dynamic imaging to assess the severity of decompensation and to detect potentially treatable symptoms.

Background Information

In order to appreciate PPS, a brief review of the original destruction by poliomyelitis virus infection may be helpful. This virus infects neurons (having a particular affinity for anterior horn cell motor neurons). It leaves a post-polio pattern of motor unit instability. Once the neuron is infected, it is either destroyed or damaged. Muscle fibers are described as having been *orphaned* by these damaged/destroyed neurons. Some motor units will be lost; yet, other orphaned muscle fibers may be reinnervated by surviving motor neurons' terminal axonal sprouting. These reinnervated *post-polio* motor units will be larger as they have more fibers per neuron. The poliovirus in effect reorganizes the motor units, leading to increased amplitude and duration of action potentials in the *recovered* enlarged motor units and decreased recruitment due to the loss of motor units. In essence, a post-polio pattern of motor unit instability emerges. Researchers have speculated that in the post-polio patient, increased metabolic demands were being placed on the enlarged motor units. It is thought that this might lead to an inability of the axon to meet the metabolic demands of all its muscle fibers, causing them to be continuously denervated and reinnervated. Furthermore, the researchers have suggested that a net denervation will eventually occur, which manifests itself as the PPS symptom: new onset of muscle weakness.

Treatment Goals

There is not one treatment for the PPS cluster of various signs and symptoms. The goal of treatment is to manage the patient's symptoms, help with comfort, and enable relative independence as much as may be possible. Several self-management strategies have been offered such as trying to maintain a healthy lifestyle while limiting activities that tend to produce fatigue and/or pain, avoiding falls, and protecting the lungs.

Nancy Jeanne Haak

See also Aspiration: Swallowing; Laryngeal Disorders: Benign Vocal Fold Pathologies; Motor Speech Disorders; Neurogenic Communication Disorders; Swallowing Disorders

Further Readings

Driscoll, B. P., Gracco, C., Coelho, C., Goldstein, J., Oshsima, K., Tierney, E., & Saski, C. T. (1995). Laryngeal function in post-polio patients. *Laryngoscope, 105,* 35–41.

Howson, C. P., Leavit, R. P., & Fiore, E. L. (Eds.). (2001). *March of Dimes International Conference on Post-Polio Syndrome. Identifying best practices in diagnosis and care.* New York, NY: The March of Dimes Birth Defects Foundation.

Jones, B., Buchholz, D. W., Ravic, W. J., & Donner, M. W. (1992). Swallowing dysfunction in the post-polio syndrome: A cinefluorographic study. *American Journal of Roentgenology, 158,* 283–286.

Soderholm, S., Lehtien, A., Valtonen, K., & Ylienen, A. (2010). Dysphagia and dysphonia among persons with post-polio syndrome—A challenge in neruorehabilitation. *Acta Neurologica Scandinavica, 122,* 343–349.

Websites

Mayo Clinic. Post-polio Syndrome. Retrieved from www.mayoclinic.org/diseases-conditions/post-polio-syndrome/home/ovc-20314505

Medicine.net. Post-polio Syndrome: *MedicineNet.com.* Retrieved from www.medicinenet.com/post-polio_syndrome/page2.htm

POSTTREATMENT RELAPSE IN STUTTERING

Stuttering is a common speech disorder that involves the repeating of sounds or words, *blocks* in speech production, and sometimes extraneous movements. Onset usually occurs during the preschool years after a period of typical speech development. Stuttering generally becomes more difficult to treat with age. Persistent stuttering can be associated with reduced educational and occupational attainment and risk for developing a range of mental health problems, particularly involving anxiety.

For young children, treatment aims to eliminate stuttering, and many will recover requiring no further treatment. However, treatment for chronic stuttering typically involves control or management strategies. There are a range of treatment approaches for adults who stutter; however, speech restructuring has the most published research evidence. This entry provides an overview of speech restructuring treatment for individuals who stutter, the rate of posttreatment relapse, the relationship between social anxiety disorder and stuttering, and the role of speech–language pathologists.

Treatment for Chronic Stuttering

Speech restructuring involves teaching clients to control stuttering by changing the way they speak. Clients initially learn a new way of talking that involves speaking with a slow and exaggerated technique that reduces stuttering. This speech is then gradually made to sound more natural (i.e., acceptable for use in everyday speaking situations), while still controlling stuttering. The Camperdown Program, developed by researchers at the Australian Stuttering Research Centre, is one of many speech restructuring programs used to treat adolescents and adults who stutter. The Camperdown Program requires around one fifth of the treatment time of other speech restructuring approaches.

Posttreatment Relapse

It is widely recognized that after speech restructuring up to two thirds of adults will have difficulty maintaining their treatment benefits. Until recently, there has been no explanation for such relapse rates; however, a 2009 report provided a compelling explanation. Around two thirds of adults who participated in a large study involving speech restructuring treatment were diagnosed with one or more mental health disorders, the majority involving anxiety. Importantly, the presence of any mental health condition was associated with an increase in stuttering severity and avoidance of speaking situations 6 months after completing treatment. In other words, the participants who had one or more mental health disorders were unable to maintain the low levels of stuttering they achieved immediately after treatment. That finding occurred in the absence of any difference in amount of stuttering for those with and without mental health disorders before and immediately posttreatment. Additionally, those results are consistent with an earlier study in which participants who had relapsed were 3 times more likely to experience high anxiety levels.

Treatment for Social Anxiety Disorder

Many studies have confirmed that the most common mental health problem associated with stuttering is social anxiety disorder. Social anxiety disorder involves extreme fear of embarrassment and negative evaluation from others during social interactions. Those with the condition avoid talking and in extreme cases will avoid social situations altogether. This can lead to social isolation and a range of other problems. One way to address the problem of relapse for adults who stutter is to target mental health disorders, in particular social anxiety disorder.

The leading psychological treatment for social anxiety disorder is cognitive behavior therapy (CBT). A CBT package has been designed specifically for adults who stutter. That package uses standard CBT procedures based on the Clark and Wells model of social anxiety as well as stuttering specific mental health assessments. Preliminary results have shown the CBT package can remove social anxiety disorder, reduce speaking situation avoidance, and improve Global Assessment of Functioning. In a randomized trial of the CBT package combined with speech treatment, the CBT treatment removed social anxiety disorder and improved psychological functioning; however, it did not improve speech outcomes. Continued research investigating the effects of CBT for anxiety and speech outcomes with adults who stutter is needed.

CBT is typically administered by a psychologist or a health professional trained in CBT procedures. However, the development of an Internet-based, interactive CBT package may mean that a live psychologist will not always be required to administer the treatment.

The Role of Speech–Language Pathologists

It is important that speech–language pathologists inform clients that the presence of mental health problems may increase the risk of relapse following speech treatment. A comprehensive assessment should involve screening for mental health problems, in particular, anxiety. The Unhelpful Thoughts and Beliefs about Stuttering (UTBAS) scale is a useful measure for this purpose. It was developed from a file audit of adults who stutter presenting to an anxiety disorders clinic. The full version contains 66 items made up of the negative thoughts of those patients. For example, "Other people will think I'm stupid if I stutter" and "I'll never be successful because of my stutter." A screening version with just six items is also available. High scores indicate the presence of negative thoughts that may impact speech treatment and alert the potential need for a referral to a psychologist.

Final Thoughts

Research since 2000 has provided insight into the problem of relapse for adults who stutter. That evidence has highlighted the need for mental health management for many who present to speech–language pathologists for stuttering treatment. Therefore, clients will require a comprehensive assessment and may require referral to a psychologist or relevant CBT program if indicated.

Robyn Lowe and Sue O'Brian

See also Cognitive Behavioral Therapy; Fluency and Fluency Disorders; Speech–Language Pathology; Stuttering and Emotional Reactions; Stuttering Treatment

Further Readings

Iverach, L., Jones, M., O'Brian, S., Block, S., Lincoln, M., Harrison, E., . . . Onslow, M. (2009). The relationship between mental health disorders and treatment outcomes among adults who stutter. *Journal of Fluency Disorders, 34,* 29–43.

Menzies, R., O'Brian, S., Lowe, R., Packman, A., & Onslow, M. (2016). International Phase II clinical trial of CBTPysch: A standalone Internet social anxiety treatment for adults who stutter. *Journal of Fluency Disorders, 48,* 35–43.

Menzies, R. G., O'Brian, S., Onslow, M., Packman, A., St Clare, T., & Block, S. (2008). An experimental clinical trial of a cognitive-behavior therapy package for chronic stuttering. *Journal of Speech, Language and Hearing Research, 51,* 1451–1464.

St Clare, T., Menzies, R. G., Onslow, M., Packman, A., Thompson, R., & Block, S. (2009). Unhelpful thoughts and beliefs linked to social anxiety in stuttering; development of a measure. *International Journal of Language & Communication Disorders, 44,* 338–351.

POVERTY AND LANGUAGE

Living in poverty can influence how an individual acquires and develops language and can determine whether or not an individual speaks with a pronounced minority or regional dialect. Poverty-related effects on language are complex and intertwined. Through socialization, a child's home environment determines the form and quantity of linguistic stimuli, thus determining the course of language development and acquisition at an early age. Patterns of language use and linguistic stimuli in the home vary by social class, creating and perpetuating a developmental language gap that leaves children living in poverty at a relative disadvantage compared with their more affluent peers. Furthermore, living in a low-income area can determine a child's access to an equitable education, which in turn can determine the trajectory and subsequent success of their development and acquisition of language.

Although patterns of language development and use among people living in poverty exist, there remain great variations in language patterns within lower social classes. People living in poverty belong to a heterogeneous social group in terms of race, ethnicity, gender, ability, first language, and education. A child's language development and use may also be impacted by dialectal differences that exist between regional language boundaries and between rural and urban areas within a region. These social factors, in addition to socioeconomic status, contribute to a complex understanding of how language is developed and used by people living in poverty.

Poverty and Language Development

Living in poverty may have adverse biological and cognitive consequences for a child's language development and cognitive processing, including delays in the development of vocabulary, phonological awareness, and understanding of grammar and syntax. These developmental delays are attributed to the daily stress of living in poverty, to home patterns of language use, and to a relative lack of language-based educational stimuli in lower socioeconomic home environments. Living in poverty is stressful, and the presence of stress in an environment can impede a child's cognitive development. Biologically, children and adults living in poverty are more likely to have increased levels of the stress hormone cortisol in their bodies. Cortisol slows cognitive development, especially in the regions of the brain responsible for the development and processing of language. The daily stress of living in poverty is significant enough to have an early impact on a child's development of language acquisition skills. From this starting point, a child's linguistic competency may continue to be negatively impacted by other poverty-related environmental and structural factors such as food insecurity and a lack of access to educational resources.

On average, by the time a child of lower income and less educated parents enters school they are two years behind their more affluent peers in overall language competency as measured by standardized language development tests. Leading research by Ann Fernald and colleagues indicate this language gap begins to appear as early as 18 months. By age 3, children from more affluent backgrounds have heard 30 million more words than the average child living in poverty. Although it is important to note that quality of language input is important, the 30-million-word gap tends to persist and can increase with time in the absence of significant educational interventions.

Class-based parenting styles and language use, as well as lower income parents' lack of access to educational resources, are additional factors that contribute to the persistence and increase in the language gap. Parents from lower income backgrounds have fewer financial resources and therefore less money to spend on children's literature as well as educational resources and enrichment activities that promote language and literacy skills. Children living in poverty are more likely to lose valuable gains in reading and writing achievement during summer breaks from school because parents cannot afford extracurricular educational programs that contribute to the maintenance of language skills. Lower income parents who work multiple jobs or long hours also have less time to dedicate to enriching the linguistic environment at home by talking and reading with their children.

Sociolinguistically, parents from lower income backgrounds are more likely to have a limited vocabulary, to engage in less word play with children, and to speak to their children with a more authoritarian tone. Authoritarian parenting styles that are more common in lower income families do not encourage children to use language as a tool to communicate and influence parents' decision-making. Affluent and educated parents engage in more word play with their children and encourage their children to use language to negotiate their needs and wants, thus influencing parents' behavior. Lower income parents' more authoritarian parenting style and relative lack of word play limits the exposure lower income children have to developing greater vocabulary and a more sophisticated use of language to negotiate their environment. A family's patterns of word play and linguistic negotiation can shape their interaction with educators.

In the early 2000s, Annette Lareau found that patterns of parents' interactions with teachers and administrators vary by social class. Parents and children from more affluent backgrounds are more likely to use language confidently to negotiate and influence the behavior of teachers and administrators. On the other hand, parents living in poverty may have limited access to and experience with K-12 educators. Many parents living in poverty work multiple jobs or have jobs with hours that prevent them from attending school functions such as parent conference night. Additionally, parents living in poverty may lack educational qualifications or have themselves struggled in school. Therefore, they may choose to defer to teachers' judgment and capitulate educational decisions to their child's teachers. For these reasons, parents are less likely to use language to influence the behavior of school faculty. Parents living in poverty value the education of their children. However, educators should be aware that parents living in poverty may not use language in the same ways that more affluent parents use language—to negotiate and influence teachers and administrators.

Poverty and Dialect

Language functions as a marker for social class in societies. How an individual uses language, which language they use, their accent, dialect, and breadth of vocabulary are often a reflection of their social class and area of geographical origin. Middle- and upper-class people are more likely to speak standard forms of a language, such as Standard American English, because socially dominant, standard dialects are more commonly spoken in middle- and upper-class home environments and because wealthier members of society have greater access to educational resources that reinforce dominant forms of speech. In the United States, Standard American English is the dialect of American English that is valued, widely accepted, and used by government employees and politicians, major corporations, the media, and institutions of formal education.

Working-class and lower class people are more likely to speak with a minority and/or regional dialect or to be English-language learners. Due to the lower social class status of people living in poverty, minority and regional dialects are often socially stigmatized forms of speech. For example, people who speak nonstandard forms of American English such as Appalachian English, African American Vernacular English, and Chicano are often perceived as being cognitively or linguistically deficient. In popular media, speakers of Appalachian English or other rural dialects are often portrayed as backward and uneducated.

Descriptive linguists acknowledge this stigma is a form of language discrimination, because all languages and dialects are equally capable of communicating needs, wants, desires, and ideas. Additionally, as with Standard American English, dialects of American English such as African American Vernacular English have a predictable grammar and syntax. Despite popular beliefs, people living in poverty who speak with regional and/or minority dialects are not linguistically deficient. However, because language is a signifier of social status in our society, people living in poverty are more likely to speak nonstandard dialects of English that do not have the same social prestige as Standard American English.

Poverty, Language, and Schooling

In schools, students' English language competency is associated with their potential for economic and social mobility. Standard American English is the form of American English that is valued, taught, and assessed in formal education in the United States. For students living in poverty, the devaluation of regional and minority dialects in schools may have negative, life-altering consequences. The social stigma or lack of social value attributed to minority or regional dialects creates further disadvantages for students living in poverty because it exacerbates the previously mentioned gap in language use between lower and upper-class families. If children are reared in a home environment where they are socialized to speak Standard American English, they are at an advantage in school because the home language is congruent with the language valued in school. Children who speak a nonstandard dialect of English, or another language, must learn to code switch between the home language and language used at school. For children living in poverty, the language gap may be exacerbated by incongruence between home and school language use. This explains why children living in poverty are more likely to be tested and placed in remedial reading and writing classes in school.

Owing to the stigma associated with nonstandard dialects of English and the language gap, students living in poverty are more likely to be identified as having language-based learning disabilities and placed in remedial reading and writing classes. Unfortunately, students living in poverty are at an additional educational disadvantage because they are more likely to attend schools that cannot adequately remediate language development problems. Schools in impoverished areas are more likely to have fewer qualified teachers, a high student-to-teacher ratio, and to have fewer resources to support language development.

Although poverty may negatively influence language development, people living in poverty are not inherently linguistically pathological. It is important to remember that people living in poverty make up a large, heterogeneous social group; the lower classes in our society are made up of people of various backgrounds, including but not limited to race, ethnicity, geographical location, gender, ability, and level of education. Critics have cautioned against the overgeneralization of research on lower class language development and language patterns in order to avoid perpetuating stereotypes about people living in poverty. For example, not all lower class people live in environments lacking linguistic stimuli or educational resources. Not all lower class people speak with a distinct minority or regional dialect. People from all social classes may exhibit idiosyncratic patterns of speech or may struggle with language and cognitive development. However, patterns of language use do vary by social class and can have a profound impact on children's language development, overall linguistic proficiency, and whether or not they were taught a socially valued and standardized form of language in the home environment.

Natalie Keefer

See also Cognitive Development; Descriptive Linguistics; Language Acquisition; Reading Fluency; Socialization; Sociolinguistics

Further Readings

Fernald, A., Marchman, V., & Weisleder, A. (2013). SES differences in language processing skill and vocabulary are evident at 18 months. *Developmental Science, 16*(2), 234–248.

Gorski, P. (2008). The myth of the culture of poverty. *Educational Leadership, 67*(7), 32–36.

Hart, B., & Risley, T. (2003). The early catastrophe: The 30 million word gap by age 3. *American Educator, 27*(1), 4–9.

Hirsch-Pasek, K., Adamson, L., Bakerman, R., Owen, M., Golinkoff, R., Pace, A., . . . Suma, K. (2015). The contribution of early communication quality to low-income children's language success. *Psychological Science, 26*(7), 1–13.

Lareau, A. (2003). *Unequal childhoods: Class, race, and family life.* Berkley: University of California Press.

Lippi-Green, R. (2012). *English with an accent: Language, ideology, and discrimination in the United States* (2nd ed.). London, UK: Routledge.

Nieto, S. (2010). *Language, culture, and teaching: Critical perspectives* (2nd ed.). London, UK: Routledge.

Perkins, S. C., Finegood, E. D., & Swain, J. E. (2013). Poverty and language development: Roles of parenting and stress. *Innovations in Clinical Neuroscience, 10*(4), 10–19.

POWER RELATIONS IN SERVICE DELIVERY

As a helping profession, speech–language pathology is an intervention-oriented endeavor. Speech–language therapists spend the majority of their professional time in therapy sessions with individuals who have been diagnosed with a communication disorder, and they may work with these individuals within the therapeutic context for months or even years. It is within these sessions (i.e., service delivery) that the central activities of speech–language pathology happens and that the successful remediation of communication impairments occurs. Therefore, investigations of all kinds of therapeutic interactions have provided an increased focus on the complexity of therapy, including power relations (i.e., how power is distributed in social settings). When considered as the social action between a speech–language therapist and a client to improve the client's communicative abilities, therapy involves verbal discourse as well as other factors such as eye gaze, proxemics, and more complex social relations such as the establishment and maintenance of power, authority, and control in therapeutic interactions. This entry provides an overview of power relations in service delivery by defining interactional power and control, highlighting the relationship between language and power relations, and finally examining power relations in speech–language therapy.

Interactional Power and Control

Interactional power is defined as the ability to influence the behaviors of others. Likewise, the definition of *control* is the act of influencing the behaviors of others, and the definition of *authority* is the right and responsibility to do so. Interactional power relations exist in every therapy session since all therapy requires at least one clinician and one client. In addition to roles adopted, power can be expressed through a variety of social actions during a therapy session. One example can be found in mediated repair. When a child fails to complete a multistep task, such as set up a board game for play, the clinician may do any or all of the following: identify the problem, provide possible solutions, complete the task correctly, and provide feedback regarding the task. All of these social actions express interactional power, and this requires clinicians to understand how to use interactional power intentionally to improve the communication abilities of the client.

The idea of interactional power and power relations becomes crucial when considering therapeutic interactions as a whole. Interactional power relations may be broadly conceptualized as a dynamic and complex social construction that is the collaboration between two or more people to determine specific roles in an interaction. It is essential to note the changeable nature of power relations. Power relations are not formal and stagnant roles and positions, but rather they vary depending on a host of interacting factors and actions. Accordingly, the participant who occupies the power position has the capacity to structure the therapy session according to his or her agenda. Terms like *power, control,* and *authority* are allocated to these relationships, and since these terms are more relational than discrete, explicit definitions are not easily constructed. Nonetheless, interactional power is an intricate social phenomenon with several observable operational characteristics.

Due to the impact and importance of interactional power as a primary mechanism for organizing therapy sessions and enforcing one's agenda, control becomes a chief aspect of power. Control can be viewed as the act of influencing another participant's behavior. Further one must acknowledge that control is both a process and a product, just like any social action. First, the processes of control may be defined as determining functions of the social structure of social occasions where the focus of control is not on the words spoken or the gestures completed, but rather on how the gestures and words come to be used. Correspondingly, products of control are defined as the mechanisms through which control is expressed. The first point of agreement is that discourse is a major component of social action. Participants frequently express interactional control through discourse. Here, the definition of discourse includes both verbal and nonverbal actions such as gestures, eye gaze, and body positioning.

Language and Power Relations

Language within discourse is often considered the principal means for the conveying of ideas, beliefs, and feelings. This includes information regarding the interactional power relationships between participants. In fact, language use can be seen as a subset of social action. Language, being the primary tool of discourse, is an essential ingredient in the employment of control in any social occasion. It is not only what is said but also how it is said that provides participants with information about the power relationship and thus how control is applied in interactions. Further, it is necessary to highlight the relationship between language and discourse as well as discourse and social action. Namely, language is an integral part of discourse and discourse is an integral part of social action. They cannot be separated from one another. Discourse, of which language use is an essential element, is a social action that imparts interactional power and control.

Power Relations in Speech–Language Therapy

Speech–language therapy sessions may be considered social occasions and consequently deal with the dynamics of power relations, while noting that control of the speech–language therapy session falls most heavily on the clinician.

One study focusing on discourse in speech–language therapy sought to account for how clinicians and children with language impairments communicate with each other in clinical settings. This study and subsequent studies revealed that clinicians dominate the therapy sessions in a variety of ways. First, clinicians tend to dominate the communicative space. That is, they speak almost twice as often as the clients do. Further, most of the clinician utterances were categorized as requests. Correspondingly, clients engage mostly in responses to these requests. Other research investigated how specific therapeutic interaction practices affected treatment outcomes, that is, how therapeutic framework creates conditions for clinician control and specifies mechanisms that may be employed within that framework.

For example, the idea of a therapeutic agenda is advanced in analysis of therapeutic discourse. Of interest is the organization of therapy sessions. Some researchers propose that speech–language therapy sessions have three main phases: an opening phase, therapy activity phase, and a closing phase. Of these, the therapy activity phase is the most central to the therapeutic agenda. Here, clinicians organize therapy to control the therapeutic interaction systematically. This, in turn, enables the clinician to assist in improving a client's communicative competence. Further, the clinician's agenda is created based upon certain nonverbal, but salient maxims: (1) the clinician begins the activity; (2) once begun, the activity must run its course; (3) the clinician is to aid the client in producing speech and language; (4) the clinician provides feedback regarding such productions; (5) other information is imparted to the client as needed. Once the framework of therapy is created to shift control to the clinician, the clinician may use other mechanisms of therapeutic interactions to maintain or modify that control.

Later research sought to understand the mechanisms at work in therapeutic interactions which leads to a deeper understanding of the complexities involved in the therapeutic process. One of the mechanisms includes discourse markers which are used to regulate speech–language therapy sessions. Discourse markers bracket units of talk and serve three purposes in therapeutic interactions. The first purpose is control, which indicates the sequencing of activities, tasks, and topics within an interaction. Second, discourse markers also play an evaluative role through response to a client's actions. Finally, discourse markers are also used as general responses to a client's informative statements. The use of discourse markers express aspects of clinician control, such as managing the sequence of therapy activities, providing evaluative feedback, and acknowledging information.

Since 1995, other researchers have gained insight into the forces that create contexts where clinicians retain much of the interactional power. One of those forces is the multifunctionality aspect of feedback. There are at least seven functions of feedback: to maximize targeted behaviors, to convey policies and procedures of therapy, to organize activity and discourse sequences, to regulate the pace of the interactions, to empower clients, to establish and maintain solidarity, and to preserve clinician control. The last function is successfully achieved through the employment of the other functions, despite the multiple specific functions of feedback in therapeutic interactions. Hence, there is an overarching purpose of feedback to foster clinician control.

Jack Damico and Sandy Damico's seminal research article on the dominant-interpretive framework is a powerful take on understanding power relations. The dominant-interpretive framework is a construct for the various ways that the dominant participant (i.e., the clinician) establishes and maintains evaluative control. Namely, how does a dominant participant exert control over the meaning making of the passive participant? Their research found that clinicians systematically and conventionally cued clients to recognize meaning making mismatches between the participants. The mismatches were then subjected to a mediated repair sequence with clinicians providing appropriate feedback given for successful repairs. The key here lies in the point that determinations of correctness belong to the participant in control of therapy (i.e., the clinician).

The saliency of interactional power and control in therapeutic discourse is not only noted in a formal analysis of these therapeutic sessions but the targets of the interventions. That is, the clients themselves may also be aware of the various types of manipulations and engage in behavior to reinforce the power relations. For example, one research study found that children, in their own words, accurately described the power relations between themselves and their clinician. Namely, the clinician is the one with the communicative competence who consequently provides evaluative feedback regarding the child's misarticulations.

In 2004, research on clinical power relations has focused on the discourse within therapeutic interactions as a reliable predictor of the therapeutic relationship. Of particular note are Request-Response-Evaluation sequences as a method educators and clinicians use to establish and maintain their role as expert. Interestingly, this discourse sequence allots the clinician two speaking turns and the client only one, which ties back to some of communication disorders earliest research on the topic as the dominant-interpretative framework.

Another key question in research is not only how therapeutic control is exerted but whether some control strategies are more efficacious in reestablishing communicative competence. Seven primary strategies are used by clinicians to create clinician control. These are dominion over the physical context, employment of a dominant interpretive framework, manipulation of timing in discourse, occupation of communicative space, use of tripartite structures, utilization of discourse markers, and manifestations of nonverbal behaviors (e.g., eye gaze and gestures). Several of these strategies have been discussed earlier including the use of tripartite discourse structures (i.e., Request-Response-Evaluation sequences), the use of a dominant interpretive framework, and the domination of communicative space (or number of turns at talk). Other strategies uncovered include control of the physical space, which includes the *ownership* of the therapy space as well as the materials used within it. Finally, aspects of control also include timing variations as well as nonverbal actions such as eye gaze and body movements. Verbal and nonverbal behaviors seek to control the activities of therapy as well as to provide evaluations of the client's performance. These interactional control strategies, when used appropriately, serve to improve the communication abilities of clients.

Holly Howat

See also Clinical Linguistics; Clinician; Constructivism; Enculturation into the Profession; Service Delivery Models; Sociolinguistics

Further Readings

Damico, J. S., & Damico, S. K. (1997). The establishment of a dominant interpretive framework in language intervention. *Language, Speech, and Hearing Services in Schools, 28,* 288–296.

Damico, J. S., Simmons-Mackie, N. N., & Hawley, H. K. (2005). Language and power in the clinical context. In M. J. Ball (Ed.), *Clinical sociolinguistics* (pp. 63–73). Oxford, UK: Blackwell.

Goffman, E. (1969). *Strategic interaction.* Philadelphia: University of Pennsylvania Press.

Kovarsky, D. (1990). Discourse markers in adult controlled therapy: Implications for child centered intervention. *Journal of Childhood Communication Disorders, 13*(1), 29–41.

Leahy, M. M. (2004). Therapy talk: Analyzing therapeutic discourse. *Language Speech and Hearing Services in Schools, 35,* 70–81.

Letts, C (1985). Linguistic interaction in the clinic: How do therapists do therapy? *Child Language Teaching and Therapy, 1,* 321–331.

Panagos, J. M. (1996). Speech therapy discourse: The input to learning. In M. Smith & J. S. Damico (Eds.), *Childhood language disorders* (pp. 41–63). New York, NY: Thieme Medical.

Prutting, C. A., Bagshaw, N., Goldstein, H., Juskowitz, S., & Umen, I. (1978). Clinician-child discourse: Some preliminary questions. *Journal of Speech and Hearing Disorders, 43,* 123–129.

Pragmatic Development

Fundamental to success as a linguistic communicator is the ability to use language appropriate to the context (i.e., pragmatics). Pragmatic *rules* are inherently variable, and they are intimately bound up with overall sociocultural development. Unlike more structurally obvious language aspects such as grammar and vocabulary, pragmatics lacks exact age norms. This entry provides an overview of pragmatic development, touching on growth over time in several broad areas of language use.

Early Social Exchanges

Experiences in infancy set the developing child on the road to pragmatic competence, as babies engage in reciprocal exchanges with caregivers. Face-to-face interaction provides rich opportunities for infants to learn about social exchange. Games such as peekaboo and daily routine interchanges with caregivers provide them experiences where they learn about influencing and being influenced by others. Some of the very earliest exchanges involve laughter, where infants frequently smile and laugh in response to adult actions, and such experiences, along with gestures, vocalizing, and, later, verbalizing, result in infants developing a repertoire of contextually appropriate communicative abilities. As children grow, they experience ever-widening contexts of communication, with opportunities to refine their understanding of how to modify what they say to meet listener needs. They learn that each context requires a different approach, as they see the contrast between peer and adult interactions, the expectations of home versus school, and unstructured play versus organized activities.

Development of Communicative Functions

An important source of growth and development in neurotypical children is the spontaneous desire for social engagement, seeking to engage caregivers by verbal and nonverbal means. As they develop communicative skills such as pointing or labeling objects with single words, they begin to be able to express a range of communicative functions. Often the most common early communicative acts of a toddler may be thought of as involving demands, but even more often toddlers use language for purely social purposes. A toddler may delightedly say *moon* gazing at the sky, look back at his or her mother, and then wait for the mother's response, out of pure joy at sharing his or her excitement with Mother. In fact, it is highly predictive of autism when a child only uses language for requesting and not for social purposes. Therefore, it is an important aspect of assessment of early pragmatic development to establish that the child uses language for a variety of purposes, both instrumental, such as requesting and refusing, and social, such as commenting and greeting.

There are a variety of approaches to documenting the development of communicative functions (sometimes called *communicative intents* or *speech acts*). Two well-known approaches were developed by scholars John Dore and Michael Halliday in the 1970s. Common labels for functions include terms such as *requesting*, *commenting*, *labeling*, *protesting*, or *greeting* often used by clinicians to analyze language samples in young children. As children develop and refine their social communicative abilities based on experience, the complexity of communicative intents becomes more difficult to categorize. Some intents are inherently complex, challenging a child's understanding of its implications—for example, a 5-year-old may know the word *promise* but not be able to grasp its true meaning. She may *promise* to clean her room as a way to be agreeable and please her parents; an 8-year-old is more likely to understand that a promise is a personal commitment that may have later consequences if not carried out.

While cataloging intents is an important tool in assessing pragmatic development, its applicability to older children and adolescents is challenged by the increasing complexity of human interactions. A particular communicative act may have more than one purpose. In preschool children, it may be sufficient to document the development of successful requesting by describing how often they make requests and for what purposes; for adolescents, one would also want to know whether they can make polite requests—that they know how to exercise tact and discretion. Politeness and tact are very context sensitive and have multiple aspects—thus a form of utterance that is totally fine to say to a sibling might be terribly rude if said to the school principal. Such distinctions can be made by looking at some quantifiable elements—longer requests are usually more polite than short ones, and indirect more than direct, as in "Gimme that" versus "May I please borrow your book." But often the elements that point to whether an utterance is appropriate in context are not amenable to simple lists of features. And it is this aspect of language that is the difference between pragmatic success and pragmatic impairment. A 10-year-old child with autism may be capable of creating complex utterances, even with a range of intents, but still be impaired pragmatically, struggling to take the listener's point of view or to adhere to social norms.

Conversational Development

Labeling the function of each child utterance is not the only way to approach analysis of pragmatic development. Looking at the child's role in a communicative exchange is equally important. One measure of growth is to count the number of turns a child can take in conversation. The percentage of time a child responds versus initiates conversation may also tell a lot about overall pragmatic competence; individual differences may lead some children to be more active and others more passive. Whether a child can ask for clarification as needed or respond when a partner asks for clarification is another area where children's knowledge of the needs of their listeners is demonstrated. By school age, children will even start self-correcting when they realize they may have been unclear—for example, "She—I mean Shontae—gave me a present."

Another way to analyze conversation is to look at topic manipulation; this looks not just at overall turns in the conversation but at whether children are able to maintain the same topic over multiple exchanges. As children move into later school age, they gain in the ability to maintain a topic over many turns and in the ability to shift smoothly and seamlessly from one to the next. For abrupt changes, new topics can be marked clearly as a shift using discourse markers, such as "by the way" or "oh and also." Another important development is the ability to successfully navigate the natural flow of conversation as it gradually shifts, with links from idea to idea until the talk has drifted to a whole new area. Pragmatic impairment leads to lopsided exchanges, often characterized by insistence on controlling the topic. In successful conversation, each speaker has to handle many details in what appears aimless but actually requires carefully but swiftly chosen phrasing, with an aim to be cooperative and meet the listener's needs.

Perspective-Taking and Referencing

Developments such as refined ability to tailor one's words to one's audience, use of discourse markers, and ability to use language that is clear to listeners all relate to a key aspect of being a successful communicator: the ability to take into account the listener's point of view. Young children are known to have difficulty with perspective-taking—also called *theory of mind*—that is, the ability to understand that other people have different information and experiences and that therefore one needs to shape communication accordingly. Such knowledge shapes many aspects of language, including the ability to know when one can use a pronoun and when it might be confusing. Elements of language such as pronouns that change with context are known as *deixis*, and these are difficult in the early years. For example, the meaning of *you* and *me* changes depending on who is speaking. Toddlers may say *you* when they mean *me* and vice versa, because they don't yet grasp that words can shift meaning with context. In other referencing challenges, a toddler may start out by pointing to objects his or her partner cannot see, or a preschooler may say nonspecific words such as *that one*. By school age, a child will be able to use highly specific references, such as "the little one that has the Batman picture on it." The gradual accumulation of such expertise—how to incorporate what you know about what the other person is likely to know and how the listener might react—allows children over time to employ linguistic details to communicate successfully in the full range of contexts they experience.

Humor

Even very young babies can be amused, but the development of humor in language is based on sophisticated language abilities. For example, one cannot recognize a pun without being able to hold two unrelated meanings of the same word in one's mind at the same time. Jokes begin to be understood as something funny long before the child quite grasps why; between early and late school age, children grasp the details of different joke forms. They also become capable of using nonverbal information such as tone of voice to distinguish sarcasm.

Narrative Development

Conversation is one important side of pragmatics, but narrative is an almost equally important aspect of communicative competence. The psychologist Jerome Bruner described storytelling as a universal human approach to organizing experience and processing information. Narrative, unlike conversation, is primarily constructed by one speaker, burdening the narrator with heavier cognitive and linguistic demands than the conversationalist. In addition to taking into account listener's point of view and using language tailored to meet listener's needs, the narrator must plan ahead and develop a structure and order that is not needed in conversation—decisions on details to leave in and exclude must be made in accordance with the overall planned structure.

Very young children have cognitive limitations that make it difficult for them to conceive of anything outside of the here and now. As preschoolers begin to develop a concept of time, they start being able to comprehend and express narratives. In the early 1990s, the work of Allysa McCabe and Carole Peterson developed the basis of age-related expectations for narratives of personal experience. The earliest stories told by preschoolers are simple two-event structures: "Jason hitted me. I fell down." Over time, children become capable of both understanding and producing lengthier descriptions of events more remote in space and time, until school-age children can narrate multievent sequences with details making them understandable to listeners who did not share the experiences being related. They also become capable of telling fictional stories, based on exposure to books, movies, and other media. Fiction has its own structure, often referred to as *story grammar* based on the work of Vladimir Propp, who analyzed folk tales to uncover recurring patterns. These story grammar elements, such as setting, initiating event, plan, and resolution, can be applied to analyze children's stories, in order to determine their quality and level of sophistication. In addition to overall structure, stories use language, including vocabulary and sentence structure, which is different from everyday speech. When reading a sentence like the following, many details point to it as likely to be fiction: "The forbidding fortress towered over the town and seemed like a predator crouched to spring, making the townspeople creep about like mice." Children's exposure to written narrative language containing these special elements is key to their ability to process fictional text. Thus, this aspect of pragmatics is intimately linked to literacy.

Final Thoughts

The ability to engage with others is critical to all aspects of life, from home to school to work.

Children's exposure to diverse speakers, linguistic models, and contexts helps them build up a repertoire of abilities permitting flexible and skillful use of language. Individuals who have pragmatic impairments, such as those with autism, face enormous personal challenges—without social communicative competence, many aspects of their daily life are impeded, and intervention to explicitly teach pragmatics is crucial. Even for children not facing such challenges, opportunities to develop pragmatic competence using language in multiple ways for multiple purposes are critical to their successful development.

Lynne E. Hewitt

See also Discourse Analysis; Language Acquisition; Language Disorders in Children; Narratives; Pragmatics

Further Readings

Cummings, L. (2009). *Clinical pragmatics*. Cambridge, UK: Cambridge University Press.

Halliday, M. A. K. (1975). *Learning how to mean: Explorations in the development of language*. New York, NY: Elsevier.

Levinson, S. C. (1983). *Pragmatics*. Cambridge, UK: Cambridge University Press.

Pragmatic Impairment

Pragmatic impairment (also known as *social or pragmatic communication disorder*) can be defined as any breakdown in the use of language across a range of communicative contexts. Deficits in the pragmatics of language pose a significant barrier to effective communication and can compromise social, academic, and occupational functioning. To mitigate these adverse consequences, individuals with pragmatic impairment are assessed and treated by speech–language pathologists. This entry examines the different etiologies that can cause pragmatic disorders and significant distinctions in the classification of these disorders. It also considers the contribution of cognitive deficits to these disorders and addresses how clinicians assess and treat pragmatic disorders.

The pragmatics of language involves a wide skill set, including the use and understanding of nonliteral language (e.g., metaphor, idiom); the introduction, development, and termination of a topic of conversation; and the contribution of relevant, informative utterances to a conversation. The abilities to repair conversational breakdown, to foreground new information in utterances, and to use a range of speech acts (e.g., promises, apologies) are also key pragmatic language skills. The developmental disorders, illnesses, and injuries, which can disrupt these skills, are very wide ranging indeed.

Classifications

Children may fail to develop pragmatic language skills along normal lines on account of genetic syndromes, which cause intellectual disability (e.g., fragile X syndrome) or neurodevelopmental disorders such as autism spectrum disorder (ASD). The impaired pragmatic skills in these individuals are *developmental* pragmatic disorders. Pragmatic language skills may develop normally only to be impaired by events that occur outside the developmental period. These events include the onset of infections (e.g., meningitis), cerebrovascular accidents or strokes, brain tumors, traumatic brain injuries, and neurodegenerative diseases (e.g., Alzheimer's disease). The resulting pragmatic impairments are *acquired* pragmatic disorders. Both developmental and acquired pragmatic disorders are assessed and treated by speech–language pathologists.

It is important to acknowledge that developmental pragmatic disorders may be found in adults, and acquired pragmatic disorders can arise in children. An adult with intellectual disability related to a genetic syndrome may be unable to make polite requests of a conversational partner or may fail to comprehend the indirect speech acts used by others. However, these difficulties have their origin in the limited acquisition of pragmatic language skills during the developmental period. Accordingly, the adult in this case has a developmental pragmatic disorder. By the same token, following a traumatic brain injury (TBI), a child of 15 years of age may be unable to relate events in a story in the causal and temporal order in which they occur. These narrative production skills may have been well developed prior to the head injury, which disrupted them. As a result, the child exhibits an acquired pragmatic disorder. A further distinction in the classification of pragmatic disorders is that between a *primary* and a *secondary* pragmatic disorder. In some of the etiological groups described previously, pragmatic difficulties are not related to deficits of structural language. For example, a child with ASD may have marked pragmatic impairments in the presence of relatively intact phonological, syntactic, and semantic skills. Because this child's pragmatic difficulties are not related to structural language deficits, they are a primary pragmatic disorder. A quite different scenario occurs in the case of an adult with nonfluent aphasia who is unable to undertake the subject–auxiliary verb inversion that is needed to produce a conventional indirect speech act (e.g., "Can you open the window?"). Because this individual's pragmatic difficulties are related to an impairment of syntax, they are a secondary pragmatic disorder. Of course, it is possible for a single individual to have both a primary and a secondary pragmatic disorder.

Shift in Thinking on Pragmatic Impairments

Since the 1970s, when researchers first began to acknowledge pragmatics as an area of clinical significance to speech–language pathology, there have been considerable developments in the understanding and management of pragmatic disorders. Pragmatic impairments are no longer treated as an area of language pathology, which (a) does not require direct intervention because these skills improve *automatically* as improvements occur in syntax and semantics (they do not) and which (b) holds less significance for a speaker's communicative competence than the formal language skills that have been traditionally dominant in speech–language pathology clinics. Clinicians and researchers in general acknowledge that clients can pass standardized language batteries and yet still exhibit marked communication difficulties that affect social, academic, and occupational functioning. There is also widespread agreement that pragmatic language skills must be assessed and treated on their own terms and not viewed as having secondary significance to formal language skills in the clinical management of clients. Indeed, it is not uncommon for clinicians to have a pragmatic focus to assessment and intervention even when other language skills are impaired, if there is little prospect of meaningful recovery of these language skills (e.g., in the case of clients with severe aphasia) or if pragmatic skills are judged to make a more significant contribution than formal language skills to a client's effectiveness as a communicator. Extensive rehearsal in a clinical setting of how to form passive voice sentences or to use relative clauses is of little benefit to clients who cannot open a conversation with a friend or make requests appropriately of those around them. The *pragmatic turn* in speech–language pathology achieved a much-needed realignment of communicative priorities for clients.

Role of Theory of Mind Deficits

The development of clinical pragmatics has occurred concurrently with a significant increase in research in the cognitive and neurosciences. This has allowed researchers to examine the cognitive and neural substrates of pragmatic disorders. Because of this research, there is growing evidence that deficits in theory of mind (ToM) and executive functions can make a substantial contribution to the pragmatic difficulties of clients. ToM is the ability to attribute mental states to one's own mind and to the minds of others. One mental state in particular, communicative intention, is the basis of all utterance interpretation. To understand the ironic intent of a speaker who produces the utterance "What a delightful child!" in the presence of a disruptive five-year-old, a listener must attribute to the speaker the belief that the child is anything but delightful and the communicative intention that the speaker wants to make this belief manifest to the listener. If such mental state attribution does not take place, as is the case, for example, in children with ASD, then utterance interpretation will be compromised. Through extensive experimental studies, researchers have clearly established a role for ToM deficits in a range of pragmatic language impairments, including failure to understand metaphor and irony and comprehend indirect speech acts.

Role of Executive Function Deficits

Executive function deficits are another significant group of cognitive impairments, which have implications for pragmatic language skills. Executive functions are a wide-ranging set of cognitive skills, which are integral to the planning, execution, and regulation of goal-directed behavior. Key executive functions include working memory, attention, mental flexibility, planning ability and organization, impulse control and self-regulation, problem-solving ability, and initiation of activity. These skills are intimately connected with the brain's frontal lobes, although other neural circuits are also implicated. The presence of frontal lobe pathology in clients who sustain a TBI places these individuals at high risk of executive dysfunction. Executive function deficits are believed to play a role in the significant pragmatic and discourse impairments of these clients. Difficulties with topic management, poor narrative cohesion and coherence, and reduced informativeness in conversation and other forms of discourse have all been linked to executive function deficits. Aside from TBI, executive function deficits have also been shown to play a role in the pragmatic and discourse anomalies of other cognitive–communication disorders such as right hemisphere language disorder and the communication difficulties that attend the dementias.

Assessment

There is a widespread agreement among clinicians that pragmatic disorders cannot be adequately assessed using the single word and sentence testing formats of standardized language tests. To a large extent, this explains the lack of pragmatic language *tests* that are used to assess clients suspected of having a pragmatic disorder. Clinicians are much more likely to use pragmatics checklists and profiles to assess this group of language skills. Following observation of recorded or real-time conversation, clinicians judge whether certain pragmatic skills are present or absent and if they are used appropriately or inappropriately. One drawback of these assessments is that ratings can vary according to the skill and expertise of the observer (e.g., teacher, parent, speech–language pathologist). Studies have also found weak correlations between ratings of pragmatic skills by parents and professionals. Also, knowing *that* a particular skill is absent from a client's pragmatic repertoire is not the same as knowing *why* this occurs.

Other pragmatic assessments are based on approaches such as conversation analysis and discourse analysis. Monologic discourse is most often examined in the context of narrative production and picture description tasks. These assessments give clinicians unparalleled insight into the pragmatic language difficulties of clients. However, they are also very labor- and time-intensive, a fact that has limited their widespread use in clinical settings. There is little evidence to date that computer-based applications have done much to increase the routine adoption of conversation analysis and discourse analysis in clinics, with clinicians in general reporting positive attitudes toward both conversation analysis and discourse analysis but still stating a lack of available clinical time as the most significant barrier to their widespread use.

Intervention

Pragmatic language intervention proceeds by means of an eclectic set of techniques and approaches. Typically, pragmatic language skills are addressed as part of a social communication intervention, which emphasizes verbal and nonverbal pragmatic skills, receptive and expressive language skills, social cognition (ToM), and social interaction. There is some evidence for the efficacy of social communication interventions for children with pragmatic impairment. Intervention may also target the training of specific conversational skills so that clients receive explicit instruction and practice in how to open and close conversations, take turns with others, and much else besides. The extent to which an intervention of this type develops an individual's pragmatic competence, rather than just trains superficial skills, is not clear. Pragmatic language skills are also part of the social skills training of the type used with clients who have schizophrenia. Behaviors such as speaker–listener proximity during conversation, appropriate use of greetings and salutations, politeness in conversation, and use and understanding of facial expressions and prosodic cues may all feature in a social skills intervention. ToM training in clients with specific ToM deficits (e.g., children and adults with ASD) has the potential to improve this key cognitive skill for utterance interpretation. Each of these interventions has as its focus the client with pragmatic impairment. Clinicians have also acknowledged the role that conversational partners can play in facilitating (and hindering) the communicative competence of adults with pragmatic disorder. Originally implemented in the treatment of clients with aphasia, conversational partner training is now used in the management of a wide range of clients with pragmatic difficulties. These training packages, several of which are now commercially available, can increase opportunities for communication for clients with dementia, aphasia, and other conditions. They can also target and help partners modify behaviors that limit a client's participation in conversation. A focus on more effective conversational repair strategies and the avoidance of protracted exchanges around a client's retrieval of a specific word are possible targets of an intervention based on conversational partner training.

Louise Cummings

See also Autism Spectrum Disorder; Conversation Analysis; Dementia; Discourse Analysis; Executive Function and Communication; Right Hemisphere Cognitive–Communication Disorders; Theory of Mind

Further Readings

Asp, E. D., & de Villiers, J. (2010). *When language breaks down: Analysing discourse in clinical contexts.* New York, NY: Cambridge University Press.

Cummings, L. (2009). *Clinical pragmatics.* Cambridge, UK: Cambridge University Press.

Cummings, L. (Ed.). (2017). *Research in clinical pragmatics.* Switzerland: Springer.

Müller, N. (Ed.). (2000). *Pragmatics in speech and Language pathology.* Amsterdam, The Netherlands: John Benjamins.

Perkins, M. (2007). *Pragmatic impairment.* Cambridge, UK: Cambridge University Press.

Pragmatics

Pragmatics can be defined as a set of rules governing the use of language within a communicative context. The ability to interpret and use these rules to share intended meaning in a social context is called *pragmatic competence*. To clearly understand what is meant by pragmatics, it is helpful to visualize language as a set of concentric circles. Phonology and its rules for describing the phonemes and the allowable combinations of phonemes of a language would be at the center. Combinations of phonemes would be used to encode words that refer to meaning, or semantics, in circle two. Additional phonemes, affixed to words, give further nuance of meaning to the words, such as time of action (e.g., verb tense) or status of subjects (e.g., plural, possessive), marking the third circle as morphology. The fourth circle, syntax, describes the word and morpheme ordering rules used to specify the relationships of meaning held between the words in a sentence. Each of these levels subsumes the ones below it, and together they provide a model of the structural and linguistic knowledge used to generate sentences. While essential for language, a sentence is a string of words without context, and therefore without communication. It is not until the fifth and outermost circle, pragmatics, that one begins to understand the communicative functions of language and the rules or conventions of use that allow for meaningful communication between individuals. This entry provides an overview of pragmatics, including speech acts, contextual variation, discourse and Grices's maxims, politeness principles, and how pragmatic competence is developed.

Understanding pragmatics can be a daunting task since there are an infinite number of ways language can be used within a given social situation. Yet everyone can identify individuals who lack pragmatic competence as well as those who excel at this ability. Pragmatics requires a broad kind of reasoning that goes beyond sentences and requires immediate inferences to be made about the who, what, where, when, and why of the communication. Although there is not a complete model or theory to explain how this complex communication is accomplished, much is known about the types of rules and processes that must be used to guide these decisions.

Speech Acts

If a sentence is an ordered string of words and morphemes encoded by phonemes, then an *utterance*, or actually speaking a sentence, entails all of this as well as the intentional acts of a speaker to influence a listener within a shared event. Key to this definition of an utterance is that language is both intentional and that it is an act or action much like pointing, grabbing, or running. In other words, an utterance is a linguistic action performed by a speaker with an intent specific to a given context or situation. This led philosophers like John Austin and John Searle to refer to utterances as *speech acts*. According to speech act theory, speakers have particular ideas or propositions to communicate and must decide how to word these propositions in order to achieve the desired effect or outcome. For the most part, this is done without conscious reflection and nearly instantaneous with the thought, although certain speech acts delivered in a context such as a speech may occur with considerable preparation. Each speech act is composed of an illocutionary act, locutionary act, and perlocutionary act.

The *illocutionary act* or *force* is the motive or intention of the speech act. These motives can include actions such as declaring, promising, querying, requesting, referring, describing, arguing, demanding, apologizing, asserting, or a myriad of other purposes. To communicate the intention, a *locutionary act* must be produced. The speaker must draw upon the phonological, semantic, morphological, and syntactic levels of the concentric circles to give the intended message linguistic form. The form must directly or indirectly correspond with the intended illocutionary force, and it must be structured as a declarative sentence that makes a statement or relays information, imperative sentence that issues commands or requests, exclamatory sentence that expresses strong emotion, or an interrogative sentence that asks a question. The sentence must contain or imply a *referring expression* that names the subject and a *predicate expression* that tells something about the subject. Thus, the locutionary act can be viewed as the words that are produced and heard when the speech act is uttered.

Speakers produce a locationary act with the intention of having a particular effect or outcome on the listener, such as directing that person's attention or obtaining a requested object. This effect is called the *perlocutionary act*. When the speech act is successful, the desired outcome is achieved, but there are many instances when what one says is not what the other person interprets. This is because of *contextual variation*.

Form-Function Mapping or Contextual Variation

Producing speech acts may appear to be a fairly straightforward process of matching the meaning and intent of a message to the correct forms. "The cookies look good" appears to be a compliment produced using a declarative sentence, with the expectation that the listener will smile and say, "Thank you." But the word choice as well as the interpretation depends on a wide range of linguistic and nonlinguistic contextual variables. If the baker had just expressed that the oven was too hot, "The cookies look good" might be produced with the intent of teasing the person about the burnt cookies.

John Searle referred to the process of deriving meaning beyond the literal expression of the words as *implicature*, that is, the propositional meaning of a speech act is inferred from the context or another proposition rather than from the literal meaning of the sentence. Implicature can be viewed as the relation between the uttered and the implied statement. Sometimes the implied function may be expressed in a manner very different from the uttered form. "The cookies look good," spoken with a hand held up toward the cookies would have a declarative form (i.e., making a comment about the cookies) but in function it would be a request (i.e., "Give me a cookie"). To use this type of *indirect speech act*, certain assumptions or *presuppositions* must be made about the listener. For example, the age and linguistic skill of the listener must be sufficient to understand indirect requests, and the listener must share the nonlinguistic context. If the listener did not notice the up-turned hand gesture, a *communication breakdown* would occur and the intended outcome would not be realized (i.e., no cookie). Nonliteral expressions are also used to add humor, interest, or excitement. Looking at the burnt cookies and saying, "May they rest in peace" only has meaning if one recognizes the expression and makes an analogy to the cookies. The choice of using direct or indirect and literal or nonliteral language depends on many variables such as the age, gender, race, dialect, social status, and role of the speaker and listener, as well as the situational context.

Discourse

Speech acts do not generally occur in isolation but rather in larger units such as conversations and narrative monologues. According to Paul Grice, the interlocutors in a conversation must adhere to the *cooperative principle* to be mutually understood. The four main cooperative principles, termed *Grice's maxims*, describe the rules for taking turns and cooperating that people assume within conversations.

- *maxim of quantity*: provide the correct amount of information, neither too much nor too little based on presuppositions about the listener and what he or she knows about the topic
- *maxim of quality*: provide information believed to be truthful and supported by sufficient evidence
- *maxim of relation*: make one's contributions relevant to the conversation and pertinent to the topic
- *maxim of manner*: deliver information in a manner that is clear, brief, orderly, and avoids vagueness or ambiguity

When the maxims are violated, communication breakdowns may occur or social sanctions may be applied. People may avoid those whom they perceive to be prevaricators or those who launch into endless monologues. But sometimes speakers purposefully violate one or more of the maxims for purposes like exaggeration or humor. Saying, "The cookies look good" in response to the burnt cookies is an example of violating the maxim of quality or truthfulness in an attempt at humor. When communication breakdowns do occur, interlocutors attempt to repair them by giving and receiving feedback or correcting conversation errors.

Geoffrey Leech proposed that conversation also requires adherence to the *politeness principle* and specified *politeness maxims*, including tact, generosity, approbation, modesty, agreement, and sympathy. There is considerable variation in these maxims between cultures, so what is perceived as polite in one culture may be rude or odd in another. The maxims *tact* and *generosity* focus on minimizing imposition on others and putting others before oneself. The *approbation* and *modesty* maxims focus on avoiding negatives or insults and instead praising others, while minimizing praise of oneself. The *agreement* maxim suggests the use of indirect language to express disagreement while maximizing points of agreement. The sympathy maxim focuses on minimizing animus and maximizing sympathy toward others. These maxims manifest in behaviors such as using more indirect speech acts in formal situations or with higher status addressees, and more neutral or positive word choices in polite exchanges.

Carol Prutting and Diane Kirchner suggested that interlocutors must adhere to other principles or rules when communicating. These include:

- *Topic control rules:* use culturally appropriate conventions for selecting, initiating, maintaining, changing, and ending the topic
- *Turn-taking rules:* use rules to initiate, respond, repair/revise, interrupt, give feedback, judge quantity, and conciseness
- *Lexical selection rules:* be specific, accurate, and maintain cohesion in word choice
- *Stylistic variation:* modify communicative style based on presuppositions about the listener and the context
- *Paralinguistic aspects:* speak intelligibly and use appropriate vocal intensity, vocal quality, prosody, and fluency
- *Nonverbal aspects:* use culturally appropriate physical proximity, physical contacts, body posture, limb movements, body posture, facial expression, and eye gaze

Development

Preschool-age children demonstrate early mastery of basic principles of pragmatics. Even single word utterances are produced with communicative intent, and children quickly acquire a wide range of illocutionary functions and the linguistic skills to express them. An extensive body of research demonstrates that the precursors to conversations are established during the prelinguistic stages of development. Elizabeth Bates, Luigia Camaioni, and Virginia Volerra described development from birth to 18 months using the properties of speech acts.

Perlocutionary Phase

During the perlocutionary phase, the child has an effect on the behaviors of listeners without the intent of communicating. Adults respond to cries, coos, and other nonlinguistic behaviors as if the child produced a request or command. The adult engages the child in reciprocal vocal turn-taking called *protoconversations*. During this phase, the child can engage with an object by grabbing, banging, or exploring it, or the child can engage in interactions with others. However, the child cannot coordinate both and will reach for a toy but not signal the adult to help retrieve it.

Illocutionary Phase

During this phase, generally beginning at about the age of 10 months, the child acquires the ability to coordinate both objects and others using communication. The child may reach for a toy but also establishes eye contact with the adult and gazes back to the toy to intentionally request assistance. The communications are done without language, and thus are called *proto-declaratives*.

Locutionary Phase

Gradually, the child incorporates more words and greater syntactic complexity to communicate needs and information. Language provides the child with a new powerful tool for accomplishing goals and controlling the environment. As the child masters the ability to coordinate objects, other people, and language into a triadic relationship, increasing pragmatic competence is demonstrated.

Final Thoughts

Pragmatics is a relatively new branch of linguistic study (although the origin of the term dates back to ancient Greece and Rome) that overlaps with many other fields, such as sociolinguistics, linguistics, philosophy, semantics, and semiotics. Grice suggested it is separate from other areas of research because of its focus on the practical or conversational aspects of meaning. The concepts of pragmatics, such as speech acts, cooperative principle, and politeness principle, have influenced the research in a broad range of disciplines, including communication disorders where these subtle nuances of language use may pose significant difficulty for children with language impairments, as well as those who experience neurological impairments across the life span.

Jan Norris

See also Cooperative Principle; Implicature; Nonverbal Communication; Pragmatic Development; Pragmatic Impairment

Further Readings

Austin, J. L. (1962). *How to do things with words*. Oxford, UK: Clarendon.

Grice, H. P. (1975). *Logic and conversation*. In P. Cole & J. Morgan (Eds.), *Speech acts: Syntax and semantics* (Vol. 3., pp. 41–58). New York, NY: Academic Press.

Hulit, L. M., Fahey, K. R., & Howard, M. R. (2014). *Born to talk: An introduction to speech and language development* (6th ed.). Boston, MA: Pearson Education.

Leech, G. (1983). *Principles of pragmatics*. London, UK: Longman.

Prutting, C., & Kirchner, D. (1987). A clinical appraisal of the pragmatic aspects of language. *Journal of Speech and Hearing Disorders, 52*, 105–119.

Searle, J. (1969). *Speech acts*. Cambridge, UK: Cambridge University Press.

Yule, G. (2010). *The study of language* (4th ed.). Cambridge, UK: Cambridge University Press.

PREMORBID LEVEL

Premorbid (from the Latin, *pre-* "before" and *morbidus* "sickly" or *morbus* "illness") refers to the functioning of an individual prior to the onset of an acquired disease or illness. While the term *premorbid level* is most often used in relation to psychological function (e.g., cognitive ability, intelligence, or personality), it can also be used in reference to physical functioning (e.g., premorbid heart rate, premorbid lung function). In the field of communication sciences, levels of speech, voice, resonance, or swallowing function may have been obtained or recorded before the illness and so are often accessible or easily estimated based on comparing the decline with *typical function*. However, it can be much more difficult to measure premorbid cognitive and linguistic skills because of the large *typical* range possible and lack of sufficient data prior to the illness. This entry provides an overview of premorbid level as it relates to cognitive and linguistic skills, examining how demographic data, neuropsychological tests, and anecdotal data are used as a basis for premorbid level and exploring the purpose of premorbid estimates.

Cognitive and Linguistic Skills

Changes in cognition and language are common in cases of acquired neurological disorders. Difficulties with production and comprehension of language, social skills, attention, memory, awareness, problem-solving, orientation, and executive function all impact communication and may result in a change in intelligence or personality. To accurately measure this change, one must have knowledge of the individual's cognitive functioning before the incident or illness. Since this information is seldom available, many clinicians use information they do have access to in order to estimate prior functioning.

Naturally, these estimates of premorbid psychological functioning are inherently uncertain, and a thorough assessment prior to the onset of the illness or event that impacted cognitive skills would provide the most accurate premorbid estimate. Without this information, premorbid level is most often based on demographic data (e.g., age, education, race, socioeconomic status), performance data (as measured by neuropsychological tests), or anecdotal information.

Demographic Data

Demographic-based regression approaches to estimate premorbid functioning use variables such as age, ethnicity, education, occupation, socioeconomic status, and urban–rural residence. Although this approach to calculation of premorbid level is objective, demographically identical individuals may demonstrate significant cognitive and intellectual differences. Familial data may be a strong predictor of premorbid abilities, and assessment of closely related family members may provide a representative picture of the client's premorbid level.

A number of studies have demonstrated positive correlations between demographic predictions and predictions of premorbid intelligence using comprehensive neuropsychological testing. These studies identified age, race, education, and occupation as the most significant indicators of premorbid level. It is important to remember that this is an estimate, and individual differences preclude a true assessment of premorbid ability based on demographics. Many researchers therefore recommend that estimations utilizing demographic data also incorporate premorbid and/or postmorbid neuropsychological performance scores.

Neuropsychological Tests

Professionals have sought to obtain premorbid scores through use of neuropsychological tests since after World War I, as they attempted to measure prewar levels of functioning. Most quantitative methods used to estimate premorbid function examine premorbid IQ rather than other cognitive skills. Many standardized neuropsychological tests have published premorbid estimation formulas. Widely accepted examples include the National Adult Reading Test-Revised, the Kaufman Brief Intelligence Test, the Wechsler Adult Intelligence Scale-Revised, and the Wechsler Intelligence Scale for Children-Revised. These formulas include demographic-based regression approaches that assume premorbid function is close to available demographic norms, current ability (hold) approaches based on independent test batteries, and approaches that use a combination of performance and demographic data.

Literature suggests that approaches combining demographic data and scores from current ability measures are most highly correlated with actual premorbid level. However, tests administered after the injury or insult examine current cognitive level, and the current abilities of the individual impact the overall premorbid score. One must also fall within the normative groups and categories in order for any of these estimates to be applicable, and if an individual is an outlier (i.e., very young, elderly, or culturally and ethnically different), this estimate may be skewed. Additionally, many of these formulae do not account for disabilities that may have existed before the injury. Finally, premorbid level as measured by neuropsychological tests may indicate premorbid intelligence but not the actual premorbid functioning of the individual.

Much of the population routinely completes standardized tests that are included in their academic records and that provide a representation of IQ and academic abilities. These may be obtained as a representation of the individual's premorbid level before the disorder or illness and do not rely on current levels of functioning.

Anecdotal Data

In the clinical setting, anecdotal data are collected as clinicians gather information and descriptions of the individual's prior abilities and occupational records, which are not accounted for by demographic data or standardized assessments. Many researchers fear this method is particularly biased, as premorbid functioning reported by individuals and their caregivers may be exaggerated; individuals may not be referencing the point of functioning directly before the injury but a reference point long before that; and the clinician may be influenced by fatigue, distraction, recent experiences, and overconfidence. Clinicians are trained to find abnormalities and thus may overemphasize expected difficulties or may fall subject to an *anchoring* bias and cling to their first impressions rather than remaining open to alternative viewpoints. This error may be reduced by the application of objective or quantitative methods.

Purpose of Premorbid Estimates

All approaches to estimating premorbid level have advantages and disadvantages, and different methods may have differential utility depending upon both the individuals studied and the disorder in question. The most accurate representation of premorbid functioning is a thorough and well-documented assessment before the event that caused the change in functioning. Premorbid levels are calculated for a number of reasons. First, it may be important that legal benefits are obtained and disability be established as significant with the appropriate authorities. In order to qualify for financial support or benefits, one must be able to indicate functioning is significantly different from premorbid functioning. Similarly, if the client is pursuing personal injury litigation due to the circumstances of the incident, one must be able to demonstrate to what degree skills were lost as a result of the incident that caused the difficulties. Finally, ascertaining premorbid levels may aid professionals in establishing diagnoses of disorders (e.g., identifying the subtle cognitive changes in the early stages of degenerative disorders) and setting achievable long-term goals for the client.

Louise C. Keegan

See also Bias; Cognition; Intelligence; Neurogenic Communication Disorders; Standardized Testing; Traumatic Brain Injury

Further Readings

Axelrod, B. N., Vanderploeg, R. D., & Schinka, J. A. (1999). Comparing methods for estimating premorbid intellectual functioning. *Archives of Clinical Neuropsychology, 14*(4), 341–346.

Crawford, J. R., Millar, J., & Milne, A. B. (2001). Estimating premorbid IQ from demographic variables: A comparison of a regression equation vs. clinical judgment. *British Journal of Clinical Psychology, 40,* 97–105.

Franzen, M. D., Burgess, E. J., & Smith-Seemiller, L. (1997). Methods of estimating premorbid functioning. *Archives of Clinical Neuropsychology, 12*(8), 711–738.

Kareken, D. A. (1997). Judgment pitfalls in estimating premorbid intellectual function. *Archives of Clinical Neuropsychology, 12*(8), 701–709.

Shinka, J. A., & Vanderploeg, R. D. (2014). Estimating premorbid level of functioning. In R. D. Vanderploeg (Ed.), *Clinicians guide to neuropsychological assessment* (2nd ed., pp. 39–68). New York, NY: Erlbaum.

PRENATAL DRUG EXPOSURE

See Speech, Language, and Learning Difficulties Associated with Prenatal Drug Exposure

PRESCHOOL LANGUAGE INTERVENTION

Preschool language intervention is a term that refers to practices that promote the development of language, including oral and written forms. The intervention is designed to improve the speech and language skills of children who are 3–5 years of age. The term applies to programs for children with poorly developed speech and language skills because of environmental factors, such as poverty, or English as second language learners. It also refers to therapy provided by a speech–language pathologist (SLP) for children with identified speech and language disabilities. Preschool language intervention provided by the SLP may be implemented within individual therapy sessions or in small and/or large groups. The approaches to invention may range from highly structured to naturalistic approaches incorporating incidental teaching. While some intervention programs include a manualized curriculum (e.g., High-Scope), most preschool language interventions are more loosely designed according to a set of principles and strategies that are individualized for each child or preschool setting.

Children with a range of disabilities may be seen for preschool language intervention. The program may focus on a specific etiology, such as hearing impairment or autism, or it may be in a preschool setting in which children with disabilities are included and receive special services. These services may be in the form of supplementary individual intervention provided by a SLP, or the SLP may be the primary instructor in a small language intervention group. Many interventions incorporate parent training, including programs primarily implemented by parents under the direction of an educator or SLP. This entry provides an overview of common preschool language disorders and then examines preschool language interventions, including structured, naturalistic, and language and literacy interventions.

Preschool Language Disorders

Children with preschool language disorders may exhibit difficulties with understanding language and/or producing age-appropriate language. Children often show concomitant disorders of speech, particularly word pronunciation (i.e., speech sound disorders). Children with intellectual disability, autism, hearing impairment, or neuromotor impairment (e.g., cerebral palsy) typically demonstrate mild to severe language impairment. Children may also present with a mild to severe specific language impairment in the absence of other disabilities. The types of difficulties shown involve understanding basic concepts; asking and answering questions; following directions; learning new vocabulary words; understanding and using appropriate word order (i.e., syntax) and word endings (i.e., morphology); telling stories, as well as engaging in and maintaining social conversations with peers and adults (i.e., pragmatics); and developing literacy skills. Preschool language interventions may address some or all of these dimensions.

Structured Approaches

Discrete Trial Training

Discrete trial training is a highly structured approach. The interventionist targets specific language forms based on developmental sequences or functional needs. Materials are selected to elicit practice responding to or producing those language forms. The interventionist controls the order in which the material is presented, the criteria for an acceptable response, and the type and schedule of reinforcement. The materials used, such as pictures of action verbs, are generally unrelated to each other except that they each represent exemplars of the targeted form (e.g., present progressive verb tense).

Benefits of discrete trial training include a guided focus on a desirable language skill, maximum practice of the skill within a short time frame, and an increased awareness of the form when it is heard or used in the natural environment.

Criticisms of this approach include that the talk is unnatural, resulting in poor generalization to real communication. The meaning and the function of communication are minimized in favor of language form since the interventionist ignores what the child said and instead only reinforces how accurately the child produced the target form. This results in the highly unnatural situation where saying, "The boy is jumping" results in receiving a random secondary reinforcer, such as blowing bubbles, that is completely unrelated to jumping. Furthermore, the topics of the series of discrete trials are unrelated (e.g., the boy is jumping, the cat is sleeping, the truck is moving), so the learning is not embedded within higher level organization, resulting in isolated skill learning. Practicing the form does not help the child understand how to share meaning or how to use the form to accomplish communication goals.

A variation of Discrete Trial Training is *Applied Behavioral Analysis* (ABA), first used by O. Ivar Lavaas in 1980 for children with autism. This is a very intensive behavioral therapy that is implemented daily for 40 hr each week. Training generally lasts 3 years or longer, with long-term retention of learned skills shown by many participants. Concerns include that claims to a recovery from autism are not based on good research, and that equal or better outcomes for social, pragmatic language are shown for more naturalistic approaches. The intervention is costly and the necessity of 40 hr of intensive weekly intervention has not been empirically established.

Focused Stimulation

Focused stimulation is similar to discrete trial training in that a specific word, phrase, or grammatical form is targeted based on developmental sequences or functional needs of the child. However, training of the targeted language occurs within an activity such as playing, storybook reading, or a structured task. The play or interactions are manipulated within the natural environment to create a setting where the target behavior is likely to occur with high frequency. The adult models the use of the target language within the sentence. For example, while playing with a dollhouse, the interventionist might target the present progressive verb form. She manipulates dolls, while emphasizing the target form, as in, "Look, the baby *is* crying. Mama *is* looking at the baby. Mama *is* picking up the baby. Mama *is* going to feed her."

The goal of focused stimulation is to heighten the child's awareness of the language form. As the child repeatedly hears the form used in context, the likelihood that the child will imitate its use in that context increases. When this occurs, the adult can respond to the child by repeating or recasting the child's sentence, as in, "You are right. The mama is picking up the baby." The reinforcement occurs as the adult recognizes the meaning and enthusiastically agrees with the child. Further, the targeted forms are produced within sentences that are related to the dollhouse play, thus providing a coherent context for the talk. While structured, the interactions maintain properties of natural communication, integrating language content, form, and use. However, the talk focusing on a specific form often becomes contrived and limits what can be talked about. It assumes that repeated use of the same form is a necessary learning process for children with language disorders, although there is no evidence to support this contention.

Naturalistic Approaches

Naturalistic approaches conduct intervention in a natural setting such as a playroom, during meals, or in the child's home. Language goals may be set ahead of time, but the interventionist responds to the child's needs in the moment. The adult attends to the child's interests and is responsive to the child's topics and needs for language structures to successfully communicate at that moment. This is referred to *as following the child's lead*.

Communication temptations are often incorporated into naturalistic approaches. For example, a desired object may be placed in a location visible to the child but too high to reach, or in a plastic container with a tight lid. Wind-up toys or other cause-effect toys may be presented that are too difficult for the child to use independently, thus creating the need for the child to make a request for assistance. Interesting games or motivating songs may be abruptly ended, requiring the child to request continuation or another turn. Activities such as sand play or blocks provide opportunities for the child to request more. These temptations provide opportunities for the child to learn how to use language to request the desired objects or actions from an adult or peer.

Milieu Communication Training (Milieu Teaching)

One approach that incorporates communication temptations is termed *Milieu Communication Training*. Training takes place in everyday environments, with the goal of building the child's ability to successfully function and communicate within familiar activities such as routines. Communication temptations are arranged within the environment, and the adult expectedly waits for the child to initiate communication. The adult watches for initiations from the child, such as gesturing, vocalizations, or interest in an object or activity, and interprets these behaviors as a request. The interventionist responds by assisting the child to access or manipulate the desired object. Thus, children learn the function of communication through the intrinsic consequences.

The overall goal is to increase the number and complexity of communication acts produced by the child. The adult's role is to be highly responsive to communicative attempts, even when those behaviors are not intentionally communicative. In the early stages, the adult may respond to the child's reaching, grabbing, or looking without communicative intent. As intervention progresses, the child is encouraged to use gestures, eye contact, vocalizations, and words to initiate communications. As the capabilities of the child increase, the adult holds out longer for words or word approximations before responding to the child. The adult also begins to use modeling, prompting, and expansions of child utterances to encourage the use of verbal language.

Incidental Teaching

Incidental teaching is another approach that makes use of communication temptations. Desired objects or activities are arranged within the environment to elicit requests or comments from the child. Before the adult provides the desired object or turn in response to the child's initiation, the adult requests more elaborated language using a carrier phrase such as "Say …" or "Tell me…" (e.g., Tell me, "I want a cookie"). The goals of incidental teaching are to increase the child's opportunities to talk, to encourage spontaneous language, and to expand the complexity of language used by the child.

Preschool Language and Literacy Interventions

Oral and written language are linked from infancy onward, developing concurrently rather than sequentially. From infancy, children make discoveries about the content, form, and function of print through experiences with storybook reading, nursery rhymes, alphabet blocks, and a myriad of toys, games, and electronic devices that encourage exploration of print. Children with preschool language disorders are at risk for long-term written language delays, especially reading comprehension. Children with language disorders also have difficulty viewing and manipulating words in the abstract, a language ability needed for rhyme, sound segmentation, sound blending, and other phonemic awareness abilities that support learning to decode written words. It is not surprising that many children identified with preschool language disorders are later re-identified with reading disabilities. Thus, it is critically important that preschool language interventions provide a strong focus on written language.

Dialogic Reading

Dialogic reading is an approach to shared storybook reading where the child is encouraged to ask questions, make comments, and respond throughout the interactive reading. The adult uses strategies to actively engage the child as both an active listener and as a costoryteller. An emphasis is placed on building vocabulary and general background knowledge as well as recognizing elements of narrative structure as the story unfolds. The adult prompts the child to retell parts of the story during the reading. Conventions of book handling and print are also pointed out and discussed as the story is read.

Topics from the story are used to develop thematic activities that are carried out in art, play, music, snack time, and so forth. For example, children reading *The Three Little Pigs* may create sack puppets in art, sing *Who's Afraid of the Big Bad Wolf* in music, build strong houses in the block center, and eat little pigs (i.e., cookies with pink frosting) for snack. The thematic approach enables children to use new vocabulary words and concepts from the story throughout the day and in varying contexts.

Dialogic reading has been shown to have large effects on vocabulary, language development, and comprehension. However, the effects on alphabet knowledge are minimal. Thus, preschool language intervention also includes a focus on phonological awareness.

Phonological Awareness

Phonological awareness is the ability to detect and manipulate the sounds of phonemes in words. A child must understand that a word can be conceptualized as an abstract object, with parts such as initial or final phonemes, and these phonemes can be deleted, substituted, or blended to form rhymes, syllables, and new words. Phonological awareness is an auditory ability that focuses on the sounds of language. However, the most effective interventions teach phonological awareness skills using print. The visual representation of sounds provided by the alphabet enables children to conceptualize and physically manipulate phonemes. Programs such as Lindamood Phoneme Sequencing and Phonic Faces speech alphabet associate phonemes with speech production cues.

Final Thoughts

Poor language development during the preschool years is predictive of reading, comprehension, writing, speaking, and social language deficits that may be long term and lead to school failure. Approaches to preschool language intervention range from highly structured to more naturalistic, but all are designed to elicit a high frequency of communications from the child and to expand the complexity of language skills the child understands and spontaneously uses.

Jan Norris

See also Academic Impact of Communication Disorders; Functional Communication Skills; Language Disorders in Children; Language Therapy and Intervention; Play Therapy

Further Readings

Gilbert, K. (2008, October). Milieu communication training for late talkers. *SIG 1 Perspectives on Language Learning and Education, 15,* 112–118.

Institute of Educational Sciences. Intervention Reports. Retrieved from https://ies.ed.gov/director/board/reports/index.asp

Lovaas, O. I., Ackerman, A. B., Alexander, D., Firestone, P., Perkins, J., & Young, D. (1980). *Teaching developmentally disabled children: The me book.* Austin, TX: Pro-Ed.

PRESCRIPTIVE AND DESCRIPTIVE APPROACHES

Grammarians, philologists, linguists, and other language scientists find different ways to communicate about the rules that make up a particular language. One very basic distinction is the approach one takes toward this goal, namely to *prescribe* how the building blocks of a language are combined for proper use or to *describe* how this is done. Since prescriptive approaches are arguably ill-suited for research purposes and theory formation, modern linguistics—generative and nongenerative alike—adopts a descriptive approach. The descriptive approach also contributes to factors of adequacy, which is of particular interest to generative grammarians. This entry provides a brief overview of the prescriptive and descriptive approaches to the rules of a language.

A prescriptive approach focuses on talking about how a language *ought* to be used—how one should speak, what type of language to avoid, and so on. As such, linguistic prescriptivism involves siding with one variety or manner of speaking a language over another and includes judgments on what usages are socially proper or politically correct. Obviously, some degree of standardization is needed in language. A standardized variety of a language is necessary if the majority of speakers are to understand television programs, newspapers, books, and other means of mass communication. There is also a need for a standardized variety of language in the context of language learning, even if it is a little stilted and formal. Hence, a prescriptive approach is commonly taken in language classes, where the aim is to teach child or adult learners how to use language in a very particular way. The main aims of linguistic prescription are then to specify standard language forms either in general or for specific purposes (e.g., appropriate style and register in respective contexts) and to formulate these in such a way as to make them easily taught or learned.

In contrast, a descriptive grammar focuses on describing the language as it is used, not saying how it should be used. A descriptive approach would thus hold that a sentence is grammatical—or, using a more adequate term, *acceptable*—if a native speaker would produce that sentence in speaking. The aim of linguistic analysis is to then try and describe how that sentence is produced through theorizing about the mental processes that lead to the surface form in order to provide a comprehensive, systematic, objective, and precise account of the patterns and use of a specific language or dialect, at a particular point in time. The aim of the descriptive approach to language study, then, is to describe the facts of linguistic usage as they are, rather than how they ought to be, with reference to an imagined ideal state.

With further relevance to theoretical linguistics, a generative grammar is said to be a set of formal rules, which projects a finite set of sentences upon the potentially infinite set of sentences that constitute the language as a whole, and it does this in an explicit manner, assigning to each a set of structural descriptions. As a theory of language, generative linguistics considers *grammar* to be a system of underlying rules that generate exactly those combinations of words, which form grammatical sentences in a given language. Among the types of grammar that are typically distinguished are *descriptive grammar* (aiming for a systematic description of a language as found in a sample of speech or writing as in, e.g., reference grammars or grammatical handbooks), *theoretical grammar* (using linguistic data as a means of developing insights into the nature of language as such, sometimes called *formal grammar*), *comparative grammar* (comparing the forms or states of a language with a combination of theoretical–descriptive methods), and *traditional grammar* (summarizing the range of attitudes and methods found in the prelinguistic era of grammatical study, usually used with a critical implication primarily at the prescriptive and proscriptive outlook).

In this context, a *rule* as used in generative grammar denotes a formal statement of correspondence between linguistic elements or structures. Generative rules are predictive. They express a hypothesis about the relationships between sentences, which will hold for the language as a whole and will reflect the native speaker–hearer's competence. Such rules may be subclassified in terms of the components of the grammar in which they appear, such as *phonological rules*, *syntactic rules*, or *lexical rules*. The linguistic sense thus contrasts with the traditional use of the term, where rules are recommendations for correct usage, as in the prescription that a preposition is not to be used at the end of a sentence (but cf. "Which city did she move to?") or that infinitives ought not to be split (but cf. "To boldly go where no man has gone before."). No prescriptive or proscriptive implication is present in the descriptive sense of *rule*.

A theory of language that achieves an exhaustive and discrete enumeration of the data points of the language is said to be *observationally adequate* (as in a very large corpus). With grammar denoting a theory of language, it is said to be *descriptively adequate* if it correctly describes the intrinsic competence of the ideal speaker–hearer (beyond the corpus). As well, a linguistic theory is said to be descriptively adequate if it makes a descriptively adequate grammar available for each language. Furthermore, a (generative) grammar should be able to get at what underlies the speaker–hearer's competence. To the extent that a theory of language succeeds in providing the right kind of strategy for the innately guided language acquisition process (primary linguistic data), it is said to be *explanatorily adequate*.

Applied to speech, language, and communication disorders, one might hold that the prescriptive approach to language would provide the rule-based framework—in the traditional sense—which the patient should attain (in a developmental impairment) or regain (in an acquired disorder). However, it is the descriptive approach that sets the real benchmark, and it does so in both ways: A good linguistic description of languages guides speech–language therapy, and sound intervention informs the descriptive linguist.

Kleanthes K. Grohmann

See also Descriptive Linguistics; Generative Linguistics; Language; Language Register; Syntax and Grammar

Further Readings

Chomsky, N. (1986). *Knowledge of language: Its nature, origins, and use*. New York, NY: Praeger.

Finegan, E. (1980). *Attitudes toward English usage: The history of a war of words*. New York, NY: Teachers College Press.

McArthur, T. (Ed.). (1992). *The Oxford companion to the English language*. Oxford, UK: Oxford University Press.

Newmeyer, F. J. (2003). Grammar is grammar and usage is usage. *Language*, 72, 682–707.

Pinker, S. (1994). *The language instinct: How the mind creates language*. New York, NY: Harper.

PREVALENCE OF COMMUNICATION DISORDERS

Prevalence (also known as *point prevalence*) refers to the number of people in a population with communication disorder(s) at a particular time. *Period prevalence* refers to the number of people with communication within a population that are receiving services over a certain period of time (typically over the past year). *Incidence* refers to the number of newly diagnosed cases of communication disorder(s) within a population over a specified time. Information about prevalence of communication disorders is used to plan and monitor the outcomes of prevention and intervention programs, and inform allocation of resources and public health policy. Population risk is also determined using prevalence data and can be used to target prevention programs for groups at risk. Epidemiological studies of communication disorders typically report prevalence, period prevalence, and/or incidence. This entry provides an overview of the prevalence of communication disorders, and then explores communication disorders in childhood, adulthood, and across the life span.

Overview

Prevalence estimates differ depending on the population studied, definition, and type of communication disorder (speech, language, stuttering, voice, and hearing); severity (mild, moderate, and severe); identification technique (reported concern and direct assessment); informant (self, parent, speech–language pathologist, doctor, educator, and psychologist); age of identification (early childhood, school age, and adulthood); and need for inclusion of a medical diagnosis (cleft palate, aphasia, traumatic brain injury, and cerebral palsy). Some studies consider the general population, whereas others consider clinical populations. Some prevalence studies only report the primary area of disability, whereas others report all areas of disability for an individual. Unsurprisingly, the use of more stringent definitions results in lower estimates of prevalence and incidence. Due to the differing definitions used in prevalence studies, *italicization* will be used in this entry for the terminology used within reported studies.

Identification of communication disorders in prevalence studies can be informed by the World Health Organization's International Classification of Functioning, Disability and Health and include difficulties with Body Structures (e.g., cleft palate), Body Function (e.g., articulation of speech sounds, fluency, language), and Activities and Participation (e.g., conversation). Environmental and Personal Factors may act as barriers or facilitators to effective communication. Thus, prevalence of impaired Body Structures (e.g., cleft palate) will be different from that of impaired Body Function (e.g., speech sound disorder) and limited Activities and Participation (e.g., difficulty communicating). The environment also impacts the prevalence of communication disorder. For example, increasingly many jobs require high levels of literacy and communication, whereas jobs requiring manual labor are increasingly mechanized and computerized. Thus, the impact of limited communicative capacity increasingly impacts participation in society, changing the significance of prevalence data.

Prevalence of Communication Disorders

There is no definitive figure regarding the prevalence of communication disorders across the world. Most studies of the prevalence of communication disorders demonstrate a higher prevalence in early childhood compared with older ages, and in males compared with females. Higher prevalence is also reported in those with a family history of speech, language, and literacy difficulties. Race, culture, and socioeconomic status are rarely reported as influencing the prevalence of communication disorders.

Approximately 15% of the world's population has some type of disability according to the World Report on Disability, published in 2011 by the World Health Organization and the World Bank. However, the World Report on Disability indicates that people with *communication difficulties* may be underrepresented in this figure, despite having difficulties in daily activities. The underrepresentation may be because communication disorders can be invisible (e.g., compared with a physical disability); communication disorders may be undiagnosed or unreported due to limited knowledge and services within communities; there may be the (mis)assumption that communication disorders must occur in conjunction with a medical cause (e.g., stroke, cleft palate, cerebral palsy); and there also may be confusion within the community between communication disorder and typical language learning by people who are multilingual.

Prevalence of Communication Disorders in Childhood

Communication disorders are one of the most prevalent childhood disabilities when compared with other types of disability. For example, in the United Kingdom, a study of children aged 5–15 conducted by the Office of Population Census and Surveys reported a higher prevalence of disability in *hearing* (18%), *communication* (14%), and *locomotion* (8%) than in other areas. In 2009, the Australian Bureau of Statistics reported that of children with a *disability* attending school (aged 5–20 years), 43.7% experienced *communication difficulties* and 34.0% experienced *speech and sensory disability*. In a longitudinal study of 14,500 Australian students (in grades K–12), *communication disorder* (13.04%) was the second most common area of learning needed after *specific learning difficulty* (17.93%), followed by *behavioral/emotional difficulty* (8.16%), *physical/medical disability* (1.52%), *intellectual disability* (1.38%), *hearing impairment* (0.96%), and *visual impairment* (0.16%). In a cross-sectional study of Jamaican children aged 2–9 years, *speech* (1.4%) was the second most common area of childhood disability after *cognitive* (8.1%); it was followed by *visual* (1.1%), *hearing* (0.9%), *motor* (0.4%), and *seizure* (0.2%).

Prevalence of Speech and Language Disorders in Childhood

The high prevalence of speech and language disorders in children has been reported in many studies. A systematic review published by James Law and colleagues in the year 2000 indicated that the prevalence of *primary speech and/or language delay* ranged from 2.0% to 24.6%, prevalence estimates for *speech delay only* ranged from 2.3% to 24.6%, and prevalence estimates for *language delay only* ranged from 2.02% to 19%. Since this systematic review, additional prevalence studies have been published. For example, across 14 studies of Australian children, the range of prevalence of communication disorders was 0.12%–41.2%, and most of these studies reported prevalence between 12% and 25%.

Period Prevalence of Childhood Speech and Language Disorders

There are a few examples of the period prevalence of childhood speech and language disorders. According to the 2015 report from the U.S. Department of Education for 2013, 17.9% of children with disabilities aged 3–21 years, who were served in the public school system, received services for *primary speech or language impairments*. This figure was higher for children aged 3–5 years, where 44.2% received services for primary speech or language impairments. In 2004, the Middlesbrough Primary Care Trust of the United Kingdom reported period prevalence of 16.3% for primary communication disability and 14.6% for speech–language disability. In order, the children were reported to have *speech difficulties* (29.1%), *receptive language difficulties* (20.4%), *expressive language difficulties* (16.9%), *dysfluency* (5.3%), and *voice or nasality disruption* (2.0%).

Prevalence of Communication Disorders in Adulthood

In adulthood, communication disorders typically are associated with a medical incident and can occur as a result of a stroke, traumatic brain injury, cancer, or onset of neurogenerative diseases such as Alzheimer's disease or Parkinson's disease. In addition, people who had a communication disorder in childhood may continue to have difficulties into adulthood, which may be influenced by the severity of the disorder and the amount and success of intervention received.

The reported prevalence of aphasia ranges from 0.1% to 0.4%, and the incidence in the developed world ranges from 0.02% to 0.06% according to Chris Code and Brian Petheram. The two most common neurogenerative diseases in adulthood are Alzheimer's disease and Parkinson's disease. In the United States, the prevalence of people with Alzheimer's disease is estimated to be 4.5 million, and it is estimated that the number will triple to 13.5 million by the year 2050. Lonneke de Lau and Monique Breteler estimated the prevalence of Parkinson's disease to be 0.3% of the population and 1% of people more than 60 years old. They reported the incidence of Parkinson's disease to be between 8 and 18 per 100,000.

Prevalence of Communication Disorders Across the Life Span

Prevalence of communication disorders across the life span is often calculated during population censuses or studies of a representative sample of the population. For example, in Lakshadweep India, 3.63% of the population (N = 22,558) was reported to have *communication disorders* in 2017. Prevalence was higher in males, and more of the population had *speech–language disorders* compared with *ear-related problems*.

The only study of the lifetime prevalence of stuttering reported prevalence of 0.72% (studying 12,131 people aged 1–99). Across studies, prevalence of stuttering is higher for children under 6 years of age than for older people; it is higher in males than females. The incidence of stuttering across the life span is commonly reported to be 5%. Ehud Yairi and Nicoline Ambrose analyzed published data since 2000 and suggested that the 5% figure may underestimate the incidence of stuttering over the life span.

Prevalence and Incidence of Hearing Loss

The prevalence of *disabling hearing loss* is 5.3% according to a 2012 review by the World Health Organization of 42 population-based prevalence studies. The "WHO Global Estimates on Prevalence of Hearing Loss" defines disabling hearing loss as "hearing loss greater than 40 dB in the better hearing ear in adults (15 years or older) and greater than 30 dB in the better hearing ear in children (0 to 14 years)" (p. 3). They indicated that the majority (91%) of people with hearing loss were adults, and hearing loss occurred in more males (56%) than females (44%). South Asia, Asia Pacific, and sub-Saharan Africa have the highest prevalence of disabling hearing loss in adults over 65 years of age. The prevalence of hearing loss can also be affected by presence of other conditions such as 22q11.2 deletion syndrome.

Prevalence and Incidence of Cleft Lip and Palate

Cleft lip and palate can be associated with communication disorders. In the United States, the prevalence of cleft lip and/or palate has been estimated to be 2.2–11.7 per 10,000 births. In Northern Ireland, the prevalence of cleft lip and palate between 1981 and 2000 was 1.47 per 1,000 live births. A study of nearly 6 million births across 14 European countries (between 1980 and 2000) identified 5,449 cases of cleft lip with or without cleft palate and reported prevalence of cleft lip and palate to be 9.1 per 10,000: 1,996 (36.6%) of cleft lip and 3,453 (63.4%) of cleft lip and palate. More males than females (1.70) had cleft lip and palate. The majority of children with cleft lip and palate (70.8%) did not have other conditions, whereas 29.2% were associated with other disabilities.

Prevalence and Incidence of Oral Cancers

Oral cancers can be associated with communication disorders. Tongue cancer is the most common oral cancer and incident rates are high in countries such as India (male incidence is 6.5 per 100,000 per year) and France (male incidence is 8.0 per 100,000 per year). The incidence of mouth cancer is relatively low in most Western countries; however, it is relatively high in Asia where the male incidence is greater than 10 per 100,000 per year. Lip cancer is rare in Asia, but higher in North America (male incidence is 12.7 per 100,000 per year), Europe (male incidence is 12.0 per 100,000 per year), and Oceania (male incidence is 13.5 per 100,000 per year). Oral cancers have been associated with smoking, solar radiation, and viruses.

Sharynne McLeod

See also Accent Modification; Comprehensibility; Multilingualism; Oral Language; Phoneme

Further Readings

Calzolari, E., Pierini, A., Astolfi, G., Bianchi, F., Neville, A. J., Rivieri, F., & EUROCAT Working Group. (2007). Associated anomalies in multimalformed infants with cleft lip and palate: An epidemiologic study of nearly 6 million births in 23 EUROCAT registries. *American Journal of Medical Genetics, Part A, 143A*, 528–537.

de Lau, L. M. L., & Breteler, M. M. B. (2006). Epidemiology of Parkinson's disease. *The Lancet Neurology, 5*(6), 525–535. doi:10.1016/S1474-4422(06)70471-9

Hebert, L. E., Scherr, P. A., Bienias, J. L., Bennett, D. A., & Evans, D. A. (2003). Alzheimer disease in the US population: Prevalence estimates using the 2000 census. *JAMA Neurology, 60*(8), 1119–1122. doi:10.1001/archneur.60.8.1119

Hutchison, T., & Gordon, D. (2005). Ascertaining the prevalence of childhood disability. *Child: Care, Health and Development, 31*(1), 99–107.

Konadath, S., Chatni, S., Lakshmi, M. S., & Saini, J. K. (2017). Prevalence of communication disorders in a group of islands in India. *Clinical Epidemiology and Global Health*. Advance online publication. doi:10.1016/j.cegh.2016.08.003

Law, J., Boyle, J., Harris, F., Harkness, A., & Nye, C. (2000). Prevalence and natural history of primary speech and language delay: Findings from a systematic review of the literature. *International Journal of Language and Communication Disorders, 35*(2), 165–188.

McLeod, S., & McKinnon, D. H. (2007). The prevalence of communication disorders compared with other learning needs in 14,500 primary and secondary school students. *International Journal of Language and Communication Disorders, 42*(S1), 37–59. doi:10.1080/13682820601173262

Moore, S., Johnson, N., Pierce, A., & Wilson, D. (2000). The epidemiology of mouth cancer: A review of global incidence. *Oral Diseases, 6*, 65–74. doi:10.1111/j.1601-0825.2000.tb00104.x

World Health Organization. (2012). WHO global estimates on prevalence of hearing loss (p. 3). Retrieved from http://www.who.int/pbd/deafness/WHO_GE_HL.pdf

Yairi, E., & Ambrose, N. (2013). Epidemiology of stuttering: 21st century advances. *Journal of Fluency Disorders, 38*(2), 66–87. doi:10.1016/j.jfludis.2012.11.002

PREVENTION OF HEARING DISORDERS

In order to determine how a hearing loss can be prevented, one needs to view the causes of hearing loss. This entry provides an overview of hearing loss across the life span: (1) before birth, (2) during birth, and (3) after birth and then explores hearing conservation programs (HCPs) at school, in the community, and in the workplace.

Before Birth

The time period involving before birth is referred to as *prenatal* in the professional community. Discussion of prenatal causes starts with the inherited genetic factors. Specifically, the genetic makeup of parents of the child plays a significant role; parents may carry genes on their chromosomes, which result in hearing loss. If the parents pass the gene on to the offspring, the child may develop hearing loss. The inheritance may be autosomal dominant or autosomal recessive. Autosomal-dominant inheritance refers to a condition where the child might receive a set of abnormal gene from one parent, which could result in hearing loss. On the other hand, for the child to manifest hearing loss with autosomal-recessive inheritance, the child will have to receive abnormal recessive genes from both the parents. In order to prevent hearing loss, one has to obtain case history from the parents and follow it up with genetic counseling. In some instances, DNA testing can be conducted to determine known genes that lead to hearing loss. Prevention of hearing loss in this instance is achieved by making a decision to not conceive. In the future, there may be an option to alter the abnormal gene by means of genetic engineering; however, at this time, such technology is not available.

Parents may also prevent hearing loss by taking precautions during the pregnancy. It should be verified that the mother has had vaccination for measles and mumps, since these and other viral infections lead to higher prevalence of hearing loss in the offspring. In addition, parents should be advised to limit or discontinue the consumption of alcohol or other drugs, which may result in hearing loss as well as other problems related to brain development.

During Birth

There is not much a parent or professionals can do during the process of birth to prevent hearing loss. Professionals such as nurse or doctor or midwife may note the conditions during birth to determine the risk of hearing loss. The current policy of universal screening that is adopted in many states within United States aids in early detection of hearing loss and its future impact.

After Birth

This time period is referred to as *postnatal*. The information pertaining to this period will be subgrouped into birth to 2 years, 2–5 years, 5–18 years, and 18 years and older.

Birth to 2 Years

The common cause of hearing loss during this period is infection and the medication used to treat the infection. One way to prevent hearing loss is to limit the exposure of the child to infecting agents. Because the probability of infection increases in a group setting, not having the child in a nursery with other children would reduce the possibility of infection and hence the hearing loss.

If the child were to have an infection, treatment using antibiotics should be monitored, since some of the medication may be ototoxic. If the medication is ototoxic, parents should seek alternate medication when feasible. If the infection results in middle ear infection, the child needs to be monitored by professionals so that the infection is kept under control. One of the recommendations to the parents would be to monitor upper respiratory infection and seek medical attention as soon as possible. If the child has allergies, with symptoms manifesting as upper respiratory infection, hearing loss can be prevented by keeping the allergy in control. Parents may reduce the risk of hearing loss by ascertaining that the child has been vaccinated for measles, mumps, and meningitis. Chances of hearing loss due to meningitis are higher, in addition, if the medication used to treat meningitis is known to be ototoxic. Chances of preventing hearing loss increase as one becomes more educated about the side effects of medication and is proactive about requesting alternate medication with no ototoxic side effects.

2–5 Years

Steps taken to prevent hearing loss in this group are not substantially different from the ones used for the younger age group. Parents and caretakers need to be informed about the possibility of hearing loss due to middle ear infection (also known as *otitis media*) and swimmer's ear (otitis externa). Symptoms indicative of ear infection are crying, slight increase in body temperature, inability to pay attention, repeated requests, or appearing distracted. One way to assure that parents have this information is by asking the primary care professional (family doctor or pediatrician) to inform the parents about the risk of ear infections and to ask them to be watchful. Another significant manner in which hearing loss can be prevented is by limiting the child's exposure to noise such as firecrackers or other loud noise makers.

5–18 Years

A major cause of hearing loss in this age group is exposure to high levels of sound. Specifically, for children from age 10–18, the major source of high level of sound happens to be personal devices, such as MP3s, iPods, smartphones, and tablets. Some of the children may be exposed to loud sounds from guns, if they participate in hunting activities. Prevention of hearing loss is achieved by HCP at schools and in the community.

18 Years and Older

The most common cause of hearing loss in older individuals is the exposure to noise at the workplace. Once again, hearing loss can be prevented by implementing HCP, both in the community setting and in the workplace.

HCP

The goal of the HCP is to reduce the risk of damage to hearing. It is achieved by educating the individuals about the agents that cause hearing loss. HCP has three components: (1) identifying existing hearing loss, (2) preventing hearing loss, and (3) educating the population to care for their hearing. The HCP program is executed in different ways in different settings.

The public-school HCP is mandated by states in the United States. State laws determine the group of children whose hearing needs to be screened. Many state regulations require screening of children's hearing in kindergarten or first grade, third grade, fifth grade, and every third year after that. Many state-mandated hearing screening levels are 25 dB HL, while American Speech-Language-Hearing Association recommends 20 dB HL. If the child fails a hearing screening, it is an early opportunity to provide education to prevent further hearing loss. If state-mandated hearing screening is not available, one may implement such a program with the assistance of academic programs in communication disorders taught at the college/university levels; academic programs in the universities may provide screening to local schoolchildren by having undergraduate/graduate students in the communication disorders (speech pathology and audiology) program volunteer and gain experience testing children under supervision. Local communities may take charge of setting up screening for schoolchildren by volunteering their time and assisting the college students in screening hearing.

In order to prevent hearing loss, it is necessary to provide education. Education in the school setting should be provided to administrative staff, teachers, and students. Education should include the following information: (1) anatomy and physiology of the hearing system, (2) definition of *hearing loss* and various degrees of hearing loss, (3) types of hearing loss, (4) impact of hearing loss on hearing in classroom and academic performance, (5) temporary and permanent nature of hearing loss, and (6) ways to reduce the probability of hearing loss specifically pertaining to noise. Students should be told that sound levels from personal systems through headphones or earbuds can exceed 115 dB HL and are known to cause permanent hearing loss. The children need to be taught how excessive noise can cause noise-induced hearing loss over time. Children need to be provided with information about protecting their hearing from excessive noise. Noise sources such as rock concerts, shooting, fireworks, woodworking class, automotive repair shops, and gymnasium need to be identified. Parents of the children need to be directed to resources available through National Institute of Health, American Speech-Language-Hearing Association, and National Institute of Deafness and Communication Disorders in the United States. Teachers and parents need to set clear rules for when hearing protectors should be worn (e.g., while attending a monster truck show or football stadium or mowing the lawn). In addition, parents and teachers need to educate children to monitor loud noises using apps available through smartphones. One of the recommendations made by National Institute of Deafness and Communication Disorders is to place red stickers on objects that can reach unsafe noise levels. Another recommendation is to set a maximum volume on the child's personal digital devices.

HCPs for older individuals can be provided in either a community setting or work setting. In the community setting, noise pertaining to recreational or leisure time activities should be addressed. It could be noise associated with snowmobiling, hunting, metal- or woodworking, lawn mowing, or using power tools around home. In particular, using a chain saw to cut wood produces dangerous levels of noise.

Health fairs are an efficient way to educate individuals about noise levels and hearing loss. Health fairs should include hearing screening, which provides an opportunity to educate the public. The public should be provided with information regarding dangerous levels of noise, exposure limits to noise, and the impact of excessive noise on the hearing system. The public needs to be informed as to the permanent nature of hearing loss. Once again, most of the support materials can be accessed through National Institute of Health, American Speech-Language-Hearing Association, or National Institute of Deafness and Communication Disorders. Health fairs should also provide printed material for individuals to take with them for future reference. If health fairs are not part of the community activity, information regarding noise levels and its impact on hearing may be provided through television (e.g., public service announcements) and billboards. In addition, information booklets may be placed in doctors' offices and other health service centers.

In addition to organizing health fairs, one may further reduce the exposure to loud noise by informing the public about zoning or noise control. Zoning codes restricting noise above specific level at certain times can be established and implemented at the city level.

HCPs for senior citizens can be provided through retirement homes or nursing homes. National consensus has indicated that 80% of individuals older than 65 years experience at least one chronic condition and approximately 50% older than 60 years have two or more chronic conditions. Some of the medications prescribed to treat these chronic conditions may be ototoxic, leading to hearing loss. While some elderly individuals tend to develop hearing loss associated with aging, some may acquire hearing loss due to the medications. One way to prevent hearing loss is to monitor the side effects and request medication that does not have hearing loss as a side effect.

The HCP in the workplace is typically associated with industrial or military settings. Federal regulations have been in place to monitor noise levels, monitor hearing, abate noise, and provide hearing protection to the employees in United States. The Occupational Safety and Health Administration (OSHA) enforces the regulations in workplace settings. For military, the regulatory agency is the Department of Defense. For mining, it is Bureau of Mines, and for transportation, it is Department of Transportation. Federal noise standards apply to the workplace. For example, OSHA and National Institute for Occupational Safety and Health have provided noise levels that indicate damage risk criteria. The damage risk criteria are based on an 8-hr workday, 5 days a week. The criteria do not take into consideration the recreational and secondary job noise exposure. The HCP at the workplace requires a noise survey in order to determine which workers are exposed to greater than 85 dBA during an 8-hr day. OSHA requires that workers who are exposed to 85 dBA during an 8-hr workday must be provided with a HCP. If the worker is in an area where the noise is in excess of 90 dBA during an 8-hr day, noise control measures must be put into place.

HCP according to OSHA involves educating the management and the workers. The purpose and process of the HCP must be explained to individuals in the management. The process of the HCP in the work setting involves not only a noise survey but also reduction of noise levels when possible, identification of hearing loss; provision of ear protectors, education, and monitoring; and management of hearing loss. Education of the workers should be done one-on-one. Because of the federal mandate and guidelines, the HCP at the workplace usually runs smoothly under the supervision of an industrial audiologist. In countries where there are no mandated HCPs in the workplace, employees should be made aware of the impact of noise on hearing through public media, so they may seek services. In addition, local groups of audiologists may provide in-services to employees and employers at various work settings that have high levels of noise; they can present information pertaining to both the impact of noise and how to prevent or alleviate the problems associated with noise.

Musicians are an adult population who needs attention. Marshall Chasin has noted that musical instruments produce sounds ranging from 70 to excess of 12 dB SPL. According to Brian Fligor, musicians may be exposed to very high levels of noise—anywhere between 80 and 130 dBA. Most musicians practice as much as 8 h a day. On the other hand, nonmusicians, who enjoy just listening to music, may be exposed to sounds as high as 100 dBA while listening to digital music players. It has been shown that some individuals listen to music longer than 4–8 h per session, almost every day. Use of hearing protectors by musicians and music industry professionals can dramatically reduce hearing loss. Musicians need protection from very loud sound levels, but they also need to hear while they play. Hence, one should not recommend traditional earplugs but rather counsel them to acquire musician's earplugs, which protect their hearing without blocking input required to perform in a group. The musician's earplugs need to be fitted by professionals in order for them to provide comfort and optimal attenuation. In addition, to provid the musicians with earplugs, one must provide baseline hearing assessment and ongoing monitoring. The same protocol that is used to prevent hearing loss in musicians should also be used with individuals in professions associated with music, such as sound engineers and DJs. One efficient manner in which to address the population would be to have a HCP program in every College of Music, so that when the students go through the educational program, they receive information pertaining to how to prevent hearing loss.

As noted previously, there are steps one may take to prevent hearing loss. The nature of the measure taken to prevent hearing loss varies depending on one's age and the agent causing the hearing loss risk. As long as professionals, caretakers, and parents are educated, hearing loss can be prevented most of the time.

Shalini Arehole

See also Genetics; Geriatric Audiology; Hearing Screening; Noise-Induced Hearing Loss and Its Prevention; Otitis Media; Ototoxicity

Further Readings

Alpiner, J. G., & McCaarthy, P. A. (2000). *Rehabilitative audiology: Children and adults* (3rd ed.). Baltimore, MA: Lippincott Williams & Wilkins.

American Speech Language and Hearing Association. (2015). *Noise and hearing loss prevention*. Retrieved from www.asha.org/public/hearing/Noise-and-Hearing loss-Prevention/

Chasin, M. (2009). *Hearing loss in musicians: Prevention and management*. San Diego, CA: Plural.

Filgor, B. J. (2009). Do headphones cause hearing loss? Risk of music induced hearing loss for the music consumer. In M. Chasin (Ed.), *Hearing loss in musicians: Prevention and management* (pp. 53–61). San Diego, CA: Plural.

Johnson, C. D., & Seaton, J. B. (2012). *Educational audiology handbook*. Clifton Park, NY: Delmar Cengage Learning.

Kelly, B. R., Davis, D., & Hegde, M. N. (1994). *Clinical methods and practicum in audiology*. San Diego, CA: Singular.

National Institute of Deafness and Other Communication Disorders. (2015). *Can noise induced hearing loss be prevented?* Retrieved from www.nidcd.nih.gov/health/hearing/pages/noise.aspx#6

Prevention of Speech and Language Disorders

Effective communication is necessary for individuals to fully participate in important life contexts: home, school, work, and the larger community. The presence of a speech and/or language disorder can negatively impact social interactions in any context. This entry provides an overview of the prevention of speech and language disorders and their causes. Next, the entry examines specific examples of ways in which the onset of speech and language disorders associated with either environmental or genetic causes have been prevented completely, or the severity of the disorders reduced through primary and, to a lesser extent, secondary prevention efforts.

Three Levels of Prevention

The American Speech-Language-Hearing Association identifies three types or levels of prevention: primary, secondary, and tertiary. Primary prevention involves taking action to ensure that a disorder does not occur in the first place. Secondary prevention refers to the early identification of a disorder and the initiation of an intervention that arrests or even reverses the impact of the disorder. Tertiary prevention denotes an intervention that reduces the rate of progression or the functional impact of a disorder. Secondary and tertiary interventions can take multiple forms including surgery, medication, prosthetic use, augmentative or alternative communication use, and behavioral intervention. It is generally accepted that the earlier secondary or tertiary prevention efforts begin, the more likely these efforts will completely prevent a speech and language disorder or the more they will reduce the negative long-term effects on speech and language, although there are exceptions to this rule. Screening programs are often used to identify the presence of factors that place speech and language development or proficiency at risk so that prevention efforts can be initiated. For example, prenatal screening is used to detect medical or genetic disorders in a fetus; neonatal screenings are used to detect congenital problems such as Phenylketonuria or hearing loss; children are screened in the preschool period or on school entry in order to identify the presence of developmental speech or language problems early. Adults may be screened for risk factors associated with a stroke or early signs of dementia.

Speech and Language Disorders

Speech and language disorders can take many forms. They occur in children and adults. They can be present at birth (i.e., developmental), or the onset can begin at some later point in time (i.e., acquired). Speech disorders include problems with spoken articulation, voice, or fluency (i.e., stuttering). Language problems can affect spoken, written, or signed modalities. A person with a language disorder can have difficulty understanding or using the semantic, morphosyntactic, or pragmatic aspects of language. Many times, the origin of the speech or language disorder is unknown, but other times, causes can be identified. If a cause is known, then prevention efforts are enhanced. Environmental causes of structural or functional problems resulting in speech and language disorders include poverty, nutritional insufficiency (e.g., cleft palate, stroke), accidents or abuse (e.g., head injuries), and exposure to toxins (e.g., fetal alcohol syndrome, mercury poisoning). Genetic or chromosomal abnormalities can also cause a structural or developmental disorder that negatively impacts speech and language acquisition (e.g., Down syndrome, fragile X syndrome). Speech and language development or proficiency can be directly impacted by sensory (e.g., hearing loss), neurological (e.g., intellectual disabilities, stroke), and motor difficulties (e.g., cerebral palsy) that, in turn, may have an environmental or genetic cause.

Environmental Causes

Poverty

Research shows that poverty radically impacts health. Indeed, the Canadian Medical Association estimates that social factors associated with poverty are attributable to 50% of all health problems. Poverty increases the risk of exposure to toxic levels of stress (which negatively impacts genetic makeup and neurocognitive development), poor nutrition and food insecurity, unsafe housing and homelessness, physical injury, exposure to toxic substances (e.g., lead and mercury), reduced access to medical care, and social isolation. These social determinants of health negatively impact children's development in utero and throughout infancy and childhood. Persons with a disability are more likely to live in poverty. Conversely, poverty puts people at a higher risk for developing or acquiring a disability, including a speech and/or language disorder. As a group, children living in poverty tend to have smaller vocabularies than peers with higher incomes, are less prepared to enter school, perform more poorly in school, and are more likely to drop out of school. Adults who experience poverty are typically less educated, under- or unemployed, and are at higher risk for mental illness and addiction.

Poverty is most directly prevented by providing families with an income adequate to meet their basic needs. Most countries do not provide social assistance at a level that allows people to escape poverty. Other primary prevention efforts are less impactful because they are designed to selectively address only one negative outcome of poverty, with an expectation there will be trickle-down effects to others. For example, inadequate or unsafe housing may be addressed through housing allowances or low-cost housing; low nutrition and food insecurity may be addressed through milk programs, food banks, or school lunch programs. Secondary prevention efforts focus upon reducing the negative impacts of poverty. For children, this includes providing parent training programs that teach parents ways to facilitate their child's language or literacy development; parent–child interactive programs that allow parents to learn and practice facilitative interaction techniques with their children; and high-quality day care and preschool programs that employ curricula specially designed to support language and preliteracy development (e.g., Abecedarian Project and Perry Preschool Project). Secondary prevention efforts such as these have been documented to positively impact children's development and school success. However, these programs typically do not completely close the achievement gap between those living in poverty and those living out of poverty. Nor do they eliminate poverty and its negative impacts for future generations.

Folic Acid Deficiency

For healthy development, a fetus requires sufficient nutrition in utero. One vitamin that has been identified as particularly important for the healthy development of the palate, brain, and spinal cord is folic acid, a B vitamin. Folic acid deficiency in the first trimester of a pregnancy is associated with the presence of cleft palate and spina bifida. Children with a cleft palate may have difficulties with speech sound articulation and voice resonance, even after surgery has closed the cleft. Spina bifida is associated with language and reading comprehension and social interaction problems. Providing adequate doses of folic acid during pregnancy, especially in the first trimester, is a primary prevention approach, which can reduce the incidence of cleft palate or spina bifida. According to estimates, administering appropriate doses of folic acid during the first trimester prevents between 50% and 70% of spina bifida cases. While there is little firm evidence that a causal relationship between folic acid deficiency and the presence of a cleft palate exists, folic acid is widely used to prevent a cleft palate. A secondary prevention approach, closure of the cleft palate, can result in the complete avoidance of the speech articulation and resonance difficulties associated with cleft palate in some children and reduce the severity of these problems in others. Outcomes are better if the palate is surgically closed between 6 and 15 months of age, rather than later. For both cleft palate and spina bifida, another secondary prevention approach is to teach parents speech and language stimulation techniques, which can be implemented starting in infancy. For example, for children with cleft palate, encouraging frequent speech sound productions through imitation routines and gently pinching the child's nose when they are phonating to contrast oral and nasal speech sounds can be useful.

Stroke

A stroke occurs when either a blood clot blocks a blood vessel in the brain or a blood vessel hemorrhages in the brain. Strokes in the left hemisphere of the brain cause aphasia (a language disorder) and/or dysarthria or apraxia (speech disorders). Strokes in the right hemisphere of the brain have less impact upon speech and language but can cause cognitive difficulties that may impact one's ability to communicate concepts logically or appropriately. While strokes are more likely in older adults (3/4 occur in adults 65 years of age or older), children and infants can also experience them. There are a number of important nutrition and other lifestyle-related risk factors for stroke. The most important risk factor for strokes is high blood pressure. Others include the presence of diabetes, high cholesterol, obesity, and high alcohol consumption. Primary prevention of stroke and its accompanying speech and language disorders includes taking high blood pressure and anticoagulant medications, exercising regularly, not smoking, and eating a healthy diet. Rapid response following a stroke is key to secondary prevention. One study indicated that those who go to a hospital within 3 h of a stroke have less debilitating symptoms later. Conventional wisdom suggests treatment should begin as early as possible, but there is currently little data to support decisions regarding optimal timing.

Toxin Exposure

Cognitive, social-interactive, speech, and language disorders can result if a fetus, child, or adult is exposed to toxic substances. Fetal alcohol spectrum disorder (FASD), for example, is caused by alcohol consumption by the mother during pregnancy. Fetal exposure to alcohol in the first trimester is particularly damaging. There are no clear guidelines for how much exposure is necessary for FASD to occur; therefore, complete abstinence during pregnancy is recommended. Primary prevention of the cognitive, speech, and language disorders associated with FASD is to educate and support mothers in the avoidance of alcohol intake during pregnancy. Treatment for alcoholism would be another primary prevention strategy. Early identification and intervention (i.e., secondary prevention) can ameliorate symptoms associated with FASD and support optimal cognitive and language development.

Vocal Abuse

Many individuals acquire voice disorders through vocal trauma or overuse. Teachers and exercise instructors may often need to speak loudly to be heard above the ambient noise in their work environments. Doing this over protracted periods of time can result in vocal nodules (i.e., growths on the vocal chords) which, in turn, cause a chronically hoarse voice and difficulty modulating voice loudness and pitch. The formation of vocal nodules and consequent voice disorders can be prevented by reducing the need for people to speak loudly over prolonged periods of time. For example, optimizing classroom acoustics and using voice amplification systems for teachers can reduce the need for teachers or exercise instructors to strain their voices when communicating at work.

Traumatic Brain Injury

A frequent cause of speech and language disorders in both children and adults is traumatic brain injury. Traumatic brain injury most often occurs as a result of vehicle accidents or falls, although a substantial proportion of head injuries in young children result from physical abuse. Primary prevention includes public education about the causes and impacts of traumatic brain injury, programs that focus on prevention of abuse such as anger management programs and positive behavior management programs, and safety regulations such as laws that require use of seatbelts in cars or helmets on motorcycles or bicycles.

Genetic Causes

The onset of some speech and language difficulties can be prevented through genetic counseling and testing. A family history of cognitive, speech, language, and/or hearing disorders may signal the presence of a heritable genetic problem, although many of these disorders have no known genetic cause or the genetic problem has occurred de novo and are therefore not part of the parents' genome. A genetic counselor can help determine whether genetic testing would be helpful to detect heritable genetic disorders. Genetic testing by potential parents can provide them with definitive information about whether heritable disorders are present and the likelihood of a particular disorder being transmitted. They may then choose to avoid pregnancy—a primary prevention option. For example, fragile X is a disorder resulting from a fragile site on the X chromosome. Mothers can be carriers of fragile X but show no symptoms themselves. A history of fragile X in the family can lead to genetic testing of a woman contemplating pregnancy to facilitate family planning.

Prenatal testing is used as both a primary and secondary prevention tool. For example, it is now routine in many locations to use blood serum tests to detect Down syndrome in a fetus in the first trimester. Combined with ultrasound, such tests can have a sensitivity of 85% or more. Sensitivity increases to a 100% with follow-up chorionic or amniotic fluid sampling. Such screenings are not without controversy. Research has indicated that, if Down syndrome is detected, many parents who are given a choice terminate the pregnancy (primary prevention). Others choose to keep the child and use the time before birth to prepare themselves and plan early intervention options (secondary prevention). Children with Down syndrome are at high risk for heart problems, gastrointestinal difficulties, and conductive hearing loss secondary to frequent middle ear infections. Early and ongoing medical care from physicians familiar with the difficulties experienced by these children is critical to primary and secondary prevention of further developmental difficulties associated with illness and hearing loss. For children with Down syndrome, similar to children with many other disorders that affect cognitive, speech, and/or language development, intervening early is associated with better outcomes (secondary prevention). Early behavioral intervention programs that facilitate speech and language development in functional contexts through parent training, starting in infancy, are of critical importance in order to optimize development in these children.

Gene editing is a primary prevention technique currently being studied but not yet available as a prevention tool for disorders affecting speech and language development. In gene editing, affected genetic material would theoretically be replaced with healthy genetic material, or genes would be *reprogrammed* to act in healthier ways. This method has proven useful in exploring disease mechanisms and may someday be available as a primary preventive approach to various genetic disorders. With its use come ethical questions, which are being debated.

Final Thoughts

This entry has provided an overview of different types of speech and language disorders that can occur and examples of primary and secondary prevention efforts directed at these disorders. The many potential causes of speech and language disorders mean that a number of factors need to be considered in their prevention. Causes include genetic differences and environmental factors, which have complex sets of correlates, such as financial resources, nutritional intake, and unsafe living conditions. It is also important to consider that genetic and environmental factors can interact, as the study of epigenetics shows. All aspects of an individual's context need to be considered in the prevention of speech and language disorders if effective communication in important life contexts is the goal. Additionally, the causes of many speech and language disorders are unknown. Consequently, providing a healthy environment where all individuals can thrive is as important as continuing to research the causes of these disorders.

Elizabeth Kay-Raining Bird and Bonita Squires

See also Epidemiology of Communication Disorders; Etiology; Genetics; Poverty and Language; Prevention of Hearing Disorders; Stroke; Teratogens; Vocal Hygiene

Further Readings

Bishop, D., & Leonard, L. (Eds.). (2014). *Speech and language impairments in children: Causes, characteristics, intervention and outcome.* London, UK: Psychology Press.

Canadian Task Force on Preventive Health Care. (2016). Recommendations on screening for developmental delay. *Canadian Medical Association Journal, 188,* 579–587.

De-Regil, L. M., Peña-Rosas, J. P., Fernández-Gaxiola, A. C., & Rayco-Solon, P. (2015). Effects and safety of periconceptional oral folate supplementation for preventing birth defects. *Cochrane Database of Systematic Reviews* (12). Art. No.: CD007950. DOI:10.1002/14651858.CD007950.pub3

Gullotta, T. P., & Bloom, M. (Eds.). (2014). *Encyclopedia of primary prevention and health promotion* (2nd ed.). New York, NY: Springer Science+Business Media.

Mate, K., Magin, P., Brodaty, H., Stocks, N., Gunn, J., Disler, P., & Pond, C. D. (2017). An evaluation of the additional benefit of population screening for dementia beyond a passive case-finding approach. *International Journal of Geriatric Psychiatry, 32,* 316–323.

Mikkonen, J., & Raphael, D. (2010). *Social determinants of health: The Canadian facts.* Toronto, Canada: York University School of Health Policy and Management. Retrieved from http://www.thecanadianfacts.org/

Thornton, R., Glover, C., Cene, C., Glik, D., Henderson, J., & Williams, D. (2016). Evaluating strategies for reducing health disparities by addressing the social determinants of health. *Health Affairs, 35,* 1416–1423.

Thurman, D. J. (2016). The epidemiology of traumatic brain injury in children and youths: A review of research since 1990. *Journal of Child Neurology, 31,* 20–27.

Primary Progressive Aphasia

Primary progressive aphasia (PPA) is a general term for a collection of clinical syndromes with onset frequently occurring prior to 65 years of age, characterized by ongoing deterioration in language abilities (speaking, comprehending, reading, and writing) caused by degenerative brain disease. This entry describes the three main clinical variants of PPA, together with a brief overview of speech pathology assessments and interventions that may assist individuals with PPA and their families.

The basic criteria for diagnosis of PPA have been described by neurologist Marcel Mesulam, who first coined the name *primary progressive aphasia*. During the early course of PPA, the most prominent difficulty is with language, not episodic or visual memory, visuoperceptual abilities, or behavior. The language difficulty is apparent on clinical investigation and during everyday activities, and it cannot be better explained by other neurodegenerative, medical, or psychiatric disorders. In all cases, the symptoms emerge because of deteriorating function in a network of brain regions involved in speech and language, due to the gradual spread of disease—typically one of the diseases on the frontotemporal lobar degeneration spectrum or Alzheimer's disease. These diseases tend to show a predilection for certain brain regions; thus, the language symptoms typically cluster into one of three recognized variants; however, there are also many individuals with a symptom profile that does not neatly fit one of these three variants.

The three variants of PPA are *nonfluent/agrammatic variant PPA*, *semantic variant PPA* (also widely known as *semantic dementia*), and *logopenic variant PPA*. They were described by Maria Luisa Gorno-Tempini and a team of 19 other neurologists, psychologists, and speech pathologists in an expert consensus paper, in 2011. Nonfluent/agrammatic PPA is characterized by agrammatic language production and/or apraxia of speech or other motor speech disorder, along with two of the following: impaired comprehension of syntax, preserved comprehension of single words, and preserved knowledge about objects. Brain imaging shows atrophy predominantly in left frontoinsular regions. Semantic variant PPA shows the core clinical features of impaired comprehension and naming of pictures and objects caused by underlying semantic memory deterioration. There may be surface dyslexia or surface dysgraphia (reading words aloud or spelling them phonetically, for example pronouncing *yacht* as [jætʃt]), with spared repetition, grammatical, and motor speech abilities. Brain imaging in semantic variant PPA shows striking anterior temporal atrophy. In logopenic progressive aphasia, there are prominent difficulties with word retrieval and sentence repetition, with three of the following additional features: phonological errors in speech production, spared comprehension of word meanings, spared grammatical abilities, and spared motor speech abilities. Brain imaging in this variant shows left posterior perisylvian or parietal abnormality.

Diagnosis of the underlying neuropathology in PPA requires microscopic investigation for atypical protein deposits (i.e., inclusions) in brain tissue, usually carried out postmortem. The nonfluent/agrammatic variant is typically associated with deposits of tau protein (i.e., corticobasal degeneration or progressive supranuclear palsy inclusions), semantic variant PPA with transactive response DNA binding protein 43, and logopenic variant PPA with Alzheimer's disease pathology that occurs in a distribution different from the one seen in Alzheimer-type dementia when there is prominent early episodic memory loss.

Diagnosis of the clinical PPA variant involves history taking and targeted assessment of each of the language features associated with each variant as noted previously and thus may include confrontation naming (to assess word retrieval); eliciting connected speech and conversation (to assess syntax, word retrieval, and spoken language comprehension); word and sentence repetition tasks (assessing repetition directly, as well as phonological errors, apraxia of speech, and motor speech disorder); and assessment of single word comprehension and object knowledge. Comprehensive neuropsychological assessment may also be conducted to exclude other neurological or psychiatric disease. The clinical assessment reveals the person's current profile of linguistic and other cognitive strengths and weaknesses, indicating targets for behavioral interventions and client and caregiver education and support. Diagnosis of PPA variant assists in predicting the most likely neuropathology, which in turn indicates the most likely clinical course, including possible later emergence of nonlanguage symptoms (i.e., movement, swallowing, behavior, and other, nonlinguistic, cognitive impairments), allowing for proactive management of these symptoms. Because of the progressive nature of the disease, clinical review should be carried out regularly.

As of mid-2018, there are no disease-modifying treatments for PPA, although research continues at pharmacological and genetic frontiers. Selective serotonin reuptake inhibitor medications can assist with behavior problems if these emerge with progression. Most attention has therefore been directed to speech pathology interventions that reduce language impairment and increase communicative activity and life participation levels. Naming therapy using familiar, personally relevant items can improve and maintain word retrieval and increase brain activation. Conversation training can help key communicative partners reveal the competence and increase the confidence of the person with PPA in everyday interactions. Alternative and augmentative communication (e.g., communication books, communication boards, synthesized speech devices) can provide support for communication as language deteriorates. People with PPA and communication partners can also be assisted with education and psychosocial support, including services provided by PPA and dementia advocacy and support organizations, and referral for psychological and coping interventions. Because the onset of PPA in many cases occurs prior to the age of 65, people with PPA and their spouses also may need support to manage ongoing financial commitments, childcare, and/or parent-caring responsibilities.

Karen Croot

See also Aphasia; Cognitive Impairment; Dementia; Neurogenic Communication Disorders; Quality of Life and Neurogenic Communication Disorders

Further Readings

Gorno-Tempini, M. L., Hillis, A. E., Weintraub, S., Kertesz, A., Mendez, M., Cappa, S. E., . . . Grossman, M. (2011). Classification of primary progressive aphasia and its variants. *Neurology, 76,* 1006–1014.

Nickels, L., & Croot, K. (2014). *Clinical perspectives on primary progressive aphasia.* Hove, UK: Psychology Press.

Sapolsky, D., Domoto-Reilly, K., Negreira, A., Brickhouse, M., McGinnis, S., & Dickerson, B. C. (2011). Monitoring progression of primary progressive aphasia: Current approaches and future directions. *Neurodegenerative Disease Management, 1,* 43–55.

Volkmer, A. (2013) *Assessment and therapy for language and cognitive communication difficulties in dementia and other progressive diseases.* Guildford, UK: J&R Press.

Priming

Priming is a cognitive process, that is, an implicit function of one's memory, in which a recent experience causes one's sensitivity to related items to be increased. As a result, while one is conducting an action or a task, particular associations or representations are already active in memory and impact the outcome of the action or the task. Priming can happen in every part of one's experience; it occurs when somebody who is expecting a BABY (Note: uppercase words represent concepts in this entry) sees babies everywhere; it occurs when a person who buys yellow shoes starts to see yellow shoes everywhere; and it occurs when those exposed to words of RUDENESS are more likely to interrupt others in their communications. Thus, in priming, a recent experience brings related objects or concepts to the surface of consciousness and makes them more accessible, in a way that they prepare an individual to perceive related items or concepts. The influence of this experience on judgment and decision making is called a *priming effect*. This entry provides an overview of the various types of priming and their uses as well as related tasks and terms.

The simplest type of priming is defined as *repetition priming*, which describes facilitation in the processing of a stimulus when it has just been encountered. One version of *word completion task* is based on this type of priming, in which a word list is given to the participant to study (e.g., *around, suit, call, low, can, pear, heat, hiss*) and then another list with word fragments is to be completed. The list is typically too long to be memorized in a short time by the participant, as he or she is not informed about the purpose of the task. The results show after encountering certain words, there is more possibility the participant will use those words than nonencountered words to complete the list of word fragments (e.g., a_round not *ground*, s_uit not *quit*, c_all not *ball*, l_ow not *row*, c_an not *man*, p_ear not *dear*, h_eat not *meat*, h_iss not *kiss*).

There are other versions of word completion tasks used to study implicit memory; however, depending on the purpose of an experiment, different processing demands and different types of priming may be involved. For example, in a task based on semantic priming, two lists are presented, and incomplete words are related to (cannot be the repetition of) the words in the first list. The results show the participant completes related words more quickly and accurately than unrelated words. The reason is because when a word like *homework* is presented, the concept of SCHOOL is activated in the mind, and this causes recall of related words, for instance, *study, exam, pencil, student, teacher, blackboard*. Later, if these words are encountered (in the second list), they are recognized more accurately than unrelated and inactivated words (e.g., *car, street, park,* also presented in the second list). Therefore, priming of the participant's performance is facilitated by a past experience, without requiring deliberate recollection of that experience.

In experimental psychology, a technique called *priming paradigm* is used to study priming effects. Two consecutive stimuli are presented to the participant, the first being the prime and the second the target, and the effect of the first stimulus on the second one is studied. There is typically a delay between the presentation of the prime and the target; this is known as *stimulus onset asynchrony* (SOA). The participant reads the prime silently and decides whether the target is a real word or nonword (i.e., lexical decision task) or merely reads it aloud (i.e., naming task). The common finding is that the participant is faster and more accurate in lexical decision or naming when the target is related to the prime. The most established type of this priming experiment is semantic priming, and it is perhaps best known because of the seminal work of David E. Meyer and Roger W. Schvaneveldt in the 1970s, when they saw participants were faster in deciding that *nurse* was a real word when it was followed by a semantically related word like *doctor*, rather than an unrelated word like *bread*. This effect provided support for the idea that semantic memory (i.e., knowledge of word meaning and related concepts) works because of a spread of the activation process.

Semantic memory is conceptualized in terms of a network in which processing is accomplished through spread of activation between connected nodes. The presentation of a prime word activates its node in memory, and then this activation spreads to highly related words and increases their accessibility. This process occurs automatically as an inherent part of word recognition; that is, the participant does not make an explicit judgment about the link between the prime and the target. It is noteworthy that when SOA is short (i.e., fewer than 400 ms), the resulting priming effect is assumed to occur via passive spread of activation in semantic memory, whereas with a long SOA (i.e., more than 400 ms), the participant actively looks for relations between prime and target words. Thus, longer response times in this condition may be seen because SOA creates an opportunity for more connections to be activated.

In priming literature, other types of priming are mentioned. In *associative priming*, two stimuli are not related, but their appearance together causes one (of the two) to have the capability of priming the other. Therefore, priming between *yellow* and *banana*, *bee* and *honey*, *cradle* and *baby*, *wave* and *ocean*, *book* and *page*, *sheep* and *wool*, *cow* and *milk* can be considered as associative priming. In *perceptual priming*, priming occurs based on the physical properties or structure of the two items. Some consider the previously mentioned simple word completion task as a type of perceptual priming. In *conceptual priming* (sometimes used interchangeably with *semantic priming*), the priming effect is the product of conceptual analysis, for example, when the participant is cued with a category label such as "animal" and is asked to generate examples of that category (e.g., *mouse, deer, aunt, tiger, snake, goat, dog, pigeon*).

In therapeutic settings, depending on the type of disorder, priming can be used by clinicians to create a more stimulating working environment, promote clients' comprehension, and positively influence their mental schemes and ideas.

Ensie Abbassi and Bess Sirmon-Taylor

See also Cognition; Meaning; Memory; Schemata; Semantic Development; Semantic Field

Further Readings

Bargh, J. A. (2006). What have we been priming all these years? On the development, mechanisms, and ecology of nonconscious social behavior. *European Journal of Social Psychology, 36,* 147–168.

Butler, L. T., & Berry, D. C. (2004). Understanding the relationship between repetition priming and mere exposure. *British Journal of Psychology, 95,* 467–487.

Chiarello, C., Burgess, C., Richards, L., & Pollock, A. (1990). Semantic and associative priming in the cerebral hemispheres: Some words do, some words don't . . . sometimes, some places. *Brain and Language, 38,* 75–104.

Meyer, D. E., & Schvaneveldt, R. W. (1971). Facilitation in recognizing pairs of words: Evidence of a dependence between retrieval operations. *Journal of Experimental Psychology, 90,* 227–234.

PROFESSIONAL ASSOCIATIONS

Professional associations for those who specialize in working with people with communication disabilities have developed over time to address multiple purposes. Membership varies between countries but always includes speech–language pathologists (or their equivalent) and may also include audiologists and communication assistants. Although associations vary in their stated goals, they all aim to maintain standards of practice and advocate for the profession. This entry provides an overview of professional associations, including their history, membership, and purpose.

History

People who have communication disorders have historically received attention to varying degrees by a range of professionals (e.g., medical doctors, psychologists, educators). However, the development of a profession specializing in communication assessment and intervention did not commence until the first and second decades of the 20th century. These developments were concentrated in the Western Hemisphere, including Europe, United Kingdom, Australia, and the United States, with professional associations following soon after.

The earliest reported multidisciplinary meeting of communication specialists to share information and practice was in Vienna, in 1924. This meeting was the genesis of the International Association of Logopedics and Phoniatrics (IALP). Associations in the Western Hemisphere developed during a similar time frame, often starting with local meetings or societies and then amalgamating nationally, for example, United States (1925), United Kingdom (1945), Australia (1949), and Canada (1964). This developmental process continues to be mirrored across the world, as the profession of speech–language pathology becomes established in new countries. The American Speech-Language-Hearing Association (ASHA) lists 50 countries that have similar associations on their website.

IALP's goals and mission are focused on facilitating quality science, education, and clinical practice by those working with people with communication and swallowing disorders. Its membership includes nationally based professional associations that take more direct action regarding standards of practice for communication specialists as well as advocacy for people with communication disorders. The Asia Pacific Society of Speech, Language, and Hearing has a similar role with a more regional focus. This entry focuses on national professional associations with an emphasis on the more established associations in the Western Hemisphere, which are informing, and indeed being informed by, the newly developing professional associations in other countries.

Membership

Membership requirements vary across the professional associations, and the terms used to identify the communication specialists also vary. Those professionals who work with or advocate for the needs of people who have communication disorders, their families, caregivers, and communities are called *speech–language pathologists*, *speech and language therapists*, *speech therapists*, and *speech pathologists* (these will all be referred to as SLPs in this entry). The scope of practice for SLPs has extended since the mid-1980s to include assessment and intervention for people with swallowing disorders.

The majority of associations are single discipline. However, some associations, such as ASHA, include audiologists who have a specific role for people who have communication needs related to their hearing. Other associations such as Speech-Language & Audiology Canada also include communication health assistants who support the delivery of speech pathology or audiology services under supervision. Membership is available to those deemed eligible and requires an annual financial contribution.

The work of associations is enabled by significant voluntary contributions of time and expertise by its membership. Associations with larger memberships, and therefore a larger financial base, also employ staff to support the work of voluntary members and to also directly provide services.

Purpose

Professional associations state their purposes in various ways and may call them missions, goals, visions, aims, to name a few. There are some commonalities between these statements. While many have overall statements that include the associations' aim to serve the interests of those who have communication disorders, the primary focus for associations is to serve their membership. All professional associations address members' standards of practice as well as represent and advocate for the interests of their membership.

Associations adopt a variety of strategies to support their members' standards of practice. These include support for professional development, research, and the establishment and regulation of practice standards. SLP associations vary to the degree in which they undertake these three major areas of activity. Newer associations with smaller memberships in countries where the profession is only recently founded may not have sufficient resources to establish and regulate practice standards immediately but usually aim to do so. For example, the Malaysian Association of Speech-Language and Hearing (formally founded in 1995) clearly states its intention to establish and regulate standards in its vision and mission statement. Therefore, quality of practice is a key concern for all associations, and regardless of size, associations aim to advocate for quality of practice as well as for the interests of their membership.

Professional Development

All associations provide members with support to maintain their professional development through formal and informal activities. This may include educational events such as workshops and conferences (e.g., Indian Speech and Hearing Association held its 50th national conference [ISHACON] in 2018). Associations facilitate networking and communication across their membership through publications such as newsletters or bulletins by special interest groups. Associations are also embracing the opportunities that technology now provides to increase members' access to professional development, for example, through social networking sites, online forums, and videoconferencing.

Research

Research is supported through facilitating networking between members and also access to research subjects by allowing researchers to notify members about current research projects. Associations may also provide research grants to members, for example, members of the South African Speech-Language-Hearing Association can apply for grants each year. Many associations have one or more journals where peer-reviewed research is published, and these are provided to members as part of their membership. For example, the Royal College of Speech and Language Therapists publishes the *International Journal of Language and Communication Disorders*; Speech Pathology Australia (SPA) publishes the *International Journal of Speech Language Pathology*; and ASHA publishes four peer-reviewed journals including the *Journal of Speech, Language, and Hearing Research*.

Standards and Scope of Practice

SLP associations are usually concerned with identifying the professional practices their members should be able to carry out, to what level, and across what scope of practice. *Scope of practice* has been described by the New Zealand Speech Language Therapists' Association as including the populations SLPs work with, services provided, rationale for practice, contexts, and models of service provision.

Associations may publish position papers and clinical guidelines to guide their members about service delivery for particular populations (e.g., people who have laryngectomies), types of practices (e.g., use of specialist equipment such as Fibreoptic Endoscopic Evaluation of Swallowing), and approaches to service delivery (e.g., evidence-based practice). Some guidelines have been rigorously developed using evidence-based practice approaches where the best available research evidence is sourced, rigorously evaluated for quality, and synthesized to inform the guideline's recommendations for practice. Guidelines are usually also made available to inform the public and policymakers.

Members also participate in developing codes of ethics or principles to guide practice. The degree to which associations engage with regulation and/or enforcement of these standards depends on their country's regulatory framework for professional practice. Given the varying size and stages of development of SLP associations, the degree to which associations are able to engage in specifying or regulating these varies.

Standards or requirements for membership also vary from country to country but do include possession of an approved qualification, which indicates the member has demonstrated relevant knowledge and skills. Some associations also require members to provide evidence that they are actively engaged in maintaining knowledge and skills required for professional practice (i.e., continuing professional development). Specifying and assessing the required standards for SLPs to meet to be eligible for association membership is challenging.

Determining the key components that ensure an SLP is able to provide a quality service is not simple. Acquiring a relevant knowledge base is important for informing professional judgment and action; however, having relevant knowledge does not mean that the SLP can apply that knowledge professionally. In addition, SLPs not only bring conceptual knowledge to their practice but also knowledge derived from their experience and also the experience of their service recipients. Skills are also necessary for good SLP practice and may include practical skills such as being able to carry out assessments or professional skills such as working in teams. However, professional practice is more than a set of skills that is learned and applied according to a set of guidelines. Personal qualities such as emotional skills (e.g., empathy and compassion), values (e.g., honesty, integrity), ethics (e.g., doing no harm), and intellectual dispositions (e.g., critical thinking) also contribute to high-quality professional practice.

Associations are increasingly adopting a competency-based standard approach that focuses on what the SLP needs to be able to do and to what level. A competency-based approach is less focused on specific knowledge, skill, and personal qualities the SLP can demonstrate and more focused on his or her ability to integrate and apply these aspects to competently provide quality services. The focus is therefore on observed competence in the way the SLP provides services.

The way in which competencies are defined and the level of performance required also varies between associations, in particular, the level of specificity and how many competencies have to be met. A balance needs to be struck between under-specifying competencies leading to gaps in competence and overspecifying them such that the holistic integration and application of competencies to create quality practice is lost. This is a challenge faced by all professions and continues to attract ongoing debate. Nevertheless, a competency-based approach to setting professional standards represents progress in identifying what is required for competent professional practice.

Regulation of Standards

Practice standards are used in varying ways to maintain the quality of SLP practice depending on the regulatory framework of the country. Many countries have a professional association as well as government-mandated registration/licensing requirements at a national or state level that must be met to legally practice as an SLP. Usually, the SLP must be eligible for practicing membership of the national SLP professional association as one of the requirements for registration. Registration protects the public through powers that include deregistering SLPs for practice should they breach the requirements for practice (e.g., incompetence) and legally precludes them from practice. However, governments have not made registration available in all countries (e.g., Australia), and in those cases, the professional associations are the only protection for the public—but only if service recipients know to ask if the SLP is eligible for membership of his or her professional association. Associations may also enforce their standards of ethics and investigate complaints made against their members regardless of whether their government registers SLPs.

Associations commonly aim to regulate or protect standards by requiring that their members engage in continuing professional development. Larger or well-established associations will require their members to maintain their membership or practicing status through accruing sufficient continuing professional development points. Members do this by providing evidence of engagement in professional development activities such as attending workshops, conferences, independent or formal study, mentoring, and/or teaching.

Professional associations use practice standards to accredit their domestic SLP education programs to ensure that the education provided adequately prepares graduates for competent practice and to determine whether graduates should be eligible for membership. Accreditors review the education program against the standards established by the professional association and determine whether they are met. Professional associations vary in the emphasis given to competency-based learning outcomes (e.g., as demonstrated by the types of assessments) versus time in training (i.e., mandated hours of supervised practice) and learning inputs (e.g., specifying curriculum content). The accreditation of programs is closely linked to registration/licensing, as SLPs applying for registration must have graduated from a government-approved program.

Governments also collaborate with SLP associations to recognize the qualifications of SLPs entering the country and allow them to engage in SLP practice. This type of recognition is becoming more crucial with the increasing international mobility of the workforce. Six associations have established a mutual recognition agreement to assist with this process between their countries (the United States, Australia, Canada, Ireland, New Zealand, and the United Kingdom). This agreement, once certain conditions are met, allows their members to become members of the other associations.

Advocacy

As stated previously, professional associations are primarily concerned with advocating for the needs of their members. This includes identifying and protecting professional boundaries by specifying who is and who is not eligible for membership and therefore who should (or should not) be providing services to people with communication and swallowing disorders. Specifying scope of practice is important for identifying and protecting these boundaries and regulation of standards, as already described, and also protects the interests of members by ensuring that members are associated with quality service.

These activities may or may not indirectly benefit service recipients, depending on whether such activities promote or restrict the access of service recipients to support. However, advocacy activities are frequently mutually beneficial. For example, a number of associations have engaged in advocating for access to SLPs by young people in the criminal justice system. If this is successful, this will increase employment or practice opportunities for SLPs and create better outcomes for young people whose offending is linked to their communication and literacy difficulties. Furthermore, freely providing information to the public on the nature of communication disorders and how to access services creates further mutual benefit.

Specific advocacy activities include lobbying the government for changes to policy, and strategies used to effectively influence policy will necessarily depend on the form of the national government and local culture. SLP associations are frequently acknowledged as the peak professional bodies and therefore are invited to comment on policy. For example, SPA was integrally involved in the coordination and provision of information to the 2013–2014 Australian Senate Inquiry into the prevalence of communication disorders and speech pathology services. Associations also seek to proactively influence government policy. For example, ASHA has a political action committee (ASHA-PAC) that aims to represent the interests of its members via lobbying and raising funds to support political candidates who support members' work.

Final Thoughts

Professional associations for SLPs are focused on the needs of their members and play a key role in maintaining standards of practice and advocating for the profession. The relationship between associations and the formal regulation of practice via registration or licensing varies, but professional associations are generally very influential in ensuring that people who have communication and swallowing disorders receive services from appropriately prepared and qualified professionals. Therefore, SLPs often choose to join and contribute to relevant professional associations.

Sue McAllister

See also Advocacy; Enculturation into the Profession; Ethics in Communication Disorders Service Delivery; Communication Disorders; Speech–Language Pathology

Further Readings

American Speech-Language-Hearing Association. Retrieved from http://www.asha.org/

Asia Pacific Society of Speech, Language and Hearing. Retrieved from http://www.apsslh.org/

Indian Speech and Hearing Association. Retrieved from http://www.ishaindia.org.in/

International Association of Logopedics and Phoniatrics. Retrieved from http://www.ialp.info/
Malaysian Association of Speech-Language and Hearing. Retrieved from http://mash.org.my/
New Zealand Speech Language Therapists' Association. Retrieved from https://speechtherapy.org.nz/
Royal College of Speech and Language Therapists. Retrieved from http://www.rcslt.org/
South African Speech-Language-Hearing Association. Retrieved from https://www.saslha.co.za/
Speech-Language & Audiology Canada. Retrieved from http://sac-oac.ca/
Speech Pathology Australia. Retrieved from http://www.speechpathologyaustralia.org.au/

Prognosis

A *prognosis* is a well-informed estimate or prediction of future outcomes. This term may also refer to the process of arriving at such estimates (something that is often called *prognostication*). It is commonly expressed in terms of likelihood or probability. In the context of communication disorders it may refer to the probability of such things as achievement of a developmental or recovery milestone, or achievement of (or regaining) typical or normal status. Such prognoses may include the outcome likelihood both with and without intervention (i.e., by comparison to the natural history of the condition), or with one intervention versus another.

A viable prognosis is essential to informed decision making by clinicians, clients, and their families, funders, and policymakers. At the level of clinicians and their clients, prognoses are integral to all three components of evidence-based practice (EBP). First, by surveying the research literature clinicians are able to objectively compare the relative prognoses of available treatment options. Second, they are able to factor in their own experience with each treatment or with the disorder in question to adjust those prognoses relative to the client under consideration. Third, by providing a set of relative prognoses, clinicians ensure that clients and their families are making informed choices; as such, client preferences and values may be more meaningfully integrated into the clinical decision process. At the funding and policy levels, the ability to generate prognoses has the potential to promote the efficient use of limited resources. As well, the absence of viable prognostic information may stimulate research efforts.

Factors Affecting a Prognosis

Many general factors likely interact with the intervention to determine both short- and long-term prognosis. The most obvious factor is the age of the client. Generally speaking, the younger the client the better the prognosis. The presumption here is that being younger means being physiologically better able to adapt and learn or relearn the necessary skill (i.e., greater plasticity). With developmental disorders (i.e., in children), being younger also means fewer long-standing habits to overcome. With acquired disorders, older adults may have less energy or motivation to participate in therapy. More specifically, adults who have retired may lack the typical motivation that comes with a desire to return to work.

Time elapsed since onset or identification of the problem is also likely to affect prognosis. Generally, the longer the delay to begin treatment the poorer the prognosis. With children, greater plasticity and reduced likelihood of developing bad habits would account for this. For example, early intervention for young children with a cleft of the palate may prevent the adoption of (aberrant) compensatory articulations. Likewise, earlier intervention for older children who stutter may allow them to develop good speech habits before they experience a large number of negative reactions to their speech from others. With adults, it is thought that intervening earlier may allow for developing new habits while the recovering nervous system is in the process of reorganizing itself. Doing so may also allow for learning compensatory strategies using a maximally functioning system in the case of degenerative disorders. Intervening earlier may also prevent development of dependence and withdrawal from social interactions, which can easily become habituated.

For adult clients, the amount of formal education is thought to affect prognosis with better outcomes usually associated with higher levels of attainment. The presumption here is that individuals with higher levels of education may have better cognitive and language abilities and thus may be more able to both comprehend instructions and fully appreciate the reasons for different aspects of the management plan. On the other hand, clients with more education may be more aware of the gap between their current state and their premorbid abilities causing them to be less motivated or to withdraw from therapy.

Prognosis is also thought to be affected by the presence of other problems. For example, reduced hearing acuity or reduced intellectual status may have a negative impact on prognosis by making it more difficult for the client to understand instructions or appreciate the goals of therapy. The presence of other health conditions (e.g., respiratory conditions, motor impairments) may negatively affect prognosis by making it more difficult to consistently attend therapy or carry out home practice exercises. The presence of other communication impairments may also negatively affect a prognosis. The child with a speech sound disorder combined with a language impairment, for example, is likely to make slower progress in therapy and is more likely to develop a reading disability compared to a child with only a speech sound disorder. Adults with a swallowing disorder who have a concurrent language impairment may have a poorer prognosis, because they either have difficulty understanding therapy directions for managing their food intake or have problems expressing their preferences for or satisfaction with details of the management plan.

The availability of environmental support from family or friends is generally thought to improve a prognosis. Such support may be practical (e.g., ensuring that the client attends therapy or carries out homework activities) or emotional (i.e., offering encouragement) in nature.

Although challenging to quantify, motivation is frequently cited as crucial to prognosis. The client who is more willing to work hard both within therapy sessions and with home practice is thought to be far more likely to develop (or relearn) the skills being taught.

A final factor that may affect a prognosis is the relative similarity between the client being considered and the populations studied in the available research or who have been previously treated by the clinician. For example, if research on a particular condition or intervention is based only on older children but the client under consideration is quite young, the relative strength of the prognosis being made must be tempered and less definite. Likewise, in much of communication disorders the vast majority of the research is grounded in studies of monolingual English speakers; extrapolating such research to generate prognoses for bilingual speakers may be quite difficult. The same is true relative to dialect. The bulk of the speech and language research is based on speakers of mainstream dialects; using such data to attempt a prognosis for a speaker of a nonmainstream dialect remains problematic.

Prognosis and Human Communication Disorders

As with many disciplines, the ability to make very precise prognostic statements remains somewhat elusive in the field of communication disorders. This should not be surprising given the above discussion on factors related to prognoses, as well as the fact that communicating with language is an inherently complex process. Perhaps most important, the available literature on prognosis, while expanding in recent years, remains limited.

Despite the limitations, speech, language, and hearing professionals continue to attempt prognoses. One well-known approach illustrates both the nature of how prognosis might be applied and some of the present limitations. Stimulability is a measure used for selecting therapy goals for individuals (particularly young children) with speech sound disorders. In its classic sense, stimulability represents the ability of individuals to successfully imitate the production of a speech sound that they are not currently producing correctly. The clinician presents the client with a model of the target sound by itself (i.e., outside the context of a real word) and asks the client to repeat it. If unsuccessful after several attempts, the client is said to be "not stimulable for [target sound]." If successful, the clinician models the sound at progressively higher linguistic levels (e.g., nonsense syllables, words, or phrases) and asks for a repetition at each level. The process is repeated until the client is unsuccessful and the highest level of success is reported (e.g., "The client was stimulable for [target sound] to the _____ level").

Most interpret the presence of some degree of stimulability as a form of readiness for therapy or an emerging ability to manage the production of the sound. Differences arise, however, in deciding on the implications of this interpretation. Many clinicians choose to work only on sounds that are at least somewhat stimulable or begin therapy with stimulable sounds as a way to ensure early success. Some clinicians and researchers argue that if stimulability for a sound suggests that the client will master the target sound without therapy, direct therapy should focus only on nonstimulable sounds. For those who work directly on stimulable sounds, the level to which the client is stimulable is also often interpreted as the point at which therapy should begin. The formal research related to stimulability has yielded mixed findings relative to these issues. While a strong relationship has been shown between stimulability and improvement on speech sounds, (a) it does not always accurately predict success in therapy, (b) it does not always accurately determine the best level to start therapy, and (c) it does not always accurately predict who will not need therapy for particular sounds.

Measures Related to a Prognosis

Aside from a straightforward probability value, a number of different measures have been associated with the formal generation of a prognosis. Three examples include relative risk, survival analysis, and cost/benefit analysis. *Relative risk* (or the more recent related measure the *odds ratio*) was developed by epidemiologists to help ascertain the probability of particular disease outcomes. It has also been applied to studies of improvement in communication disorders. Relative risk is effectively a comparison of the proportion of individuals in two groups who end up with a particular outcome. For example, imagine two groups of children with delayed speech development who each receive different treatments. Of 100 children who receive treatment A, 80 end up with fully normal speech skills, but only 40 of the 100 who receive treatment B achieve the same outcome. In this case, the risk (or odds) of achieving normal speech is two times greater with treatment A compared to treatment B. In other words, treatment A appears to be twice as effective as treatment B. Confidence intervals are typically calculated around both relative risk and odds ratios measures.

Survival analysis (or life tables analysis) was originally developed by the life insurance industry but has been applied in the field of communication disorders. It requires some complex statistical analysis of longitudinal data, which yield a prediction of the amount of time before a particular outcome is likely to be achieved. For example, imagine two hypothetical groups of children born with unilateral clefts of the palate. The children in group A undergo surgical repair of the palate at approximately age 12 months, but surgery is delayed for group B until age 36 months. Following the groups longitudinally, it is observed that children in group A tend to be rated as fully intelligible by approximately age 5 years, while this milestone is not achieved by those in group B until age 7 years. Thus, a child whose palate is surgically repaired at age 12 months is likely to achieve this important developmental milestone approximately 2 years earlier than the child whose repair occurs at 36 months.

A third example of a measure associated with a prognosis is a *cost-benefit analysis* (sometimes called the *net benefits* approach). This involves comparing groups that are exposed to different treatments and examining as many of the possible costs involved and weighing those against all the possible benefits that might be accrued over the lifespan. An example of where this might be applied is the choice of one versus two cochlear implants for children born with severe or profound bilateral hearing loss. Adding a second implant involves additional risk of a second surgical procedure and significant extra costs for both the surgery and the extra hardware. These risks/costs are then balanced against findings of children with two implants who demonstrate better ability to localize sound in emergencies, better communication skills, and better educational and quality of life outcomes. Each of these risks/costs and benefits can be quantified and an estimate can be made as to whether the benefits outweigh the risks for these children.

Peter Flipsen Jr.

See also Causation; Outcome Measures; Prevention of Hearing Disorders; Prevention of Speech and Language Disorders; Recovery From Aphasia; Research; Statistics: Predictive; Stimulability

Further Readings

Asch, D. A., Patton, J. P., & Hershey, J. C. (1990). Knowing for the sake of knowing: The value of prognostic information. *Medical Decision Making, 10*(1), 47–57.

Bichey, B. G., & Miyamoto, R. T. (2008). Outcomes in bilateral cochlear implantation. *Otolaryngology–Head and Neck Surgery, 138*, 655–661. https://doi.org/10.1016/j.otohns.2007.12.020

Casarett, D. (2016). The science of choosing wisely—Overcoming the therapeutic illusion. *New England Journal of Medicine, 374*(13), 1203–1205. https://doi.org/10.1056/NEJMp1516803

Croft, P., Altman, D. G., Deeks, J. J., Dunn, K. M., Hay, A. D., Hemingway, H. . . . Timmis, A. (2015). The science of clinical practice: Disease diagnosis or patient prognosis? Evidence about "what is likely to happen" should shape clinical practice. *BMC Medicine, 13*(20), 1–8. https://doi.org/10.1186/s12916-014-0265-4

Gruber, F. A. (1999a). Tutorial: Survival analysis—A statistic for clinical, efficacy, and theoretical applications. *Journal of Speech, Language, and Hearing Research, 42*(2), 432–447. https://doi.org/10.1044/jslhr.4202.432

Gruber, F. A. (1999b). Probability estimates and paths to consonant normalization in children with speech delay. *Journal of Speech, Language, and Hearing Research, 42*(2), 448–459. https://doi.org/10.1044/jslhr.4202.448

Powell, T. W., & Miccio, A. W. (1996). Stimulability: A useful clinical tool. *Journal of Communication Disorders, 29*(4), 237–253. https://doi.org/10.1016/0021-9924(96)00012-3

Shriberg, L. D., Flipsen, P. Jr., Thielke, H., Kwiatkowski, J., Kertoy, M. K., Katcher, M. L., . . . Block, M. G. (2000). Risk for speech disorder associated with early recurrent otitis media with effusion: Two retrospective studies. *Journal of Speech, Language, and Hearing Research, 43*(1), 79–99. https://doi.org/10.1044/jslhr.4301.79

PROMPTS

The term *prompts* refers to the way a desired response/behavior is elicited, and it is often used interchangeably with the term *cues*. Prompts can take many forms and vary in regards to the level of support provided to a client during a course of treatment. Initially, the clinician identifies the target response/behavior, and then writes a long-term goal and an accompanying set of short-term objectives that define the level and type of prompts that will support learning in treatment. Often referred to as a *prompting* or *cueing hierarchy*, this usually follows a *most* to *least* support approach, as the client typically needs significant support when first learning the targeted response/behavior, but then requires less support as treatment progresses and associated learning occurs.

Many speech–language objectives are initially targeted following a *verbal prompt*. Most support in regards to this type of prompting would consist of a verbal model, with the client required to produce the desired response/behavior in direct imitation of the clinician. The client's performance accuracy is monitored, and the verbal prompt is eventually faded or discontinued. This fading or discontinuing of the prompt is necessary, to ensure that the client does not become prompt dependent and learns to produce/perform the desired response/behavior independently and spontaneously. Verbal prompts are often used when teaching speech sounds, language forms, and other specific verbal output, but in some cases they could be used to teach other nonverbal responses/behaviors. An example short-term objective at this prompting level might read, "The client will produce /r/ in the word-initial position in response to picture stimuli and following a verbal model in 80% of opportunities across two consecutive sessions." This measurable objective allows the clinician to use data taken during client sessions to guide when to decrease the support provided via prompting, thus making the client's treatment as efficacious as possible. Specifically, when the initial short-term objective's scoring criteria are met, the clinician automatically shifts to a new short-term objective providing less prompting of the target response/behavior. In some cases, a verbal prompt can also be used to shift from most prompting to least prompting. For example, the verbal prompts "Ask me a question" or "Tell me more" might be used to elicit responses that were initially targeted in direct imitation.

Another common type of prompt is a *visual prompt*. Visual prompts typically consist of picture stimuli or orthography (for clients who can read). Although some speech–language objectives may begin at this prompting level (i.e., *most* support), it is more common for visual prompts to be used as a lower level of support for the client who had previously required a verbal prompt to elicit the desired response/behavior. In those cases, this type of prompting is classified as *least* support. Referring back to the previous short-term objective example, the prompting level could be adjusted to fade support, with the resulting new short-term objective reading, "The client will spontaneously produce /r/ in the word-initial position in response to picture stimuli in 80% of opportunities across two consecutive sessions." In this way, the original verbal prompt is now removed, with response to a visual prompt (picture stimuli) providing less support while also still facilitating learning. Stimuli that can serve as a visual prompt vary (print, photographs, picture symbols, line drawings, etc.) depending on the needs of the client.

A final common type of prompt is a *physical prompt*. As this implies, actual physical intervention (usually in the form of hand over hand support) is provided, which can be faded first to a *partial physical prompt* (e.g., touching the client's elbow), and eventually to a *gestural prompt* (e.g., physically pointing). This type of prompting is often used when teaching a client nonverbal behaviors such as following a picture schedule or completing a hands-on task (e.g., picking up a specific block when requested to demonstrate language comprehension). Again the approach used is often *most* to *least* support, with client performance data guiding when a specific short-term objective is met, and support reduced in subsequent objectives. Example short-term objectives implementing physical prompts might read, "Provided hand over hand prompting, the client will remove picture symbols representing therapy activities upon their completion in 80% of opportunities across two consecutive sessions" followed by "Given a partial physical prompt (elbow touch), the client will remove picture symbols representing therapy activities upon their completion in 80% of opportunities across two consecutive sessions," and terminating in a short-term objective targeting the desired response/behavior without a prompt. Although the preceding example includes a hierarchy of only physical and gestural prompts, it should be noted that physical and gestural prompts may also be used in a hierarchy that includes verbal prompts (serving typically as least support in those cases).

In contrast to the specific prompt types reviewed above, some clinicians may prefer to choose a more flexible approach in their targeting and scoring of performance related to treatment, and therefore choose to focus more on the *hierarchy* or *level* of prompting versus stating a particular *type* of prompt. Prompting typically still follows a *most* to *least* approach, with the terminology used reflecting that approach. The terms *maximal prompts* (or prompting), *moderate prompts* (or prompting), and *minimal prompts* (or prompting) are common and allow clinicians to provide their own interpretation of what each term means (e.g., perhaps a more broad definition, with more than one type of prompt considered maximal, moderate, or minimal). As the terms imply, maximal prompting is associated with most support, while minimal prompting is associated with least support.

There are a variety of prompts that can be used to elicit a desired response/behavior, and those reviewed above represent the major types and levels that are commonly seen in the treatment of speech and language goals and objectives. It is the responsibility of the clinician writing the goals and objectives for a specific client to determine the appropriate prompt type and level that will result in the most effective and efficacious treatment.

Annette Champion

See also Clinician

Further Readings

Hegde, M. N. (1998). *Treatment procedures in communicative disorders*. Austin, TX: Pro-Ed.

McCauley, R. J., & Fey, M. E. (Eds.). (2006). *Treatment of language disorders in children*. Towson, MD: Brookes.

Wolery, M., Ault, M. J., & Doyle, P. M. (1992). *Teaching students with moderate to severe disabilities: Use of response prompting strategies*. London, UK: Longman.

Prosodic Disorders

Prosodic disorders are disruptions to the features of speech that are typically responsible for conveying a range of information about, for instance, the grammatical status of an utterance, relative stress and emphasis in words and longer stretches of speech, structures of discourse and interaction, and aspects of speaker mood and emotion. In normal speech, alterations in pitch, amplitude, and duration constitute the core framework for implementing prosodic variation and distinctions, with those alterations being largely determined by particular vocal tract configurations and sequencing and timing of articulatory events. While the segmental level of speech production consists of a phoneme-by-phoneme activation process on the part of the speaker (notwithstanding the ways in which successions of speech sounds affect and change one another), the term *suprasegmental* is used to encompass pitch, amplitude, and duration. It is not unusual for *suprasegmental* and *prosodic* to be used interchangeably. Unlike the case for segmental aspects of speech, where investigators tend to agree on analytic models and methods, there is relatively less consensus with respect to the most productive frameworks for approaching prosodic analysis, whether in the case of normal or disordered speech. As suggested above, prosodic patterns are generally responsive to and vary according to contextual aspects such as relative formality and emotion, although speakers may exploit standard patterns for ironic purposes. This entry focuses on providing core information on the clinical conditions in which prosody production is known to be problematic for patients. The following sections offer underpinning accounts of why and how prosodic problems occur in given conditions, discuss breakdowns in prosodic perception among patients, and summarize effects of disordered prosody upon listeners' judgment of affected speakers.

To date, accounts of prosodic disorders have focused on dysarthric conditions, principally Parkinson's disease (PD): Reductions and exaggerations in pitch variability, for instance, affect the perceived naturalness of PD speakers. In the speech of those with cerebral palsy, the disturbances can be significant enough to interfere with the intelligibility of the speech in question. Effects of prosodic disorders upon listeners are discussed later in this entry. Considerable attention has also been paid to apraxic and dyspraxic disorders, with studies of speech in autism constituting the main focus of research effort in these areas.

Available research underscores the contribution made by prosody to overall communicative success: If it is sufficiently impaired, then it can be responsible for damaging and even obscuring the semantic content of the intended message.

Causes and Manifestations of Prosodic Disorder

When an individual is affected by a neurological, sensorineural, or motoric condition that impedes normal vocal tract state or activity or by auditory processing difficulties that affect either acquisition or maintenance of normal speech, it is reasonable to expect a corresponding prosodic effect. It is also known that cognitive problems, ranging from temporary to longer term interferences, can impinge upon prosodic realization. In all cases, the term *dysprosody* is appropriate, and while *aprosody* is also used, it is rare: The latter implies the complete absence of prosodic distinctions, but where it used, it tends rather to denote deterioration.

For patients with PD, the accumulation of acoustic information shows that there is a reduction in overall pitch range among affected speakers, resulting in an inability to exploit pitch range for signaling contrastive stress. In the case of apraxic patients, common evidence for prosodic disorder derives from the studies of developmental verbal dyspraxia and, as indicated above, autism. Most studies of speech characteristics in individuals with developmental verbal dyspraxia highlight both expressive and receptive prosody as causes for concern, to the extent that both areas often constitute the most notably disordered elements of communication in the condition. In the case of expressive aspects, the normally documented traits are exaggerations of pitch height, pitch range, and pitch movement.

The literature on prosody disorder also indicates that age-related cognitive deterioration may lead to problems in realizing prosody. In the case of Alzheimer's patients, for instance, it is known that specific problems exist in terms of using prosody to signal elements of conversation interaction and management.

Not all accounts of prosodic disorder offer explanations that can be directly linked to motor system impairments. Among apraxic children where autism spectrum disorder (ASD) is the main focus of enquiry, there exist unusual patterns of prominence deriving from misplaced stress, not all of which are consistent with behavior in non-ASD apraxia. The differences for ASD children are considered to be driven by particular breakdowns in their social and pragmatic calibration of their speech, and unusual prominence patterns are the result of misapplied or excessive loudness and high pitch on utterance elements that are not usually emphasized. Disorders of prosody, therefore, are often a consequence of a complex set of related pragmatic, social, and clinically relevant variables.

In addition to the prosodic problems that have been documented for a range of speech-disordered patients, there is evidence to indicate similar issues in cases of specific language impairment and developmental delays. Typically, children in these categories exhibit difficulties in assigning appropriate prosodic patterns in their speech, and experiments designed to target prosody usually report improvements in the area, not least in terms of children's overall awareness of prosodic variation and its function.

A further condition not mentioned thus far, but one whose manifestations tend to include strong elements of prosodic disorder, is the aphasic condition known as *foreign accent system*. The perceptions of foreignness documented in foreign accent system tend to cite problems with handling of pitch and stress assignment as being the main triggers for listeners' perception of odd or inconsistent accents.

The prosodic aspects of speech among patients with hearing impairment are known to suffer as a result of an ability either to acquire or maintain the sensorineural feedback systems, which support normal production of stress, loudness, and pitch. Although research focuses on children's speech, there is ample information to confirm that the speech of the postlingual deaf (i.e., those whose hearing loss postdates their acquisition of language) exhibits prosodic deterioration, albeit with intersubject variation. Most recent and current work relating to prosody and hearing impairment has been undertaken in the context of charting improvement after cochlear implantation (CI), with the general conclusion being that prosodic production improves post-CI.

Intersubject Variation in Disordered Prosody

Caution should be exercised with regard to assuming straightforward relationships between clinical conditions and the existence and manifestations of prosody disorder. Notwithstanding the apparent global improvements following prosodic intervention mentioned above, it is clear that significant intersubject variation exists in the extent and type of dysprosody present. Such base-level differences among affected individuals are likely to determine the level of improvement, or otherwise, one might expect following therapeutic intervention. For patients with PD, for example, deep brain stimulation has been used a means of exciting the areas of the brain associated with prosodic production: While this intervention results in overall improvements, changes observed are not always positive and may even result in worsening of prosodic performance. The preexisting state of given patients' speech is therefore known to have a strong influence on the potential for improvement.

Patients' Understanding of Prosody and Listener Assessment of Disordered Prosodic Patterns

Existing work on prosodic disorders focuses on the physical, physiological, and cognitive aspects underlying the production of relevant patterns and on the auditory manifestation of those disorders. Nonetheless, increasing attention is paid to two additional areas, namely (1) patients' own ability to receive and process prosodic information and (2) judgments made by listeners when they encounter unusual prosodic patterns in clinical speech varieties and the effect of those judgments upon interaction.

Sufficient evidence exists to confirm that patients who encounter problems in assigning prosody to their own speech may also have difficulties in perceiving prosody correctly, in deriving correct functional information from the perceived patterns, and reacting accordingly. Several studies investigate the effect of right hemisphere damage on patients' ability to process intonation patterns for the purpose of decoding emotion in interaction, and the core finding indicates that the right hemisphere damage poses significant difficulty for prosodic processing. Nonetheless, what might look like an ambivalence in the literature regarding whether a strong association does or not exist, there are obvious explanatory features for such superficially anomalous results, namely the particular stylistic content of data and lack of homogeneity among the group under investigation. Available discussions in this area confirm the basic presupposition that prosodic processing in right hemisphere damage is problematic and indicate the need for further systematic research to identify relevant variables that affect the degree of processing disorder in this condition. For speakers with ASD, processing problems also exist: Typically, the perception of stress poses difficulty, with lexical stress being particularly problematic.

As noted previously, the choice of test data used to access patients' prosodic skills impacts upon conclusions drawn about speaker ability, and this point is also pertinent where speakers' own perceptions are being investigated. The role of data choice in helping to uncover trends in patients' ability to decode prosody is frequently emphasized by means of PD studies. Here, studies evidence varying ability in recognizing prosodic patterns and indicate that in addition to group heterogeneity as an explanatory factor, the semantic context of test material also determines recognition success: The more nonsensical the carrier sentences are, for example, the lower were the identification of success rates.

Patients with bipolar disorder as a result of auditory cortex deficits also exhibit prosody perception difficulties. In particular, problems with tone discrimination are highlighted and these, in turn, are responsible for impaired abilities in recognizing emotional content in utterances and interactions.

With regard to CI speakers, research focuses on the extent to which implantees improve in their recognition of speech prosody. The conclusion from work undertaken is that unilateral CIs do not permit any appreciable improvement in the ability to perceive affect in speech, and this lack of improvement is attributed to the need for binaural coordination in recognizing and interpreting prosody.

For cognitive disturbances, there is evidence that patients' backgrounds in terms of their exposure to past negative or positive experiences can exert a priming effect upon their ability to perceive negative or positive emotions by way of prosodic cues. One suggestion, for instance, is that trauma suffered during childhood stunts the ability to recognize positive aspects of emotional prosody.

A significant body of work has been devoted to the ways in which listeners judge disordered prosody and how those judgments contribute to interactive success and perceptions of speaker naturalness. The Prososdy–Voice Profile developed by Lawrence Shriberg and his colleagues, in 1990, has driven a great deal of experimental work on the contribution of prosody to evaluations of patients' communicative and social ability, most notably for ASD. All studies that have used the protocol confirm that a positive correlation exists between prosodic ability and perceptions of social communicative skills.

On the basis of available findings summarized here, there is a clear rationale for focusing on therapeutic methods for ameliorating prosody as a means for enhancing communicative efficiency.

Joan Rahilly

See also Fluency and Fluency Disorders; Intonation; Phonological Disorders; Pitch; Prosody

Further Readings

Bellon-Harn, M. (2011). Targeting prosody: A case study of an adolescent. *Communication Disorders Quarterly, 32,* 109–117.

Lenden, J. M., & Flipsen, P. (2007). Prosody and voice characteristics of children with cochlear implants. *Journal of Communication Disorders, 40* (1), 66–81.

Nazarov, A., Frewen, P., Oremus, C., Schellenberg, E. G., McKinnon, M. C., & Lanius, R. (2015). Comprehension of affective prosody in women with post-traumatic stress disorder related to childhood abuse. *Acta Psychiatrica Scandinavica, 131*(5), 342–349.

Paul, R., Augustyn, A., Klin, A., & Volkmar, F. R. (2005). Perception and production of prosody by speakers with autism spectrum disorders. *Journal of Autism and Developmental Disorders, 35*(2), 205–220.

Peppé, S. J. E. (2009). Why is prosody in speech-language pathology so difficult? *International Journal of Speech-Language Pathology, 11*(4), 258–271.

Shriberg, L. D., Kwiatkowski, J., & Rasmussen, C. (1990). *Prosody-voice screening profile (PVSP)*. Tuscon, AZ: Communication Skill Builders.

Skodda, S., Grönheit, W., Schlegel, U., Südmeyer, M., Schnitzler, A., & Wojtecki, L. (2014). Effect of subthalamic stimulation on voice and speech in Parkinson's disease: For the better or worse? *Frontiers in Neurology, 4* (Article 218), 1–9.

Prosody

Prosody is the melody and rhythm of speech. It is suprasegmental in nature, meaning it relates to the features of an utterance that are above the phonological level (i.e., consonants, vowels). Prosody conveys a wide range of information in the speech signal, including linguistic and affective, meaning differences. The primary prosodic components consist of speech melody (or intonation), phrasing distinctions, lexical stress, phrase-level accentuation, rhythm, and tempo. Linguistic prosody may express lexical stress or tone distinctions, semantic form (e.g., declarative, interrogative), pragmatic intent, syntactic structure, and information about emphasis, focus, or contrast. Affective prosody conveys emotional information via the speech signal (e.g., sadness, happiness). Changes in prosody can also be used to express sarcasm or irony. Not all languages employ prosody and express meaning differences in the same way. Nevertheless, the prosodic characteristics of speech are highly interactive and essential for successful communication.

Prosodic features play a critical role during language acquisition, aiding early word segmentation and word learning. In many communication disorders, aspects of the prosodic system may be impaired. This can affect how a listener perceives the prosody (or lack thereof) of an individual with a communication impairment, leading to a breakdown in understanding. This entry first defines the different aspects of prosody as they relate to speech and language. Following a general definition, this entry discusses the primary correlates of prosody, the role of prosody in early language acquisition, and prosody in relation to communication disorders.

Components of Prosody

Cadence, melody, intonation, rhythm, and pitch are just some of the words used when asked to define prosody. This is a difficult task to complete in one word since prosody encompasses a variety of different features. To begin, it is important to define the prosodic hierarchy—the different levels of constituents that govern many aspects of a speech signal. At the lowest level is the syllable unit (or sometimes the mora); syllables can be grouped into successively higher level units like the foot, prosodic word, phonological phrase, intonational phrase, and finally the utterance. Different prosodic features affect different levels of this hierarchy to create variations in meaning. The main features defined here are speech melody, phrasing, lexical stress, accentuation, rhythm, and tempo.

Speech Melody

The rise and fall of pitch over the course of an utterance creates speech melody distinctions (i.e., intonation), which can signal semantic meaning differences. For example, in English, a speaker can vary the intended meaning of an utterance from a declarative to a yes–no interrogative by altering the overall speech melody (e.g., *Paul loves skiing.* vs. *Paul loves skiing?*). A declarative typically has a falling final pitch boundary tone. Alternatively, the exact same utterance produced with distinct intonational contour and a rising final tone indicates that the speaker is asking for information, creating a yes–no interrogative. Other differences in the overall melody can indicate that the speaker is calling out to someone (vocative) or commanding something (imperative).

Phrasing

Dividing speech into units modifies the phrasing of an utterance. Changing where phrase breaks are placed cues a boundary and can modify the interpretation of an utterance. For example, saying *Julian loves chocolate cookies, and cake* differs from *Julian loves chocolate, cookies, and cake*. In the first utterance, Julian loves two distinct things (*chocolate cookies* and *cake*), while in the second, he loves three things (*chocolate, cookies*, and *cake*).

Creating phrase breaks in speech can also be used to avoid ambiguity. For example, the first interpretation of the utterance *They know you realize your goals* is one without phrase breaks, where "your goals" is the object of the verb "realize." A second interpretation is *They know, you realize, your goals*, where "your goals" is now the object of the verb "know." Depending on the intended meaning, a speaker can vary their prosody to create unique phrasing structures.

Lexical Stress and Accentuation

Highlighting a syllable within the word is lexical stress and highlighting at the higher utterance or phrase level is accentuation. Crosslinguistically, languages differ on whether lexical stress location changes the meaning of a word and whether stress placement is predictable. A language with fixed stress places the stress in the same position for each word (e.g., nearly all words in Finnish stress the first syllable). On the contrary, English does not have fixed stress, meaning that the location of the stressed element varies by word (e.g., LEXical, disTINguished, incomPLETE). While English does not generally alter the meaning of a word based on stress, there is a group of disyllables that change between a noun and a verb depending on stress location. When the first syllable is stressed, it generally indicates the noun interpretation, and when the second syllable is stressed, it indicates the verb interpretation (e.g., pérmit (n.), permít (v.)). Stress patterns often shift for compound words in English, indicating a change in structure and meaning (e.g., *bláckboard* [classroom chalkboard] vs. *black bóard* [board that is black]).

Accentuation differs by highlighting a unit at a higher level, in the phrase or utterance. A speaker can signal a different pragmatic interpretation for the same word string simply by changing which word in the utterance receives accentuation. For a sentence produced out of the blue in English (broad focus), the final word usually carries the primary accentuation (John hid the *candy*). But this accentuation can be moved around to change the meaning that a listener extracts from the utterance. For example, the implied contrast is different for these four locations of accentuation: (1) *JOHN hid the candy* (and not Jim), (2) *John HID the candy* (and did not eat it), (3) *John hid THE candy* (and not some other candy), and (4) *John hid the CANDY* (and not the drinks). This is also referred to as *contrastive or narrow focus* and makes a particular portion of the utterance more prominent. While this is the case for English, languages differ greatly in how they use stress and accentuation to highlight words, phrases, or utterances.

Rhythm

Rhythm is the marking of prominence relations in a language. Generally, languages fall into one of three different rhythmic classes. Syllable-timed languages, like French, have syllables that are relatively equal in length. Stress-timed languages, like English, have a more uneven pattern, with stressed syllables often produced with a greater duration than unstressed syllables. Mora-timed languages, like Japanese, base their timing and rhythm patterns on the mora instead of the syllable (a phonological unit that is lower in the prosodic hierarchy than the syllable). Individual words of a language also contribute to its rhythmic pattern, with some languages having more words with final versus initial stress or vice versa. In English, many words are trochaic (disyllables with stress on the first syllable) rather than iambic (disyllables with stress on the final syllable). For these rhythmic patterns, languages most likely exist along a continuum with some being closer to purely stress-timed, syllable-timed, or somewhere in between, and individual utterances in almost any language can have any of these rhythmic shapes. Exploiting these types of patterns is also common in poetry. For example, the rhythm of a poem in iambic pentameter relies on a weak–strong stress pattern across lines.

Tempo

Tempo is the variation in speech rate. Speech rate has many influencing factors that largely reflect affective information over linguistic information. Factors that affect speech rate between speakers include dialect, age, and gender. Factors that can vary speech rate within a single speaker include context (speaking in front of a group), physical factors (fatigue), and emotion. For instance, emotion can vary tempo via happiness or sadness, where the latter may provoke a slower speaking rate. This can vary substantially across speakers, and individuals express emotion in a variety of ways through prosody. Emotional information can also be expressed in ways other than tempo, such as pitch, loudness, and segmental quality.

Primary Correlates of Prosody

Prosody relays a vast amount of information via the speech signal. Through variation in the acoustic correlates of prosody, a speaker can signal lexical stress, semantic meaning, pragmatic intent, and affect. These messages are relayed by the main perceptual correlates of prosody (and their primary acoustic counterparts) that include pitch (fundamental frequency or F_0), length and timing (segmental/pause duration), loudness (intensity), and segmental quality and reduction (spectral features). Importantly, this set of correlates does not have a one-to-one correspondence to signal structural or affective meanings. The same acoustic features may simultaneously vary to express a structural difference in meaning (e.g., an utterance-final pitch rise to signal a yes–no interrogative) and an affective state (e.g., larger pitch excursion on an utterance-final rise to express nervousness).

Prosody and Language Acquisition

Sensitivity to prosody begins before a baby is born. In the womb, the fetus is exposed to and learns the prosodic features of their native language. A series of studies conducted soon after birth demonstrate that infants prefer their native language over another language, their mother's voice over another woman's voice, and a familiar story read to them in the womb over an unfamiliar one.

As infants begin to learn language, they take advantage of prosody to uncover patterns in the speech they hear. Infants use stress, rhythm, and speech melody to aid in segmenting a continuous speech stream into meaningful units. For example, in English, 9-month-olds first segment trochaic (strong–weak) structures from the speech signal before iambic (weak–strong) ones, owing to the frequency of this pattern in the input. Prosody is critical throughout the word learning process, aiding in word segmentation, referent identification, and the mapping between linguistic form and meaning. Infant-directed speech, certain pitch accent structures, and phrasal structure are some of the prosodic features that guide these early processes. When children begin to speak, they are able to capture many adultlike characteristics of speech melody.

Prosody and Communication Disorders

Prosodic deficits accompany a number of communication disorders. In many of these disorders, prosodic impairments persist even after other language issues have been addressed. Research shows that a motor speech disorder such as dysarthria is typically characterized by abnormalities in pitch and rhythm as well as tempo. Recent work highlights how prosody may differ even within subtypes of a disorder. For example, congenital dysarthria is described as having exaggerated prosodic cues and nonstandard acoustic cue combinations. In turn, acquired dysarthria is defined as having dampened prosodic cues such as monopitch, monoloudness, and slower tempo. Prosodic perception and production are also distinct in individuals with autism spectrum disorders. For affective prosody, aprosodia is a neurological condition that impairs expressive and receptive emotional prosody, including difficulty modulating pitch and loudness.

Overall, prosody is a critical component of speech and language. It signals many types of meaning differences including lexical, semantic, pragmatic, and affective. Prosody plays an essential role in early language acquisition by helping infants with the task of early word learning. Furthermore, successful communication relies on being able to produce prosodic contrasts as well as understand them. Difficulties arise when an impairment due to a communication disorder may inhibit this process. Continued research in speech prosody will provide insights into how best to intervene and diagnose prosodic impairments, increasing our foundational knowledge of this complex component of language.

Jill C. Thorson

See also Information Structure; Intonation; Paralinguistic and Prosodic Impact on Stuttering; Pitch; Prosodic Disorders

Further Readings

Jun, S-A. (Ed.). (2005). *Prosodic typology: The phonology of intonation and phrasing*. Oxford, UK: Oxford University Press.

Jun, S-A. (Ed.). (2014). *Prosodic typology II: The phonology of intonation and phrasing*. Oxford, UK: Oxford University Press.

Jusczyk, P. W., Houston, D., & Newsome, M. (1999). The beginnings of word segmentation in English-learning infants. *Cognitive Psychology, 39*, 159–207.

Ladd, D. R. (1996). *Intonational phonology*. Cambridge, UK: Cambridge University Press.

McCann, J., & Peppé, S. (2003). Prosody in autism spectrum disorders: A critical review. *International Journal of Language and Communication Disorders, 38*(4), 325–350.

Nespor, M., & Vogel, I. (2007). *Prosodic phonology: With a new foreword*. Berlin, Germany: Mouton de Gruyter.

Selkirk, E. (1981). On prosodic structure and its relation to syntactic structure. In T. Fretheim (Ed.), *Nordic prosody II* (pp. 111–140). Trondheim, Norway: Tapir.

Shattuck-Hufnagel, S., & Turk, A. (1996). A prosody tutorial for investigators of auditory sentence processing. *Journal of Psycholinguistic Research, 25*(2), 193–247.

Prosthetics for Structural Deficits

Prosthetic speech management is a viable treatment option for selected patients with structural or neurogenic speech disorders. Structurally based disorders typically require a prosthesis that will obturate the space of an oropharyngeal defect. Disorders of neurogenic origin, resulting in dysarthria that affects velopharyngeal (VP) function, may be managed by lifting the soft palate into position. The two most common prosthetic devices include the palatal obturator (also known as a speech bulb) and the palatal lift, both of which aim to improve VP closure for speech. Overall, the goal of prosthetic management is to assist with function of the oral and VP structures to improve speech intelligibility and quality. Swallowing difficulties may also be improved in selected cases. While there are only a few types of speech prostheses, it is important to recognize that patient care and prosthetic design must be individualized.

Patients with various causes of velopharyngeal dysfunction (VPD) may benefit from prosthetic management. VPD is defined as the inability to separate the nasal cavity from the oral cavity during speech and/or swallowing. See Table 1 for a list of types of congenital and acquired conditions that can result in VPD and may be treated with a palatal lift or obturator. Patients who have undergone partial glossectomy are a special case that may benefit from a palatal drop appliance. The best prosthetic results are generally found in patients with isolated structural palatal defects. Outcomes tend to be less predictable in patients with multi-subsystem dysarthria and significant language/cognitive deficits.

Table 1 Conditions associated with velopharyngeal dysfunction (VPD) that may be managed with a prosthesis

Structurally based conditions (resulting in velopharyngeal insufficiency):

- Cleft palate
- Short soft palate (congenital or after palate repair)
- Symptomatic palatal fistulae
- Iatrogenic oropharyngeal defects (such as after cancer resection or trauma)

Neurogenic conditions (resulting in velopharyngeal incompetence):

- Flaccid dysarthria
- Neurofibromatosis Type 1
- Stroke
- Traumatic brain injury
- Parkinson's disease
- Amyotrophic lateral sclerosis (ALS)
- Palatal paralysis or paresis

Note: Structurally based conditions are typically managed with a palatal obturator (speech bulb). Neurogenic conditions are often managed with a palatal lift.

Assessing Patient Candidacy for a Prosthesis

It is critical to consider medical, speech, swallowing, dental, behavioral, and psychosocial factors when assessing a patient's candidacy for prosthetic management. Based on all available diagnostic information including the patient's medical history, current speech and swallowing difficulties, the oral and dental examination findings, and oral/velopharyngeal imaging results (e.g., nasopharyngoscopy or videofluoroscopy), if VP closure is not possible and surgical management is not feasible (or contraindicated), then prosthetic management should be considered. The treatment team should then discuss the degree to which improvement of VP closure will likely impact the patient's overall speech (and swallowing) disorder. The speech effects can be reasonably simulated by plugging the patient's nose and having the patient produce speech stimuli loaded with oral-only consonants (e.g., "Pet a puppy"), then contrasted with production of these stimuli without the nose plugged. The degree of perceived improvement when the nose is plugged is comparable to that which could be achieved by an optimized speech prosthesis. If the perceived degree of improvement is minimal, then the patient may not stand to benefit sufficiently from prosthetic treatment to offset the burden of care (multiple dental visits, time off work, transportation and insurance costs, etc.).

In some pediatric cases, the patient-family may be uneasy about proceeding with surgical management. Even if the child has been deemed a safe and reasonable candidate for VP surgery, some families may see a prosthetic as a lower risk alternative. While this may be the case, the family should be counseled on the anticipated benefits and the burden of care of prosthetic management. Parents should also be given realistic expectations about device tolerance if the child is known to have a "sensitive" gag reflex. In cases in which the child's medical condition or the family's religion excludes surgery as a treatment option, prosthetic management may be the only available treatment for VPD. In cases where surgery is possible and deemed safe, but the prognosis is guarded or unclear, prosthetic management may offer the benefit of serving as a temporary treatment that can simulate the effects of the surgical outcome so that providers and patient-families can evaluate the relative risk-benefit ratio of later surgical management.

Some of the most important considerations for determining if a child is able to tolerate a speech prosthesis are behavior and psychological factors. If a child is anxious or unable to cooperate for standard dental visits or oral exams, that child will be unlikely to tolerate the impressions and dental visits needed to fit and adjust the prosthesis. The treatment team should also make sure the patient-family has adequate understanding of the number of visits, expected cost, and duration of treatment to successfully complete the prosthetic treatment plan. This should include all preliminary dental restorations, possible placement of molar bands or other tooth modifications to support device retention, speech evaluation costs, and device-related costs from start to finish. In addition, patients should be aware of the financial implications of a lost or broken device.

Dental hygiene is another critical factor for determining candidacy for an intraoral appliance. If dental hygiene is poor, wearing an intraoral device on a daily basis is likely to worsen hygiene and increase caries risk. Current tooth eruption status is also critical for pediatric patients. If the first permanent molars have not yet erupted, then the child may not yet be a candidate since the child lacks the adequate dentition to retain the device in place. Speech prostheses cannot be retained by baby teeth or teeth that are unstable. It is also important to discuss any current or upcoming orthodontic treatment such as expanders or braces that will prevent (or delay) use of the device.

Types of Speech Prostheses

The most common indication for prosthetic management is to improve VP closure for speech or swallowing. A palatal lift or palatal obturator can achieve this goal, but patient selection and device design are critical. It is also important to manage patient-family expectations of what a prosthetic speech device can and cannot do, especially in cases with complex speech or swallowing disorders. The prosthetic device is designed with the goal of having a targeted impact on the speech parameters affected by VPD. It is important for treatment team to counsel the patient-family on prognosis for improvement and determine the degree of anticipated benefit from the device. In general, patients receiving a speech prosthesis should expect a reduction in hypernasality and audible nasal emission, an improvement in intraoral pressure for articulation, and a reduction in nasal regurgitation.

The palatal lift is a good option for patients with normal palatal length but reduced palatal elevation (known as *velopharyngeal incompetence*). The device is usually made out of an acrylic base, similar to a standard orthodontic retainer but with an extended "tail" to support the soft palate (see Figure 1). In essence, this device lifts the soft palate up into position to contact the posterior pharyngeal wall to assist with VP closure.

The palatal obturator (also known as a speech bulb) is most appropriate for patients with a tissue deficiency such as a short soft palate, unrepaired or dehiscent palate, or palatopharyngeal defect (i.e., after surgical resection) in which the anatomic structures cannot contact the posterior pharyngeal wall for speech or swallowing (known as *velopharyngeal insufficiency*). In this case, the device must be custom shaped to fit the size, shape, and location of the tissue defect in order to fully obturate the VP space sufficiency. Examples of palatal obturators are depicted in Figure 2. In some cases, a patient may require a combined palatal lift and obturator appliance or a palatal prosthesis that includes false teeth. There are also palatal obturators that can be designed to address a fistula of the hard or soft palate. In these cases, the prosthetic team must custom design the device to cover and plug the fistula to ensure an adequate seal to eliminate nasal escape of food, liquids, and airflow (during speech).

A lesser known prosthetic device that may be helpful for improving swallowing function and oral articulation is the palatal drop. This device may be beneficial for patients who have undergone partial glossectomy with limited tongue mass or function. This device is intended to assist the tongue with moving the food bolus back in the

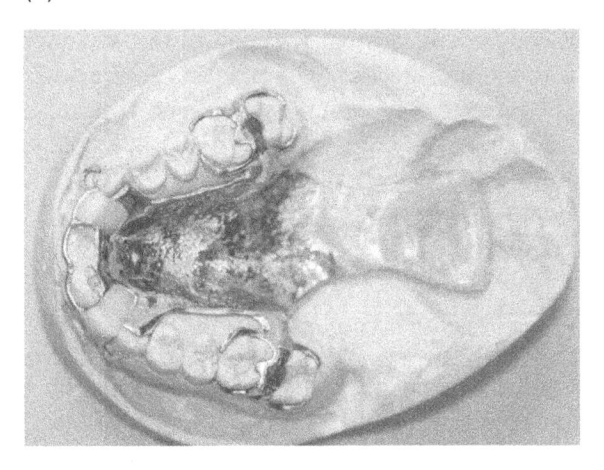

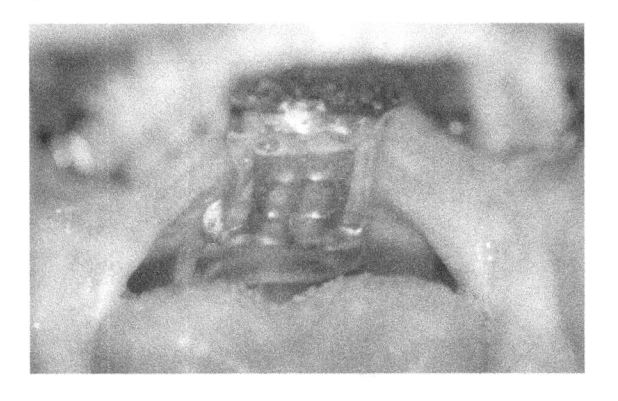

Figure 1 (a) Example of a palatal lift. (b) Example of a palatal lift inserted intraorally

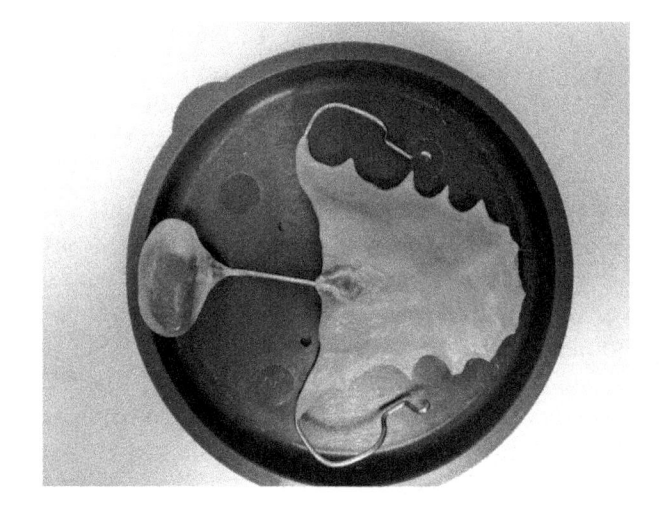

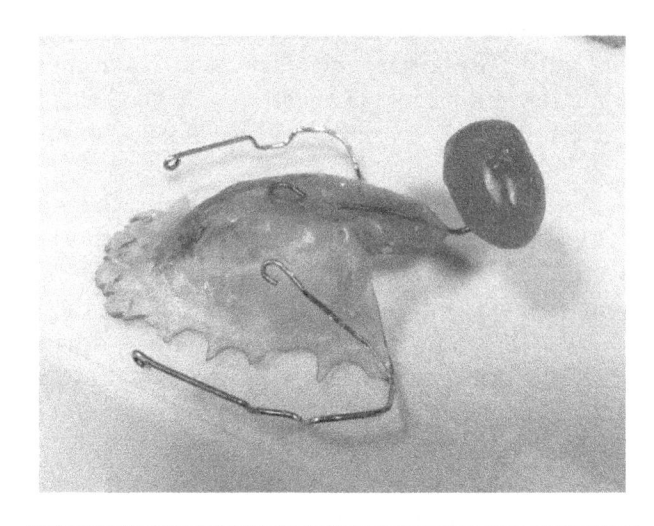

Figure 2 Examples of palatal obturators

oral cavity and to provide an enhanced contact point for articulation of alveolar, palatal, or velar consonants. The palatal drop is a maxillary appliance that is selectively thickened to facilitate tongue-to-palate contact on the affected side/sites.

Interdisciplinary Management

An interdisciplinary approach is key to successful management and optimization of outcomes. This typically includes a speech–language pathologist (SLP) and a dental specialist, often a prosthodontist, who work closely to evaluate patient candidacy, design the prosthesis, and coordinate the treatment. The patient and family should also be viewed as part of the team. The role of the SLP is to evaluate the patient's speech, swallowing, and VP function. The SLP works closely with the prosthodontist to help optimize the design of the speech prosthesis based on the patient's speech characteristics, with a focus on resonance, nasal emission, and perceived pressure for oral consonants. The SLP first conducts a perceptual speech evaluation followed by instrumental evaluation (e.g., nasalance measurement) and VP imaging, such as nasopharyngoscopy or videofluroscopy. They are also responsible for ongoing dynamic assessment, patient and family counseling, and collaboration with the community-based SLP, if the patient also requires speech therapy. The SLP should help differentiate what speech symptoms will respond to prosthetic management, if speech therapy is indicated, and determine the prognosis for improvement. The form and function of the lips, tongue, dentition, palate, and posterior pharynx must also be carefully inspected to determine what deviations may impact speech production. Palatal length, elevation, and symmetry should also be noted.

While the perceptual evaluation of speech is the gold standard for evaluating patients with suspected VPD, direct visualization of the VP mechanism is invaluable when determining a prosthetic treatment plan. Nasopharyngoscopy during speech is the preferred method of visualization since it provides information about palate elevation, posterior pharyngeal wall motion, and lateral wall motion. Videofluoroscopy is also a useful technique as it provides information regarding palatal elevation and length.

The role of the prosthodontist or other related dental professional (such as an orthodontist) is to evaluate patient's dental health, guide dental modifications to facilitate device retention, build the speech appliance and make modifications, and coordinate any ongoing dental care with a community-based dentist. The prosthodontist builds the speech appliance based on results of the speech evaluation, VP imaging, and dental exam findings. The prosthodontist will assess candidacy for the device including the occlusal relationship, tooth stability, and health of the soft tissue. Adequate dentition is needed for optimal retention, typically the permanent molars or premolars, although advances in technology and the availability of osseointegrated implants may allow for novel approaches to device retention.

Prosthetic Device Selection, Fabrication, and Modifications

After the initial speech and dental evaluation, the SLP and prosthodontist will determine which type of prosthetic is needed. For palatal lifts or obturators, the appliance generally consists of two parts created in succession: first, the oral appliance (the palatal retainer) and then the posterior extension (the tail or obturator). The orthodontist will take impressions of the patient's dentition and fabricate an acrylic appliance. To help acclimate patients to the device, they are instructed to wear it several hours per day, gradually increasing their tolerance of the appliance. The goal is for the appliance to feel comfortable enough to wear during all waking hours. For some patients, this may take a matter of days and for others, this may take weeks.

For a palatal lift, the ideal candidate will have adequate dentition to allow for proper retention of the device; however, the length and flexibility of the palate will also be taken into account to ensure adequate retention and lift. After the oral appliance is made, the posterior lift is gradually increased in length (and width, as needed) until speech is sufficiently improved, while maintaining comfort during swallowing.

After the initial palatal retainer is created for a palatal obturator, a wire extension and then the initial posterior portion (a "minibulb") is added. Once the minibulb is fitted, the team will work collaboratively to modify the bulb's shape and size over several visits, balancing speech improvement with comfort for swallowing and nasal breathing.

Modification of the posterior portion of the device involves joint visits with the prosthodontist and SLP. Nasopharyngoscopy is the best way to visualize the nasopharynx during speech production and tailor the size and shape of the appliance. When imaging is not available, systematic revisions/additions can be guided by close SLP monitoring of resonance, nasal air emission, and oral pressure changes during speech, combined with careful oral examination for signs of discomfort, tissue pressure, or ulceration. Temporary additions are usually done with wax or other thermoplastic substance. Once the device shape/size is determined to be optimal, it is then permanently converted to acrylic. This modification process may be repeated over several visits until adequate VP closure is achieved.

For most patients, slow and systematic additions work well to adequately desensitize the oral structures (and gag) to the device and allow for a comfortable fit. In more challenging cases, or in the case of very young patients, a more structured and paced approach may be necessary. General behavioral modification principals apply in these instances. Creating a structured schedule of wear is recommended, with positive reinforcement provided at scheduled intervals. The child may begin by wearing the device during speech therapy and gradually increase the duration of wear an hour each day for the first few weeks. In children who are still growing and transitioning from mixed to permanent dentition, the oral appliance will need to be remade every few months to year, depending on growth and changes in dentition.

A well-fitting speech prosthetic should not cause any discomfort. If the appliance causes pain or ulceration, the prosthodontist can adjust the fit or shave away acrylic to decrease size and increase comfort. In the case of loose-fitting appliances in adults, a dental adhesive may help to improve retention. Speech prostheses may be a temporary or permanent treatment approach. Even in cases where permanent use of the prosthetic is intended, all speech prostheses are removable to ensure adequate nasal airflow for sleep breathing and to promote dental health. In addition, patients should be reminded that since a speech appliance does not permanently change structure, its effects are only realized when the device is being used with the expectation that speech returns to baseline when the device is taken out of the mouth.

Patients should continue to be followed by their prosthetic team on a yearly or biannual basis in order to ensure adequate speech outcome, comfort, retention, and dental health. Additionally, continued follow-up with the patient's medical team or cleft/craniofacial team is also recommended.

Collaboration between the prosthetic team and the medical/craniofacial team can help streamline care. Similarly, collaboration between the community SLP and the prosthetic team SLP should occur throughout the treatment process. While the prosthetic team SLP's role is to guide VP management, the community SLP typically provides speech–language therapy, encourages the patient to wear the prosthesis, and reports any concerns back to the prosthetic team.

Speech Prostheses as a Temporary Training Device?

A prosthetic device may be used in a child with VPD with a severe articulation disorder who is not yet a surgical candidate, in order to provide improved VP closure for speech to facilitate progress in speech therapy. A prosthetic can also be trialed following traumatic brain injury or other abrupt neurologic insult resulting in dysarthria, if symptoms of VPD are severe. In the latter case, there is the possibility that the device may be phased out as neuroplasticity and the effects of rehabilitation improve overall speech function. Past studies have also shown that in patients with VPD of structural origin, a structured approach to lift or bulb reduction can stimulate lateral pharyngeal wall motion. This can also lead to the possibility of lift or bulb size reduction or rarely, the potential for elimination of the entire device.

Evaluating Outcomes and Patient Satisfaction

The perceptual speech evaluation is the primary mode of assessing the outcome of prosthetic speech management. Assessing speech both with and without the device in place is also helpful for determining outcome. It is equally important to assess patient satisfaction. The VPI Effects on Life Outcome tool (known as the VELO), created by Jonathan Skirko in 2013, is a tool that can be administered prior to use of the prosthetic and again after a reasonable period of use in order to quantify improvements in quality of life.

In sum, every management option has unique benefits and challenges, though the risks of prosthetic management are relatively low. Prosthetic management is a reasonable and effective treatment for VPD in select patient populations for whom surgical intervention is not feasible.

Adriane L. Baylis and Kaylee Paulsgrove

See also Cleft Lip and Palate: Speech Effects; Dysarthria; Resonance Disorders

Further Readings

Leeper, H. A., Charles, D. H., & Sills, P. S. (2009). Prosthetic management of maxillofacial and palatal defects. In K. T. Moller & L. E. Glaze (Eds.), *Cleft lip and palate: Interdisciplinary issues and treatment* (2nd ed., pp. 601–634). Austin, TX: Pro-Ed.

Light, J. (1995). A review of oral and oropharyngeal prostheses to facilitate speech and swallowing. *American Journal of Speech-Language Pathology, 4*(3), 15–21. https://doi.org/10.1044/1058-0360.0403.15

Peterson-Falzone, S. J., Hardin-Jones, M. A., & Karnell, M. P. (2010). *Cleft palate speech* (4th ed.). St. Louis, MO: Mosby Elsevier.

Pinto, J. H. N., & Pegoraro-Krook, M. I. (2003). Evaluation of palatal prosthesis for the treatment of velopharyngeal dysfunction. *Journal of Applied Oral Science, 11*(3), 192–197. http://dx.doi.org/10.1590/S1678-77572003000300007

Reisberg, D. K. (2016). Prosthetic management of velopharyngeal dysfunction. In J. Losee & R. Kirschner (Eds.), *Comprehensive cleft care* (2nd ed., pp. 1299–1308). Boca Raton, FL: CRC Press.

Sell, D., Mars, M., & Worrell, E. (2006). Process and outcome study of multidisciplinary prosthetic treatment for velopharyngeal dysfunction. *International Journal of Language & Communication Disorders, 41*(5), 495–511. https://doi.org/10.1080/13682820500515852

Skirko, J., Weaver, E., Perkins, J., Kinter, S., Eblen, L., & Sie, K. (2013). Validity and responsiveness of VELO: A velopharyngeal insufficiency quality of life measure. *Otolaryngology-Head and Neck Surgery, 149*(2), 304–311. https://doi.org/10.1177/0194599813486081

Yorkston, K., Spencer, K., Duffy, J., Beukelman, D., Golper, L., & Miller, R. (2001). Evidence-based practice guidelines for dysarthria: Management of velopharyngeal function. *Journal of Medical Speech-Language Pathology, 9*(4), 257–273.

Proxemics

Proxemics is the study of the social and physical aspects of an individual's personal space. It can be conceptualized in terms of our input senses (eyes, ears, and nose), which make judgments regarding the amount of space between ourselves and the persons or things we interact with. However, these judgments are not straightforward. A substantial body of research into proxemics illuminates the almost innumerable factors that inform the interactants' judgments regarding the personal space of themselves and their interlocutor.

Understanding proxemics in communication requires a complicated dance that embraces the shifting influences of the immediate communicative environment and the larger physical environment in which interaction occurs. The physical environment shapes the communicative interactional space through both fixed and semifixed features. Fixed feature spaces are constrained by immovable constituents such as rooms within a larger space, dividing walls, or any fixed object that obstructs your line of sight. Semifixed spaces are those with movable objects such as the chairs and tables in clinic rooms or meeting spaces that can be arranged to achieve a desired effect, enforcing a power hierarchy or creating an egalitarian workspace. These features can encourage interaction (sociopetal), or they can support isolation or privacy (sociofugal). For example, increased interaction occurs with seating arranged in a circle or U-shape with reduced barriers such as tables, while less interaction is present when sitting in rows where a person's body orientation restricts gaze. This has important implications for the development of therapeutic alliance between a clinician and client, enough so that Irvin Yalom and Molyn Lesczc (2005), in their book *The*

Theory and Practice of Group Psychotherapy, attend to both the fixed and semifixed features of the physical space for treatment when they state:

> Group meetings may be held in any room that affords privacy and freedom from distractions ... The first step of a meeting is to form a circle so that members can see one another ... If members are absent most therapists prefer to remove the empty chairs and form a tighter circle. (pp. 281–282)

The interactants forming the immediate communicative environment create an additional space, the informal space, so named by E. T. Hall in his 1966 book, *The Hidden Dimension*, because it operates on a level that is seemingly unconscious. However, the informal space is regulated by a multitude of factors that dictate the distance zone and body orientation between interactants. Prior to the discussion of these factors, an overview of the continuum of distance zones in personal space is in order. Hall conceptualized a model of the interaction between social, kinesthetic, and sensory input factors that identifies four zones of social distance from the most to least proximal; they include intimate, personal, social, and public. An intimate zone extends about 46 cm from an individual's person and as the name implies, is reserved for those persons to which she feels close. The distance of the personal zone can span between 46 to 122 cm from the individual and typically familiar friends approach this social distance. The third most proximal distance is social distance, spanning 122 to 366 cm from the individual, and this distance can be either formal (beginning around 243 cm) or informal. The final distance classification is the public zone, which ranges from 366 cm to the limits of an individual's sight. A common example of this zone is that between a speaker and audience in a large auditorium.

As stated above, the distance zones are governed by physical characteristics that we experience through our senses, such as sound and lighting, and the physical space features (fixed and semifixed). For example, sound affects the interaction distance in that an expectation of quiet will encourage close proximity, and acoustic constraints mandate proximal positioning to overcome loud background noise. Similarly, the lighting in our environment will influence our choices for spatial proximity, which, like sound, is tied to sociocultural conventions and the physical limitations of our senses. Furniture arrangements, as an example, can promote cooperation when individuals are seated side by side or catty-corner at a table. However, when placed facing each other with no table between, there is increased likelihood of intimacy, expressed as therapeutic alliance.

Factors Influencing Social Distance

While familiarity between interactants plays a significant role in the proxemic behaviors, decisions on interactional proximity are subject to many additional influences. Gender differences exist, with females maintaining reduced personal space zones when interacting with others of either gender. Age affects proximity with social distance zones progressively expanding from age 6 until around age 10. Even the topic of conversation can result in proximity differences with negative topics being associated with greater conversational distance. The setting in which people interact influences proximity and body orientation through the setting-associated norms, such as those attendant to a library, or the setting's noise or lighting, such as in a crowded pub. An important contributor to distance zones is the attitude or emotions of either interactant, requiring greater or lesser distance, greater or lesser touch, and greater or lesser gaze. Additionally, one's personality influences their proxemic behavior with extroverts being more likely to position themselves facing their interlocutor with closer proximity and introverts preferring to avoid direct gaze and close proximity.

Culture, be it ethnic, social, or socioeconomic, becomes a large contributor to proxemic behavior as uniformity in the proxemics of one's informal space becomes enculturated within a community. For example, Latin-Americans and Southern Europeans, the so-called contact-cultures, are more likely to have closer personal spaces characterized by increased proximity, touch, and gaze, whereas noncontact cultures, such as those of Asia, Canada, and the United States, maintain greater distances with reduced touch and gaze. Each community cooperatively recognizes and adheres to prescribed distances. Then, when encountering an individual from another community, each will still project their own expectations and norms for appropriate proxemic behavior. A mismatch of proxemic expectations between interactants can occur due to differences, whether real or perceived, in any of the factors that inform decisions of interactional spaces. Proxemic interference can result in discomfort and, more often, misunderstanding. Furthermore, because interactants are not making decisions about these informal spaces at a conscious level, they often cannot identify the source of their discomfort. This discomfort encourages one of the interactants to distance himself from his interlocutor, both physically and psychosocially.

Proxemics and Communication Disorders

Proxemic interference can become quite problematic in communication-disordered populations. There has been limited research in proxemics as it relates to communication disorders, but the findings have indicated that many communication-disordered individuals, such as persons with traumatic brain injury, autism spectrum disorder, and even Parkinson's disease, have difficulty attending to proxemic cues. Clinical research in autism spectrum disorder points to the foundation of social competence formed through play, whose context supports understanding the expectations for observing distance zones, of when and how to enter someone else's personal space and allow others to enter yours. However, a credible researcher and clinician will acknowledge that one contributor to interactants' proxemic behaviors can mitigate others, thus confounding the conclusions that can be drawn from proxemics research focused on both typical and disordered communication.

Proxemics and Clinical Interaction

Regardless of the complex interaction between influences on proxemic behavior, attending to these factors is paramount in establishing a productive, collaborative relationship. The therapist must attend to cultural expectations and sensory limitations of their client by observing and then respecting their client's personal space needs related to distance, gaze, and touching. This consideration extends to a client's personal effects, a semifixed feature. While the therapist is sometimes required to violate a client's personal space in carrying out clinical tasks, an accounting of and permission for entering a client's intimate, or even social, distance zone will reduce potential distress.

Therapists can exploit the fixed and semifixed features of the clinic setting to achieve desired levels of alliance and power. Smaller spaces, with comfortable lighting and minimal extraneous noise, will encourage increased proximity. Sitting catty-corner at a table will afford increased mutual gaze opportunity and sharing of work materials. These physical aspects of treatment delivery have the power to increase therapeutic alliance and thus collaboration. Conversely, very brightly lit, cavernous rooms and seating arrangements with the table acting as a barrier between the therapist and client will enforce a power differential that places the therapist in a superior role. In summary, by understanding and employing interaction principles learned from proxemics, therapists can maximize treatment benefits gained from clinical interactions.

Jennifer Thompson Tetnowski

See also Autism Spectrum Disorder; Conversation; Counseling in Speech–Language Pathology; Gaze; Group Therapy; Traumatic Brain Injury

Further Readings

Hall, E. T. (1966). *The hidden dimension*. Garden City, NJ: Doubleday.

Knapp, M. L., & Hall, J. A. (2010). *Nonverbal communication in human interaction* (7th ed.). Boston, MA: Wadsworth Cengage Learning.

Yalom, I., & Lesczc, M. (2005). *The theory and practice of group psychotherapy* (5th ed.). New York, NY: Basic Books.

PSYCHIATRIC DISORDERS WITH COMMUNICATION DISORDERS

Psychiatric disorder, mental illness, mental disorder, and psychological disorder generally refer to a pattern of behavioral and/or psychological symptoms that cause distress to an individual and significantly impact on their usual functioning or activity. Psychiatric disorders are common and are considered to affect about a third of the world's adult population, with subsequent high rates of disability. Psychiatric disorders are less well understood in developing countries, where religious and cultural beliefs can influence how psychiatric disorders are understood and managed. In this entry, *communication disorders* refer to children and adults who present with a range of speech, language, and communication impairments which may be (a) an intrinsic part of the psychiatric disorder, such as the language and communication abnormalities in schizophrenia or (b) a secondary consequence of the psychiatric disorder due to side effects of medication or associated with the psychiatric disorder, for example, a childhood communication disorder as a risk for later psychiatric disorder. The neuropsychiatric disorders whereby communication is affected such as Alzheimer's disease, dementia, and Parkinson's disease are not included here.

This entry describes how communication can be affected in psychiatric disorders; how childhood communication disorder can be a risk factor for psychiatric disorders; and finally, how communication with people with psychiatric disorders can be facilitated to enable their optimal engagement in therapeutic interventions and overall management.

Communication in Common Adult Psychiatric Disorders

Psychiatric disorders are diagnosed by the medical field of psychiatry according to the *International Classification of Diseases* (World Health Organization) and the *Diagnostic and Statistical Manual of Mental Disorders* (American Psychiatric Association). Within psychiatric disorders, a long-standing distinction is made between organic and functional disorders. *Organic* indicates there is a biological cause for the psychiatric disorder, such as the brain changes and subsequent cognitive difficulties found in dementia, whereas *functional* does not implicate a clear biological cause. The overlap between organic and functional disorders is fully acknowledged. A further distinction is made between psychoses and neuroses. *Psychoses* are psychiatric disorders, for example, schizophrenia, where the person is considered to lose contact with reality, and the symptoms are not easily understandable (e.g., hallucinations, delusions, and difficulties maintaining insight in his/her thinking and behavior). *Neuroses*, for example, depression and anxiety, are psychiatric disorders, where the person is considered to maintain contact with reality and insight into their thinking and behavior. The symptoms, although severe, are more easily understandable than the symptoms found in psychoses.

A psychiatric disorder often has a significant impact on a person's communication. Changes in the person's speech and language, and in how the person communicates, are of importance for the diagnostic process. Speech will be observed in terms of the rate of speech, volume, and overall intelligibility. Aspects of language such as the amount of language the person uses, how well he/she understands, the types of words he/she uses, how the person puts words together into phrases and sentences to express meaning are also considered. How the person relates socially to, and communicates with, others combines with their speech and language ability to give a holistic view of their overall communicative competence.

Depression is a very common psychiatric disorder. It is a functional mood disorder that can be transient and recurrent or much more chronic and pervasive over the life span. Symptoms are grouped into biological or somatic, mood and cognitive and expected to persist for a period of 3 months or more with significant distress caused to the individual as well as a change of functioning in their usual everyday activity such as not being able to work. Biological symptoms can include disruption to sleep patterns, changes to appetite with subsequent weight loss, and in severe cases, psychomotor retardation, where there is a slowing of movement. Mood symptoms range across feelings of sadness, loss of interest in usual activities, and low mood. Feelings of guilt, worthlessness, and suicidal thought constitute some of the cognitive symptoms. In depression, a person's communication may become slow and effortful with a reduced desire to communicate with others. The *pressure* or rate of speech may be described as slow, and there may be a *poverty of content* to describe the person's lack of communication.

Alexithymia is often present, and this refers to the person's difficulties in being able to talk about the emotions they are experiencing. This can lead to reduction in the amount of communication he/she is able to engage in.

Depression can occur as a reaction to an acquired communication disorder such as aphasia resulting from a stroke. The complexity of not being able to communicate effectively while experiencing depression with the addition of the communication difficulties characteristic of depression will be challenging and distressing to the individuals and their family/carers. In contrast to depression, the term *mania* refers to an episode of very high or excited mood and is a feature of bipolar disorders, in which the episode of mania will contrast starkly with episodes of depression. In mania, the pressure of speech is often fast, sustained, and difficult to interrupt, in contrast to communication during a depressive phase.

Schizophrenia is a severe psychiatric disorder where a psychosis is present. This means the person is not always able to differentiate his or her own thinking from consensual reality. This loss of contact with reality is referred to as *psychosis*. Symptoms in schizophrenia can be differentiated into positive and negative. This distinction refers to the negative symptoms such as apathy, poverty of speech, and anhedonia as a lessening of the person's usual activity (psychological deficits). The positive symptoms such as hallucinations, delusions, and disorganized thinking/thought disorder are viewed as additional activity the person experiences (psychological additions). Cognitive symptoms can include inattention, disorganized thinking, and memory difficulties. Speech, language, and communication abnormalities are common symptoms in schizophrenia and can severely impair the person's ability to communicate.

Thought disorder is a positive symptom of schizophrenia and is broadly defined as thinking that is not logical or coherent and shows a loss of contact with reality. This thinking is observed through the person's speech, language, and communication, where abnormalities of language are identified and make it difficult to understand the thoughts the person is expressing. Detailed descriptions of these abnormalities have been formulated, such as:

poverty of speech: a significant reduction in the amount of spontaneous talking the person engages in so the person will give little if any response to questions, not offer information, and any communication given is very brief;

pressure of speech: the person talks much more quickly than usual and is difficult to interrupt or slow down: Tangentially, it is difficult to see the relevance of what the person is saying;

distractible speech: the person may stop in the middle of what they are saying and pause or not continue or be distracted to talk about something else and perseveration;

persistent repetition of a word or topic or idea: The extract below is from a 43-year-old man with schizophrenia who replies to a question asking how he is feeling. The extract shows evidence of thought disorder and the language abnormalities described in schizophrenia including perseveration, repetition, distractible speech, and derailment.

er (. . .) for instance (. . .) you (. . .) you (. . .) you (. . .) get pain (. . .) er (. . .) er (. . .) for instance (. . .) heavy exercise for instance (. . .) er (. . .) there's black (. . .) er (. . . you get (. . .) er (. . .) for instance (. . .) with suffering from black depression in fact for seven years in fact er (. . .) you you not (*mumbles*) take somewhere over (. . .) er (*pause of 15 seconds*) headaches (*pause of 19 seconds*) headaches are (. . .) internal (. . .) er (. . .) internal (. . .) er (. . .) nurses I think come from in fact you can't leave out a set of nurses in fact make sure you operate on the scalp for instance it's impossible to (*mumbles*) (. *pause for 1 second*)

Communication in Common Child Psychiatric Disorders

Communication disorders are prevalent in the population of children with psychiatric disorders such as attention deficit hyperactivity disorder (ADHD) and conduct disorder. ADHD is one of the most common psychiatric disorders in children. Symptoms of ADHD are grouped into inattention, impulsivity, and hyperactivity with a distressing and significant impact on the children and their family/carers. Children and young people with conduct disorders engage in persistent patterns of antisocial behavior, again with consequences for their development and functioning. A wide range of speech, language, and communication difficulties are reported in children with ADHD and conduct disorder with a tendency to social communication difficulties rather than structural language difficulties, although many do also have structural language difficulties as well. Yet, to be consistently identified are specific profiles of communication ability and disorder that will be attributable to other contributing factors such as family and social background, school attendance, level of learning ability, and comorbidity with other developmental disorders. Selective mutism is a child psychiatric disorder where there is a persistent refusal to speak in certain situations such as school, compared with home, where the child talks as usual. The child experiences such high levels of anxiety about talking at school that they become unable to talk and rely on nonverbal communication or are not able to consistently communicate verbally or nonverbally. This makes learning in school and being part of the school community very challenging. Addressing the anxiety these children experience in talking is an important component of their management.

Longitudinal research confirms that children with developmental communication disorders such as specific language impairment are at greater risk of emotional and behavioral difficulties and psychiatric disorders in later childhood, adolescence, and adult life. Various developmental mechanisms have been proposed to explain this. One of these focuses on the psychosocial rejections, victimization, and lack of success some of these children experience, which lead to difficulties with psychosocial adjustment. Other mechanisms focus on a shared neurodevelopmental cause, explaining the cause of the communication disorder and the psychiatric disorder as well as shared common antecedents such as low intelligence and environmental deprivation. These are complex developmental interactions, and it is most helpful to consider how a developing child's communication ability contributes to their social and emotional competence rather than viewing language and communication as a specific causal factor in the development of psychiatric disorder.

Communication and People With Psychiatric Disorders

The diagnosis of and management of children and adults with psychiatric disorders involves assessment and review of their mental state as well as interviewing or asking patients to describe their symptoms. Hearing should be checked to make sure there are no new or long-standing hearing impairment that is impacting on communication, nor should it be assumed that the person can read. Communication between patient and professional is crucial in this interaction, and the professional needs to be mindful as to how to encourage effective communication in this exchange. For example, a person who is experiencing auditory hallucinations will be distracted, will take much longer to understand what they are being asked, and may need information to be repeated or presented in another way. Listening to the patient, minimizing misunderstandings, encouraging him or her to talk about their symptoms, and maximizing effective communication in a patient with thought disorder are all valuable communication skills. Good practice should aim to (a) speak slowly and calmly while making time to listen fully to any responses given, (b) reduce the person's anxiety so he or she feels comfortable to talk, (c) make careful use of open and closed questions, and (d) reflect back to the person rather than directing him/her. Accurate diagnosis and management of people with psychiatric disorders can be compromised by ineffective communication. For example, professionals have historically been encouraged not to collude with a patient in their psychosis; yet, recent research shows it can be beneficial for patients to talk about their psychosis. Effective communication with the person is essential to promote their full understanding of and engagement in their therapeutic intervention and management.

Judy Clegg

See also Attention Deficit/Hyperactivity Disorder (ADHD); Cognition; Depression; Diagnostic and Statistical Manual of Mental Disorders (DSM); Language Disorders in Children; Psychosocial Issues Associated With Communication Disorders; Selective Mutism

Further Readings

Brownlie, E., Bao, L., & Beitchman, J. H. (2016). Childhood language disorder and social anxiety in early adulthood. *Journal of Abnormal Child Psychology, 44* (6), 1061–1070.

Bryan, K., & Cummings, L. (2015). Psychiatric disorders and communication. In L. Cummings (Ed.), *The Cambridge handbook of communication disorders*. Cambridge, UK: Cambridge University Press.

Hawkins, E., Gathercole, S., Astle, D., The CALM Team, & Holmes, J. (2016). Language problems and ADHD symptoms: How specific are the links? *Brain Sciences, 6*(4), 50.

Salmon, K., O'Kearney, R., Reese, E., & Fortune, C. A. (2016). The role of language skill in child psychopathology: Implications for intervention in the early years. *Clinical Child and Family Psychological Review, 19*, 352.

Psychoacoustics

Psychoacoustics is a branch of psychophysics that studies auditory perception. From its inception, psychoacoustics has been a multidisciplinary field that is closely related to acoustics, audiology, biophysics, cognitive psychology, neuroscience, and signal processing.

Most psychoacoustic studies gain insights about auditory perception by conducting behavioral experiments. In a typical psychoacoustic experiment, acoustic stimuli are presented to human subjects and the subjects are instructed to perform a behavioral task and generate responses accordingly. For example, in order to study the subject's hearing sensitivity at a certain frequency, a pure tone at this frequency could be presented to the subject, and the subject's task is to indicate whether the pure-tone stimulus is audible by either raising his or her hand or pressing a corresponding button. This way, the level of the pure tone could be related to a response probability, which reflects the subject's hearing sensitivity.

Knowledge gained from psychoacoustics has been widely adopted in many hearing-related applications. Psychoacoustic principles contributed to the creation of surround-sound technology that is used to create virtual sound environments during movies. Most digital audio files are coded with the help of psychoacoustic models, so that the parts of the original audio signals that are inaudible to human listeners would not occupy storage space. Manufacturers of home appliances often rely on psychoacoustics, so that sounds emitted from their products would achieve a desirable quality.

The field of audiology has a deep connection to psychoacoustics. Behavioral audiometric testing uses many experimental techniques developed in psychoacoustics. Psychoacoustics also directly impacted the development of both analog and digital hearing aids.

Hearing Sensitivity

The human auditory system is very sensitive to acoustic stimuli. The sound pressure level (SPL) required for a stimulus to be audible to a listener is the listener's absolute threshold for the stimulus. Lower absolute thresholds indicate greater hearing sensitivity.

To describe a listener's hearing sensitivity, it is common to measure the absolute threshold for pure tones (also called hearing threshold) as a function of frequency. This function is often called minimum audible curve. In the free field, normal-hearing human listeners are sensitive to pure tones between 1 kHz and 4 kHz. The absolute threshold in this frequency range is close to 0 dB SPL. The lowest threshold in the minimum audible curve could be found at approximately 3–4 kHz, associated with the acoustic resonance of the outer ear. Above 4 kHz, the absolute threshold rises quickly as frequency increases, which sets an upper limit to the audible frequency range at about 20 kHz. Below 1 kHz, the absolute threshold rises gradually with decreasing frequency, forming a lower frequency limit at about 20 Hz.

Besides frequency, the absolute threshold also depends on the duration of the stimulus. For pure tones, the absolute threshold decreases by 3 dB for every doubling of duration, until the duration reaches approximately 500 ms. Beyond 500 ms, further increases in duration do not affect threshold.

Loudness and Dynamic Range of Hearing

When presented above the absolute threshold, a sound stimulus tends to give rise to a loudness percept. Generally speaking, stimuli with higher sound pressure levels are perceived as louder. This relationship between sound pressure level and loudness can be described by Stevens' power law. According to Stevens' power law, every 10 dB of increase in sound pressure level approximately corresponds to a doubling of loudness.

Loudness can be quantified using the unit *sone*. One sone corresponds to the loudness of a 40 dB SPL, 1 kHz pure tone. In many applications, the interest is to quantify the relative loudness between two stimuli rather than to measure the loudness per se. For such situations, loudness level is often used. The unit for loudness level is *phon*. A loudness level of 40 phon means the stimulus is equally loud as a 40 dB SPL, 1 kHz pure tone. As the frequency of a pure tone varies, the sound pressure level associated with a certain loudness level would vary. The function describing this relationship is called equal-loudness-level contour, or simply equal-loudness contour. The shape of the equal-loudness-level contour follows that of the minimum audible curve. That is, a pure tone of very low (e.g., < 100 Hz) or very high (e.g., > 8000 Hz) frequency would require a higher sound pressure to reach the same loudness level compared to a 1 kHz tone.

When the sound pressure level exceeds a certain criterion, listeners would start to experience discomfort, and the criterion level is called the loudness discomfort level. For a certain frequency, the range of sound pressure level from the absolute level to the loudness discomfort level defines the dynamic range of hearing. Between 1 kHz and 4 kHz, the dynamic range of hearing is approximately 120 dB.

Although the dynamic range of hearing is very broad, the auditory system is able to achieve very fine resolution in sound intensity. The minimum difference in sound pressure level required to discriminate two pure-tone stimuli, or the intensity discrimination threshold, is between 0.5 dB and 2 dB throughout the dynamic range of hearing.

Frequency Selectivity and Masking

One fundamental aspect of auditory perception is frequency selectivity, which means that the auditory system can process sounds of different frequencies separately. Frequency selectivity of the auditory system is closely related to the masking phenomenon.

Masking refers to the phenomenon that the detection threshold of a target sound is elevated by the presence of another masker sound. For a pure-tone target, the masking effect is greater when the masker is closer to the target frequency. On the other hand, when the masker is distant from the target frequency, little masking effect would be observed. This can be well explained by the power spectrum model of masking, which assumes that the detection is made through a band-pass filter centered at the target frequency. The target is detected when the signal-to-noise ratio at the output of the filter exceeds a certain criterion.

This hypothetical filter is called the auditory filter. Narrower auditory filters correspond to finer frequency resolution. The shape of the auditory filter can be experimentally estimated using masking experiment. It has been found that the bandwidth of the auditory filter increases with frequency. For frequencies above 1000 Hz, the auditory-filter bandwidth is approximately 11–13% of the filter's center frequency. The shape of the auditory filter is also dependent on sound intensity. At low levels, the filter is relatively symmetric, while at high levels the filter becomes asymmetric, usually associated with the emergence of a shallow low-frequency tail. These properties of the auditory filter resemble the tuning property of the cochlea; therefore, frequency selectivity of the auditory system is mainly governed by the physiology of the peripheral auditory system.

Temporal Processing

The auditory system is capable of handling fast-varying acoustic signals. One of the well-studied approaches to assess temporal acuity of the auditory system is to estimate listeners' ability to detect the presence of a brief silent gap in a continuous carrier sound. For broadband noise carriers, listeners can detect gaps as short as 2–3 ms. For pure-tone carrier, 6–8 ms is required to detect the gap, except for very low frequencies or very low intensities.

Another approach to assess temporal acuity is to impose amplitude modulation on a carrier sound and have the listener detect the presence of the amplitude modulation. For sinusoidal modulators, as the modulation rate increases the listener's ability to detect the amplitude modulation degrades, exhibiting a low-pass characteristics. The cut-off frequency of this low-pass shape is typically between 50 Hz and 150 Hz.

The limited ability to detect very short gaps and very fast amplitude modulation is mainly due to the sluggishness of the central auditory nervous system, which can be effectively modeled as a temporal integrator. The temporal integrator integrates envelope fluctuations within a sliding time window. This process smoothens the stimulus envelope, making gap detection more difficult when the gap duration is shorter than the duration of the temporal integrator. Similarly, high-rate amplitude modulation would be more difficult to detect when the envelope of the amplitude-modulated stimulus fluctuates at a faster time scale compared to the duration of the integration window.

Pitch

Pitch is a perceptual property of sounds. Listeners can often rank-order pure tones from "low" to "high" in terms of their pitch. This provides a basis for the perception of musical melodies.

For pure tones, lower frequencies correspond to lower pitch percept. It has been hypothesized that the pitch perception for pure tones is governed by the tonotopic organization of the auditory periphery. That is, the pitch of a tone may be related to its corresponding location along the length of the cochlea. The above hypothesis is called the place coding theory of pitch perception.

However, the place coding theory cannot explain the observation that pitch perception is very weak or absent for frequencies above 4–5 kHz. When measuring the frequency difference needed to discriminate two pure tones of closely spaced frequencies, that is, difference limen for frequency, the resulting difference limen is about 0.1–0.3% across a wide frequency range, except that the different limen degrades sharply with increasing frequency for frequencies above 4–5 kHz. One explanation for this phenomenon is that the pitch of a tone is related to the periodicity of the tone's waveform, and the periodicity information is coded in the auditory nerve by synchronized firing patterns of action potentials. This ability to synchronously respond to the acoustic waveform is called phase-locking. At frequencies above 4–5 kHz, the phase-locking ability of the auditory nerve begins to degrade, which provides an explanation for the degraded difference limen for frequency observed for the same frequency region. The above hypothesis is the temporal coding theory of pitch perception. It is very likely that pitch perception for pure tones relies on both place and temporal coding mechanisms.

Complex sounds with multiple frequency components can also give rise to pitch percept if the sounds exhibit periodicity. Periodicity in the time domain is equivalent to a harmonic structure in the frequency domain, which means that all frequency components on the spectrum of a periodic stimulus are integer multiples of a common fundamental frequency. The pitch of the stimulus is determined by the fundamental frequency.

Binaural Hearing

Binaural hearing provides listeners with an acute ability to localize sound sources in space. To achieve this ability, the auditory system makes use of various acoustic cues.

When identifying horizontal sound source locations, the listener's two ears receive different acoustic inputs. When the sound source is on the left side of the listener, the sound wave would have to travel farther to reach the right ear compared to the left ear. Therefore, the acoustic signal received by the left ear leads that in the right ear, causing an interaural time difference. The auditory system is sensitive to the interaural time difference for stimuli at low frequencies. In addition, a sound source on the left side may also cause a higher sound pressure level in the left ear than the right ear, that is, an interaural level difference. Interaural level difference is only present when the wavelength is comparable or shorter than the distance between the two ears; therefore, it is a high-frequency cue.

Combining the interaural time difference and interaural-level difference, human listeners can achieve highly accurate sound localization. The minimum amount of angle difference between two sound sources required for a human listener to discriminate the two sources, that is, minimum audible angle, is as small as 1 degree when the sources are in front of the listener. The minimum audible angle increases as the source location moves to the side.

The vertical position (i.e., elevation) of a sound source is reflected in the spectra of the acoustic inputs received at the two ears. These spectral features are results of sound reflections from the listener's pinna, head, and torso and can be captured using the head-related transfer function.

Summary

Psychoacoustics aims to establish quantitative links between the acoustic properties of stimuli and perception. Psychoacoustic studies do not only provide descriptions of human listeners' basic hearing capability but also contribute to the understanding of the acoustical, physiological, and cognitive mechanisms underlying auditory perception.

Yi Shen

See also Binaural Hearing; Frequency Resolution; Loudness; Masking; Perception; Pitch; Sound Localization; Temporal Processing

Further Readings

Moore, B. C. (2012). *An introduction to the psychology of hearing.* Leiden, The Netherlands: Brill.

Plack, C. J. (2013). *The sense of hearing.* New York, NY: Routledge/Psychology Press.

Yost, W. A. (1994). *Fundamentals of hearing: An introduction.* Cambridge, MA Academic Press.

Psychogenic Voice Disorders

Many regard the larynx as the "valve of emotion" —the control valve that regulates the release of intense human emotions such as fear, anger, grief, and joy. The English language is replete with expressions describing the connection between voice and intense emotion. For instance, colloquialisms such as "I got all choked up," "I tried to scream, but nothing would come out," "My heart was in my throat," "I was so nervous my voice was shaking," and "I broke down in tears and couldn't speak" are just a few familiar examples. Because the human voice is the carrier of intense emotion, when it becomes disordered (in pitch, loudness, or quality) it is not infrequent for clinicians to offer psychological factors, emotional states, or inhibitory processes as primary causal mechanisms. This is true in the case of *psychogenic or functional* voice disorders, wherein no visible structural or neurological pathology of the larynx exists to explain the partial or complete voice loss. "Psychogenic" implies that the voice disorder is a manifestation of some *confirmed* psychological disequilibrium. It is believed that the larynx, by virtue of its neural connections to emotional centers within the brain, is vulnerable to excess or poorly regulated musculoskeletal tension arising from stress, conflict, fear, or emotional inhibition. Such dysregulated laryngeal muscle tension can interfere with normal voice and give rise to complete aphonia (i.e., whispered speech) or partial voice loss (dysphonia).

Psychogenic or functional voice disorders may account for more than 10% of cases referred to specialty voice clinics, occur predominantly in women, and commonly follow cold-like symptoms. In clinical circles, the terms *psychogenic* and *functional* voice disorder are often used interchangeably. The label "functional" suggests a voice problem of physiological function rather than anatomical structure. That is, the larynx is functioning abnormally despite displaying normal structure and vocal fold mobility. However, *functional* is commonly contrasted with *organic* and often carries the added meaning of psychogenic. Stress, emotion, and psychological conflict are frequently presumed to cause or exacerbate functional symptoms. Thus, a psychogenic voice disorder is roughly synonymous with a functional one, but has the advantage of stating unambiguously, after an exploration of its causes, that the voice disorder is a manifestation of one or more forms of psychological distress.

It is important to recognize that "psychogenic voice disorder" is not to be used as a de facto diagnosis for a voice problem of undetermined etiology. Rather, at least three criteria need to be satisfied before such a diagnosis is made: (1) symptom psychogenicity, (2) symptom incongruity, and

(3) symptom reversibility. *Symptom psychogenicity* refers to the finding that the voice disorder is logically linked in time of onset, course, and severity to an identifiable psychological antecedent, such as a stressful life event or interpersonal conflict. These interpersonal conflicts typically often involve someone important in the individual's family or work life and are believed to center around a conflict over speaking out or voicing one's genuine emotions or opinions. Such information is typically acquired through a psychosocial interview that aims to survey any possible sources of psychological distress or communication breakdown that might have preceded the onset of the voice disorder. *Symptom incongruity* refers to the observation that vocal symptoms are physiologically incompatible with existing or suspected disease, are internally inconsistent, and are incongruent with other speech and language characteristics. A frequently cited example of symptom incongruity is complete aphonia (whispered speech) in a patient who also demonstrates a normal throat clear, cough, laugh, or hum, whereby the presence of such normal nonspeech vocalization is clearly at odds with assumptions regarding the neural integrity and function of the larynx. Finally, *symptom reversibility* refers to the complete, sustained alleviation of the voice disorder with brief voice therapy (usually within a couple of treatment sessions) or through psychological abreaction. Furthermore, maintenance of voice improvement following treatment requires no compensatory effort on the part of the patient. Psychogenic dysphonia should be *suspected* when strong evidence exists for symptom incongruity and symptom psychogenicity, but *confirmed only* when there is convincing evidence of symptom reversibility.

Psychological Factors in Psychogenic Voice Disorders

A wide array of psychopathological processes contributing to voice symptom formation in psychogenic voice disorders has been proposed. Historically, the prevailing psychological explanation for psychogenic dysphonia is conversion disorder. Conversion disorder involves unexplained symptoms or deficits affecting voluntary motor or sensory function that suggest a neurological or other general medical condition. In conversion voice disorders, psychological factors are judged to be associated with the voice symptoms because conflicts or other stressors preceded the onset of the dysphonia. In short, patients are believed to *convert* psychological distress into a voice symptom. The voice loss, whether partial or complete, is also often interpreted to have symbolic meaning. That is, the voice loss symbolizes the breakdown in communication between patients and someone important in their life or their inability to express particular feelings. In some cases, primary or secondary gains are thought to play an important role in maintaining and reinforcing the conversion disorder. Within the theory of conversion, primary gain refers to anxiety avoidance accomplished by preventing the psychological conflict from entering conscious awareness. Secondary gain refers to the avoidance of an undesirable activity/responsibility and the extra attention or support conferred to the patient.

When the larynx is involved, the voice disorder is referred to as conversion dysphonia or aphonia. In *aphonia*, patients typically lose their voice suddenly and completely and articulate in a whisper. The whisper may be pure, harsh, or sharp, with occasional high-pitched squeaklike traces of voicing. In *dysphonia*, some phonation is preserved, but disturbed in quality, pitch, or loudness. Myriad dysphonia types are encountered including hoarseness (with or without strain), breathiness, and high-pitched falsetto, as well as voice and pitch breaks that vary in consistency and severity.

While conversion disorder has enjoyed a relatively prominent place as an explanatory construct for psychogenic voice disorders, certain authorities have recently argued that there is actually little research evidence to support conversion as the central explanation. Instead, a number of alternative models to account for psychogenic voice loss have been offered. In these models, the exquisite sensitivity of the larynx to emotion and the related adverse effects of laryngeal musculoskeletal tension are highlighted. These explanatory models emphasize both the inhibitory effects of excess laryngeal muscle tension on voice production and the role of life stress or interpersonal difficulties that stimulate internal conflict (particularly in situations involving conflict over self-expression or speaking out). This inner conflict or stress (especially in individuals who have difficulty expressing emotions or opinions) becomes channeled into musculoskeletal tension in or around the larynx, which physically inhibits voice production. Unlike in conversion disorder, these theories discount the role of primary and secondary gain, and instead they emphasize the inhibitory effects of laryngeal muscle tension on voice production.

In a similar vein, other researchers have proposed a theory that links personality to the development of functional dysphonia (FD). The trait theory of FD shares the theme of inhibitory laryngeal behavior, but it attributes this muscularly inhibited voice production to specific personality typologies. In brief, the authors speculate that the combination of personality traits such as introversion and neuroticism (trait anxiety) leads to predictable and conditioned laryngeal inhibitory responses to certain environmental signals/cues. For instance, when undesirable punishing or frustrating outcomes have been paired with previous attempts to speak out, this can lead to muscularly inhibited voice. The authors argue that this conflict between laryngeal inhibition and activation (that has its origins in personality and nervous system functioning) results in elevated laryngeal tension states and can give rise to incomplete or disordered vocalization in an otherwise structurally and neurologically intact larynx. Thus, the trait theory highlights the role of specific personality traits (introversion and neuroticism) that when combined may predispose an individual to functional voice loss.

In an investigation designed to test the trait theory and assess whether personality factors play a role in common voice disorders, researchers compared a vocally normal control group and four groups with voice disorders—functional dysphonia (FD), vocal nodules (VN), spasmodic dysphonia (SD), and unilateral vocal fold paralysis (UVFP)—using the Eysenck Personality Questionnaire (EPQ). The EPQ generates scores for the personality superfactors extraversion (E) and neuroticism (N). Extraversion involves the willingness to engage and confront the environment, including the social environment. Extraverts (i.e., high E) tend to be dominant, sociable, and active, whereas introverts (i.e., low E) tend to be quiet, unsociable, passive, and careful. Neuroticism, the second personality dimension, can be likened to emotionality and is related to anxious, depressed, tense, and emotional characteristics. High N individuals tend to be emotionally unstable, worried, and highly reactive to environmental stimuli. The results showed that distinct personality characteristics were present within the FD and VN groups, and were noticeably absent in the other groups. Comparisons revealed that the majority of FD and VN subjects were classified as introverts and extraverts, respectively. As compared to the other groups, the FD group scored significantly higher on the neuroticism dimension thereby providing robust evidence to support the role of elevated N in FD development. Comparisons involving the SD, UVFP, and control subjects did not identify any consistent personality differences. On the whole, these differences in personality were compatible with the predictions of the trait theory. The authors concluded that the results largely support the contention that individuals with certain personality traits may be susceptible to developing FD. More recently, researchers have shown that in vocally normal speakers, specific personality traits such as introversion (and constraint) appear to lead to increased laryngeal muscle tension states in response to stressful conditions, thereby supporting the potential role of personality and stress in the development of FD.

Finally, some researchers have observed that patients with psychogenic dysphonia and aphonia often have an abnormally high number of reported allergy/asthma/upper respiratory infection symptoms, suggesting a link between psychological factors and respiratory and phonatory disorders. They speculated that organic changes in the larynx, pharynx, and nose facilitate the appearance of a functional voice problem; that is, they direct the somatization of psychodynamic conflict. Similarly, it has been asserted that a relatively minor organic change in the larynx such as swelling, infection, or laryngitis may trigger muscle misuse of the voice, particularly if the individual is exceedingly anxious regarding his or her voice or health. The same authors proposed that anticipation of poor voice production in hypochondriacal, dependent or obsessive-compulsive individuals leads to excessive vigilance over sensations arising from the throat (larynx) and respiratory system that may lead to altered voice production.

While numerous theories have been offered to explain psychogenic voice loss, the precise mechanism underlying such psychologically based disorders remains unclear. Research evidence to support the various psychological mechanisms offered is limited. The empirical literature evaluating the voice disorder–psychology relationship in psychogenic voice disorders is characterized by a lack of consensus regarding the frequency and degree of specific personality traits, conversion disorder, psychopathological symptoms such as depression and anxiety, and the salience of stressful life events including interpersonal conflict.

Part of the variability in findings is likely related to the absence of strict inclusion and exclusion criteria related to the patients included in many studies. For instance, confusion surrounds the diagnostic category of "functional dysphonia," because it may include an array of medically unexplained voice disorders: psychogenic, conversion, hysterical, tension-fatigue syndrome, hyperkinetic, muscle misuse, or primary muscle tension dysphonia. Although each diagnostic label implies some degree of etiologic heterogeneity, whether these disorders are qualitatively different and etiologically distinct remains unclear. When applied clinically or in research, these various labels often reflect clinician supposition, bias, or preference. Voice disorder taxonomies have yet to be adequately operationalized; consequently, diagnostic categories such as psychogenic voice disorder, functional dysphonia, or primary muscle tension dysphonia often lack clear thresholds or discrete boundaries to determine patient inclusion or exclusion. This diagnostic imprecision combined with methodological inadequacies may contribute to some of the conflicting results regarding the presence and degree of emotional maladjustment in patients with so-called psychogenic or functional voice disorders.

Despite these methodological shortcomings, several general patterns have emerged from the research literature regarding functional voice disorders with a trend toward elevated levels of (a) state and trait anxiety, (b) depression, (c) somatic preoccupation/complaints, and (d) introversion in patients with functional/psychogenic voice disorders. Patients have been described as inhibited, stress reactive, socially anxious, and nonassertive and with a tendency toward restraint. However, further research is needed to better understand the precise mechanism contributing to psychogenic voice loss.

Management of Psychogenic Voice Disorders

Despite uncertainty surrounding exact causal mechanisms, there is ample evidence in the clinical voice literature that direct symptomatic voice therapy for psychogenic voice disorders can often result in remarkable voice improvement. Symptomatic voice therapy involves using voice facilitating techniques aimed at correcting the voice symptoms (i.e., restoring normal voice) without necessarily targeting the psychological adjustment issues that ostensibly underlie the voice disorder. Before symptomatic therapy is undertaken, the patient is typically reassured regarding the absence of any structural laryngeal pathology and some discussion surrounding the untoward effects of excess or dysregulated muscle tension on voice production, and its possible link to stress, situational conflicts, or other psychological precursors may be undertaken. Because laryngeal muscle tension is frequently offered as the proximal cause of the psychogenic voice disorder, many voice therapies that aim to reduce, re-coordinate, or rebalance such muscle tension are employed including yawn-sigh, resonant voice therapy, Accent Method, visual and electromyographic biofeedback, stretch and flow, and progressive relaxation. Prolonged hypercontraction of the paralaryngeal muscles is often associated with elevation of the larynx and associated structures, with accompanying pain and discomfort (when the circumlaryngeal region is palpated). Thus, a number of clinicians have described manual circumlaryngeal techniques to determine the presence and degree of paralaryngeal musculoskeletal tension, as well as methods to relieve such tension during the assessment and management. These manual techniques, including circumlaryngeal massage, have been reported to be particularly effective in the management of functional/psychogenic voice disorders and are described in detail in a related entry (see Manual Circumlaryngeal Therapy).

In addition to excess laryngeal musculoskeletal tension, some patients with psychogenic dysphonia and aphonia appear to have lost kinesthetic awareness and volitional control over voice production for speech purposes. Yet, they display normal voicing for vegetative or nonspeech acts (i.e., symptom incongruity). For instance, some aphonic and severely dysphonic patients may be able to clear their throat, grunt, cough, sigh, gargle, laugh, or hum or produce a high-pitched squeak with normal or near normal voice quality. In symptomatic therapy, then, the patient is asked to produce such vocal behaviors. The goal of these voice maneuvers is to elicit even a brief trace of clearer voice so that it may be shaped toward normal quality or extended to longer utterances. If established, the restored voice is typically maintained without much compensatory effort (i.e., symptom reversibility) and may improve further during conversation. Depending upon the clinicians' beliefs/biases regarding the importance of psychological factors in the development of the disorder, they may explore possible psychological antecedents once the voice has returned to normal.

Certainly, symptomatic therapy for psychogenic voice disorders can produce rapid improvement; however, voice therapy can also be a challenging and protracted experience. Because there are few studies directly comparing the effectiveness of specific therapy techniques, not much is known about whether one voice therapy approach for psychogenic aphonia/dysphonia is superior to another. In some particularly recalcitrant patients, novel approaches involving bathing the vocal folds in lidocaine (a substance that reduces sensation within the larynx) have been reported to provide relief in patients who had previously failed traditional voice therapy.

The long-term effectiveness of direct voice therapy for psychogenic voice disorders also has not been rigorously evaluated. Of the few investigations that exist, the results regarding the stability of voice improvement following therapy are mixed. Following direct symptomatic voice therapy, it is important to recognize that only the voice symptom has been eliminated, not the underlying cause of the disturbance itself. Therefore, the nature of precipitating and perpetuating factors, including possible psychological dysfunction, needs to be better understood. If the situational, emotional, or personality features that originally contributed to the voice disorder remain unchanged following behavioral treatment, it is logical to expect that such persistent factors would increase the probability/risk of future recurrences. Therefore, in some cases, posttreatment referral to a psychologist may be advised to achieve more enduring improvements in the patient's emotional/life adjustment and voice function. This is especially appropriate in cases where dysphonic relapses are frequent and protracted. In this regard, cognitive behavioral therapy (CBT) approaches appear to have the most empirical support. CBT also offers the patient training in conflict resolution and assertiveness skills, which may be deficient in this patient population.

Summary

Psychogenic voice disorders provide compelling evidence of the connection between mind and body. Perhaps more than any other structure in the body, the larynx is a site for tension arising from stress, emotional inhibition, fear/threat, communication breakdown, and certain personality typologies. Direct symptomatic therapy for psychogenic voice disorders can often restore normal voice. There remains, however, much to be learned regarding the underlying bases of these disorders, the long-term fate of direct therapeutic interventions, and the role of supportive psychological counseling.

Nelson Roy

See also Anatomy of the Human Larynx; Manual Circumlaryngeal Therapy; Muscle Tension Dysphonia (MTD); Voice Disorders; Voice Therapy

Further Readings

Butcher, P., Elias, A., & Raven, R. (1993). *Psychogenic voice disorders and cognitive-behaviour therapy*. San Diego, CA: Singular Publishing.

Morrison, M. D., & Rammage, L. A. (1993). Muscle misuse voice disorders: Description and classification. *Acta Oto-Laryngologica, 113*(3), 428–434. https://doi.org/10.3109/00016489309135839

Roy, N., & Bless, D. M. (2000). Personality traits and psychological factors in voice pathology: A foundation for future research. *Journal of Speech, Language, and Hearing Research, 43*(3), 737–748. https://doi.org/10.1044/jslhr.4303.737

Roy, N., & Bless, D. M. (2000). Toward a theory of the dispositional bases of functional dysphonia and vocal nodules: Exploring the role of personality and emotional adjustment. In R. D. Kent & M. J. Ball (Eds.), *Voice quality measurement* (pp. 461–480). San Diego, CA: Singular Publishing.

PSYCHOLINGUISTICS

Psycholinguistics is the use of psychology to understand linguistics. It is an intriguing area of study because it investigates how language becomes a tool for cognitive functions such as thinking, problem solving, and remembering. It is also a major area of research in neurolinguistics that studies brain functioning and language. Psycholinguistics is important for human communication sciences and disorders because it connects psychological functioning and brain behavior, linguistics, and the communicative use of language in special populations. Theories that drive and are transformed by psycholinguistic research provide ways to understand normal language and cognitive development as well as developmentally different and acquired disorders of language and thought. Psycholinguistics contributes through research to the social and neurobehavioral sciences and is used by therapists such as speech–language pathologists during assessment and intervention for persons of all ages.

This entry summarizes key elements of psycholinguistics beginning with its historical foundations in philosophy, psychology, linguistics, and speech–language pathology. Links between the emergence of clinically useful applications of theory and research, such as psychometrics and child language analyses, inform how psycholinguistics was and is used by speech–language pathologists in assessment and intervention.

Historical Foundations

Psycholinguistics grew from ideas and research in several scholarly fields over the course of the 20th century, including philosophy, linguistics, psychology, as well as speech–language pathology. Philosophers study language in order to understand values, beliefs, and logic, whereas linguists study and document languages to uncover the rules used to organize elements of sounds, words, sentences, and texts that preserve and share meaning among people. Whereas linguists are interested in language, psychologists are interested in language as a phenomenon that influences social interactions and as a stimulus that leads to mental, cognitive, and behavioral responses to sensation and perception. Speech–language pathologists use and expand findings from linguistics and psychology to better understand and treat the cognitive linguistic–communicative challenges faced by special populations. Overviews of selected topics addressed by these fields provide a time line for the emergence of psycholinguistics as an interdisciplinary behavioral science.

Philosophy

Studies related to psycholinguistics began with philosophical questions that explored the relationship between language and human reasoning. The writings of Wilhelm Wundt, a German philosopher intensely interested in language and the internal states of individuals, shaped psychological theory at the turn of the 20th century. He used observation, experiments, and logical argument to demonstrate that only humans could develop language, which in turn shaped intellect. This resulted in debates and public lectures across fields of scholarship that touched on the topic with regard to humankind and nonhuman animals. Wundt's contributions were the beginning of a psychological rather than philosophical approach to the topic of language and the mind.

Linguistics

Like philosophy, linguistics is a very old field of study. Linguists have studied and continue to study the languages of the world whether they are gestural, visual, or spoken. Their goal is to uncover what is systematic about each language. Rather than begin with a question such as is language innate in humankind or learned, they dissect what is said and/or written to find the rules that govern the construction and use of languages. Comparing and contrasting languages has helped them devise a linguistic tree, whereby the elements of sounds, words, parts of words, and use of words illustrate which languages are related to each other.

Among the most influential linguists in modern times is Noam Chomsky (b. 1928). With a specialty in syntax, he was hired by the Massachusetts Institute of Technology as they began to develop computer languages. Chomsky was instrumental in providing a theoretical framework that credited both an innate biological mechanism in humans and universal linguistic rules that could apply to language learning. This was expanded in response to changes in the field of linguistics to include aspects of thinking and human interaction rather than just syntax. Although Chomsky began his career as a linguist, his writings have bridged psychology, philosophy, and artificial languages over his long and productive career.

Child Language

Child language development is a specialty within linguistics. Just as linguists found rules and compared languages spoken by adults using these, some scholars took interest in child language development because it was not fully formed. Pivotal questions included whether child language was its own language or a miniature version of adult language, whether child language follows the same patterns of development across languages, and whether the ability to learn language is innate or driven by the use of language within cultures. Roger Brown conducted studies on child language acquisition at Harvard University. His research established an ordinal sequence of early morphosyntactic development in young children that remains in use today. Other child language researchers, such as Susan Ervin-Tripp and Dan Slobin at the University of California-Berkeley, challenged Noam Chomsky's conclusions about how underlying and universal rules are used by humans to learn and organize language. They contended that Chomsky's morphosyntactic theories did not explain child language acquisition. Their case studies and longitudinal data collections contributed to the semantic revolution that opened up and propelled the study of psycholinguistics forward.

Psychology

In psychology, two conflicting perspectives on language and the mind contributed to the emerging field of psycholinguistics. John B. Watson, an American psychologist in the early 1900s, was opposed to Wundt's methods and conclusions about language and consciousness. He believed that the conclusions reached in psychological studies should be based on observable and objective data obtained through controlled experiments. His writings and research set the foundation for American behaviorism, which was popularized by B. F. Skinner. Skinner's prolific writings, including a book written to illustrate how language is a learned behavior, established behavioral approaches as part of mainstream psychology by the mid-20th century.

In contrast to behaviorism, other scholars interested in child behavior were using nonexperimental approaches to study language and mind. Edward Sapir, best known for his work in cultural anthropology, used descriptive linguistics to study language and cultures. His methods were social rather than experimental and useful to researchers studying social contributions to language. Jerome Bruner was a cognitive psychologist influenced by the work of Jean Piaget and Lev Vygotsky. His research with children, child learning, and social context established a theoretical base and methods for examining language and thinking in the context of culture.

Speech–Language Pathology

The field of speech–language pathology has roots in psychology, linguistics, and communication. Whereas linguists are interested in language and psychologists are interested in mental, cognitive, and behavioral responses to sensation and perception, speech–language pathologists seek to better understand and treat the cognitive linguistic–communicative challenges faced by special populations.

Speech–language pathology was primarily known as a *therapeutic profession* at the time psycholinguistics was emerging as a scholarly field. Students were trained to be speech therapists. They provided therapy for voice, stuttering, and articulation disorders; taught speech and language to individuals who were deaf or who were blind as well as deaf; helped individuals with cognitive differences such as intellectual disability gain functional communication skills; and worked with individuals after stroke or head trauma so that they could regain speech and language. Speech pathology scholars used theories from and built upon research in psychology, linguistics, aphasiology, and communication, each of which were part of the body of knowledge that was becoming psycholinguistics.

Situating critical questions from each field in the context of application helped speech–language pathology enlarge theories and perspectives on language development and use, cognition, and neurobiological processing. At the same time, contributions from speech–language pathology provide a distinct focus for in-depth investigations of studies being pursued by linguists seeking to understand child language development and psychologists seeking to isolate the way the brain processes language. Examples of this are reflected in the assessment tools and interventions used by speech–language pathologists in the mid- to late 1900s.

Assessment and Intervention

The integration of psycholinguistic theory into clinical practice happened naturally since speech–language pathology faculty working on critical issues in psycholinguistics had clinical populations available to them. Key examples reflect how psycholinguistic research led to discrete diagnostic and intervention tools for three clinical populations: child language, language and learning, and acquired disorders of language and cognition. A 20th-century history of assessment and intervention in these areas illustrates the links between linguistics, psychology, and speech–language pathology and serves to illustrate how clinical practices responded to theoretical changes with practical solutions.

Child Language

Both linguists and psychologists were working on specific theoretical problems from their own perspectives or from joint perspectives in the 1960s and 1970s. This was especially prevalent in the area of child language. The Stanford Child Language Research Forum, which has been meeting annually since 1967, provides the opportunity for scholars across interdisciplinary fields to talk, listen, and think together about child language. The interrelationship of topics was prevalent as psychologists investigated linguistic questions and linguists used psychology to explain language. Brian MacWhinney and Catherine Snow regularly attended these meetings and in 1984 gave a presentation on the development of a child language database. Researchers were asked to contribute language transcripts collected in their research studies to form an expansive pool available to all researchers. This collection of child language samples continued to grow in the 21st century and came to include dialects and languages other than English. Various linguistic analyses from application of *Brown's Stages* of syntactic and morphological development to turn-taking, examination of how mothers versus fathers talk to their children, and other communicative markers became research papers that in turn challenged and changed the field of child language.

Speech–language pathologists during this same time were increasingly assessing and providing intervention to younger children. Therapists were expected to determine the developmental language status of children as young as 2 years of age, and by the 1990s, as early as 10 months of age. Clinical questions and the planning of interventions flowed from the linguistic and psychological studies of mid-20th-century research. One such instrument was the MacArthur-Bates Communicative Development Inventories, which can be used for children between the ages of 8 and 30 months. Input for development and field-testing included child language researchers, clinicians, and parents. Gesture, vocabulary items, functional uses of language, and morphosyntactic elements were included to capture linguistic changes that form the basis of assessment and guide intervention with young children. This assessment remains in use and has expanded to numerous world languages as an assessment instrument that is culturally and linguistically valid.

Language and Learning

Critical arguments about child language acquisition that moved psycholinguistics forward also became important to therapists working with preschool children who were not talking and school-age children with learning disabilities. Tests of intelligence as well as speech, language, and hearing were part of psychoeducational assessment. As a result, therapists including speech–language pathologists and psychologists needed assessment tools that could profile cognitive linguistic skills for intervention planning.

This shift in speech–language pathology is reflected in the 1968 publication of a book on preschool language and learning by Tina Bangs, director of the Speech and Hearing Center in Houston, TX. Her book built on changed perspectives about child language acquisition as well as an awareness of the growing field of learning disabilities. It addressed the importance of language, particularly early language development, for academic success. The assessment and curriculum were constructed using key linguistic—language-based disorders of speaking, listening, reading and writing—and psychological aspects of development related to learning such as memory, attention, and perception. While assessment results were reported by maturational age, much like the Stanford-Binet Test of Intelligence, qualitative descriptions of language including reading and writing as they relate to attention, memory, and perception were included and related to classroom learning situations.

Speech–language pathologists serving school-age children in the United States required definitive and predictive evaluation tools to document disability and change. The goal was to have batteries of tests that were psychometrically constructed so an individual's scores could be reliably compared with a valid set of normative scores, much like the Wechsler Intelligence Tests. For intervention purposes, they wanted such tests to provide patterns of strengths and weaknesses so therapy could be individualized and yield measures of change. The Illinois Test of Psycholinguistic Abilities is an example of such a test; it was used extensively for nearly 30 years as a diagnostic instrument for children with language, learning, and cognitive differences. Samuel Kirk, a psychologist by training who specialized in special education, developed the test with colleagues as a tool for delineating specific difficulties children might have with communication, be it spoken or written, and cognitive abilities that support such communication. Rather than focusing on word knowledge, verbal subtests require children to manipulate language. Subtests that focus on perception, sequencing, and organization of visual and auditory materials were designed to target nonlinguistic aspects of learning. Although the name remained the same, the test was revised in 2001 to assess only spoken and written language, perhaps reflecting shifts in the clinical utility of psycholinguistic testing within the field of speech–language pathology.

Acquired Disorders of Language and Cognition

David Wechsler, a psychologist who first began a psychometric approach to intelligence testing in the 1930s, had constructed a series of intelligence tests for children and adults by the 1950s. Psychometrically normed verbal and nonverbal scales included tasks with psycholinguist parameters such as processing speed, spatial abilities, word knowledge, and problem solving. This allowed results for both normal and individuals with cognitive differences to be compared across subtests and with other psychometrically normed tests in fields such as psychology and speech–language pathology. His tests became a standard part of psychological assessment, neuropsychological assessment, and rehabilitation planning. While this test could identify differences in cognitive functions, it was less effective for intervention planning since even the nonverbal subtests incorporated language.

Bruce Porch, a speech–language pathologist working in a countrywide hospital system, developed a test, the Porch Index of Communicative Ability, that yielded descriptive results about communication rather than an IQ score. His goal was to use a multidimensional scoring system that was reliable and valid and would form the basis for therapeutic planning. Reading, writing, listening, and speaking were assessed with the same 10 items over various levels of difficulty, which gave a profile of abilities that involved linguistic and psychological manipulation. Performance on the test could be used to decide the level at which to begin intervention. Subsequent administrations measured change in response to therapy. While clinically useful, results could not be profiled with normative tests such as the Wechsler Adult Intelligence Test. Edith Kaplan layered the descriptive Boston approach to neuropsychological assessment onto the Wechsler Adult Intelligence Test as an alternative to the Porch Index of Communicative Ability.

Other applications of psycholinguistics assessment that can be used as the foundation for intervention have emerged over the last 20 years in speech–language pathology. In the 1990s, the Psycholinguistic Assessment of Language Processing in Aphasia was introduced as a psychometrically designed assessment of auditory processing, semantics, language comprehension, and reading. The instrument grew out of research that informed clinical practice. While not all sections of the instrument are standardized, it is credited as being a clinically useful instrument for assessment of adults with language impairment secondary to stroke or traumatic brain injury. A review of the assessment instrument in 2010 suggested that it remains a useful clinical tool that can be adapted for international use.

Future Directions

By the turn of the 21st century, psycholinguistic research included volumes of studies that focused on pragmatics, second-language learning, special populations, computer languages, the brain and language, semiotics including music and cognition, and neurobehavioral research made possible by the increased availability of technology to image the brain's activity during language functioning. Advances such as these coupled with changes in the ways individuals function in everyday life will continue to expand research and application of psycholinguistics. As seen at the beginning of the movement, the challenges of living in more complex and technologically linked and dependent cultures will be reflected in theories and practices within linguistic, psychological, and speech–language pathology. Building on this, psycholinguistics has a long and rich history of development that is likely to continue for decades as new technologies become part of how humans live, communicate, and think. Speech–language pathology as a client-centered profession has contributed to and profited from research in psycholinguistics. This vital aspect of human functioning will continue to inform practices that serve the communicative needs of individuals from birth to death.

Fran Hagstrom

See also Diagnosis of Communication Disorders; Intelligence; Learning Disabilities; Linguistics

Further Readings

Anastasi, A., & Urbaina, S. (1997). *Psychological testing* (7th ed.). Boston, MA: Pearson.

Bangs, T. E. (1968). *Language and learning disorders of the pre-academic child.* Englewood Cliffs, NJ: Prentice-Hall.

Brown, R. (1973). *A first language.* Cambridge, MA: Harvard University Press.

Chomsky, N. (1972). *Language and the mind.* San Diego, CA: Harcourt Brace Jovanovich.

Fenson, L., Marchman, V. A., Thal, D. J., Dale, P. S., Reznick, J. S., & Bates, E. (2007). *MacArthur-Bates communicative development inventories: User's guide and technical manual* (2nd ed.). Baltimore, MD: Brookes.

Kay, J., Colthear M., & Lessor, R. (1992). *Psycholinguistic assessment of language processing in aphasia (PALPA): Auditory processing.* Mahwah, NJ: Erlbaum.

Levelt, W. J. M. (2013). *A history of psycholinguistics, the pre-chomskyan era.* New York, NY: Oxford University Press.

Loritz, D. (1999). *How the brain evolved language.* New York, NY: Oxford University Press.

Macwhinney, B., & Snow, C. E. (1990). The child language data exchange system: An update. *Journal of Child Language, 17,* 457–472.

Milberg, W. P., Hebben, N., & Kaplan, E. (2009). The Boston approach to neuropsychological assessment. In I. Grant & K. M. Adams (Eds.), *Neuropsychological assessment of neuropsychiatric and neuromedical disorders* (3rd ed., pp. 42–65). New York, NY: Oxford University Press.

Paraskevopoulos, J. N., & Kirk, S. A. (1969). *The development and psychometric characteristics of the revised Illinois test of psycholinguistic abilities.* Chicago: University of Illinois Press.

Porch, B. E. (1971). *Porch Index of Communicative Ability.* Palo Alto, CA: Consulting Psychologists Press.

Wechsler, D. (2008). *Wechsler Adult Intelligence Scale-fourth edition (WAIS-IV).* New York, NY: Pearson.

Psychological Stress and Speech Disorders

Psychological distress can be defined as an unpleasant condition that can have undesirable effects on a person's functioning, usually including symptoms that are worrying and unsettling, such as anger, irritability, confusion, elevated anxiety, and depressive mood, while a *disorder* is defined as a condition in which disruption occurs to typical physical or mental function. According to the American Speech-Language Hearing Association, a speech disorder occurs when a person is not able to speak correctly or fluently or has problems with his or her voice. This is opposed to a language disorder, where a person has trouble understanding others due, for instance, to neural damage following a stroke. A speech disorder therefore occurs when typical speech is disrupted. Speech disorders include disruption to articulation (e.g., phonological disorders), fluency (e.g., stuttering or cluttering), and voice (e.g., dysphonia). While psychological distress is not considered one of the core criteria in the definition of speech disorders, research since 2008 has revealed that a substantial proportion of older adolescents and adults who stutter, perhaps up to 40%, will have elevated levels of psychological distress resulting in substantially lowered quality of life and well-being. Research in this area has also demonstrated that a significant risk of developing a psychological disorder exists for people who stutter. For these reasons, this entry focuses on what is known about psychological distress associated with stuttering. It is important that this risk is recognized in society, so that people who stutter are aware they may need to take remedial action to address their distress, and that clinicians treating stuttering are aware of the risk so they can treat the distress or refer patients who stutter to a suitably qualified clinician.

Definition and Epidemiology of Stuttering

Stuttering (or stammering) can be defined as a disorder affecting the rhythm of speech, and while the person knows what he or she intends to say, the person cannot do so because he or she experiences involuntary, repetitive prolongations or blocking of sounds. Developmental stuttering is not a rare condition, occurring in all cultures. The prevalence of stuttering is around 1% of the population, while the risk (incidence) of stuttering has been found to vary between 3% and 5%. It is usually first diagnosed in children around the ages of 2–5 when speech is developing; however, stuttering occurs across all age groups, with a 4:1 ratio of males to females by adulthood. Stuttering has also been found to have a genetic cause. Stuttering usually runs in families, and if an identical twin stutters, there is a much higher risk that both twins will stutter compared to nonidentical twins (about 60% to 20%, respectively). Exceptions to a developmental diagnosis include acquired stuttering, that is, those who have a sudden onset of stuttering in adulthood, for example, as a result of injury to the brain in the speech areas.

Psychological Theories of Stuttering

Mid-20th-century theories concerning the causes of stuttering contended it was psychogenic in origin, that is, stuttering was caused by psychological distress. Freudian theory suggested the distress was caused by dysfunctional unconscious psychosexual processes resulting in frustration and anxiety, due to repressed unresolved needs during childhood. Theories in the mid- to late 20th century abandoned a Freudian view of stuttering and argued that stuttering was caused by learned fears leading to elevated anxiety. For example, stuttering was believed to be associated with a fear of speaking due to role conflicts experienced in childhood. This fear of speaking led to an anticipatory struggle, in which the person who stuttered became highly worried (i.e., anticipating trouble and experiencing embarrassment, frustration, anger, and so on) about the consequences of stuttering (i.e., failure to be fluent) and struggled to avoid it. The worry and internal struggle led to elevated anxiety that caused the speech system to break down, resulting in stuttering. Other learning theories argued stuttering was a behavior acquired through classical or operant conditioning. Theories in the late 20th century suggested it is the temperament or personality of the person that could cause the stuttering. However, there is no convincing evidence available to support a theory that stuttering is caused by psychogenic or learning dynamics.

Multifactorial Theories of Stuttering

Theories in the early 21st century suggest stuttering has a multifactorial cause. Stuttering most likely occurs when the many demands associated with speaking fluently exceed the cognitive, linguistic, motor, and emotional capacity to speak fluently. Demands include many factors, such as an inherited predisposition to stutter, gender, age, rate, and complexity of speech (e.g., reading vs. spontaneous talking, talking on the telephone, giving a speech); context of the social interaction; expectations of control (i.e., self-efficacy); anxiety and mood status; and presence of neurophysiological abnormalities. All these factors contribute to a complex equation that explains the etiology of stuttering.

Anxiety in the Stuttering Moment Versus Chronic Levels of Psychological Distress

Importantly, it is believed that the struggle and distress often associated with the stuttering moment may, over time, in some individuals, result in elevated psychological distress, and that this psychological distress is a result of the impairment imposed by a chronic speech disorder. The emotions involve complex psychophysiological reactions to anticipated threats such as stuttering. This is normal, as fear encourages survival-based behavior, enhancing adaptive coping. However, fear can also disrupt functioning. In a stuttering event, fear of speaking can overload the capacity of the speech system and lower the speech processing capacity. It is entirely normal to experience fear when a person is stuttering in a context where he or she could be embarrassed or where it is believed that it is important he or she be fluent. Increased fear of speaking will often increase the severity of the stuttering moment. Fear and anxiety will generally disrupt adaptive coping in a wide variety of situations. People who stutter will experience psychological distress when they stutter; however, most will not develop chronically elevated psychological distress. Conversely, others who become distressed and anxious during the stuttering moment will go on to develop elevated levels of psychological distress that will become chronic with time.

Psychological Distress in Children Who Stutter

Younger children who stutter have been shown to be more likely to have typical levels of psychological distress; however, by late adolescence, psychological distress has been shown to be significantly elevated compared to similar aged people who do not stutter. Fears associated with verbal communication are significantly elevated in children who stutter (aged around 9 years) compared to children who do not stutter, and these fears have been shown to become elevated by adolescence. Children aged around 5 years with a speech disorder have also been found to have an increased risk of developing an anxiety disorder by early adulthood. Therefore, this suggests that as a child grows older, the risk increases that the experience of stuttering will increasingly be associated with problems like shyness, bullying, and discrimination; lowered self-esteem; self-consciousness; avoidance of social contexts in which he or she has to speak; and mood decline, potentially leading to psychological disorder.

Psychological Distress in Older Adolescents and Adults Who Stutter

A major methodological problem with research that has investigated psychological distress in people who stutter is the nature of the sample. Most studies have employed potentially biased nonrandomized convenience samples (e.g., a survey of people being treated for stuttering attending a clinic). To address this problem, between 2000 and 2002, Ashley Craig conducted a randomized population study in which 4,689 households (over 10,000 people) were randomly selected from New South Wales, Australia. A representative from each family was interviewed by telephone to determine whether anyone in the family stuttered and also to determine the level of psychological distress in anyone who stuttered and did not stutter living in the household. The results showed that those who were diagnosed as someone who stuttered had significantly elevated psychological distress compared to those who did not stutter. There is now extensive evidence supporting the conclusion that chronic stuttering is associated with elevated psychological distress, resulting, for instance, from difficulties gaining employment due to stuttering, experiencing discrimination when employed, and low self-esteem and poor perceived attractiveness when seeking a sexual partner. Additionally, stuttering was found to be associated with a significant lower quality of life in domains such as vitality and social, emotional, and mental health functioning. The extent of the negative impact of stuttering on quality of life has been suggested to be comparable to the impact of a neurological disorder such as traumatic spinal cord injury or diseases such as diabetes and coronary heart disease.

Controlled research, with 200 adults who stuttered since childhood and 200 adult controls (who did not stutter) of similar age and sex, found that adults who stuttered were more likely to have considerably elevated levels of psychological distress compared to those who did not stutter. Psychological distress domains affected included anxiety, somatization, interpersonal sensitivity, depressive mood, hostility, and paranoia. A meta-analysis of 19 studies, published in 2014, examined psychological distress reported in methodologically high-quality studies, comparing anxiety in adults who stutter with anxiety in adults who did not stutter. The 19 studies involved 1,268 adults who stuttered and 1,664 adults who did not stutter. Medium to large overall differences in psychological distress were found (i.e., in trait and social anxiety). Results of meta-analyses are believed to provide the highest levels of evidence in science, so this finding provides very persuasive confirmation that chronic stuttering in older adolescents and adults is associated with abnormally elevated psychological distress.

Psychological Distress and Social Anxiety Disorder

Social anxiety disorder (also called *social phobia*) is an anxiety disorder in which a person experiences excessive and unreasonable fear of social situations, and this arises from a self-consciousness of being closely watched, judged, criticized by others, embarrassed, or humiliated in front of others. People who stutter and experience elevated psychological distress have a very high risk of developing social anxiety disorder. The rate of social anxiety disorder in adults who stutter is very high (around 40%) compared to the risk in those who do not stutter (4%). Social anxiety disorder can be highly debilitating and generally results in decreased social functioning.

Final Thoughts

Many people who stutter have a greatly increased risk of developing abnormally elevated psychological distress. Evidence from a variety of studies strongly indicates that the majority of people who stutter will experience some level of psychological distress (e.g., trait and social anxiety), with up to 40% developing severely elevated levels that may progress into a psychological disorder. This means that many adults who stutter will experience symptoms such as frequently feeling nervous and tense; feeling like a failure; often feeling exhausted; feeling like they want to avoid social contact; feeling inadequate, insecure, disturbed, and frequently worrying about things; frequently feeling embarrassed about social interactions; constantly feeling nervous about social scrutiny; frequently afraid of social disapproval; constantly worried about appearing stupid in social interactions; and feeling very distressed when they believe they have made a social error (e.g., stuttering severely).

Treatments do exist that can improve fluency as well as the psychological stress associated with the stuttering. An effective approach to stuttering treatment is to combine fluency-enhancing skills with behavioral and cognitive behavior skills, as this has been shown to reduce stuttering and psychological distress. People who stutter should be offered such treatment, at least by late adolescence, if any sign of increased distress is observed.

It is also critical that treatment include strategies designed to address psychological distress, as quite often, treatment is only aimed at improving fluency, ignoring the symptoms associated with of psychological stress. This is quite common if only speech pathologists are involved in the treatment. Involving both speech pathologists and clinical psychologists in treatment optimizes chances of helping people who stutter develop healthy fluency as well as positive emotional and cognitive expectations. For example, the development of a strong belief of control over their fluency (e.g., robust self-efficacy) can have a beneficial influence on their anxiety and mood and boost their resilience to manage their speech disorder. Importantly, stuttering treatment should also promote stronger social support networks, resulting in more effective social engagement. Stuttering should not be ignored but treated when first observed to help people who stutter to manage their disorder in a resilient manner.

Ashley Craig

See also Psychiatric Disorders With Communication Disorders; Resilience; Self-Management; Stuttering and Emotional Reactions; Stuttering Treatment

Further Readings

Blood, G. W., Boyle, M. P., Blood, I. M., & Nalesnik, G. R. (2010). Bullying in children who stutter: Speech-language pathologists' perceptions and intervention strategies. *Journal of Fluency Disorders, 35*, 92–109.

Craig, A., & Tran, Y. (2006). Chronic and social anxiety in people who stutter. *Advances in Psychiatric Treatment, 12*, 63–68.

Craig, A., & Tran, Y. (2014). Trait and social anxiety in adults with chronic stuttering: Conclusions following meta-analysis. *Journal of Fluency Disorders, 40*, 35–43.

Craig, A., Blumgart, E., & Tran, Y. (2011). Resilience and stuttering: Factors that protect people from the adversity of chronic stuttering. *Journal of Speech, Language, and Hearing Research, 54*, 1485–1496.

Craig, A., Hancock, K., Tran, Y., Craig, M., & Peters, K. (2003). Anxiety levels in people who stutter: A randomized population study. *Journal of Speech, Language and Hearing Research, 46*, 1197–1206.

Ezrati-Vinacour, R., & Levin, I. (2004). The relationship between anxiety and stuttering: A multidimensional approach. *Journal of Fluency Disorders, 29*, 135–148.

Mulcahy, K., Hennessey, N., Beilby, J., & Byrnes, M. (2008). Social anxiety and the severity and typography of stuttering in adolescents. *Journal of Fluency Disorders, 33*, 306–319.

Tran, Y., Blumgart, E., & Craig, A. (2011). Subjective distress associated with chronic stuttering. *Journal of Fluency Disorders, 36*, 17–26.

PSYCHOSOCIAL IMPACT OF APHASIA

Many qualities define human beings, but emotions are central to what humans are as a species and as individuals, and emotional responses to social events make up a large chunk of human lives. This entry first defines *psychosocial life* and then examines the negative impact of aphasia on the psychosocial lives of people living with a devastating disability, aphasia. Those professionals engaged in therapeutic and rehabilitation work spend significant amounts of their time with people whose emotional and social lives are knocked sideways by significant and catastrophic circumstances.

What Is Psychosocial Life?

Psychosocial refers to the social context of emotional experience. Emotions are closely tied up with interactions with others, either directly or indirectly, through books, movies, songs, and so on, and this interactive experience is what produces most of the average person's happiness, sadness, anxiety, and disgust. How many distinct emotions exist is a matter of controversy, but at least five can be identified, based on their presence across diverse cultures, the existence of distinctive facial expressions, and the physiological changes that accompany them. These are happiness, sadness (when significantly sad, depression), anxiety, anger, and disgust.

There have been a number of approaches to the investigation of psychosocial state in people with aphasia, such as examining the prevalence and the impact of emotions like depression and anxiety and factors like overall well-being and quality of life (QoL). Much of this work centers on a number of broad parameters that define psychosocial well-being, and the list of six parameters in Table 1 is influential. They are listed together with an indication of how they can be affected by aphasia. These parameters relate to having autonomy and self-acceptance in one's life and control of one's environment, enjoying a sense of purpose and a sense of personal growth and enjoying and maintaining positive relationships.

Depression is common in those who have experienced a stroke and have aphasia, and there are three principal considerations concerning the emotional and psychosocial impact of brain damage on the individual with aphasia. These are the *direct* or *primary* effects of neurological damage, which impact on the neurophysiological and neurochemical substrate of emotional processing, and the *indirect* or

Table 1 Ryff's Six Parameters of Adult Well-Being and How They Can Be Affected by Aphasia

Parameters of Well-Being	Aphasia
Autonomy	Significantly reduced
Self-acceptance	Significantly affected
Purpose in life	Significantly reduced
Positive relationships	Negatively affected
Control of own environment	Significantly reduced
Personal growth	Opportunities reduced

Source: Ryff (1989, pp. 1069–1081).

secondary effects, which should be seen as natural reactions to a set of calamitous personal circumstances and events, and the preexisting psychological balance, constitution, and the ways of coping that the individual can harness and bring to bear on those circumstances. A further effect, *tertiary*, has been suggested that can establish itself in the chronic stages after the individual has made some recovery from the damage to the brain and comes to a fuller appreciation of the long-term realities of living with aphasia. Existing knowledge and understanding of the impact of the primary and secondary factors is improving, but little is known about the effect of the preexisting psychological constitution of the individual. The signs of these forms of emotional responses to brain damage are summarized in Table 2.

However, as Ryff notes, one should question the validity of using purely clinical criteria to identify depression observed poststroke because changes in energy levels, weight, appetite, and sleeping patterns result not only from depression but also commonly from other neurological and neuropsychological conditions associated with stroke and hospitalization. As well, neurological deficits often impair facial expression and emotional expression, through motor speech and vocal tone and body posture, mistakenly suggesting the presence of depression.

Table 2 Primary, Secondary, and Tertiary Signs of Depression Following Brain Damage

Primary

- Significant weight loss or gain when not dieting or decrease or increase in appetite
- Insomnia or hypersomnia
- Psychomotor agitation or retardation
- Fatigue or loss of energy

Secondary and Tertiary

- Feelings of worthlessness or excessive or inappropriate guilt
- Diminished ability to think or concentrate or indecisiveness
- Recurrent thoughts of death or suicide or a suicidal attempt

Source: Herrmann, M., & Wallesch, C. W. (1993). Depressive changes in stroke patients. *Disability and Rehabilitation* 15, 55–66.

The Size of the Problem

Loneliness and low satisfaction with life and with social networks are particularly important and contribute to long-term psychological distress, depression, and anxiety in people with poststroke aphasia. Depression is known to be very common in survivors of stroke. One study, for instance, conducted a longitudinal study over 3 years in 79 survivors of stroke and found that at discharge from hospital 25% had major depression; at 3 months, this had increased to about 33% but reduced at 12 months to around 17%. However, at 3 years postonset of stroke, the percentage of those with major depression had crept up again to 25%. Major depression has been documented in 10% of spouses of survivors of stroke at 3 months postonset, increasing linearly to 50% at 3 years. Clearly, depression increases in survivors of stroke and their spouses over time, making a major case for intervention. A large study used the Hospital Anxiety and Depression Scale to measure depression and anxiety in 220 survivors of stroke at 2, 4, and 6 months and 5 years after stroke in four European centers. Anxiety and depression increased significantly between 6 months and 5 years. The prevalence of anxiety was 29% and depression 33% at 5 years poststroke. Severity of anxiety and depression significantly increased between 6 months and 5 years poststroke. Higher anxiety and depression scores at 6 months were significantly associated with anxiety and depression at 5 years. A systematic review of studies of poststroke depression produced 5,400 informants from 37 cohorts. An association was found between early depressive symptoms and the continuation of depression 12 months poststroke, and a significant correlation between depression and mortality at 12 and 24 months.

QoL in people with aphasia is significantly lower than in people without aphasia, affecting social integration, social networks, and social activities. Over 60% of people with aphasia report having less contact with prestroke friends, and 30% were unable to name even one close friend. Health-related QoL (HRQoL) is concerned with the impact of a health state or a health condition (e.g., aphasia) on a person's ability to lead a fulfilling life. It incorporates the individual's subjective evaluation of his or her physical, mental/emotional, familial, and social functioning. HRQoL scales are often used to assess a person's QoL and also incorporate other domains that are relevant to the population. This broad definition incorporates a person's culture and value systems encompassing factors like a safe environment and material well-being. Health-care systems and providers usually do not take responsibility for these global human concerns, even though they can be adversely and significantly affected by a condition like aphasia.

An important large-scale study of HRQoL in hospital-based long-term care in Canada used the Minimum Data Set Health Status Index, a universally employed measure based on a range of clinical assessments in North American long-term care facilities. It examined HRQoL in 66,193 residents. Analysis estimated the impact of 60 diseases and 15 conditions on HRQoL. Aphasia showed the largest negative relationship to Minimum Data Set Health Status Index, followed by cancer and Alzheimer's disease. This is a dramatic demonstration that aphasia has one of the most extensive negative effects on an individual's QoL and the individual's ability to engage in and with his or her family, friends, and the wider community.

Research has shown that both recovery and response to rehabilitation in individuals with aphasia are significantly influenced by emotional and psychosocial factors. Emotional state and well-being have a significant impact on motivation and cognitive and language processing. Good motivation is particularly important to successful rehabilitation: Cognitive, memory, and language performance are known to improve with positive mood and a sense of well-being. Depression has a negative effect on recovery and cognitive resources in people with aphasia, and the outcome of rehabilitation is worse in depressed than in nondepressed survivors of stroke.

The psychosocial impact of aphasia entails the individual with aphasia coming to terms with an exceptional constellation of negative life events. Because the aphasia affects others too, it has consequences for the individual's whole social network, especially the immediate family. The disabling experience of having aphasia, rather than the impairment itself, is of special significance. Research investigating how the psychosocial impact of aphasia is experienced have found that people with aphasia and their families experience significant stressful changes as a result of professional, social and familial role changes, decreases in social contact, significant depression, loneliness, and frustration.

There has been increased attention to the primary emotional disorders, as defined previously, as interest in the representation of emotion in the brain and its association with language impairment has grown. Poststroke depression correlates significantly with anterior lesions, and research has demonstrated that with time since onset of a stroke, there is an increase in the interaction between the extent of cognitive and physical impairment and depression. But little research has aimed to identify secondary reactive emotional states following stroke and to separate them from primary effects. No differences have been found in overall depression between people with acute and chronic aphasia but marked qualitative differences in its manifestation. In participants with more acute aphasia, significantly higher ratings for physical signs of depression and disturbances of cyclic functions like sleep patterns, usually considered direct effects, have been observed. In addition, an association between severity of depression and anterior lesions close to the frontal pole has been found in participants with aphasia. These findings suggest that the symptoms of depression in people with acute aphasia may be caused more by the primary effects of the damage, rather than as a reaction to those effects. It may be that a secondary, more reactive, depression emerges at more chronic stages. While many of the classic symptoms of depression may not change, the cause of the depression may be a direct effect of brain damage early on, and as swelling and edema reduce, as well as the person with aphasia begins to be aware that his or her circumstances may not change any time soon, a natural reaction to the experience is what causes the depression. Factors judged to be symptomatic of depression have been used in studies of individuals following brain damage, like diminished sleep and eating and restlessness and crying. These are the factors included in popular depression questionnaires often used in research, although, as suggested previously, these symptoms may be caused by physical illness and hospitalization and directly unrelated to mood state.

While the most reliable method of gaining information on how someone feels seems to be to ask the individual directly, language plays a special role in the problem of identifying and measuring mood for individuals with aphasia. The effects of language impairment further complicate examination of mood in people with aphasia because an individual's mood is often interpreted through his or her facial expression, voice quality and intensity, rate and amount of speech, gesture and body posture, as well as through the individual's report of his or her mood through linguistic expression and comprehension, all of which can be affected in impaired mood and all of which can be affected by central nervous system damage.

Therefore, determining mood in an individual with aphasia presents many problems, although relatives and friends can help in verifying accuracy. A useful approach to determining inner feelings is to use nonverbal methods, like the nonverbal *visual analogue mood scale*. Despite its simplicity, the visual analogue mood scale has been shown to be reliable and valid. It has been made more relevant to severely aphasic people by substituting schematic faces for words. Facial expression is the most direct method of communicating emotion and an ability that should be preserved in most people with aphasia.

How Should Psychosocial Factors Be Incorporated Into Aphasia Rehabilitation?

This brief review has shown that the psychosocial life of a person with aphasia is not only significantly affected by the aphasia but also that the issues raised need to be incorporated into rehabilitation programs.

Depression following brain damage responds to specific pharmacotherapeutic intervention, and a range of antidepressants have been trialed with stroke survivors with depression. What is less clear is whether pharmacotherapeutic intervention may be more appropriate at acute stages when individuals may be experiencing primary depression, and counseling more preferred at chronic secondary or tertiary stages.

An approach that has been widely applied to psychological counseling, including to the emotional changes accompanying aphasia, is *the grief model*. According to this model, individuals grieving for the loss of the ability to communicate move through various stages of denial, anger, bargaining, depression, and acceptance. It is not claimed that all people with aphasia go through all of these stages, but it is suggested that some get stuck at a stage. Denial, bargaining, and acceptance are less amenable to more objective forms of measurement, but they have been investigated in people with aphasia through interpretive assessments, like personal construct therapy techniques, where it is argued that the impact of becoming aphasic is an event of such magnitude as to affect a person's *core-role construing* and that the grief the person experiences concerns loss of the essential element of oneself as a speaker. Self is intrinsically tied up with language, which is essential to every person for expressing and revealing the self. However, it is frequently observed that changes in an individual are seen following brain damage, and anger and denial are common. Whether they are indirect or direct, in the sense discussed previously, raises issues with the stages that occur as part of grief. Again, methods of therapy that are less dependent on language are required.

Counseling is an important approach that all therapists working with people with aphasia should engage in. It entails a number of unique features that allow the therapist to help individuals identify issues in their lives associated with living with aphasia where they would like to see change and positive moment forward and to provide help and support to clarify ways to achieve their aims. An important element is clear information giving, so that individuals with aphasia and their families have clear knowledge about the aphasic condition and ways to live with the condition. The counselor is a listener and, generally, utilizes what is called a *nondirective* approach to help and guide, rather than a directive or prescriptive approach. The aim is to guide the individuals in their quest, rather than instruct them or direct them on ways to achieve their goals. Another approach entails helping the individuals with aphasia, and family members, toward a situation where they can engage fully in life, despite having aphasia. This may require some acknowledgment of the realities of their circumstances, guiding them toward resolution and acceptance of their situation so that they can move on from disabling aphasia to involvement, engagement, and participation. People with aphasia themselves have become involved in the process of providing counseling support.

There are several types of support groups available in most communities in the developed world for people with aphasia and for their families. These range from self-help groups, which are run by people with aphasia themselves, often supported by helpers without aphasia who may or may not be professionals, to psychosocial support groups, providing a base for social reintegration. Participation in a self-help group can be a powerful approach to social reintegration and reengagement for people with chronic conditions like aphasia, contributing to the development of confidence and psychosocial reintegration and autonomy. These groups seldom entail working through impairment-based programs, but they may enable people to run their own groups, taking all decisions and taking on responsibilities like being the treasurer, secretary, or chairperson for the group. Such roles are seen as empowering for those who take them on. They can also entail active advocacy and lobbying within a community. A group may simply involve social gatherings, where new friends can be made, autonomy encouraged, and confidence boosted. Some groups are activity based, for example, painting can be used to explore issues arising from aphasia, and choral singing can be utilized to encourage a joint group approach involving all members of the group irrespective of severity and confidence levels. Some support groups have guest speakers or organize outings to restaurants or parks that form the basis for social exchange and engagement. Such groups play an important part in addressing issues of psychosocial adjustment for individuals with aphasia. Groups have also long been established as a means for providing counseling.

Chris Code

See also Aphasia; Aphasia Assessment; Attention

Further Readings

Code, C., Eales, C., Pearl, G., Conan, M., Cowin, K., & Hickin, J. (2003). Supported self-help groups for aphasic people; development and research. In I. Papathanasiou & R. de Bleser (Eds.), *The science of aphasia: From therapy to theory*. London, UK: Elsevier.

Code, C., & Herrmann, M. (2003). The relevance of emotional and psychosocial factors in aphasia to rehabilitation. *Neuropsychological Rehabilitation, 13*, 109–132.

Herrmann, M., Bartels, C., & Wallesch, C. W. (1993). Depression in acute and chronic aphasia—Symptoms, pathoanatomo-clinical correlations, and functional implications. *Journal of Neurology, Neurosurgery, and Psychiatry, 56*, 672–678.

Herrmann, M., & Wallesch, C. W. (1993). Depressive changes in stroke patients. *Disability and Rehabilitation 15*, 55 -66.

Hilari, K., Northcott, S., Roy, P., Marshall, J., Wiggins, R. D., Chataway, J., & Ames, A. (2010). Psychological distress after stroke and aphasia: The first six months. *Clinical Rehabilitation, 24*, 181–190.

Lam, J. M. C., & Wodchis, W. P. (2010). The relationship of 60 disease diagnoses and 15 conditions to preference-based health-related quality of life in Ontario hospital-based long-term care residents. *Medical Care, 48*, 380–387.

Ryff, C. P. (1989). Happiness is everything, or is it? Explorations of the meaning of psychosocial well-being. *Journal of Personal & Social Psychology, 57*, 1069–1081.

Psychosocial Issues Associated With Communication Disorders

Being able to communicate is essential to a person's psychosocial well-being. The term *psychosocial well-being* refers to a person's psychological, social, and emotional functioning and how this contributes to his or her overall quality of life. Psychosocial issues arise when a person's psychosocial well-being is compromised in some way through a significant change in circumstances, such as a serious illness. The person experiences challenges in adapting to his or her changed circumstances, and this is often manifested in a range of psychosocial difficulties, such as a loss of confidence, reduced self-esteem, and increased anxiety and depression. *Psychosocial adaptation* is the process by which a person adjusts his or her psychosocial functioning to his or her changed circumstances. Psychosocial well-being is challenging to conceptualize and measure, as it varies according to an individual's environment and his or her response to and adjustment to this environment. A psychosocial approach to understanding communication disorders in both children and adults seeks to understand how a communication disorder impacts their psychosocial well-being. This impact can be at one point in time as well as understanding how the person manages the impact to achieve effective psychosocial adaptation over the life span and therefore maximize his or her quality of life. Typical measures of psychosocial functioning and well-being include independence, employment, relationships and friendships, and physical and mental health. A communication disorder can have a significant impact on all these aspects, resulting in psychosocial difficulties and challenging the person to adjust to the communication disorder to maximize his or her psychosocial functioning.

A distinction is made between an *acquired communication disorder* where the communication disorder results from a medical condition, such as a stroke, a traumatic brain injury, or a progressive neurological disorder, and a *developmental communication disorder*, where a child is born with a communication impairment as part of a medical or other condition or the communication disorder becomes apparent in the child's early years of development. Stammering is a communication disorder where psychosocial issues are intrinsic to the development and continuation of the disorder. This entry describes the psychosocial impact of and psychosocial issues associated with developmental and acquired communication disorders as well as stammering, with reference to specific examples.

Psychosocial Issues in Acquired Communication Disorders

In adults, an acquired communication disorder results in the loss of previous communicative functioning with a life-changing impact on the person's psychosocial functioning and resulting quality of life. Examples of acquired communication disorders include aphasia due to a stroke, a traumatic brain injury, and progressive neurological disorders. A stroke can cause major change and disruption to the individual's everyday life with significant implications for his or her quality of life. The loss of communication ability often co-occurs with a loss of physical health and mobility, resulting in increased dependence on professionals and the family unit (if there is one). Losing communication ability often results in changes to key relationships such as a partner and family as well as friendships, reduced social networks and social isolation, unemployment, and the inability to carry on with everyday activities such as pastimes and hobbies. These aspects of daily life contribute to a person's self-identity since the person defines him- or herself according to his or her everyday activities. Employment, family, and belonging to a social group or network are all compromised by an acquired communication disorder. These life changes impact the person's self-identity, leading to difficulties in adjusting to these changed circumstances and the subsequent emerging of psychosocial difficulties.

These life-changing losses not only impact the person and the family at the time of the event but also on the person's recovery process in terms of how he or she is able to participate in the recovery process, make the psychosocial adjustments to enable his or her recovery, and accept the limits of his or her recovery. The role of the communication disorder in this process is important but often neglected. Impairments in understanding and communicating with others will hinder the person's recovery in terms of his or her motivation and engagement in the process. Understanding the expectations of health and other professionals and meeting these is challenging. Assisting service professionals, family, and friends to understand the individual's perspective is compromised by the communication disorder. When the individual finds the psychosocial adjustment too difficult and is unable to adjust to his or her new and often unwanted life, the result is often increased anxiety and depression. These are frightening mental health difficulties to experience. Identification of mental health is dependent on communication, both the individual being able to understand questions about his or her mood and emotional functioning and being able to recognize and communicate his or her mood and changes to others. Facilitating communication through supported communication such as nonverbal means with a reduced reliance on spoken input is an essential component of the recovery process since it enables the person to understand and to be able to participate in the process.

Psychosocial Issues in Children With Communication Disorders

In contrast to adults with acquired communication disorders, children with communication disorders do not usually lose previously acquired communication ability (of course, there may be some exceptions here, such as a child who has a traumatic brain injury). Instead, children's speech, language, and communication development integrates with their psychosocial functioning and well-being. A communication disorder will change through development and impact a child's psychosocial functioning including learning, behavior, and social–emotional functioning, as well as his or her ability to initiate and maintain friendships and relationships and therefore engage with peers.

In the early years, before the age of 5, there is a dynamic relationship among children's speech, language and communication development, and their social–emotional functioning. Five aspects of social–emotional functioning are highlighted: *social functioning*, where the child is able to engage in social interactions appropriate to the context; *attachment*, where the child has established a secure attachment or connection with a primary caregiver usually from birth which then enables the child to develop secure attachment and relationships with key people in his or her life; *emotional functioning*, where the child is aware of not only his or her emotions but those of others and is able to manage or regulate how he or she expresses or show these emotions to others; *self-perception*, where the child is aware of his or her own strengths and weaknesses in relation to his or her peers and is then able to use this awareness to drive his or her own motivations to engage and achieve; and finally *temperament*, which refers to the child's intrinsic personality in how he or she reacts to experiences and then manages these experiences. Disruptions to these dimensions can put the child without a communication disorder at greater risk of psychosocial difficulties.

Two important issues need to be examined here: to what extent children's developing communication skills are needed for social–emotional functioning and then to what extent social–emotional functioning is necessary for children to be competent communicators. There is very limited theoretical evidence as to the interaction involved here, but more anecdotal evidence and experience supports how closely linked these are. In social functioning, children need to be competent communicators with adequate and appropriate social communication skills or pragmatic language skills in order to engage appropriately in social interaction. The process of attachment necessitates infants to have the prerequisite intent to be communicative and to encourage their caregivers to communicate with them as well as caregivers who are able to communicate and have the capacity both communicative and emotional to communicate with their infant. To have emotional functioning, the children need to learn the vocabulary of emotions and how this vocabulary maps onto their emotions in order to be able to understand and express these to others. To develop self-perception, children need to be effective communicators who can then have strengths in effective interactions, friendships, and relationships. Children all have different temperaments often expressed through being shy, quiet, or more talkative and communicatively confident. It is proposed that these interactions are dynamic, involving factors within the child and factors external to the child, and it is likely the interaction among all these factors that is most important in understanding the association between communication competence, social–emotional competence, and effective psychosocial adjustment and subsequent mental health.

Given this dynamic relationship, it is now important to consider the impact of a communication disorder on a child's developing psychosocial functioning and well-being. Two child communication disorders are used to illustrate this.

Cleft Lip and Palate

A cleft lip and/or palate happens when the structures that form the upper lip or palate fail to join together when a baby is developing in the womb. The baby is born with the cleft lip and/or palate. The cause is unknown but has been linked to genetics and smoking in pregnancy. Cleft lip and/or palate can also be part of syndromes such as DiGeorge syndrome (also known as *velocardiofacial syndrome* or *22q11 deletion*), Pierre Robin Sequence, and Edwards syndrome. A cleft lip and/or palate can cause feeding difficulties in the early weeks and months, hearing difficulties, speech difficulties, and dental difficulties. A surgical repair is usually made in the first year of an infant's life and/or at a later stage. A surgical repair is not always completely successful, and an infant can be left with an unresolved cleft palate where there is still a gap in the palate. This has significant implications for speech development, as the developing infant is unable to effectively control the airflow through the mouth needed to make some speech sounds. Instead, some of the airflow escapes into the nasal cavity and it becomes very difficult for the child to learn and produce these speech sounds. When the child is born, the child may be unable to form an adequate seal in order to feed effectively, and the child and parent will need support to enable the child to feed effectively. Hearing difficulties are also common as the child is more prone to developing ear infections resulting in otitis media with effusion and therefore transient and recurrent conductive hearing loss. Teeth may not develop as expected and can have implications for speech development. Children with cleft lip and/or palate are at risk of a communication disorder due to speech difficulties and language delays due to hearing difficulties. In addition, for some children, despite a surgical repair being made, scarring and an unaligned repair can affect their facial appearance. Some children will find their facial appearance difficult to accept and experience negative reactions to this.

The resulting communication disorder, facial appearance, and other experiences related to the cleft lip and/or palate can result in psychosocial difficulties for some children. Communication is affected by not only unclear speech but also the compensatory behaviors children use to try and achieve more intelligible speech. The velopharyngeal inadequacy causes air to escape from the mouth into the nasal cavity, thus making some speech sounds difficult to produce. To try and prevent the air escaping from the mouth, some children will strain other speech muscles, resulting in grunt or growl noises; or the child will attempt to stop air escaping from the nose and will make a grimace-type facial expression (i.e., nasal grimacing). To try to build up more air pressure for speech, the child may put additional strain on the vocal folds, leading to a hoarse or breathy voice. Sounding different, being unable to communicate effectively, and engaging in behaviors that others may perceive as negative, as well as their facial appearance, will impact the child's psychosocial functioning. As a consequence, these children are at risk of low confidence and low self-esteem as well as issues related to the development of their self-concept and identity and peer relationships.

Developmental Language Disorders (DLDs)

In contrast to cleft lip and/or palate, a life-span perspective is needed to understand the psychosocial issues associated with children with communication disorder where the communication disorder is not identifiable from birth. Children with DLDs do not develop their speech, language, and communication abilities in the early years as expected. These children may initially present with delayed language development, but this delay does not resolve over time with or does not resolve without support. Children with DLD have a range of impairments across speech, receptive and expressive language, and social communication. These can be lifelong impairments that impact psychosocial functioning and adaptation over the life span. In childhood, the psychosocial impact of the communication disorder is observed in learning, literacy, educational progress and attainment, friendships, social–emotional development, and behavior. In later childhood and adolescence, these children are susceptible to bullying and victimization, educational underachievement, reduced peer relationships, and mental health difficulties. In adult life, psychosocial outcomes are limited and described in terms of high unemployment, reduced independent living and financial independence, and increased mental health difficulties. Criminal offending behavior is also associated with young people with DLD. Over the life span, some children will be more resilient than others to psychosocial difficulties. It is not clear what makes some children more resilient than others but the child's environment, level of support received, and severity of the communication disorder all will play a role.

Adolescence as a period of psychosocial adaptation should be considered here. For young people with a communication disorder, this transition time can be particularly challenging. The demands of adolescence involve being more independent, less support in education and more self-directed learning, increased language and communication demands of education for learning, and the complex communication skills needed to understand and negotiate peer relationships. Adolescence is viewed as a formative period in the psychosocial adaptation of young people and particularly those with a communication disorder. Where the demands of adolescence exceed the capacities of the young person, psychosocial adjustment can be challenged, leading to psychosocial difficulties.

Psychosocial Issues and Stammering in Children and Adults

Stammering is a communication disorder affecting the fluency of speech. Speech is characterized by a set of primary behaviors including repetitions of words or sounds, words or sounds are produced to sound longer (i.e., prolongations) than they usually are, and speakers get stuck on a word and are unable to say it in full (i.e., blocking). In addition to these primary speech behaviors, secondary behaviors are likely to occur, which develop through experiencing significant feelings of fear and anxiety in relation to talking. As a result, people who stammer engage in avoidance behaviors where they avoid having to speak in situations where they believe they will stammer, for example, talking on the phone. Avoidance behaviors also extend to not saying certain words or not talking to certain people as these situations also increase the risk of stammering. Additionally, secondary behaviors can also include escape behaviors such as head nodding or closing of an eye or tapping a hand on a table, which the person uses to overcome the primary speech behavior (e.g., to prevent repetitions, prolongations, and blocking). Every person with a stammer will have his or her set of individual secondary behaviors. Some people who stammer are referred to as *covert*, as it is very difficult to detect from their speech that they have a stammer. Instead, they have become very adept in their avoidance behaviors and therefore present as more fluent than they actually are.

Stammering usually starts in childhood and can persist into adult life. Many children experience a period of typical nonfluency where a child will repeat sounds or words or elongate sounds. For most children, this period resolves over time. For others, this period marks the start of a stammer. Psychosocial issues play a role in the development and maintenance of a stammer. In typical nonfluency, there is no marked effort or tension associated with the nonfluency. However, over time, these primary speech behaviors become associated with negative experiences of communication leading to the development of the secondary avoidance behaviors. The psychosocial impact of a stammer is considerable. Avoiding communication will contribute to low confidence, reduced self-esteem, reduced opportunities, and social withdrawal and isolation. These psychosocial difficulties are then viewed as a contributory factor in the continuation of the stammer, reinforcing the very negative experiences of communicating and increasing the fear and anxiety associated with talking.

Addressing the psychosocial impact of a stammer can reduce the stammering behaviors. Intervention can focus on the psychosocial impact of the stammer as well as supporting the person to reduce the primary speech behaviors. Such intervention might involve enabling a person to stammer in front of others and for the person to understand that the perceived negative reaction he or she expects does not happen; he or she experiences acceptance instead. This can then reduce the fear and anxiety which in turn can reduce the stammering behavior. While stammering is a communication disorder where there is a psychosocial impact, the psychosocial impact itself affects the development and maintenance of the stammer.

Final Thoughts

A range of psychosocial issues are associated with communication disorders in children and adults.

Adults with acquired communication disorders experience a loss in communicative ability which then impacts their psychosocial functioning and well-being. For children, the communication disorder impacts their developing psychosocial functioning with implications for psychosocial well-being throughout the life span. For some communication disorders such as stammering, psychosocial issues are intrinsic to the development and maintenance of the communication disorder. Understanding communication disorders must involve consideration of the associated psychosocial issues.

Judy Clegg

See also Adolescent Language Disorders; Aphasia; Cleft Lip and Palate: Speech Effects; Emotional Impact of Communication Disorders; Language Disorders in Children; Learning Disabilities; Psychiatric Disorders With Communication Disorders; Psychosocial Impact of Aphasia; Stuttering and Emotional Reactions

Further Readings

Beilby, J. (2014). Psychological impact of living with a stuttering disorder: Knowing is not enough. *Seminars in Speech and Language, 35*(2), 132–143.

Brumfitt, S. (Ed.). (2009). *Psychological wellbeing and acquired communication impairment.* London, UK: Wiley-Blackwell.

Clegg, J., Ansorge, L., Stackhouse, J., & Donlan, C. (2012). Developmental communication impairments in adults: Outcomes and life experiences of adults and their parents. *Language, Speech and Hearing Services in Schools, 4,* 521–535.

Howard, S., & Lohmander, A. (Eds.). (2011). *Cleft palate speech: Assessment and intervention.* London, UK: Wiley-Blackwell.

Roulstone, S., & McLeod, S. (Eds.). (2011). *Listening to children and young people with speech, language and communication needs.* London, UK: J&R Press.

PUBERPHONIA

The term *puberphonia*, also referred to as *mutational falsetto*, is a voice disorder in which childlike, higher pitched prepubescent speaking fundamental frequency is continued after completion of puberty such that the voice does not transition to a normal adult voice. In the classification manual of voice disorders, puberphonia is considered a functional voice disorder in adolescents and adults who have undergone normal growth, with no delayed puberty and no organic or endocrine disorder. Individuals with the disorder typically present to the clinic with complaints of high-pitched voices, dysphonia, vocal weakness, and fatigue.

Puberty is a period during which adolescents undergo a process of sexual maturation and develop secondary sexual characteristics. This occurs between the ages of 12 and 16 in boys and 10 and 14 in girls. Bone growth and mineralization, changes in body weight and composition, and significant hormonal changes take place. Rapid growth and transformation include not only physical changes and *growth spurts* but emotional changes as well. The first sign of puberty in girls is the beginning of breast development, and in boys, the increase in size of the testicles.

Voice also changes during this time, becoming more adultlike as the larynx grows. There is a lowering of the vertical position of the larynx in the neck, cartilage growth, and thickening of the vocal fold mucosa. One characteristic change in the male larynx is the growth of the thyroid cartilage in the anteroposterior dimension, resulting in the characteristic protrusion of the Adam's apple in the neck. The vocal folds adjust by increasing length and mass, making them heavier, and therefore slower in vibration. Anatomical studies by Joel Kahane showed that the length of the vocal folds increases about 11 mm in males and 4 mm in females. Other relevant changes include growth in the lungs and rib cage, increasing the vital capacity.

In boys, the process of vocal change is associated with pitch instability, dysphonia, and a gradual one-octave lowering of speaking fundamental frequency. Subsequently, pitch and voice quality stabilize. The entire process takes approximately 6–12 months, and the voice is fully stabilized by the age of 17. In contrast, female vocal mutation lowers the speaking fundamental frequency by only three semitones and does not hold a dramatic change in the laryngeal framework.

Puberphonic speaking fundamental frequency is produced in the falsetto register, whereas prior to mutation, this frequency falls within the modal register. As such, puberphonic voice production is characterized by reduced thyroarytenoid muscle engagement, elevated laryngeal position, reduced subglottal pressure and amplitude of vocal fold vibration, and incomplete or *touch* closure along the entire length of the glottis. Vocal folds are stretched and tense. Consequently, loudness dynamics are limited, and voice quality is somewhat breathy. Pitch breaks into the modal register as well as diplophonia may be observed.

Early reports of changes in voice quality in adolescent males go back to the Greek philosopher Aristotle (384 BCE), who wrote on "certain methods used by singing teachers" to preserve the childlike characteristics of voice. The practice of castrating young boys to prevent sexual development and hormonal changes of puberty artificially preserved the soprano or contralto voice quality and pitch range, whereas the vocal tract achieved normal growth. This tradition continued through the 1800s, particularly in Europe, where *castrati* constituted a large percentage of male opera singers.

Where puberphonia is primarily considered as a male phenomenon, cases of female puberphonia have been documented and discussed clinically. Female puberphonia may be underidentified because the characteristics of elevated pitch, increased breathiness, and reduced loudness are common characteristics of normal female voices, particularly in early adulthood. As such, female puberphonia may be misperceived as a greater degree of femininity. Limited social stigma and possible cultural–social reward may be associated with use of a "little girl's voice." Conversely, adolescent young males with a high-pitched voice may be perceived as feminine and more prone to ridicule and bullying.

The standard treatment for puberphonia is behavioral voice therapy. The primary goal across treatment is to break the habit of speaking in the falsetto or head register by establishing modal register phonation, characterized by a comparatively lower laryngeal position, increased glottal closure, and increased amplitude of vibration and subglottal pressure. Many therapy techniques in the literature have claimed successful results, including manual circumlaryngeal techniques, digital laryngeal manipulation, vegetative tasks (e.g., throat clearing, coughing, yawning), and hard glottal attacks. Singing a descending scale or producing increasingly loud vocal fry can also elicit normal modal voice production.

Once modal phonation is achieved through any of these strategies, a traditional treatment hierarchy of sustained phonation, syllables, words, sentences, and conversation can progress. Treatment goals may be achieved in as little as one to two sessions. Real-time visualization of pitch as biofeedback can be useful in maintaining a target fundamental frequency range during speech practice. Negative practice—volitionally switching between the puberphonic and *new* voice—can clarify the perceptual and kinesthetic difference between these two phonation modalities and provide patients with the ability to code switch as needed.

Occasionally, behavioral voice therapy has been shown to fail. Surgical approaches such as medialization thyroplasty, vocal fold augmentation injections, and onabotulinumtoxinA (Botox) injections have been reported as alternative treatments to improve voice. Other more esoteric methods, such as a laryngoscopic maneuver of applying pressure in the valleculae, have also been reported. It should be noted that these alternative options should be used as a last resort, only when behavioral intervention has failed.

The etiology of puberphonia remains unknown. The phenomenon may be explained as physiological in nature, illustrating an inability to adapt to the anatomical changes of the larynx. Given the efficacy of purely physiological treatment, this is indeed plausible. Psychosocial causes have been put forth, but a psychophysical theory of puberphonia has not been established. After establishing normal voice production in therapy, some patients may benefit from counseling support to assist them in the transition to the new voice in their daily lives.

Claudio F. Milstein and Eva van Leer

See also Dysphonia; Muscle Tension Dysphonia (MTD); Pitch; Voice Disorders; Voice Therapy

Further Readings

Boone, D. R., McFarlane, S. C., Von Berg, S. L., & Zraick, R. I. (2013). *The voice and voice therapy*. Pearson London, UK.

Hammarberg, B. (1987). Pitch and quality characteristics of mutational voice disorders before and after therapy. *Folia Phoniatrica et Logopaedica, 39*(4), 204–216. Retrieved from https://doi.org/10.1159/000265861

Kahane, J. C. (1982). Growth of the human prepubertal and pubertal larynx. *Journal of Speech, Language, and Hearing Research, 25*(3), 446–455. Retrieved from https://doi.org/10.1044/jshr.2503.446

Roy, N., Peterson, E. A., Pierce, J. L., Smith, M. E., & Houtz, D. R. (2017). Manual laryngeal reposturing as a primary approach for mutational falsetto. *The Laryngoscope, 127*(3), 645–650. Retrieved from https://doi.org/10.1002/lary.26053

Weiss, D. A. (1950). The pubertal change of the human voice (mutation). *Folia Phoniatrica et Logopaedica, 2*(3), 126–159. Retrieved from https://doi.org/10.1159/000262578

PULMONIC INGRESSIVE SPEECH

Of the six possible airstream mechanisms available for human speech production—pulmonic, glottalic, or velaric initiation, each of which could occur egressively or ingressively—the overwhelming majority of speech sounds occur on pulmonic egressive airstream. Glottalic egressive airstream is used to produce ejectives, glottalic ingressive airstream is used to produce implosives, velaric ingressive airstream is employed to produce clicks, velaric egressive airstream is not found in any speech known speech sounds and might be impossible to produce. Pulmonic ingressive airstream, that is, when sound is produced by lung expansion that causes air to be sucked in through the speech apparatus, is commonly believed to be rare, and is anecdotally said to be a characteristic of Scandinavian speech, but is in fact found in many languages from all over the world and appears in taxonomically different language groups. Setting deliberate and pathological occurrences aside, pulmonic ingressive speech is mainly used paralinguistically.

Pulmonic Ingressive Phonation in Animals

On the face of it, there is nothing that a priori would indicate that speech should only occur on egressive airstream, and the animal kingdom exhibits many examples of ingressive phonation, as observed already by Charles Darwin. Already in 1848, Charles Robin Segond observed that dog, foxes, cats, horses, donkeys, and birds employ pulmonic ingressive phonation. Since then, many others have listed many other species, but perhaps the most well-known examples of mammal ingressive phonation are cat purring and monkey/ape pant-hoots, both performed on alternating egressive and ingressive airstream. It is noteworthy that while monkey/ape laughter occurs on alternating egressive/ingressive airstream, human laughter is done exclusively on pulmonic egressive airstream.

The Physiology of Pulmonic Ingressive Speech

That ingressive phonation to some extent is part and parcel in the animal kingdom is illustrated by the fact that human infant cries frequently are produced on ingressive airstream, as commented upon by both Charles Darwin in 1872 and Victor Ewings Negus in 1929. It has been said that ingressive speech in infant cry constitutes one of four characteristic types of infant crying, the other three being phonation, hyperphonation, and dysphonation. That humans, as they grow older, abolish involuntary use of ingressive phonation might to some degree be explained in terms of physiology in that the vocal folds are not perfectly symmetrical and do not lend themselves as easily to phonation initiated ingressively as egressively. In fact, certain speech sounds such as sibilants, for example [s], cannot be produced ingressively in a satisfactory way.

Ingressive Speech in Speech Pathology and Speech Pathology Therapy

Pulmonic ingressive phonation has been discussed in the speech pathology literature, both as a pathology per se but also as a form of therapy or treatment. As a *speech pathology*, pulmonic ingressive fricatives have been observed in the speech of deaf children and in children with cerebral or hyperkinetic bulbar palsy. In adults, both psychogenic ingressive phonation has been reported, and it has also been observed in pathological laughter and as a part of stutter.

Pulmonic ingressive phonation has been used as a *diagnostic tool* from at least the early 19th century. Early on, it was stated that inspiratory phonation made diagnosis easier since the ventricles was more widely dilated and the medial aspect of the hypopharynx thus more easily identified. This way, for example, it was claimed, a clinician could more easily distinguish between helophytic and invasive tumors.

Ingressive phonation has also been used in *speech pathology therapy*, for both patients who stutter or who suffer from dysphonia, but also for other illnesses such as recurrent palsy, vox fistulosa, ventricular voice, and other diseases. It has been reported that one patient who suffered from adductor spastic dysphonia more or less converted to the use of ingressive speech to overcome his communication problems, with great success. However, it has also been reported that one patient who resorted to ingressive phonation to avoid stuttering fainted because of badly synchronized breathing. It should, finally, be pointed out to anyone attempting ingressive speech—whatever the rationale might be—that ingressive airstream quickly dries out the vocal folds.

Historical Evidence for Ingressive Phonation

Given that both several species of animals, notably mammals, and infants exhibit ingressive phonation, there is the question, how far back in time can we find mentions of ingressive phonation in human speech? Curiously, it was long—and erroneously—believed that ventriloquists *did their trick* by using ingressive phonation, but it seems clear that both ventriloquists and shamans in general, for example, the Pythea (Oracle) at Delphi, made use of both ventriloquism and pulmonic ingressive speech—totally different speech modes—in order to sound *outworldly*.

The oldest, unambiguous, mention of pulmonic ingressive speech seems to be David Cranz's observation in 1765 that "Greenlandic" women used it as a way to affirm something, that is, and interestingly exactly the kind of paralinguistic affirmation that today is very frequent in Iceland, Norway, Sweden, and Denmark.

Paralinguistic Use of Ingressive Speech and Phonation

Ingressive phonation used paralinguistically has been observed in the literature since at least the late 1800s. Examples include ingressive [t] or [f] to express doubt, ingressive palatal [t] to express surprise or to call horses, ingressive [1] to express delight in eating and drinking, and so on. A loud and rapid inbreathing, without any intent to produce a specific phon(em)e indicates surprise, pain, or hurt. In European languages, for example, the Scandinavian languages, English, German, and so on, there is a clear paralinguistic difference between egressive and ingressive versions of the same word, for example, *yes*. As has been pointed out (by Louis Pitschmann), no one would answer the question "will you marry me" with an ingressive *yes*. While the exact paralinguistic functions of ingressive productions of, for example, the words *yes* and *no* might vary between language, a very common function is to signal turn-taking by acting as a topic-closer or topic-changer. Another example is the well-known Japanese *hiss*, which is used as an honorific marker. It must be pointed out, however, that there is a multitude of different ingressive productions, ranging from, for example, simple breathing-in, Jamaican *kiss-teeth*, and so on, all with their own characteristics.

Pulmonic Ingressive Phonemes?

There have been at least two contenders for ingressive phonemes, or at least ingressive allophones. Initial claims that the Taiwanese language Tsou included two ingressive allophones were later discarded as idiosyncratic traits of a specific speaker. An undisputable case of ingressive phonemes, however, was the ritual language Damin, a variety of the Lardil language spoken on Mornington Island in the Gulf of Carpenteria in Australia. When Lardil men underwent subincision, they also learned a special secret language, Damin. The basic grammar was identical to Lardil, and the full vocabulary counted only 250 words, but Damin differed phonologically from Lardil—and all other known languages—by including several unique phonemes, including, an ingressive lateral fricative /L/. It must be noted that Damin was an *invented* language, and it seems that the inclusion of unique phonemes was a deliberate design feature. Also, the last speaker died decades ago so this is no longer a living language.

Other, and Deliberate, Uses of Ingressive Phonation

Besides the aforementioned *invented* phonemes and deliberate uses of ingressive phonation in speech pathology therapy, there are several other deliberate uses of ingressive phonation to be observed.

Pulmonic ingressive singing is found in modern music compositions, both in art music and as a means of achieving humorous effects, as used by Tenacious D in "Inward Singing." The use of ingressives in musical form, however, has a longer standing and was a part of vocal games both in *rekukarra* used by the Ainu people in Japan and the *kattajaq* used by the Inuit. In both these cases, ingressive phonation occurred when two singers sat close to each other, face-to-face, and sang "on each other's breaths," thus producing an alternating egressive–ingressive airstream.

Ingressive phonation has also been employed in whistled languages—a form of long-distance communication—where some types of whistles are produced on pulmonic ingressive airstream.

Another form of completely conscious use of ingressive occurs in voice disguise where it is employed the cloak the identity of the speaker. Examples of this use are found in *mumming* (or *mummering*) in Newfoundland and in *Fensterle* in Switzerland.

An exceptional use of ingressive language is Tohono O'dham, a southern Arizona Indian language, where ingressive speech was frequently used throughout in all-women groupings, with only very rare instances of male ingressive phonation. Ingressive speech in Tohono O'dham had an intimacy-building function, somewhat similar to whispering, with which it sometimes it was sometimes replaced.

Prevalence and Distribution

A common misconception is that pulmonic ingressive phonation is unique to Scandinavia—especially Sweden and Norway—and it has even been referred to as a *highly marked* feature in the literature on those languages. However, research has established that ingressive speech exists in at least 50 languages, spread across the entire globe, and that it appears in genetically unrelated language groups. Moreover, ingressive speech in all those languages exhibits striking similarities with regard to function and is most commonly associated with paralinguistic particles, for example (extra) affirmative versions of *yes* or on *no* and other short interactional linguistic items. However, although the distribution of ingressive phonation is universal, there is a very marked belt that stretches from the Baltic states (Estonia, Latvia), over Finland, Sweden, Norway, Denmark, across the northern Atlantic and the British Isles (Scotland, Faroe Islands, Iceland) into Newfoundland and Maine (although ingressive speech seems to have disappeared in the latter some decades ago) that not only exhibits an unusually high *frequency* of ingressive phonation—it has been shown that around 10% of the spontaneously produced "ja" ("yes") in Swedish are ingressive—but also a more marked qualitative usage of ingressive phonation in that ingressive speech production is not merely used on non-lexical, paralinguistics, exclamations but is found on entire *words* or even *phrases*. This latter phenomenon is most notably the case in Finnish and Icelandic where entire sentences can be produced ingressively. Since this observed belt to a large degree corresponds to (northern) Viking raids, this area has been labeled "the Viking expansion" in the literature.

A Linguistic Universal?

Given the widespread distribution of ingressive speech, it has been suggested that rather than being considered a *highly marked* characteristic of human language, ingressive speech could instead be considered a linguistic universal, perfectly matching one of William Croft's universals classes: "widespread but relatively sporadic within genetic groups may be frequent but unstable."

Phonetic Annotation

A wide variety of symbols have been employed over that past 150 years or so to indicate that individual phones are produced on pulmonic ingressive airstream, and annotation of ingressive speech still differs between, for example, conversation analysis and phonetic analysis. The extIPA symbol for pulmonic ingressive airstream is a downward pointing arrow placed to the right of the phone in question, for example, [a]⁻.

Robert Eklund

See also Anatomy of the Human Larynx; Articulatory Phonetics; Atypical Speech Sounds; Bernoulli Effect; Breathing Exercises; Clinical Phonetics; Clinical Phonology; Diagnosis of Communication Disorders; Dysphonia(s); Linguistics; Markedness; Phonetic Transcription; Pragmatics; Speech Production, Theories of; Vocal Production System: Evolution; Voice Disorders

Further Readings

Ball, M. J. (1991). Recent developments in the transcription of non-normal speech. *Journal of Communication Disorders, 24*, 59–78.

Ball, M. J. (1991). Computer coding of the IPA: Extensions to the IPA. *Journal of the International Phonetic Association, 21*(1), 36–41.

Ball, M. J., Code, C., Rahilly, J., & Hazlett, D. (1994). Non-segmental aspects of disordered speech: Developments in transcription. *Clinical Linguistics and Phonetics, 8*(1), 67–83.

Ball, M. J., Esling, J. H., & Dickson, C. (1995). The VoQS system for the transcription of voice quality. *Journal of the International Phonetic Association, 25*(2), 71–80.

Ball, M. J., & Müller, N. (2007). Non-pulmonic-egressive speech in clinical data: A brief review. *Clinical Linguistics & Phonetics, 21*(11–12), 869–874.

Catford, J. C. (1977). *Fundamental problems in phonetics.* Edinburgh, Scotland: Edinburgh University Press.

Catford, J. C. (1988). *A practical introduction to phonetics.* Oxford, UK: Clarendon Press.

Croft, W. (2003). *Typology and universals* (2nd ed.). Cambridge, UK: Cambridge University Press.

Eklund, R. (2008). Pulmonic ingressive phonation: Diachronic and synchronic characteristics, distribution and function in animal and human sound production and in human speech. *Journal of the International Phonetic Association, 38*(3), 235–324.

Halpert, H., & Story, G. M. (Eds.). (1969). *Christmas mumming in Newfoundland: Essays in anthropology, folklore, and history.* Toronto, Canada: University of Toronto Press.

Harrison, G. A., Davis, P. J., Troughear, R. A., & Winkworth, A. L. (1992). Inspiratory speech as a management option for spastic dysphonia. *The Annals of Otology, Rhinology & Laryngology, 101*, 375–382.

Pitschmann, L. A. (1987). The linguistic use of the ingressive air-stream in German and the Scandinavian languages. *General Linguistics, 27*(3), 153–161.

Van Riper, C. (1982). *The nature of stuttering* (2nd ed.). Englewood Cliffs, NJ: Prentice Hall.

Web Resources

Robert Eklund's Ingressive Phonation and Speech Page. Retrieved from http://ingressivespeech.info

PURE-TONE AUDIOMETRY

Pure-tone audiometry (PTA) is a standardized procedure used to measure detection of quiet tones of varying frequency. The test is commonly used by health-care professionals, such as audiologists, to quantify hearing loss in each ear. It can also provide information on the anatomical site (and sometimes the cause) of the hearing loss. The measurements are also used when prescribing a hearing aid. The procedure is relatively quick and easy to perform but requires a degree of skill on the part of the tester to ensure accuracy and validity of the measurements. The test procedure can be modified for use in preschool children and difficult-to-test populations. This entry discusses the underlying scientific principles of the test, how it is performed, and how the results are displayed and interpreted.

Principles of the Test

The defining principle of the test is to measure hearing sensitivity (i.e., the detection of quiet tones) to a range of pure tones that vary in frequency. The standard range of pure tones include 250, 500, 1000, 2000, 4000, and 8000 Hz, as this generally covers the most important frequencies in human speech. Hearing sensitivity at intermediate frequencies can also be measured when warranted. The clinical equipment used to perform PTA is known as a *pure-tone audiometer*.

The listener is seated in a sound-treated room to avoid any distracting environmental sounds that may mask the test tone. The tester may be located in the same room, or in a different room connected by a glass window, so that he or she can check the listener's attention and comfort throughout the test procedure. The tester controls the pure-tone audiometer, selecting the frequency and level of the tones presented to the listener via earphones. The listener is asked to attend to the tones and to indicate every time he or she hears one, irrespective of the level. The test aims to determine the minimum level the listener can detect each pure tone. The minimum level of detection is known as the *hearing threshold*, and this may vary with frequency (and differ between ears).

Unit of Measurement

Sound pressure level is measured in decibels (dB). The dB scale is logarithmic, allowing a large range of numerical values to fit into a more easily readable range of numbers. The minimum sound level detected by a group of normal hearing young adults varies across frequency. The pure-tone audiometer is calibrated so the dial reading matching this minimum level is 0 and is referred to as 0 dB hearing level (dB HL). Poorer hearing sensitivity results in measured thresholds that have positive values (e.g., 40 dB HL), while better than average hearing results in measured thresholds that have negative values (e.g., −10 dB HL). Any measured hearing threshold worse than 15 dB HL (higher threshold, lower sensitivity to sound) is considered abnormal. A classification nomenclature is used to describe the severity of a hearing loss. The classification terminology varies between the standards used.

Table 1 contains the classification systems for the American Speech-Language-Hearing Association (ASLHA) used in the United States, the British Society of Audiology used in the United Kingdom, and the World Health Organization system, which aims to define the grade of impairment. The World Health Organization explains the level of difficulty expected within each grade of hearing loss. The *slight* category is explained as a listener having difficulty hearing and understanding quieter speech, speech at a distance, and in speech the presence of background sounds. The *moderate* category is explained as a listener having difficulty hearing normal everyday speech, even at a close distance. The *severe* category is explained as a listener who may hear very loud speech and loud environmental sounds but not most conversational speech. The *profound* category is explained as a listener perceiving very loud sounds as vibrations. The World Health Organization warns that although the descriptors can be of use to summarize the hearing loss, they should not be the sole determinant in hearing aid provision (see below).

Table 1 Commonly Used Hearing Loss Classifications: American Speech-Language-Hearing Association (ASLHA), British Society of Audiology (BSA), and the World Health Organization (WHO)

Classification	Lower Limit dB HL	Upper Limit dB HL
ASLHA		
Normal	−10	15
Slight	16	25
Mild	26	40
Moderate	41	55
Moderately severe	56	70
Severe	71	90
Profound	91+	
BSA		
Mild	20	40
Moderate	41	70
Severe	71	95
Profound	95+	
WHO (grade of impairment)		
0 No impairment	≤25	
1 Slight	26	40
2 Moderate	41	60
3 Severe	61	80
4 Profound	81+	

Earphone Types

The pure tones can be delivered to the listener via two types of transducer. The first earphone type produces sound by generating vibrations of air, which are transmitted to the listener's ear through the normal route that everyday sound reaches the ear. This is air-conduction (AC) audiometry in which sounds are presented through earphones placed over the listener's ears (supra-aural earphones), or placed in the ear canal (insert earphones). Sounds reach the organ of hearing, known as the *cochlea*, within the inner ear bony labyrinth of the skull through the ear canal (outer ear), eardrum, and the ossicular chain (a series of bones in the middle ear). A hearing loss anywhere in the auditory pathway will affect the hearing threshold obtained by AC. The second type of transducer, known as a *bone vibrator*, directly transmits sound energy to the inner ear (cochlea) through the skull, largely bypassing the outer and middle ear. This is bone-conduction (BC) testing. The bone vibrator is a small vibrating device, which resembles a cuboid with rounded corners, with a disk shape protruding on one side. The disk shape is held in place by a metal spring-like band against the listener's mastoid bone just behind his or her external ear (pinna). The disk pressing against the mastoid bone transmits vibrations to the cochlea. Since BC stimuli largely bypass the outer and middle ear, hearing thresholds obtained by BC primarily reflect the hearing status of the inner ear.

A hearing loss can be classified as sensorineural, conductive, or mixed. A hearing loss is classified by comparing AC and BC thresholds within each ear. Abnormal BC thresholds indicate the presence of *sensorineural hearing loss* (SNHL). SNHL is caused by deficit of hearing function within the inner ear or the nerves or structures of the brain responsible for hearing. Higher AC threshold (poorer sensitivity) compared to BC threshold at any frequency within an ear, known as an *air-bone gap*, indicates *conductive hearing loss* (CHL). CHL loss is caused by a deficit in the outer or middle ear function. *Mixed hearing loss* is found when a combination of SNHL and CHL exist within an ear. Normal, conductive, mixed, and sensorineural hearing thresholds are visualized in the example audiogram described below.

Displaying the Results

The results of PTA are plotted on to a chart known as a *pure-tone audiogram*. The x-axis of the chart represents the frequency of the pure tone. The y-axis of the chart represents the hearing threshold level. It is an inverted scale in which lower thresholds (better hearing) appear at the top of the chart. Thresholds measured by AC and BC are plotted using different symbols. The symbols used in the United States are defined by the American National Standards Institute and adopted for use by ASLHA. The symbols commonly used in the United Kingdom are defined by the British Society of Audiology–recommended procedures.

A hypothetical audiogram plot containing only thresholds for the right ear, for simplification purposes, is shown in Figure 1. The figure depicts a

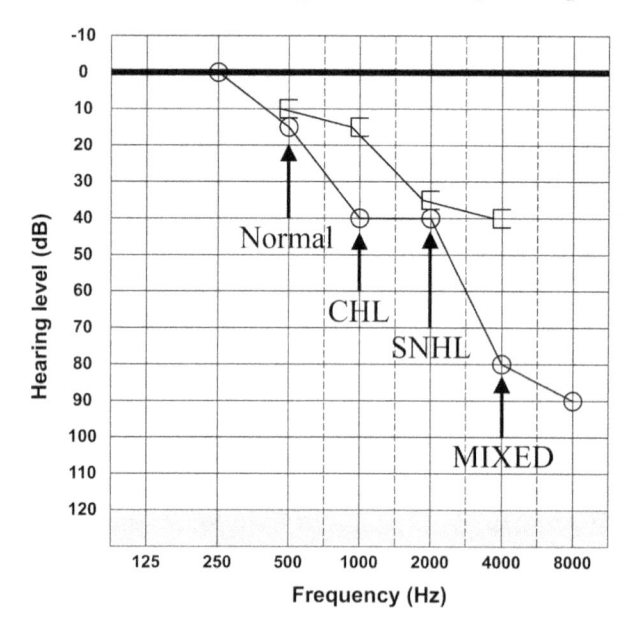

	Right ear	Left ear
Not-masked AC	O	X
Masked AC	△ (BSA O)	□ (BSA X)
Not-masked BC	< (BSA △)	> (BSA △)
Masked BC	[	]

Figure 1 An example hypothetical audiogram for a right ear that has regions of normal hearing, conductive hearing loss (CHL), sensorineural hearing loss (SNHL), and mixed hearing loss. Figure legend depicts PTA symbols used by ASLHA (British Society of Audiology differences in parenthesis)

right ear that has normal (250 Hz, 500 Hz), CHL (1000 Hz), SNHL (2000 Hz), and mixed (4000 Hz) hearing loss components at the different test frequencies as shown by the arrow markers.

Performing the Test

Hearing threshold, at each test frequency and for each ear separately, is established in a standardized way under controlled conditions. The listener is asked to respond when any sound is audible for as long as it is audible, no matter what it sounds like, or which ear it is perceived in (which ear is important and is described below).

The precise procedure used to measure threshold of hearing varies between the different national standards used. Most national standards are identical to, or based upon, the international standard entitled "Acoustics - Audiometric test methods. Part 1: Pure-tone air and bone conduction audiometry (ISO 8253-1:2010)." The test usually proceeds following standardized instructions with AC audiometry in the listener's better hearing ear (if known). The first step, known as the *familiarization stage*, begins by presenting the pure tone to the listener at a level estimated to be clearly audible. If the listener responds to the sound (by pressing a response button), then the level (amplitude) of the tone is decreased in 10-dB steps (descending trial) until the listener no longer responds. When the listener stops responding, the level of the tone is increased in 5-dB steps (ascending trial) until the listener again responds. Ascending and descending trials of tones are presented with duration and intertone interval randomized between 1 and 3 s. The hearing threshold is defined as the minimum sound level that the listener can hear in at least half of the ascending sound trials. Variations in response method can be used when required (e.g., a child may be asked to raise hand instead of pressing response button for the full duration the tone is heard), but verbal responses are avoided as the sound of the listener's voice may interfere with detection of the test tone. Once the hearing threshold to the first test frequency (usually 1000 Hz) has been established, the result is recorded and the test operator moves on to the next pure-tone frequency. This process is repeated until AC hearing thresholds have been established for all of the pure-tone frequencies. This process is repeated in the other ear and then using the bone conductor.

Untangling the Response From Each Ear

It is normal to assume that if sounds are presented to the right ear, the measured thresholds are attributed to the right ear. However, this is not always correct if the hearing is much better in the non-test ear. Cross-hearing can occur when there is a difference in AC threshold between the ears or a difference between AC and BC threshold at any individual frequency within either ear. The tester performing the PTA must carefully examine the threshold results to determine whether cross-hearing may have been present. Errors in diagnosis and patient management can occur if an audiogram is incorrectly interpreted when cross-hearing has occurred. This is because measured thresholds due to cross-hearing appear to be more acute than the true threshold of that ear.

Cross-hearing can happen because there are sound transmission pathways between the transducer placed on the test ear and the inner ear of the opposite non-test ear. In BC audiometry, almost equal levels of sound reach both ears regardless of which mastoid the BC headphone is placed behind. In AC audiometry, sound reaches the non-test ear at a reduced level to the audiometer dial setting, which is presented to the test ear. The amount by which the sound is reduced between the two ears is known as the *interaural attenuation* (IA), measured in dB. The IA differs between headphone type, frequency, and listener. Experimenters have found the minimum expected level of IA in the adult population for each headphone type. The minimum IA for the bone conductor is 0 dB (no sound lost), whereas the minimum IA for the supra-aural headphones and insert earphone used in AC audiometry is 40 and 55 dB, respectively. The possibility of cross-hearing exists if the difference in measured AC threshold of the worst ear and the cochlear threshold (BC) of the better ear, at any frequency, is greater than or equal to the minimum IA for the AC transducer used. The possibility of cross-hearing exists for BC measurements if there is a difference between AC and BC thresholds at any frequency within either ear, this is, because BC thresholds represent the threshold of the better hearing ear. If cross-hearing is suspected either for BC or AC audiometry, an additional threshold measurement procedure (called *masking*) is performed to establish true threshold of the worst ear. Masked thresholds are measured by presenting a distracting sound to the better non-test ear to prevent it from detecting the test sounds presented to the test ear.

Limitations

It is important to note that although PTA is a widely used and accepted test, it has a number of limitations. The principle limitations are summarized below.

Technical Limitations

Despite widespread use of PTA as the *gold standard* hearing test, there are some technical limitations that are worthy of note. BC audiometry is confined to a narrower range of pure-tone test frequencies (500–4000 Hz) compared to AC testing. This is because the physical characteristic of the BC headphones limited its useful output range. The maximum sound intensity that the BC headphone can produce is more limited than the AC headphones. This can result in difficulties classifying the hearing loss (SNHL/CHL) when the AC thresholds measured are higher than the maximum sound output level of the BC headphones. Misleading thresholds can also be measured when presenting high sound output levels through the BC headphone. This can occur when the listener's vibrotactile threshold (feeling the BC vibration) is lower than their hearing threshold. It was stated earlier that BC testing bypasses the outer and middle ear, but this is a simplification. The outer and middle ear structures have some involvement in sounds reaching the cochlea during BC testing. This further complicates result interpretation as middle ear disorders can also impact BC thresholds.

Other listener-dependent technical test limitations exist that can result in poorer than expected performance in hearing rehabilitation outcomes. Researchers have found that there are sometimes areas in the cochlea that are so poorly functioning that the sound presented at frequencies normally detected in that region is more efficiently detected elsewhere in the cochlea. These regions are known as *dead regions*. In other words, when presenting an 8-kHz pure tone, the subject might hear the sound using an area of their cochlea normally responsible for detecting a 4-kHz pure tone. This off-frequency hearing is thought to occur during PTA testing in about 50% of listeners whose thresholds are greater than 70 dB HL. Dead regions cannot be detected by PTA thresholds.

General Limitations

It is important to note that there is no strong association between hearing loss classification, based on PTA, and difficulties experienced in real life. The most frequent complaint of hearing-impaired listeners is an inability to follow speech in noisy environments. Although there is a correlation between measured PTA thresholds and speech detection ability in quiet situations, this correlation is much weaker in noisy situations. It is known, for example, that the ability to understand speech in background noise diminishes with age even while PTA thresholds remain relatively stable. Therefore, although the thresholds measured by PTA are of clinical use, they do not provide a comprehensive assessment of the listeners hearing difficulties. For example, a mild hearing loss does not always imply mild difficulties. It is possible that two individuals with near identical audiograms have quite different degrees of communication difficulty caused by their hearing loss.

Future Directions

PTA, the detection of quiet tones of varying frequency, has been used as the gold standard hearing test for many years. The test procedure involves determining the hearing threshold level, across a range of frequencies, in each ear separately. The hearing loss is then quantified by comparing to a group of normal-hearing young adults (represented by the 0 dB HL line on the audiogram). The use of AC earphones and a bone conductor allows the anatomical site of lesion to be identified so that the hearing loss can be categorized as conductive or sensorineural. Despite the wide spread use of PTA, it has a number of technical limitations. In addition, it does not reflect the difficulty of understanding speech in background noise, the most frequent complaint expressed by people with hearing difficulties.

Researchers in the field of audiology aim to find new ways to assess hearing loss looking beyond the PTA, particularly in the cases of listeners who report diminished hearing function but have normal measured PTA thresholds (hidden hearing loss). Researchers are also considering the efficacy of performing PTA using an extended frequency range above the present standard 8-kHz pure tone. There is also emerging evidence that the PTA, as currently measured, may not be required when prescribing and fitting hearing aids. However, it is likely that, for the foreseeable future, PTA will remain universally accepted among hearing professionals as one of the first key tests to perform in care pathways diagnosing and managing hearing loss.

Timothy S. Wilding and Kevin J. Munro

See also Hearing Disability and Disorders; Hearing Screening; Hearing Tests; Physiological Basis for Hearing; Psychoacoustics; Speech Audiometry

Further Readings

American Speech-Language Hearing Association. (2005). *Guidelines for manual pure-tone threshold audiometry* [Online]. Retrieved June 19, 2017, from http://www.asha.org/policy/GL2005-00014.htm

British Society of Audiology. (2011). *Pure-tone air-conduction and bone-conduction threshold audiometry with and without masking* [Online]. Retrieved June 19, 2017, from http://www.thebsa.org.uk/resources/pure-tone-air-bone-conduction-threshold-audiometry-without-masking/

Gelfand Stanley, A. (2016). *Essentials of audiology* (4th ed.). New York, NY: Thieme Medical Publishers.

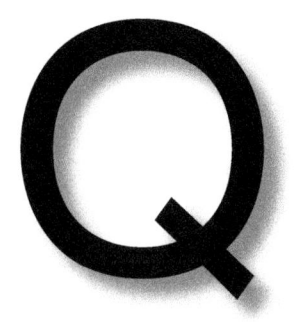

QUALITATIVE RESEARCH

The discipline of human communication sciences and disorders (HCSD) has a long history of research into the nature, development, and use of normal communicative processes, as well as the investigation of communicative impairments. Although a majority of this work has been conducted using experimental or quantitative research, there has always been some percentage of research conducted through qualitative research methods. Across the history of HCSD, much of this qualitative research involved longitudinal investigations and case studies; however, this has been changing since the 1990s as a greater diversity of qualitative approaches and methodologies has been employed in the discipline. This increased application of qualitative research is understandable, when the strengths and advantages of this research paradigm are explored. This entry will discuss a definition and description of qualitative research, a brief history, and detail some of its primary traditions of inquiry.

Defining Qualitative Research

As a research paradigm, there are many positive facets of qualitative research. It has a strong history of success when investigating social phenomena, it is based upon defensible epistemological theory, and it possesses a set of design characteristics and methodological assumptions different from other research approaches. These characteristics enable it to be well suited for investigating social action in authentic contexts.

To be accepted and to function as a valid research paradigm, it is important to understand what is meant by qualitative research and to determine how it fills a gap that other research approaches might miss. Qualitative research is often differentiated from quantitative research based upon the superficial meaning of the terms *qualitative* and *quantitative*. That is, according to this differentiation qualitative research is dependent on descriptions, such as spoken narratives, while quantitative research is based upon numbers and mathematical/predictive calculations. Although this distinction creates a limited contrast between these two research paradigms, it is too simplistic. It is true that when focusing on social actions within authentic contexts, the numeric data and predictive statistical procedures employed by quantitative research are often insufficient to examine the behaviors in question. The numbers cannot discern human motivations or operational mechanisms, and predictive statistics is not designed to seek answers to questions that stress how social actions and social experiences are created and sustained. A more formal definition is required.

Although there are many acceptable definitions of qualitative research in the literature, Jack Damico and Nina Simmons-Mackie advanced the definition of qualitative research in HCSD as a variety of analytic procedures that function as methods of inquiry designed to systematically collect and describe authentic, contextualized social phenomena with the goal of interpretive adequacy.

This definition provides several important criteria that differentiate qualitative research from other research paradigms and position it as advantageous when investigating complex social phenomenon. The terms *analytic* and *describe* characterize the procedures available under the rubric of qualitative research and their role in the research enterprise. Each of the traditions of inquiry is designed to analyze the phenomena under scrutiny so that a detailed description of the social actions observed and their interpretation are possible. Importantly, these analytic techniques possess as their primary objective *interpretive adequacy*; that is, attempting to understand how the social phenomena of interest function and why, determining what actions are produced by targeted individuals, and determining how these actions are accomplished and for what reasons. Other operational terms in this definition, such as *social*, *contextualized*, and *authentic*, highlight the scope of qualitative research: authentic social phenomena. These phenomena are guided by intentionality according to the beliefs and values that the social actors have constructed. Furthermore, the data of interest, social action, are produced in natural contexts and are significantly influenced by these operational contexts. To understand these phenomena, therefore, the research procedures must be flexible and reflexive so that the variables influencing the social actions may also be discovered, detailed, and analyzed. Understanding the behavior of interest, therefore, starts with a focus on these unconstrained social phenomena, and qualitative methods of inquiry are designed for this purpose. Finally, the phrase "systematically collect" is crucial to this definition since, as in all scientific research endeavors, there must be a defensible rationale for which procedure is employed for investigation, and the design characteristics of the procedure must be carefully and deliberately deployed.

The History of Qualitative Research

The history of qualitative research is tied to the history of the social sciences. As investigators became more interested in society and culture, discovery procedures evolved to meet the needs of emerging social scientists. Although anthropology began as a discipline in the 1840s and early researchers like Joseph François Lafitau, Lewis Henry Morgan, and Frank Hamilton Cushing have been credited with the development of early versions of ethnography and participant observation, a sufficient overview of qualitative research should begin at the turn of the 19th and 20th centuries. This particular time period was characterized by colonialism undertaken by various Western nations, and emerging social scientists were interested in exotic cultures and societal practices observed in these colonized portions of the world. In anthropology, there were efforts to understand and document the different, foreign, and unusual. For example, early anthropologists like Franz Boas conducted research on Baffin Island and produced *The Central Eskimo* in 1888, and Maria Czaplicka conducted fieldwork in Siberia and published *Aboriginal Siberia* in 1914. Although these were important books in establishing field work and cultural anthropology, one of the first universally credited versions of qualitative research was an account of field experiences written by Bronislaw Malinowski about his investigations of the cultures of New Guinea and the Trobriand Islands. Published as *Argonauts of the Western Pacific* in 1922, many commentators view this book as one of the best early ethnographies. In anthropology, numerous similar studies heralded the arrival of classic ethnography as an early tradition of inquiry, including ethnographies by Ruth Benedict, Margaret Mead, Gregory Bateson, Ruth Bunzel, Oscar Lewis, Oliver LaFarge, and Zora Neale Hurston.

Parallel to the emergence of qualitative research in anthropology, some centers within the discipline of sociology also emphasized the qualitative paradigm. As the great immigration waves occurred in the United States from the 1890s to the 1920s, there was an opportunity to study different groups and their societal differences in the large cities of the United States. In the University of Chicago's Department of Sociology in the 1920s and 1930s, the discipline of urban sociology was established, and many of the works that came from the *Chicago school* were qualitative in nature. These included *The Polish Peasant in Europe and America: Monograph of an Immigrant Group* and *The Ghetto*. Qualitative research continued through the middle of the 20th century with ethnographies structured through participant observation, narratives, artifact analysis, and interviews. Students drawn to qualitative research (regardless of their discipline) usually learned these research methods through an apprenticeship approach to learning.

In the 1960s and 1970s, however, there were significant changes in the social sciences. First, the social disciplines became more firmly anchored in theoretical principles (e.g., symbolic interactionism, constructivism, labeling theory, ethnomethodology, phenomenology, critical theory) that were applied within the disciplines. Second, there was the development of additional qualitative traditions of inquiry, often based upon these theoretical principles. Third, there was a trend to formalize and standardize the learning and application of qualitative methods. For example, Howard Becker produced a study of medical students, *Boys in White*, in 1961 that became a model for rigorous qualitative analysis. Based upon a hybridization of social positivism and quantitative research principles advocated by the *Columbia School of Sociology* and the constructivist principles and qualitative focus required with the *Chicago School of Sociology*, Anselm Strauss and Barney Glaser established *grounded theory* as another tradition of inquiry while investigating dying in hospital settings. Based upon this study, they wrote *Awareness of Dying*. They then published a more important book in 1967, *The Discovery of Grounded Theory*. This book focused on systematically detailing how to use the methodological strategies that defined grounded theory as a qualitative procedure.

During this period, Harvey Sacks and colleagues, such as Emanuel Schegloff and Gail Jefferson, created and championed conversation analysis; European scholars introduced methodological phenomenology; and linguists, sociolinguists, and anthropological linguists developed various analysis procedures. By the end of the 1970s, there was increasing use of qualitative research in all of its manifestations. To accommodate this research, numerous journals devoted to qualitative research in the social sciences were founded, such as *Anthropology & Education Quarterly*, *Cultural Anthropology*, *Discourse Processes*, *Language in Society*, *Qualitative Sociology*, *Quality and Quantity: International Journal of Methodology*, and *Urban Life and Culture*.

Since the mid-1970s, qualitative research has established itself within disciplines like anthropology, sociology, linguistics, social psychology, education, medicine, nursing, business, marketing, and political science. It is also gaining a foothold in related areas, such as second language acquisition, literacy studies, and HCSD.

The Strengths of Qualitative Research

One essential requirement for credible research is that the methods of study employed must be appropriate to the subject matter. When engaging in social science research, qualitative research fits this requirement. Throughout the history of the social sciences, the traditions of inquiry have been designed and modified to address the complexity of social action, and these design characteristics may be viewed as the strengths of qualitative research. Several of these strengths are detailed in the following subsections.

Natural Settings

The research methods are devised to collect and study phenomena in their natural settings. It is a foundational truth in the social sciences that one's actions are always influenced by the extended context within which social actions are performed. This means that to understand the phenomenon of interest and its actions and interpretations it is necessary to attend to the contextual variables that influence them. Qualitative methods are oriented to data collection techniques and interpretive analyses that enable scrutiny of natural and authentic phenomena. Rather than try to control potential extraneous variables (as experimental designs do), these variables are identified and described as they function during the ongoing give-and-take of social action.

Open and Unstructured Research Designs

There is a preference for open and relatively unstructured research designs. In concert with the first strength, it is necessary to ensure adaptability regarding when and how the data collection and analyses are applied. Since the natural context(s) being studied are dynamic and multifaceted, the ability to adjust the focus of the research, the opportunity to return to data collection even after analyses have been initiated, and the particular way the data are collected must enable sufficient attention and explication of the variables that comprise the phenomena being examined. Without such openness, the impact of the context and the complexity of the overall phenomena could not be adequately investigated.

The Researcher as Data Collector

The researcher is the key agent of data collection. To adjust to the necessity of being open to changes in decision making while collecting naturalistic data, the researcher must be able to make required adjustments as the circumstances warrant. Consequently, the researcher is expected to be on-site and to function as the primary data collection instrument. Of course, this means that the researcher must be trained in various data collection strategies so that real-time and online adjustments can be accomplished.

Descriptive, not Numeric, Data

Qualitative research is designed to collect descriptive data rather than numeric data. Since this research paradigm is interested in understanding procedural affairs, rather than investigating the relationship between variables or merely predicting the occurrence of a variable, the mechanisms or processes by which social action is accomplished are the primary objective. Qualitative research using descriptions of behavioral phenomena (e.g., interactional strategies, interactional frames, conversational devices, grammatical structures, discourse markers, social assumptions, social activities) or pictures that can be detailed and understood according to their design and usage as social patterns are required. The rich description of the actions while they are embedded within their contexts is essential to determine how the social activity is created and sustained. Although there are times when numerical data are beneficial within the qualitative research paradigm, this quantitative data should be used in accordance with actual descriptions of the social phenomena.

Focused Rather Than Broad Description

Focused description is preferred over broader description. Since the emphasis is on descriptive data obtained from authentic and complex situations, this thick description requires that data be collected with few cases and more variables than other research paradigms. A focused description of few, rather than many, facilitates the focus on the interdependence of social actions within the context and provides for sufficient time and focus to understand the complexity of social phenomena being investigated.

Investigation of Social Action

Qualitative analysis is designed to investigate the process of social action rather than its product. Consistent with the understanding of procedural affairs, the tantalizing questions in qualitative research focus on how things happen, rather than that they happened. This is accomplished in this research paradigm because the analyses target the mechanisms of action and the processes that occur to produce and sustain the investigated social phenomenon.

From the Participant's Perspective

Finally, the primary focus during data collection and interpretation is the participants' perspectives, rather than the researcher's perspective. The meanings that a social event or action have on an individual are constructed by that individual. Since appropriate interpretation and understanding is the goal of the research, it is necessary to incorporate the conceptual frameworks of the participants into one's analysis. This is the only way to understand how participants interpret and react to what is happening in their social world.

Qualitative Traditions of Inquiry

The maturation of the qualitative research paradigm, especially since the 1970s, has resulted in many methods or procedures that can be employed to study social phenomena. These range from various naturalistic data collection procedures (e.g., participant observation, semistructured interviews, video and audio recording, focus groups, artifact analysis) to general research methods (e.g., bibliographic study, critical qualitative analysis, historical methodology, and narrative, discourse, linguistic analyses). However, there are several well-established methodologies that may be referred to as *traditions of inquiry* due to their unique history of development across the social science disciplines. Some of the primary traditions of inquiry are listed below. Although certain procedures may be better suited to study a phenomenon, as an analytic paradigm, qualitative research does not favor one single methodology over any other. Instead, one's preferred use of one method over another should be dependent on the nature of the social phenomenon investigated, the context in which data collection occurs, and the familiarity and ease with which the investigator can employ the potential procedures.

Case Studies

The most widely employed qualitative tradition of inquiry is the case study. As the name suggests, the focus is on a case as an object of investigation. This focus is often an individual, but it could also be a specific topic, event, or location. Since this tradition of inquiry is identified based upon the concentration on a specific case and not the data collection techniques utilized, many of the procedures used in other traditions of inquiry are employed within case studies as well.

Conversation Analysis

Influenced by the theoretical and methodological concept known as *ethnomethodology*, conversation analysis examines conversations to study social action and interaction though the description and understanding of various interactional and linguistic devices and resources. Recognizing that there is a structural organization of talk, that this organization of talk is oriented to principles of sequential ordering, and that conversational actions are dependent upon local interpretation of conversational moves and strategies (i.e., actions project next actions), this tradition of inquiry investigates how speakers produce their own behaviors and how they interpret the behaviors of others during time at talk.

Ethnography

Having evolved from the field of anthropology in the mid-1800s, ethnography has undergone numerous modifications. However, it remains a procedure designed to investigate social life and culture in their ongoing complexity. The investigator immerses him- or herself within the culture for an appropriate period so that contextually sensitive behaviors and patterns of behaviors can be collected and analyzed using a variety of techniques like participant observation, interviewing, and the analysis of artifacts. These procedures and the subsequent analyses are discovery driven; facts, patterns, and concepts are identified and interpreted, and the result is a better understanding of the nature of specific facets of the culture through the perspective of those living within that culture.

Grounded Theory

Using what was termed *theoretical sensitivity*, the grounded theory tradition of inquiry is designed to observe, code, collect, and analyze data so that various kinds of analytic questions can be asked and answered about the social phenomenon under investigation. This process provides the researcher with a method to separate pertinent from nonpertinent data so that an insightful understanding of how various social actions are created and interpreted is the product. The data collection approaches are similar to other traditions (e.g., interviews, observation, artifact analysis), but the analysis and interpretation is different. Using several unique techniques (e.g., constant comparative method, conditional matrix), this tradition is designed to produce a *substantive theory*, an understanding of the targeted phenomenon that can predict how the observed social actions, their interactions, consequences, and subsequent related conditions operate within designated contexts.

Phenomenology

Phenomenology determines how a social action or activity is experienced as meaningful by the participants in a context of interest, usually using individual interviews as the database. Through these interviews, the researcher obtains a recollection of the lived experiences from the participants as they were subjected to a specific context or condition. Because individuals act and react to events and experiences based upon the meanings they have constructed about these phenomena, these *lived experiences* ground one's knowledge to the actual conscious perceptions one possesses and the consequential social actions that result.

Qualitative research has established greater attention and interest in HCSD, and there are progressively more applications to developmental and clinical questions being identified, especially among those questions that are not well suited for investigation within the experimental paradigm. However, it should be remembered that within the qualitative paradigm, explication is the crucial objective. The social actions of individuals, including those with communicative deficits, can be better understood by providing rich or detailed descriptions of what is occurring during their social actions. There is also, however, another facet of this dynamic process: the reality that it is the contextualizing of communication within the social–cognitive fabric that establishes people as meaningful social actors. Qualitative research is best positioned to collect and understand these complex datasets.

Jack S. Damico

See also Case Studies; Constructivism; Conversation Analysis; Focus Groups; Grounded Theory; Interviewing; Phenomenology; Research

Further Readings

Agar, M. (2013). *The lively science. Remodeling human social research*. Minneapolis, MN: Mill City Press.

Ball, M. J., Müller, N., & Nelson, R. (Eds.). (2014). *The handbook of qualitative research in communication disorders*. London, UK: Psychology Press.

Charmaz, K. (2006). *Constructing grounded theory. A practical guide through qualitative analysis*. Thousand Oaks, CA: Sage.

Creswell, J. W., & Poth, C. N. (1998). *Qualitative inquiry and research design: Choosing among five approaches* (4th ed.). Thousand Oaks, CA: Sage.

Damico, J. S., & Simmons-Mackie, N. N. (2003). Qualitative research and speech-language pathology: Impact and promise in the clinical realm. *American Journal of Speech Language Pathology*, 12, 131–143.

Denzin, N. K., & Lincoln, Y. S. (Eds.). (2008). *The landscape of qualitative research* (3rd ed.). Thousand Oaks, CA: Sage.

Maxwell, J. A. (2012). *A realist approach for qualitative research*. Thousand Oaks, CA: Sage.

Smith, J. S. (Ed.). (2003). *Qualitative psychology. A practical guide to research methods*. Thousand Oaks, CA: Sage.

Spradley, J. (1980). *Participant observation*. New York, NY: Holt, Rinehart and Winston.

Quality of Life and Neurogenic Communication Disorders

Neurogenic communication disorders not only cause impairments of speech, language, and communication in adults but also substantially impact individuals' lives and the lives of family, friends, and others around them. Historically, much of speech pathology research and clinical practice has focused on the identification and remediation of the impairments of aphasia, dysarthria, and dyspraxia, with the functional communication consequences of these impairments not considered until the 1980s and 1990s. It was not until the 1990s that the psychosocial impact of these communication disorders was formally recognized and considered, and from 2000 onward, specific consideration was given to individuals' quality of life (QOL) or well-being. QOL is, however, an ultimate outcome of speech pathology rehabilitation for adults with communication disorders, but progress has been hampered by difficulties in determining which aspects are appropriate for assessment and intervention and in considering how to undertake QOL evaluation with clients with impaired communication abilities. This entry provides a brief overview of QOL and then discusses the relevant aspects of QOL in the conditions of aphasia, dysarthria, and dyspraxia, with a particular focus on QOL assessment.

Overview

Speech–language pathologists are familiar with the World Health Organization's (WHO) International Classification of Functioning, Disability and Health as a framework for practice. However, the International Classification of Functioning, Disability and Health does not consider QOL. The WHOQOL Group, a separate entity, was tasked with defining and developing a QOL assessment. QOL as outlined by the WHOQOL Group con-context, culture, value systems, as well as how the person lives (e.g., an individual's goals and expectations). The WHOQOL Group considers QOL to be a broad concept that includes health, psychological state, independent, social relationships, and the person's environment Although the WHO-QOL Group's definition and the domains of the assessment are considered relevant to all adults regardless of health or clinical background, the assessment is extensive and not standardly used in communication disorders research or clinical practice. Other definitions of QOL include maximizing functioning and well-being or considering external context (e.g., number of social contacts in one's social network) and internal perceptions (e.g., whether an individual is satisfied with this situation and feels supported and connected to others). Generally speaking, QOL can be interpreted in two ways: health-related QOL or well-being. Regardless of interpretation, QOL is typically considered multidimensional and composed of a range of domains: That is, physical health, mental/emotional health, and social health (health-related QOL), or life satisfaction and positive and negative affect (well-being). Evaluating QOL is either undertaken qualitatively, via asking the client and family to respond to questions regarding their QOL, or quantitatively, using formal patient-reported questionnaires. These QOL assessments are either multidimensional or unidimensional assessing one domain only. QOL assessments are also considered either generic (for the general population) or condition-specific.

Aphasia

The psychosocial impact of aphasia is the most understood of all of the adult neurogenic communication disorders, having been well-documented since the mid-1990s. QOL has been investigated quantitatively and qualitatively, in both early time poststroke and chronic stages. It has also been considered from both the perspectives of health-related QOL and psychological well-being. Research undertaken by Madeline Cruice has shown that various quantitative factors statistically predict QOL with chronic aphasia, including emotional health (mood), social health, and communication disability. When people with aphasia are asked to discuss their QOL, they consider the following factors: activities, verbal communication, relationships with people, body functioning, stroke, mobility, positive personal outlook, independence versus dependence, home, and health. In terms of assessment, although people with aphasia have difficulty with the standard means of reading and reporting QOL questionnaires, family members acting as proxy respondents show bias in ratings. Thus, it is preferable and possible to support the client using interviewer-administered methods and supported communication techniques, enabling them to self-complete. There are several assessments for evaluating QOL and related areas in aphasia, including the Stroke and Aphasia Quality of Life Scale (SAQOL-39), the Visual Analogue Self-Esteem Scale, the Communication Disability Profile, the Assessment of Living with Aphasia, the American Speech-Language-Hearing Association Quality of Communicative Life Scale, and the Burden of Stroke Scale. Two are described in more detail here.

The SAQOL-39 was devised by Katerina Hilari and colleagues and is the best known and most used measure in aphasia research and practice. It contains 39 items across four subscales of Physical, Psychosocial, Communication, and Energy, using a five-point scale of difficulty with each item. It has been well tested with 83 people with primarily mild–moderate aphasia, shown to have good psychometrics, and is acceptable and highly relevant to people with aphasia. The SAQOL-39 has been translated into many languages. The authors developed an alternative version of the SAQOL-39 that is appropriate for use in a generic stroke population. This means the same generic version can be used to collect data in hospitals from patients with stroke as well as those with stroke and aphasia and also used in a similar way in research studies. The SAQOL-39g contains the same 39 items, organized in three domains.

The Assessment of Living with Aphasia was developed by Aura Kagan and colleagues and is specifically for people with the range of aphasia severity. It is pictographic, accessible, and measures aphasia-related QOL. The Assessment of

Living with Aphasia is a relatively new assessment that is likely to be of increasing use in research and practice in coming years. It is based on the Living with Aphasia: Framework for Outcome Measurement and as such covers language, participation, personal experiences, and the environment. It contains 37 items rated on a five-point scale and five items that provide descriptive information. It has been psychometrically tested on 101 participants with aphasia and has acceptable test–retest reliability, internal consistency, and construct validity and is acceptable to people with aphasia and speech pathologists.

In clinical practice, an international survey published by Hilari and colleagues found that between 10% and 27% of clinicians use QOL measures for initial assessment, outcome measurement, or both. Remaining clinicians don't assess QOL or do it informally through discussion. This is a concern because clinicians are not holistically assessing the needs and concerns of their clients, might develop treatment goals and deliver therapies that are not a priority to the client, and cannot demonstrate the value of their treatment as impacting on the client's QOL. In research, QOL is now more frequently included as an outcome and measured across a range of aphasia rehabilitation research studies; however, the actual evidence base for which treatment is more effective, or how to improve QOL most efficiently, is still emerging. Meanwhile, treatments that address what is core in QOL to people with aphasia (i.e., mood and meaningful activities, relationships, and communication) should be considered in clinical practice.

Dysarthria

Dysarthria (poststroke acquired and progressive) has broad implications for everyday life, which have only relatively recently been recognized in the literature. Dysarthria can cause changes in mood (depression and anxiety), life participation (social isolation, social exclusion, changes in employment, leisure, and social activities), and self-concept (self-perception, identity) and contribute to changes in well-being and QOL. There are no known QOL assessments for adults with dysarthria; however, there are three assessments that explore the *insider perspective* and in some way provide insights into the broader impact on people's lives. These include the Dysarthria Impact Profile, the Communicative Participation Item Bank, and the Living with Neurologically Based Speech Difficulties questionnaire. The first assessment explores psychosocial impact, and the remaining questionnaires explore individuals' perceived communication difficulties.

The Dysarthria Impact Profile was developed by Margaret Walshe and colleagues and was designed to assess the psychological and social consequences of dysarthria that can affect adults' participation. It was developed from several sources, including findings from in-depth interviews with 10 adults with chronic acquired dysarthria and a review of existing communication profile questionnaires of relevance. The Dysarthria Impact Profile comprises 48 statements, rated on a five-point scale of agreement, across the following five sections: the effect of dysarthria on me as a person; accepting my dysarthria; how I feel others react to my speech; how dysarthria affects my communication with others; and a final question regarding areas most concerned about. It has been tested on 31 adults with acquired dysarthria and found to have some good reliability and validity.

The Communicative Participation Item Bank was developed by Carolyn Baylor and colleagues and is based on the self-report of 701 individuals from across four diagnostic groups, including multiple sclerosis, Parkinson's disease, amyotrophic lateral sclerosis, and head and neck cancer. The resultant 10-item General Short Form is consistent across clinical conditions and robustly psychometrically tested. Although it provides clinicians and researchers with the individual's perception of their communicative participation, the Communicative Participation Item Bank does not consider social, emotional, or QOL/well-being aspects of living with dysarthria.

The Living with Neurologically Based Speech Difficulties self-report questionnaire was developed by Lena Hartelius and colleagues and was developed following a review of published and unpublished scales and questionnaires for individuals with speech and language disorders and a qualitative study of 18 individuals with multiple sclerosis. The questionnaire has two parts. The first part is demographics, and the second includes 50 statements in 10 categories: How communication is influenced by problems pertaining to speech, language, or cognition and fatigue; how emotions, persons, and situations affect communication; roles in which the individual feels restricted as family member, in social, or professional situations; what contributes to communication changes; how it is affected; and different strategies the individual may use to improve their communicative function.

Similar to aphasia, clinicians practicing with patients and clients with dysarthria infrequently use these assessments, and many clinicians assess QOL and psychosocial impact informally through discussion with the client. This gives rise to the same concern as mentioned above. With respect to rehabilitation, there are no known evidence-based and specific treatments for QOL in dysarthria. Clinicians typically provide treatment for dysarthria that is focused on the impairment and functional communication in both acquired and progressive fields. Research published in the mid-2010s suggests that studies are starting to consider QOL as an outcome measure from impairment-focused treatment, such as Be Clear (intensive treatment for acquired dysarthria) and Lee Silverman Voice Treatment (Parkinson's disease). It is also likely that group treatment that provides communication practice, education, peer support, and professional support for clients with dysarthria (and potentially carers, too) could have a positive impact on QOL.

Dyspraxia

The psychosocial impact and QOL in acquired dyspraxia or apraxia of speech is almost entirely absent from the English-published research literature. Nonetheless, dyspraxia has a similar impact on individuals as aphasia and dysarthria, causing distress, frustration, and reduced confidence, and impacting on all aspects of life. The American Speech-Language-Hearing Association Practice Portal on Acquired Apraxia of Speech encourages clinicians to adopt a WHO approach for comprehensive assessment in dyspraxia. The typical components outlined consider functional communication, barriers, and facilitators. They fall short, however, of considering assessment of psychosocial aspects, QOL, or well-being. Treatment outlined according to the Practice Portal is restorative (i.e., speech production and intelligibility) or compensatory (i.e., alternative and augmentative communication), and there are no specific treatments that attempt to improve QOL or consider QOL in the portal or in the English-published research literature. There is a clear need for more research and clinical practice to be undertaken and published in the area of considering psychosocial impact and QOL in adults with apraxia of speech.

Final Thoughts

In conclusion, the achievement of effective communication is a core rehabilitation and recovery goal for all adults with neurogenic communication disorders, regardless of the nature of the impairment. However, the social, emotional, and broader life consequences of aphasia and dysarthria are known to be substantial and must also be considered in speech pathology assessment and treatment. There is a clear evidence base for factors that influence QOL with aphasia in both early time postonset and long term, and robust assessments available that can be used in clinical practice. QOL treatment in aphasia is a field of rapidly growing evidence. Much more research (in general, and specifically in much larger participant samples) and attention to QOL in both dysarthria and dyspraxia is needed to ensure that individuals' needs are identified and met appropriately through speech pathology services.

Madeline Cruice

See also Aphasia; Dysarthria; Psychosocial Impact of Aphasia; Recovery From Aphasia; Rehabilitation

Further Readings

Brown, K., Worrall, L., Davidson, B., & Howe, T. (2010). Snapshots of success: An insider perspective on living successfully with aphasia. *Aphasiology, 24*(10), 1267–1295.

Cruice, M., Hill, R., Worrall, L., & Hickson, L. (2010). Conceptualising quality of life for older people with aphasia. *Aphasiology, 24*(3), 327–347.

Cruice, M., Worrall, L., Hickson, L., & Murison, R. (2003). Finding a focus for quality of life with aphasia: Social and emotional health, and psychological well-being. *Aphasiology, 17*(4), 333–353.

Hilari, K., Klippi, A., Constantinidou, F., Horton, S., Penn, C., Raymer, A., . . . Worrall, L. (2015). An international perspective on quality of life in aphasia: A survey of clinician views and practices from sixteen countries. *Folia Phoniatrica et Lodopaedica, 67*(3), 119–130.

Van der Gaag, A., Smith, L., Davis, S., Moss, B., Cornelius, V., Laing, S., & Mowles, C. (2005). Therapy and support services for people with long-term stroke and aphasia and their relatives: A six-month follow-up study. *Clinical Rehabilitation, 19*(4), 372–380.

Worrall, L., Hudson, K., Khan, A., Ryan, B., & Simmons-Mackie, N. (2016). Determinants of living well with aphasia in the first year post-stroke: A prospective cohort study. *Archives of Physical Medicine and Rehabilitation, 98*(2), 235–240.

QUALITY OF LIFE AND STUTTERING

Stuttering is a complex condition that can affect all aspects of an individual's life. Although listeners tend to identify stuttering primarily as a disorder involving disruptions in the production of speech (or disfluencies, such as repetitions, prolongations, and blocks), the difficulties that a person who stutters experiences in producing sounds and words can have a much broader impact on their communication abilities and on their lives as a whole. For example, people who stutter may experience negative emotional and cognitive reactions to stuttering, including feelings of embarrassment, shame, anxiety, depression, isolation, loneliness, or frustration. They may experience behavioral reactions, such as physical tension and struggle prior to or during moments of stuttering, as well as avoidance of sounds, words, or speaking situations as they attempt to minimize the occurrence of stuttering behaviors. Individuals might experience negative reactions from other people, such as discrimination, bullying and teasing, a lack of understanding, impatience, and time pressure. People who stutter may also experience difficulties with social interactions or performing other tasks that involve speaking, such as introducing oneself, engaging in conversations, talking on the telephone, asking or answering questions, reading aloud, and giving presentations at school or work. All of these various characteristics and consequences can be described as part of the adverse impact that stuttering can have on a person's quality of life (QOL). This entry provides an overview of QOL as it relates to stuttering, highlights the ways in which stuttering can adversely impact QOL, and briefly discusses how QOL can be addressed in stuttering therapy.

Impact of Stuttering on QOL

QOL is a multidimensional construct that is influenced by a wide range of issues related to how people experience their daily lives. Numerous definitions of QOL have been offered; such definitions typically involve the discussion of several key constructs, including satisfaction with life (and, in the case of stuttering, satisfaction with communication), functional status (e.g., the ability to perform daily activities, involving schooling and vocational or occupational endeavors, as well as social interactions), and capacity for achieving one's goals in life (relating to factors such as family interactions, socioeconomic status, religious participation, civic endeavors). Health-related QOL measures also examine factors such as physical and emotional well-being, often in response to the experience of a health condition, disorder, or disease. Definitions of QOL are also strongly related to societal factors such as the availability of support and resources for those experiencing health issues and risk factors associated with health conditions within a community or society. QOL is defined as a patient-reported outcome measure, which is required by many agencies in clinical trials or other assessments of treatment efficacy.

QOL measures have been used throughout the field of health and rehabilitation either to assess the general experience of health and well-being or to evaluate specific experiences that individuals may have as a result of living with a particular health problem. In the field of communication disorders, QOL measures have been used to examine conditions such as aphasia, attention deficit/hyperactivity disorder, autism spectrum disorders, cognitive communication disorders, hearing impairment, voice disorders, and more. Such measures are particularly relevant for considering the consequences of stuttering on people's lives, for the broader impact of stuttering is well-documented, and many approaches to stuttering therapy explicitly seek to minimize the adverse impact of the disorder. Moreover, the scope of practice for speech–language pathologists, developed by the American Speech-Language-Hearing Association, specifically states that the goal of intervention by speech–language pathologists is to improve QOL.

One way of viewing the overall consequences of stuttering is in terms of the World Health Organization's International Classification of Functioning, Disability, and Health. This framework represents the experience of a condition such as stuttering (or any other health issue) as involving (a) an impairment in body function or structure (in this case, the underlying neurological differences that lead to the difficulties with speech production and the production of speech disfluencies themselves) and (b) the effect of the impairment(s) on a person's ability to perform daily activities or participate in life as they would like to do. These activity limitations and participation restrictions constitute the adverse impact associated with the impairment as outlined previously. Individual differences in the experiences of a disorder are influenced by the so-called contextual factors, that is, the individual person's reactions to the disorder (including affective, behavioral, and cognitive reactions) as well as the reactions of those in the person's environment (such as lack of understanding of stuttering and negative public opinions about the condition). Viewing stuttering in terms of the International Classification of Functioning, Disability, and Health highlights the fact that the experience of the disorder involves more than the disruption in speech. The experience of stuttering can involve negative personal and environmental reactions, difficulties with functional communication, and adverse impact on one's satisfaction with and participation in life.

QOL and Stuttering Assessment

Researchers and clinicians in the field of fluency disorders have long acknowledged the varied problems that stuttering can cause, and numerous measurement instruments have been developed over the years that have attempted to assess various aspects of the experience of stuttering. Examples include tools examining attitudinal reactions to stuttering, communication difficulties in specific speaking situations, the relationship between locus of control and the experience of stuttering, ratings of self-efficacy and self-stigma, qualitative measures of stuttering severity, and more. In the late 1990s, such measures began to explicitly examine QOL in people who stutter as an independent (though multifactorial) construct. QOL research on stuttering has included both general measures of health-related QOL (such as the Medical Outcomes Study Short Form 36) and measures of QOL that were developed specifically for the study of stuttering (such as the Overall Assessment of the Speaker's Experience of Stuttering). Regardless of the measure that is applied, research consistently shows that many people who stutter experience adverse impact on their QOL, particularly in areas related to social and emotional well-being, satisfaction with communication, functional communication in key situations, and ability to interact freely with others. The impact of stuttering on QOL has been shown to be related to a variety of factors, including self-esteem and support from family members. Thus, QOL is not solely related to the level of stuttering that an individual exhibits.

Interestingly, the negative consequences of stuttering are not commonly seen in very young children who stutter. Certainly, some children who stutter do experience adverse impact on their QOL, even at a very young age. Overall, though, the adverse impact of stuttering appears to increase as a consequence of living with stuttering and experiencing difficulties in communicating as the child develops. Adverse impact on QOL has also been observed in the family members of those who stutter (e.g., spouses, siblings) indicating that the disorder can lead to negative consequences for more than just the speaker. The entire family is involved in coping with the stuttering disorder. To account for this broad influence of stuttering, many approaches to therapy also include strategies for minimizing the consequences that stuttering can have on the family unit as a whole.

Adverse impact on QOL is not an obligatory feature of living with stuttering. Some people who stutter are not negatively affected by their speaking difficulties. Moreover, many people who stutter can learn to overcome the effects of the disorder, typically through treatment with a speech–language pathologist or other professional, self-treatment, or participation in support and self-help organizations. Nevertheless, most people who stutter do report experiencing negative consequences at some point in their lives. Due in part to the variability of the stuttering behavior, the impact of stuttering on QOL can increase and decrease over time, as people's experiences and perceptions change. Therefore, QOL evaluation is recommended as a valuable baseline and outcome measure for clinicians who work with people who stutter. Documenting changes in QOL provides clinicians with an important guide for setting goals in treatment, while supporting the evaluation of treatment efficacy and determining the true effect of treatment on a person's life.

QOL and Stuttering Treatment

Treatment to minimize the impact of stuttering on QOL can take many forms. Some researchers attribute the negative consequences of stuttering primarily to the presence of stuttered speech itself. In this view, reducing stuttering (through fluency-enhancing or stuttering modification strategies) should yield a reduction in the impact of stuttering on QOL. Studies reveal that the link between observable stuttering severity and adverse impact is not a direct one, however. Thus, many other researchers and clinicians highlight the value of a broader approach to treatment that takes into account all components of the stuttering disorder (e.g., as described through the International Classification of Functioning, Disability, and Health model cited previously). For example, treatment can directly address the speaker's negative reactions to stuttering (personal context), through educational and desensitization activities designed to help the person who stutters become less concerned about stuttering and less physically tense during the moment of stuttering itself. Many clinicians also implement the methods of psychologically based treatments, such as cognitive behavior therapy, acceptance and commitment therapy, and mindfulness to supplement traditional speech therapy methods. Treatment can also incorporate activities designed to educate others about stuttering (environmental context), through activities such as being more open about stuttering or *advertising* or disclosing stuttering to reduce uncertainty about the behavior, in order to reduce the negative environmental reactions. Treatment can also directly address the adverse impact itself, by helping speakers minimize the activity limitations and participation restrictions they experience and ensuring that speakers are able to communicate freely and effectively, regardless of whether or not (or how severely) they stutter. Together, these strategies can help to minimize the impact of stuttering on QOL.

Understanding the complex nature of the stuttering disorder has important consequences for speech–language pathologists who seek to help people who stutter through therapy. Because stuttering involves more than just disruptions in speech production, assessment and treatment for the disorder should address more than just the disruptions in speech production. Considering the impact of stuttering on a person's life can help to ensure a comprehensive approach to the disorder that can result in meaningful improvements in a speaker's communication abilities and in his or her overall QOL.

J. Scott Yaruss and Robert W. Quesal

See also Attitudes in Stuttering; Bullying and Teasing; Circumlocution and Avoidance in Stuttering; Covert Stuttering; Emotional Impact of Communication Disorders; Fluency and Fluency Disorders; Psychosocial Issues Associated With Communication Disorders; Stuttering, Response to; Stuttering and Emotional Reactions

Further Readings

Beilby, J. M., Byrnes, M. L., Meagher, E. L., & Yaruss, J. S. (2013). The impact of stuttering on adults who stutter and their partners. *Journal of Fluency Disorders, 38*, 14–29.

Boyle, M. P. (2015). Relationships between psychosocial factors and quality of life for adults who stutter. *American Journal of Speech-Language Pathology, 24*, 1–12.

Craig, A., Blumgart, E., & Tran, Y. (2009). The impact of stuttering on the quality of life in adults who stutter. *Journal of Fluency Disorders, 34*, 61–71.

Cummins, R. A. (2010). Fluency disorders and life quality: Subjective wellbeing vs. health-related quality of life. *Journal of Fluency Disorders, 35,* 161–172.

De Sonneville-Koedoot, C., Stolk, E. A., Raat, H., Bouwmans-Frijters, C., & Franken, M.-C. (2014). Health-related quality of life of preschool children who stutter. *Journal of Fluency Disorders, 42,* 1–12.

Klompas, M., & Ross, E. (2004). Life experiences of people who stutter, and the perceived impact of stuttering on quality of life: Personal accounts of South African individuals. *Journal of Fluency Disorders, 29,* 275–305.

Yaruss, J. S. (2010). Assessing quality of life in stuttering treatment outcomes research. *Journal of Fluency Disorders, 35,* 190–202.

Yaruss, J. S., & Quesal, R. W. (2004). Stuttering and the International Classification of Functioning, Disability, and Health (ICF): An update. *Journal of Communication Disorders, 37,* 35–52.

Quantitative Research

As a well-practiced research paradigm, quantitative research has been discussed and employed across a range of scientific disciplines. Since at least 1954, when the psychologist Robert Sessions Woodworth published his influential text, *Experimental Psychology,* one type of quantitative research (experimental) has been a leading research methodology not only in the natural sciences but also in the psychological and social sciences. There have been many descriptions and definitions of quantitative research, and most of these definitions have focused on four features of quantitative research: quantification, control, comparison, and manipulation.

Based upon these features, quantitative research is defined as a set of procedures designed to investigate phenomena in controlled settings using numerical data and statistically based analyses. These research designs involve systematic manipulation of the targeted variables and objective data collection to make comparisons across the variables or to predict the occurrence of one variable when linked with another. By using measurement tools that can operationalize the human variables (e.g., traits, abilities, and behaviors) into numeric scores, statistical interpretation of the phenomenon under investigation is possible. In this way, quantitative research procedures attempt to measure social reality in such a way that an empirical description can occur; often, this description focuses on whether there is a relationship between variables (e.g., correlation or cause-and-effect relationship). Typically, quantitative research accomplishes one of the following functions: to test hypotheses, to answer research questions, to determine relationships between variables, and/or to predict the frequency of occurrence of phenomena. This entry discusses the characteristics, advantages, types, and process of quantitative research.

Characteristics of Quantitative Research

Since prediction of change in variables based upon their relationships to one another is crucial in quantitative research, the research enterprise requires that there are clear distinctions between potential causal factors (independent variables) and their effects (dependent variables). Additionally, there must be careful management of each potential operational component of these variables so that each one can be differentiated and manipulated to determine its impact. Consequently, the research design must be able to control and reduce the influence of all but the targeted variables. The following characteristics assist in this requirement.

The most frequently mentioned characteristic for quantitative research is the *quantification* of data; that is, converting variables and their changes into numerical values so that statistical analyses can be applied. Measurement is used to quantify the independent and dependent variables through operationalism so that attitudes, opinions, behaviors, and other variables can be counted and mathematically manipulated. The results of these manipulations can be interpreted to formulate findings and patterns in research. These results can then be used to generalize to a larger sample or population.

Another explicit characteristic of quantitative research is the level of *control* (how well the research design has been constructed to reduce systematic error due to uncontrolled variables). All aspects of the study are carefully designed before data are collected to ensure that variables are either held constant or systematically manipulated so that their effects can be eliminated from having any impact in the study or they can be compared to other treatment conditions. The extent to which the investigator has control over the research design typically increases the degree of internal validity. That is, by careful control, the possibility that a change in the dependent variable is the result of some causes other than the targeted independent variable in the experiment is believed to be greatly reduced. The greater control of the variables, the higher the internal validity; this provides greater confidence in the research results. Although one version of quantitative research (experimental) requires greater control of the research design than the other two quantitative versions, each of these versions still require more control than do the other research paradigms (i.e., qualitative research, mixed methods research).

A third defining characteristic deals with *measurement*. Unlike qualitative research, where the actual data collected are constructed from observations and descriptions of various actions and reactions during the research activity, quantitative measurement is accomplished using standardized and predetermined instruments that involve numbers and counting. This is necessary because the variables of interest need to be objectively measured since mathematical analysis as a process is essential for interpretation. Numeric measurement and statistical analysis connect data collection and empirical observation with mathematical expressions of quantitative relationships.

A fourth characteristic of all versions of quantitative analysis involves *generalization*. This refers to the extent to which the conclusions of the investigation would hold as well for other subject samples or for settings outside of the research design. Generalization can be approached in two ways. First, there is the *sampling model*, designed to focus on the representativeness of your sample to the population from which it was drawn. Strong generalization here allows for conclusions to adapt from a small sample to a population. Most predictive statistics are employed to predict this small-to-many possibility. The second kind of generalization is the *proximal similarity model*, which focuses on generalizing to contexts or settings different from your controlled research context. This type of generalization is not based on predictive statistics but on some implicit determination of how similar the context of interest is to the research context. The extent to which generalization occurs (from either model) is referred to as the *external validity* of the research design.

It should be noted that, when considering the integrity of the research design, it is the internal and external validity that must be determined. Although internal validity helps to support and validate a causal conclusion by reducing concerns about the approximate truth of the stated statistical inferences regarding the variable relationships, external validity is related to the ability to generalize and apply the findings to other samples and/or settings. When designing a quantitative study, it should be remembered that internal and external validity are inversely related; as one increases or strengthens, the other is reduced or weakened.

Advantages of Quantitative Research

The advantages of quantitative research are numerous. This paradigm focuses on a logical progression of explanation, a numeric description that enables the application of statistical data analysis for predictive and comparison purposes, and an objective stance. Each of these components of the research paradigm creates advantages not necessarily noted in other paradigms. In terms of logical progression, the overarching aim of a quantitative research study is to classify features, count them, and construct statistical models to explain what is observed. This is done by identifying variables of interest, structuring a way to isolate those variables critical to the research hypothesis, and then systematically comparing the relationship between the targeted variables. Since this paradigm is dependent on convergent reasoning, rather than divergent reasoning, the known facts and determined results are collected and combined to provide specific answers to predetermined questions or hypotheses. Research questions can be asked and answered, and this can be accomplished in a relatively short period of time.

Numeric descriptions are advantageous because they appear to be objective and clear-cut (at least as operationalized) such that results are not as easily misinterpreted as they might be in some other research paradigms. The statistical analyses are straightforward and allow the comparison of results (and effects) across conditions and subject groups, and numerical results can be displayed graphically and through charts, tables, and other formats that best allow for interpretation. Other advantages of numeric data include the fact that both data collection and data analysis tend to occur more rapidly in quantitative research than in qualitative or mixed methods research. This is primarily due to the fact that the interpretation is less subjective and more mathematical; decisions and results can be documented and shared efficiently. Due to the numeric data collected, documenting change is not descriptive, so detailed analysis and description is not necessary. With more efficient data collection, data from large sample sizes can be collected. Finally, statistical analysis allows for greater objectivity when reviewing results, and therefore, results are independent of the researcher.

Types of Quantitative Research Designs

There are generally three types of research designs employed in quantitative research: the experimental design, the quasi-experimental design, and the nonexperimental design. The first and most powerful is the *experimental design*. This research type exerts more control than the other two design types; there is control of extraneous variables, manipulation of the independent variable(s), and at least two subject groups for comparison purposes. Importantly, however, in the experimental design, there is also random assignment of subjects to the experimental conditions or treatment. The primary advantage of randomized selection also involves control. The backgrounds and histories of the subjects cannot be controlled as potential extraneous variables, and the assumption is that since each subject has an equal chance of being assigned to the experimental or the control group, any potential extraneous or confounding variable in the form of different backgrounds and experiences should then have an equal chance of being assigned to one treatment/experimental condition as the other. Therefore, uncontrolled variance within the subjects will be diminished. As a consequence of these components, experimental designs have greater internal validity, and the conclusion that the effect on the dependent variable is likely due to changes in the independent variable can be more confidently advanced. Within the experimental design format, there are (at least) six kinds of experimental designs:

- Posttest Only Design: This has an experimental group and a control group, but neither group is given a pretest before treatment is introduced to the experimental group. After the completion of the treatment condition, both groups receive a posttest to determine the impact of the independent variable.

- Pretest–Posttest Only Design: This is similar to the posttest only design except that both groups receive a pretest before the treatment condition, and then both receive a posttest after the treatment condition is completed.

- Solomon Four Group Design: This includes four groups in the experimental design: two experimental and two control groups. One experimental and one control group are pretested but all four receive the posttest after the treatment condition is completed. As is obvious, this is actually a combination of the first two methodologies and is usually used to eliminate error bias.

- Factorial Design: This method is employed when the investigator wants to utilize and manipulate two or more independent variables or factors simultaneously to determine their effects on the dependent variable. Consequently, two different hypotheses may be tested in the same experiment.

- Randomized Block Design: This method is used to reduce variability among treatment groups. The investigator divides the subjects into subgroups or blocks to reduce within block variability. Subjects within each block are then randomly assigned to treatment and control conditions.

- Repeated Measures Design: Subjects serve as their own control within this method because each subject is exposed to each treatment condition and the method is structured to determine (measure) how each subject responds to all of the treatment conditions.

The second quantitative research type is the *quasi-experimental design*. Although this design uses participants with the treatment condition, measures outcomes, and strives to determine whether outcome differences are related to the treatment(s), quasi-experimental studies do not use randomized assignment of participants to experimental or control groups. Consequently, there are not the same types of controls on the backgrounds and experiences of the subjects, and there is greater possibility of uncontrolled variation as a result. Since there is a greater chance of extraneous or confounding variables due to the lack of participant control via randomization, experimental manipulations and their effects on the dependent variable may not be the only explanation for the observed and measured results. Internal validity is reduced within this design.

The third quantitative research type is the *nonexperimental design*. As with the quasi-experimental design, there is no randomization of participants; however, there is also no use of either multiple groups or multiple types of measures. Consequently, there is no manipulation of the variables for comparison purposes or to determine the impact of an independent variable on a dependent variable. Often nonexperimental designs are employed in natural settings rather than in controlled settings. Examples of nonexperimental quantitative designs are the following:

- surveys, which are used to describe a population and to determine whether there are trends between variables (respondents are asked a set of structured questions and their responses are tabulated);
- correlational studies, to determine whether there are relationships between demographic data and behavior;
- comparative studies, to determine whether variables change over time or in response to another variable;
- cohost studies, which follow a targeted group over time; and
- longitudinal studies, which look at changes in variable over a period of time.

The Process of Quantitative Research

Although there are various types of quantitative research designs, each of these designs follows a general set of steps when initiating the research process. The first step is recognizing that there is a problem or a phenomenon that one wants to investigate. To examine whether the problem is due to one kind of variable influencing another, the investigator simply wants to better understand the relationship between two or more variables, or there is a need to measure (and even predict) the frequency of occurrence of a phenomenon, problems concerning attitudes, behaviors, opinions, or other defined variables are identified.

The second step is formulating a research question. The formulated question may be general or exploratory at this stage. Asking about the relationship among variables is often sufficient to get started. The question must be specific enough to identify variables to be studied, but little else is required.

Third, the investigator must do a literature review to learn more about the identified problem, where there is a gap in knowledge, the potential variables to be reviewed, and whether other investigators have recognized the same problem and already provided some research in response. Above all, the literature review enables an investigator to learn enough about the variables in question to be able to complete step four.

This fourth step is crucial; it is the formulation of a testable hypothesis. To be testable, this hypothesis should be formed as an answer to a question and should state the presumed relationship (i.e., association, correlation, causation) between the targeted variables. That is, is there a certain relationship that exists among variables? Since the hypothesis leads to selection of the research design employed, the more precise and well defined the hypothesis, the easier it will be to design the methods for testing.

Step 5 focuses on the research design. This step is important to establish the integrity and validity of the research. Since quantitative research primarily involves which variables will be scrutinized and how they will be handled, the control issue is important. Once the investigator, guided by the testable hypothesis, decides which variables to investigate (selection of independent and dependent variables), then procedures to control confounding and/or extraneous variables must be designed. For the variable(s) that can be manipulated (independent variable), this step also determines if there are assignments to different levels of this variable, how the manipulation occurs, and what methods will be used for this purpose. Another important aspect of the design involves determining the population of interest to test the hypothesis, how the subset of the population will be chosen (sampling) to help ensure representativeness (i.e., probability sampling or nonprobability sampling), and how this population is assigned to one group or another.

Step 6 is planning and implementing data collection. Considerations are focused on the selection of instruments to operationalize or quantify changes in the dependent variables within the sampling groups, where and how to collect the data of interest, and how to operationalize the independent variables. Due to the orientation to numeric data that can be used statistically, data collection methods employ structured data collection instruments that are easy to compare and manipulate statistically.

Step 7 involves sorting and analyzing the data for interpretation purposes. Since the purposes of quantitative research are classifying and counting features to test hypotheses, answering research questions, determining the relationships between variables to describe trends, and measuring and/or predicting the occurrence of the variables being studied, statistical models are typically used to explain what has been observed. Not only can some statistical procedures help control the effects of confounding and/or extraneous variables and discern the impact of multiple variables, they also enable group and/or variable comparisons about the individuals or groups in the quantitative study (experiments, correlational studies, and surveys). However, the testable hypothesis or stated question requires quantification so the data can be converted into usable statistics for interpretive purposes.

The eighth and final step in conducting quantitative research is preparation and dissemination of the research findings. Preparation for publication in peer-reviewed journals or for presentation at professional conferences allows the results of the study and its implications to be reviewed, evaluated, and employed by others in the discipline.

In the natural sciences, quantitative research may be considered the predominant research paradigm used. In the social sciences, however, it is often joined by qualitative research and mixed methods research approaches, with the crucial determiner of which approach to use based upon the questions that the researcher asks. When focusing on comparative research, treatment research, or to objectively determine the strength and effect of one or more variables (independent) on another (dependent), the quantitative approach is preferred.

Jack S. Damico

See also Behaviorism; Experimental Research; Operationalism; Outcome Measurement; Reliability; Research; Validity

Further Readings

Borbasi, S., & Jackson, D. (2012). *Navigating the maze of research*. Chatswood, Australia: Mosby Elsevier.

Campbell, D. T., & Stanley, J. C. (1963). *Experimental and quasi-experimental designs for research*. Chicago, IL: Rand McNally.

Creswell, J. W. (2014). *Research design: Qualitative, quantitative and mixed methods approaches*. Thousand Oaks, CA: Sage. (Original work published 1994)

Frankfort-Nachmias, C., & Nachmais, D. (2008). *Research methods in the social sciences* (7th ed.). New York, NY: Worth.

Kerlinger, F. N., & Lee, H. B. (1999). **Foundations of behavioral research** (4th ed.). Belmont, CA: Wadsworth.

Mills, J. A. (1998). **Control. A history of behavioral psychology**. New York, NY: New York University Press.

Robinson, D. N. (1995). ***An intellectual history of psychology*** (3rd ed.). Madison, WI: University of Wisconsin Press.

Solomon, P., & Draine, J. (2010). An overview of quantitative methods. In B. Thayer (Ed.), *The handbook of social work research methods* (2nd ed., pp. 26–36). Thousand Oaks, CA: Sage.

Spector, P. E. (1981). *Research design*. Sage University Paper Series on Quantitative Applications in the Social Sciences, series no. 23. Newbury Park, CA: Sage.

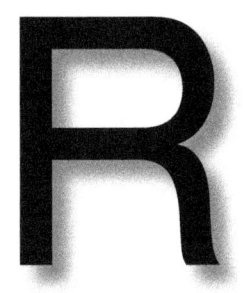

Radiation Therapy and Communication Disorders

A ubiquitous phenomenon is that humans are surrounded by radiation in some form during their day-to-day lives. Basking in the sun's rays and listening to the crashing waves on the shore are both examples of radiation. The term *radiation* originates from the word *radiate* and as such refers to the transmission of energy in the form of waves or particle movement through space or a material. There are multiple forms of radiation existing in nature, some of which are harmless and others that can be harmful depending upon exposure, and even curative, such as radiation therapy (RT).

It is the varying types of electromagnetic radiation and particle radiation that are most relevant to persons studying human behavior. Forms of radiation differ with respect to wavelength and energy emission, which impact how people safeguard themselves from ill effects and harness its power for therapeutic purposes. This entry focuses on those forms of radiation and the attendant deleterious effects that can impact human communication and quality of life.

Electromagnetic Radiation

There are multiple sources of electromagnetic radiation such as heat, microwaves, radio waves, ultraviolet (UV) light, X-rays, and gamma rays. All electromagnetic radiation consists of both waves and particles; therefore, it is the length of the waves that allows scientists to differentiate between them. As a general rule, a smaller wavelength relates to a higher energy. UV radiation, emitted by the sun, is characterized by wavelengths from 10 to 125 nanometers (a nanometer is one billionth of a meter). This high-energy radiation ionizes the surrounding air.

Ionization occurs when the energy is sufficiently powerful to knock electrons off of atoms to create positively charged ions. The surrounding air and ozone (O_3) in space absorb about 98% of the UV radiation, so what reaches the earth is nonionizing UV-B and UV-C rays. Although such nonionized radiation will not alter atomic structure, it is far from harmless depending upon exposure and sensitivity. The energy propagated via radiation can still result in electron excitation in biological molecules, resulting in cellular chemical reactions. Sunburned skin, for example, is evidence of the destructive effect of nonionized radiation.

X-rays are a form of electromagnetic radiation used routinely by the medical community, including speech–language therapists. X-rays' wavelengths average 1,000 picometers, trillionths of a meter, and carry enough energy to ionize smaller atoms while being absorbed by larger ones. It is this difference in absorption between the smaller atoms that make up soft tissue and the larger calcium atoms found in the bones that create the contrast that allows physicians and speech therapists to examine structures of the human body. Common applications of this are computed tomography scan and videofluoroscopic swallow study used to diagnose dysphagia. X-rays are additionally used to destroy cancerous cells and treat vascular defects using external beam RT. In this process, a linear accelerator, using powerful generators, creates a high-energy X-ray beam that is focused and directed to the tumor through a set of lead shutters called collimators.

Gamma radiation is also used curatively to treat tumors. Characterized by an even shorter wavelength, 30 picometers, gamma radiation transmits approximately 33 times the amount of energy as that found in an X-ray. Gamma radiation emission is the result of the decomposition of radioactive elements such as radium, uranium, and cobalt-60. In RT such as Gamma Knife® procedures, over 200 beams of radiation intersect to focus on the targeted abnormal tissue while sparing the contiguous healthy tissue.

Particle Radiation

Newer techniques in the treatment of tumors involve the use of particle radiation, alpha and beta, which are charged particles emitted from naturally occurring radioactive materials such as uranium, radium, and strontium-90. These particles are 20 times more effective for cell damage as gamma rays and X-rays. Referred to as brachytherapy, a radiation oncologist places radioactive particles within metal seeds in or near the tumor. Over several months, the radioactivity level eventually diminishes or decays to nothing. The seeds remain in the body with no lasting effect, other than the possible annoyance of occasionally triggering a metal detector at airport security checkpoints. Additionally, radioactive materials are often injected into the bloodstream and then monitored through radiographic instruments to detect disease or enhance the image captured through diagnostic imaging.

Although radiation is a powerful tool for eradicating or reducing tumors and promoting healing, extended exposure to radiation can be quite harmful.

Radiation Precautions

By understanding the physical properties of the differing forms of radiation, health-care workers can effectively treat their patients and protect their own bodies from the adverse effects of protracted exposure. Perhaps the greatest risk of the deleterious effects of radiation is among speech–language therapists who conduct videofluoroscopic swallow studies. The relatively longer wavelengths of the X-rays used in these studies can permeate paper and thin layers of wood or aluminum, but are unable to penetrate lead. This is why medical personnel involved in radiographic exams wear lead vests and usually attach a monitoring device to track their monthly exposure. Similarly, using a lead vest or moving behind a lead wall protects technicians who provide gamma radiation–based treatment. Due to their extremely short wavelength, alpha particles are unable to pass through even paper. Beta particles are only slightly more piercing, passing through paper but not aluminum, which explains why these particles are most suited to brachytherapy.

Complications in RT

Radiation treatment is designed to kill targeted unwanted cells, and, despite advances to isolate them, a common side effect is damage to surrounding tissue or changes in body systems. The risk of radiation-induced debilitating side effects is a complex issue dependent upon a person's underlying health and concomitant treatments such as chemotherapy, radiation dose, and fractionation schedule. Radiation dose refers to the effective dose that takes into account the overall sensitivity of a tumor cell toward radiation, specifically the tumor cell's ability to absorb the energy deposited in a cell or a tissue (*absorption dose*) and the amount of dose required to achieve the desired cell damage (*equivalent dose*). The dose is administered in strategic fractions to optimize its effectiveness. It is a fine line between enough radiation to destroy cancerous cells and too much radiation that results in complications. Radiation-induced complications can occur as acute, early delayed, or late depending upon the time of onset. Acute changes, occurring during treatment, are often reversible when managed correctly. Early–delayed onset complications, occurring a few weeks to a few months posttreatment, are also not permanent in most cases. However, late complications that occur months after the cessation of treatment are often irreversible and sometimes progressive.

Depending upon the tumor site, subsequent radiation treatment dose, the patient's sensitivity to radiation, and overall health, he or she can experience damage to the central nervous system, bones and sinuses, or head and neck tissues. Damage to any of these systems can negatively impact communication and/or swallowing. Damage to the central nervous system can result in focal necrosis or tissue death. This most commonly occurs at the site of a treated tumor where surrounding tissue has been compromised through edema, making it vulnerable to damage. The patient usually presents with a specific neurologic deficit. Additionally, treatment complications can include diffuse white matter injury as a result of radiation-induced demyelination, which most often occurs in the periventricular white matter. Diffuse white matter injury can also occur after chemotherapy either alone or in combination with RT.

Central nervous system atrophy is another radiation-induced complication with documented decreases in patient's intelligence quotient and neurologic function. A possible complication of RT in children is mineralizing microangiopathy, characterized by deposits of calcium within the small vessels of cerebral or cerebellar tissue that has been irradiated. Radiation-induced vascular changes within the brain can also occur, such as telangiectasia, dilation of capillaries within the irradiated white matter associated with subclinical hemorrhage, and the less common large vessel vasculopathy, characterized by accelerated atherosclerosis and thrombosis.

Radiation treatment can cause changes in bone tissue. These include fatty replacement of bone marrow, bone tissue death called as osteoradionecrosis (to which the mandible is particularly susceptible), and sinus inflammatory disease wherein acute inflammation occurs in the mucosal lining of the paranasal sinuses and mastoid air cells. The latter condition has implications for potential conductive hearing loss.

Radiation-induced changes to the head and neck pose challenges for voicing and swallowing. Changes to the superficial soft tissues, such as edema and fibrosis, result in neck tissue that is hard to touch, restricted in movement, and less responsive to vibration. For persons undergoing laryngectomy with subsequent radiation, this radiation-induced complication limits their options for establishing alternate voicing by reducing the volume and pitch variability they can achieve with electrolaryngeal devices.

Edema and thickening in the soft tissues of the larynx and pharynx are also frequent postradiation changes. The effects of these changes can include difficulty breathing, dysphonia, and swallowing deficits. Salivary glands are particularly sensitive to radiation with posttreatment reports of xerostomia, reduced saliva production being one of the most commonly reported side effects of head and neck RT. Changes to the deep tissues of the neck and xerostomia often result in severe dysphagia that impacts the patient's quality of life. Research has identified that almost a third of patients with the head and neck cancer treated with RT sustain moderate acute symptoms associated with later-developed impaired swallowing ranging from minor/mild dysphagia to dependence upon tube feeding. Research has shown that, similar to other radiation-induced complications, the risk of dysphagia post-RT is multifactorial depending upon the patient's overall health, co-occurring treatments, and the radiation dose and schedule. Further, a probability model based upon a large sample of persons diagnosed with chronic dysphagia found that earlier onset of oral mucositis, xerostomia and diagnosed dysphagia, and symptom severity and persistence were indicators of a high risk of developing chronic dysphagia.

Treating Postradiation Impairment

The recognition of the potential deleterious effects of radiation can support the mitigation of changes as a result of RT. Responsive changes in the dose or fractionation schedule, as well as adjuvant pharmacological treatment, can reduce the occurrence or severity of complications. Compensatory training programs have been shown to improve attention, memory, and language. Speech therapy has also proved successful in reducing the impact of radiation-induced changes on communication and swallowing through interprofessional approaches where the speech therapist works with radiation oncologists, dentists, occupational therapists, and dieticians initiating exercises and strategies prior to, during, and following radiation treatment. This approach has resulted in improved mobility for swallowing and decreased the incidence and severity of dysphagia and aspiration pneumonia.

Through exercise-based dysphagia therapy programs, an individual's swallowing can improve from requiring tube feeding to maintaining health and quality of life through independent swallowing ability. Understanding what radiation is, how it is used to diagnose and treat medical conditions, the important safeguards to reduce harmful exposure, and treatments that address radiation-induced complications promotes the best possible practices for treating patients with radiation-induced communicative and/or swallowing impairment.

Jennifer Thompson Tetnowski

See also Cancer of the Head and Neck; Conductive Hearing Loss and its Treatment; Dysphagia; Dysphonia(s); Videofluoroscopic Swallow Study

Further Readings

Crary, M. A., & Carnaby, G. D. (2014). Adoption into clinical practice of two therapies to swallowing disorders: Exercise based swallowing rehabilitation and electrical stimulation. *Current Opinion in Otolaryngology & Head and Neck Surgery*, 22(3), 172.

Rabin, B. M., Meyer, J. R., Berlin, J. W., Marymount, M. H., Palka, P. S., & Russell, E. J. (1996). Radiation-induced changes in the central nervous system and head and neck. *Radiographics*, 16(5), 1055–1072.

Villari, C. R., & Courey, M. S. (2015). Management of dysphonia after radiation therapy. *Otolaryngologic Clinics of North America*, 48(4), 601–609.

Ward, E. C., & van As-Brooks, C. J. (Eds.). (2014). *Head and neck cancer: Treatment, rehabilitation, and outcomes*. Plural. San Diego, CA.

Readability

Readability refers to the ease with which a written text is understood by a reader, usually reported as an index such as *grade level*. A text with a readability of 2.0 (second-grade level) is thought to be easier to read than a text with a readability of 8.5 (corresponding to eighth grade midway through the year).

Studies of text difficulty as judged by the number of uncommon words in a text were undertaken as long ago as the 1920s. In the decades that followed, educators and psychologists developed a variety of reading formulas meant to either guide writers and editors in composing a text to fit the needs of an intended audience or organize groups of texts (text leveling) as part of an instructional scheme aimed at teaching reading. Providing guidance for the writer was the original intention of readability. The development of reading materials associated with programmed instruction constitutes the majority of recent applications of the readability concept, initially through grade-level anthologies and more recently in the process of *leveling books* (i.e., sorting children's literature selections into A–Z levels).

To derive a readability score, readability formulas use measures of text features such as average number of words per sentence and average number of syllables per word. In addition, some formulas also include word frequency information drawn from a large collection of written texts. While some formulas are free, widely available, and easy to use (such as the Fry Readability Graph), others (such as the Lexile score formula) are proprietary and require payment for use.

Critics of text readability note that the original intent was to aid writers rather than to focus on the reader's experience. There are also concerns about the validity and reliability of readability formulas. Because different formulas register unacceptable disparities when applied to the same text, readability suffers from concerns about concurrent validity. For example, calculations of the range of readability scores of eight different available formulas showed that scores varied as widely as fifth-grade levels on picture book texts typically used in first or second grade and sixth-grade levels on picture books suited to middle school readers. In addition, discrepancies in readability measures when excerpts are scored in different places within the same text have raised questions about the reliability of readability as a construct.

The concept of readability is seated in a word-oriented theory of reading that is ultimately nonproductive because it fails to account for the wide variety of reader behaviors during uninterrupted readings of authentic texts. Sociopsycholinguistic studies have shown that reading involves a dynamic transaction between a reader and a text, situated in a social context, and comprehension involves interpretation or active meaning construction. From this perspective, any reading transaction involves factors related to readers (such as purpose, knowledge, motivation, experiences, and interests) and factors related to social context (e.g., physical and social environment, nature of task) as well as text-related factors.

Pedagogical Applications of Readability

In education in general, and with word-oriented views of reading specifically, readability information is used to match individuals assigned a specific reading level to a text of corresponding complexity with the goal of providing effective reading instruction. Precise matching of reader to text is done for the purpose of having readers produce accurate and fluent readings. This view diminishes the reader's role in making sense of the text and disregards sociocultural as well as developmental factors. Auto magazines are comprehensible to car mechanics but not to lawyers who negotiate legal contracts. An Australian news report describing a cricket match is incomprehensible to most American readers (although none of the words are unfamiliar). Immigrants may lack experiences to understand cultural references in *easy* texts.

If readability is extended to take into account the reader's experience, the concept fails to account for multiple layers of meaning or nuances in theme available to readers of varying ages and experiences. The practice of assigning levels to readers, as well as to texts, can be limiting and even harmful. Readers considered *below level* may take on negative views of their abilities and of reading.

Readers' interpretations of a specific text overlap due to textual cues and shared cultural experiences. However, readers have unique interpretations as they draw upon schemas including conceptual information, linguistic and cultural understandings, and prior experiences with texts.

Predictability, a pedagogical alternative to readability, reflects the role of the reader in text interpretation. Predictability addresses the supports and constraints that a text may provide for readers. Books with repetitive events and language (e.g., folktales such as *The Three Billy Goats Gruff*) are highly predictable. Illustrations, diagrams, and other graphic information that supports the text will increase the support for readers. Everyday familiar language, as opposed to controlled vocabulary, makes texts more predictable.

Predictability of a text varies depending on the reader's schemas, conceptual knowledge, cultural background, and interests. For this reason, readability formulas do not provide useful information for supporting readers or reading instruction. Reading instruction that supports developing readers includes (a) *predictable* texts that support reading development; (b) frequent read-alouds to enable students to experience a range of texts with varying genre, content, and complexity; (c) opportunities to reread familiar texts; (d) assistance in selecting texts that build upon interests and experiences; (e) firsthand learning experiences that extend background knowledge; and (f) support for readers in developing strategies that address the challenges of increasingly complex and diverse texts.

Debra Goodman and Alan Flurkey

See also Applied Linguistics; Comprehensibility; Psycholinguistics; Sociolinguistics; Texts

Further Readings

Goodman, K., Fries, P. H., & Strauss, S. L. (2016). *Reading: The grand illusion; how and why readers make sense of print*. New York, NY: Routledge.

Hiebert, E. (2009). *Interpreting Lexiles*. Apex Learning. Retrieved April 14, 2016, from http://www.apexlearning.com/documents/Research_InterpretingLexiles_2009-02.pdf

Krashen, S. (2001). The Lexile framework: Unnecessary and potentially harmful. *CSLA (California School Library Association) Journal, 24*(2), 25–26.

Smith, F. (2012). *Understanding reading: A psycholinguistic analysis of reading and learning to read* (6th ed.). New York, NY: Routledge.

READING AND READING DISORDERS

Reading as a human activity is a ubiquitous and complex linguistic ability involving numerous functions, applications, and concepts. While one frequent definition of reading is the process of deriving meaning from print, this definition is not sufficient. Although as a linguistic ability the construction of meaning from a text is typically the primary function of reading, the term can refer to a host of functions ranging from the perfunctory utterances produced by a newsreader to the detailed interpretation of any written text. Similarly, *reading* has been applied across a wide array of phenomena, from reading facial expressions, tea leaves, and pressure gauges to reading package labels, novels, and philosophical tomes. The concepts involved in reading as a human activity are also varied. Within the study of reading, it is necessary to recognize that there are different levels of reading: as a societal practice and as a personal skill; differences also exist in the overall conceptualizations about how reading is developed and how it operates as a human aptitude.

An Integrated and Pragmatic Definition

Although the various usages of the term *reading* are often based upon common expressions such as "reading the weather" or "reading the crowd's reaction to the speech," in the more specific psycholinguistic and educational usage of the term, it is a cognitive process employing multiple strategies to make sense of visual representations. That is, humans as symbolic creatures strive to ask and answer the questions, "what is going on here (with visual representations)?" and "how do these visual representations relate to what I already know?" Reading is *sense making* constructed by taking the text and interpreting it in relation to the knowledge base that the reader already possesses. In this definition, reading as a process takes the text and juxtaposes it with one's background knowledge and information by integrating it into the larger meaningful context. The result is comprehension. The literacy theorist Marie Clay defined reading as a problem-solving activity involving visual text, which becomes more powerful the more it is used; she stressed its complexity as a human aptitude because it is typically goal-directed to ask and answer questions (depending on the context) by extracting a sequence of cues from a text to yield meaningful and specific comprehension that can be used for knowledge acquisition, communication, and other social actions. Added to this operational definition is the recognition that when one reads for comprehension, the meaning does not reside in the printed marks on the page. Rather, comprehension is a cognitive process of meaning construction by the reader.

Two Levels of Reading

Based upon our awareness of reading as a pervasive activity, reading (and its more inclusive term *literacy*) functions on two different levels. First, it is a *societal practice*. This level of analysis is typically of greatest interest to sociologists, educational reformers, policymakers, and philosophers. Literacy (i.e., reading and writing) affects the social lives of individuals in modern bureaucratic societies where it is the group rather than the individual that garners attention. At this level, consideration is oriented to the role that reading (and writing) plays in the creation and maintenance of social processes and institutions such as government, education, religion, and jurisprudence. David Olson refers to this societal practice as *the invention of a world on paper* since he believes that our modern conceptions of ourselves and the world in which we operate are by-products of how written text has invented and then entrenched these conceptions.

The second level of literacy attention is as a *personal skill* that involves individuals and how they use reading and writing within specific contexts. At this level, the focus is on how reading (and writing) creates learning, psychological change, and social action within those individuals who acquire and employ the various aspects of literacy. Basically, the focus is directed toward what individuals can do with reading to advance their awareness, knowledge, and understanding of the world. This level of functioning is especially important because of the societal practice wherein reading and writing (i.e., literacy) have become so crucial to functioning in our modern bureaucratic societies. This is the level at which most educational and therapeutic concerns about reading exist, in the individual reader and his/her ability to adequately perform this acquired skill.

When addressing reading as a human aptitude, both of these levels of functioning are essential; they are closely intertwined, and the awareness, conceptualization, and application are based one upon the other. For example, due to societal practices, the definition of what it means to be a reader and writer (i.e., literate) has changed over the centuries as different societies and cultures employ literacy and its benefits differently. Similarly, the specific theoretical and practical descriptions of reading as a personal skill can greatly impact various societal treatments of literacy in terms of educational policy and research funding, as was noted during the presidency of George W. Bush in the United States. For the purposes of this entry, the remainder of this discussion will focus primarily on reading as a personal skill.

Models of Reading

There are currently two models of reading as a personal skill that are frequently discussed in the theoretical, pedagogical, and research literature. Based upon the two predominant theories of human learning that were applied during the 20th century (i.e., behaviorism and constructivism), these models have strong proponents and are both currently in active use. The first is a *skills-based model* that is based upon behaviorism as the explanation of human learning. Within this model, there is a focus on component skills such as phonemic awareness, phonetics, word identification, and fluency that typically are learned independent of one another via various learning formats. Once these component skills are learned, they are then combined into a cognitive process to assist the child in translating the visual cues into oral language for comprehension purposes. That is, this model views reading as a straightforward process of decoding visual text and then encoding it through one's oral language system. Consequently, reading is seen as a secondary skill that utilizes oral language coding so that proficient reading is primarily conceptualized as the identification of words on the page so that they can be translated.

Jeanne Chall, an early proponent of the skills-based approach, suggested that there were five successive stages in reading as a learned and acquired skill. The initial stage was termed *decoding*, and it focused on the linkage between letters and sounds; components of this stage involved how the alphabetic principle is learned and applied and whether the learner becomes aware of the relationship between sound–symbol correspondences. The focus here is on the visual code and not some attempt at understanding the text; in this model, comprehension will come later with the translation into oral language. This stage is typically the heart of the *learning to read* process as it covers the first and second grades (ages 6–7) in average children. The second stage was termed *confirmation and fluency*, and it focuses upon practicing the skills learned in stage one to increase efficiency and fluency so that the decoding skills can be effectively used for word recognition within the printed text. This stage generally covers the second and third grades (ages 7–8). These two stages, therefore, emphasize decoding and single-word recognition rather than comprehension. The third stage, *reading to learn*, stressed reading texts and practicing so that additional decoding strategies could be developed as the visual material changed and became more complex, and simultaneously, fluency was increased to aid the translation process. This stage, covering the fourth to ninth grades (ages 9–14), has been termed the *ungluing from print*, meaning that as children gain confidence and fluency, their reading becomes more automatic so that the readers don't have to focus as much on the print and can now focus more on gaining understanding via oral language translation. *Multiple viewpoints* is the fourth stage in this developmental scheme. During this stage (high school, ages 14–18), since the translation process is generally completed, the reader learns to handle increasingly difficult concepts and can consider multiple viewpoints based upon how the visual text is translated. The final stage is termed *construction and judgment* and refers to integrating new information with prior knowledge and dealing with higher levels of abstraction.

The component skills model lends itself to a teaching approach that breaks the reading process into separate components, arranged according to a developmental order and explicitly taught in a decontextualized manner. In this behavioristic approach, reading is conceptualized as a set of discrete skills that can be applied incrementally to work toward eventual comprehension based upon the process of intermodal transfer through the oral language system.

The second model of reading is the *meaning-based model*, and it is founded upon a constructivist approach to human learning. This model does not focus on translation or intermodal transfer from the written codes to oral language. Instead, reading is conceptualized as a primary meaning-making system parallel to all other functioning symbolic systems (e.g., oral language, memory, cognition), and the process of learning to derive meaning from the visual text is similar to how active processing occurs in all other meaning-making systems. When an individual reads the visual text, this visual input is juxtaposed with one's previously acquired knowledge base using internalized strategies to construct meaning. For example, during the process of reading, the child uses a sampling strategy to process enough of the visual text to make predictions (a second strategy) about the meaning of the text. These predictions are based upon the visual input being compared (a third strategy) to the reader's knowledge of how language works and about his/her knowledge of the world. Once a meaning prediction is made, the individual then continues processing the visual text to confirm or disconfirm (a fourth strategy) the previous and ongoing meaning derived from the text. This iterative process continues and results in comprehension of the written text.

In this model, reading is a sufficient system of meaning making dependent on a socially constructed process involving the need to learn how to derive meaning from the immediate visual text with assistance from more accomplished readers. Within a learning/acquisition context, the developing reader can learn various strategies to comprehend the visual text by being recurrently exposed to authentic literacy skills that are modeled by proficient readers who can mediate for the child while he/she attempts to construct meaning. It is expected that the successful developing reader is exposed to excellent models of reading and writing and that the child learns by example and then employs specific strategies that enable the construction of meaningfulness from the visual text itself rather than translate to another (oral) language system; reading, consistent with all other forms of meaning making, is a natural social process that is continually being developed through usage.

Based upon this model, reading has been referred to as a *psycholinguistic guessing game* by the theorist Ken Goodman since the competent reader has established a process of using his/her background knowledge to construct the meaningfulness of the text; these internalized processes primarily occur at a subconscious level, allowing for a reader's focus to remain on comprehension. From a teaching perspective, the emphasis is not the development of component skills or even on the letters and words (i.e., the code) on the page; the focus is on helping the child acquire the various strategies to construct meaning though active engagement with the text and with more competent readers who can model, mediate, and inform. So, for example, during the period of emerging literacy, a child and his/her caregiver may pick up a book together and engage in the social act of reading. When this occurs, there is an underlying (and meaningful) social interaction that is employed so that the caregiver collaborates with the child to construct meaning from print.

Reading Disorders and Dyslexia

As the importance of reading has increased in our modern society, more attention has turned to reading as a personal skill; particularly, there has been a focus on individuals manifesting reading difficulties. Two types of reading problems have been emphasized in the literature. The first type involves difficulty in learning or developing reading abilities. This type usually focuses on children and their preschool and school experiences. The second type of difficulty involves acquired reading deficits—that is, individuals who were competent readers, but, due to brain damage, are no longer able to read or have demonstrably reduced reading abilities.

Within the first type of problems, while this increased attention on struggling readers (and writers) has been especially noticeable since the 1960s, there has been an awareness of extreme difficulty in learning to read since the early decades of the 20th century. In 1925, Samuel Orton, a physician, employed the term *dyslexia* when discussing apparent reading disorders, and this term has continued to be applied to describe a disability in learning to read despite adequate intelligence, normal oral language skills, and sufficient instructional opportunity. While there has been debate regarding how difficult it might be to determine the exclusion conditions, especially sufficient instructional opportunity, the term has continued to be employed. Additionally, those researchers and theorists studying this condition have provided various causal explanations for dyslexia ranging from visual system deficits (the *perceptual-deficit hypothesis*) to neurological problems based more upon intersensory integration of visual and auditory input (resulting in sound–symbol associations deficits) and, finally, deficits in various aspects of verbal/linguistic processing, especially phonologic deficiencies. However, little actual data exist in support of any of these explanations.

Within the second problem type, acquired reading deficits, cognitive neuropsychologists have engaged in experimental research attempting to discover the fundamental processes that underlie this condition (also termed *dyslexia*), and two major psycholinguistic models of reading have been proposed. The first, the *dual-route cascaded* model, proposes that reading is supported in the brain by two different routes providing access to literacy skills—the lexical route and the nonlexical route. The lexical route is necessary to handle regular and irregular words, whereas the nonlexical route is used to read regular nonwords or foreign words. In this model, orthography, phonology, and semantics are disassociated with one another in the lexical route, allowing for the possibility of deficits in one area and not in any of the others. The dual-route cascaded model proposes that the mental representation of the lexicon is local (all in one place) and word processing is serial (left to right). This model is usually rendered using boxes and arrows with the boxes representing the cognitive systems and the arrows representing processes. Deficits occur in this model when a cognitive system is damaged or a process is isolated from the necessary cognitive system due to focal brain damage. The second model within acquired deficits is the *parallel distributed processing* model. This model hypothesizes that the lexicon is distributed throughout the brain and that processing goes on in parallel fashion. The parallel distributed processing model posits the semantic system as the overarching determiner of ability and that a deficit in this system (semantics) would be displayed in all areas of reading. Again, different damages due to focal brain lesions will result in different manifestations of acquired dyslexia. Each model is based upon behaviorist or neobehaviorist concepts and has not actually focused on authentic reading. Rather, these models have been established through tightly controlled experiments focusing on reading single words, nonsense words, and short phrases. Studies have been conducted to determine the viability of both models, with conflicting evidence presented on both sides. Although these models may provide us with partial insights, because these theories have been tested using decontextualized tasks measuring, at the most, single-word knowledge in carefully controlled experiments, and because they cannot replicate all that happens in a human brain, they are inadequate explanations of what happens when the reading aptitude is diminished due to brain damage.

Since dyslexia is a label that has been constructed and generally employed to stand for reading difficulties at certain levels of severity, and given that such labels are typically reflective of contemporary social conditions and the *received knowledge* of the time, care should be taken with such terminology. Brian Street has suggested that literacy difficulties are more complex than labels like dyslexia indicate. He advocates that any reading difficulties be viewed along a continuum rather than stated as a dichotomous condition of *have or have not*. Such a continuum can more easily account for the complexity of this symbolic process and can enable the differentiation of severity levels, potential causal factors, and other variables that more effectively describe the reading difficulty. In concert with this idea, Connie Weaver has proposed a reconceptualization of dyslexia as simply a condition of ineffective use and/or coordination of strategies for constructing meaning from visual text.

While the term *dyslexia* is still employed, especially in those disciplines with a medical emphasis (e.g., pediatricians, neurologists, medically based speech–language pathologists, and neuropsychologists), there have been other terms used to place children in special education programs (e.g., reading impairments, reading disorders, learning disabilities) and in other less intensive remedial programs (e.g., struggling readers). Typically, struggling readers are those who have difficulty learning to read, but they have either not received a diagnosis or, when assessed, there are other variables that may contribute to the learning difficulties (e.g., poor previous instruction, little or no accessibility to competent and engaged readers as models, low cognitive or intellectual ability, social, linguistic, or cultural differences).

Jack S. Damico

See also Academic Impact of Communication Disorders; Comprehension; Emergence and Human Communication; Miscue Analysis; Phonological and Phonemic Awareness; Reading Fluency; Writing and Writing Disorders

Further Readings

Chall, J. (1983). *Learning to read: The great debate (updated)*. New York, NY: McGraw-Hill.

Clay, M. (1991). *Becoming literate: The construction of inner control*. Portsmouth, NH: Heinemann.

Damico, J. S., & Nelson, R. L. (2010). Reading and reading impairments. In J. S. Damico, N. Müller, & M. J. Ball (Eds.), *The handbook of language and speech disorders* (pp. 267–295). Oxford, UK: Blackwell.

Goodman, K. (1994). Reading, writing, and written texts: A transactional sociopsycholinguistic view. In R. B. Ruddell, M. R. Ruddell, & H. Singer (Eds.), *Theoretical models and processes of reading* (4th ed., pp. 1093–1130). Newark, DE: International Reading Association.

Olson, D. R. (1994). *The world on paper: The conceptual and cognitive implications of writing and reading*. Cambridge, UK: Cambridge University Press.

Smith, F. (2006). *Reading without nonsense* (4th ed.). New York, NY: Teachers College Press.

Street, B. (1995). *Social literacies: Critical approaches to literacy in development, ethnography, and education*. London, UK: Longman.

Weaver, C. (Ed.). (1998). *Practicing what we know. Informed reading instruction*. Urbana, IL: National Council of Teachers of English.

READING FLUENCY

Reading fluency is a construct used in educational psychology and educational assessment to characterize skilled reading. Reading fluency is a component in models of reading-as-word-recognition and is defined as the ability to read a text correctly and quickly with appropriate expression. It is thought that when word recognition is fast, accurate, and effortless, then more attention can be diverted to comprehension. Reading fluency usually relates to oral reading, but it is thought to be an aspect of skilled silent reading as well. It is used interchangeably with *automaticity* (fast, accurate, and effortless word recognition), but the literature stresses that appropriate phrasing and inflection should be included in definitions of reading fluency. It is assessed both as a rate measured in words per minute or correct words per minute depending on the assessment being used and as a quality of oral reading as assessed on a fluency rubric. Reading fluency is frequently mentioned in the literature pertaining to remediation of reading difficulties and as a component of direct instruction.

Sociopsycholinguistic Transactional Model

The sociopsycholinguistic transactional model of reading is an alternative explanation that does not employ the construct of reading fluency. In this model, readers sample visual cues and assign wording and syntax as they construct a personal meaning in a particular social context. Reading is viewed as a language process in which the strategies of sampling and selecting, predicting and inferring, and confirming and self-correcting operate on the graphophonic, lexicogrammatical, and semantic–pragmatic cues in a text. During an uninterrupted oral reading of a whole, authentic text, a reader can produce either the expected response or a miscue (if the reader's response is not what was expected). *Reading accuracy* has no place in a sociopsycholinguistic transactional model because miscues are seen as by-products of the process of making sense of text. However, if *reading fluency* had a counterpart in a sociopsycholinguistic transactional model, it would be described in terms of mature control over a particular text wherein reading is both effective (successful at making sense) and efficient (using the least number of print cues necessary to maintain making sense).

Reading Flow

Processing text happens in time. Reading flow refers to the flexible and dynamic nature of reading strategy employment during a reading. Reading flow analysis is used with miscue analysis to extend the sociopsycholinguistic transactional model by illustrating observable instances of reading strategy use as happenings in time during a reading event.

Reading flow is reported in words per minute, but because this analysis takes into account pauses, repetitions and self-corrections, omissions, insertions, substitutions, and the assignment of alternate syntactic structures such as conjoining independent clauses or shifting clause dependencies, as well as the reading of words—in short, anything a reader does during a reading—it is more useful to think of reading flow in terms of *words processed per minute*.

Reading flow analysis is used to document within-text variation in reading rate. Levels of analysis can focus on either the paragraph or the sentence level of text. Analysis at the sentence level results in finer detail and clearer insights into how readers use time as they read.

To perform flow analysis, a desired unit of text is selected. The time taken to read each unit is divided by the number of words in that unit. In essence, reading flow documents the time it takes for a reader to cross from one unit's boundary to the next and coverts it to reading rate.

When sentence rates are charted sequentially from first to last, a stair-stepped, up-and-down pattern of reading rate variation emerges (Figure 1).

When sentence rates are paired with corresponding miscues, explanations of why readers speed up and slow down within a text come to mind. When readers are confident of their predictions and are assimilating information with little effort, they process text more quickly and efficiently. These schema-driven productions either contain no miscues or contain miscues that do not alter the meaning of the text. By comparison, readers slow down when they need to make accommodations that require additional attention such as encountering new concepts, making initial predictions that require additional scrutiny or correcting, pausing to reflect on what was just read, pausing to anticipate what might be coming next, resolving ambiguity at any level of text, or dealing with unfamiliar or unanticipated wording. Miscues typically found in these schema-forming structures are marked as single or multiple attempts at correction (both successful and unsuccessful), single or multiple repetitions, or pauses. Laughter and commentary can accompany these moments.

Variation in reading rate results from the interplay of the production of schema-driven and schema-forming structures. In other words, reading rate varies because of tension between tentativeness and certainty.

As an alternative to the construct of reading fluency, reading flow analysis demonstrates that

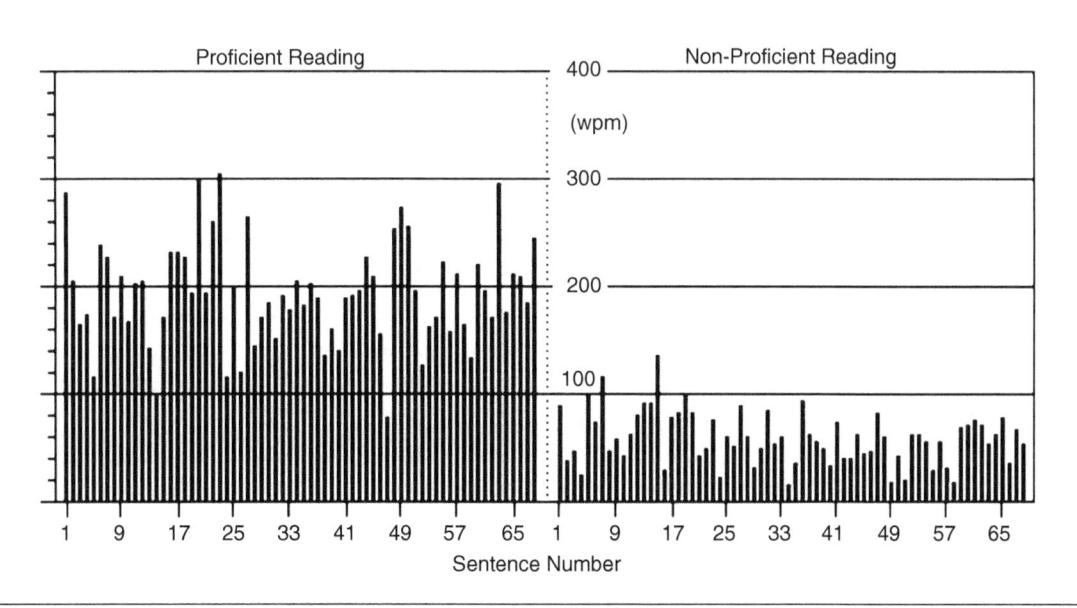

Figure 1 Successive sentence reading rates for proficient and nonproficient readings. Genre: Folktale. Length: 790 words in 68 sentences

pauses, repetitions, substitutions, insertions, omissions, syntactic restructuring, self-corrections, speeding up, slowing down, and even commentaries and laughter provide information about the strategies that readers are using as they make sense of text.

Alan Flurkey

See also Applied Linguistics; Miscue Analysis; Reading and Reading Disorders; Revaluing; Scientific Realism; Self-Correction

Further Readings

Flurkey, A. (2008). Reading flow. In A. Flurkey, E. Paulson, & K. Goodman (Eds.), *Scientific realism in studies of reading*. New York, NY: Erlbaum Associates.

Goodman, K., Fries, P. H., & Strauss, S. L. (2016). *Reading: The grand illusion; how and why readers make sense of print*. New York, NY: Routledge.

Goodman, Y., Watson, D., & Burke, C. (2005). *Reading miscue inventory: From evaluation to instruction* (2nd ed.). Katonah, NY: Richard C. Owen.

Pikulski, J. J., & Chard, D. J. (2005). Fluency: Bridge between decoding and reading comprehension. *The Reading Teacher, 58*(6), 510–519. doi:10.1598/RT.58.6.2

Receptive Language

See Expressive and Receptive Language

Recovery From Aphasia

Any communication disorder has significant negative effects on the lives of people with the condition. Research shows, however, that acquired aphasia has a more devastating impact on individuals with the condition and their families than any other condition, including cancer and Alzheimer's disease. Aphasia is a disorder in the use of language expression and comprehension and reading and writing, most commonly caused by stroke. It is well known that many people with aphasia from stroke recover, and many can recover significantly. Operational definitions, such as a change in a total score on a psychometric battery, have been widely used, even in contemporary research, but do not explain much about the cognitive and neurological processes underlying recovery. However, contemporary research is providing a deeper understanding of the processes underlying recovery from a perspective beyond aphasia battery scores or aphasia *type*. This entry discusses what is known and what is not known about recovery from aphasia.

Aphasia Battery Studies

Many group studies have used operational definitions of recovery, based on a groups' improved performance on a standardized aphasia test battery. These large-group test battery studies have shown that the most rapid recovery takes place in the first 3 months following a stroke and becomes progressively slower as time since the stroke passes, with recovery plateauing after about 12 months poststroke. When participants in these studies are grouped into the classical aphasia *types*, those with less severe forms (e.g., anomia) can recover to relatively normal levels, and those with very severe forms (e.g., global aphasia) recover the least. Those with Broca's and conduction aphasia can recover the most, from relatively severe to relatively mild. In addition, aphasia types can evolve and change over time. Nonfluent Broca's and fluent Wernicke's aphasia can improve and change the type to anomia. Conduction and transcortical aphasias and anomia often recover to normal levels. Language comprehension tends to recover better than expressive language. A problem with using aphasia type as a prognostic indicator is that research has shown that 30–70% of speakers with aphasia are not classifiable and, as noted above, many change type with recovery. Many do not recover in predictable ways.

A related group of studies in the 1980s and 1990s used a statistical approach to predicting likely recovery entailing a detailed analysis of scores on a standardized aphasia test. Using multiple regression analysis, they demonstrated that an overall score at 1-month poststroke can predict an overall score at 3, 6, and 12 months postonset with correlations ranging from .74 to .94. Research has also examined the application of intelligent neural networks, capable of learning over time, to predicting recovery based on aphasia battery scores. Similar to the multiple regression approach, the studies inputted aphasia battery totals of a large group of individuals with aphasia at 1 month poststroke and 12 months poststroke and through learning were able to predict totals at 12 months to be within 4–5%. Contemporary uses of such intelligent networks afford the possibility of comparing a range of possible aphasia recovery models through lesioning various aspects of the network (i.e., damaging components of the network to simulate real damage in a real neural network).

People with aphasia, their families, and clinicians are not just interested in psychometric recovery but are also concerned with the ability to cope, adjust, and function. After all, this is what really matters to individuals and their families. There has been little research into the recovery of these aspects of communication disability. The few studies completed suggest a complex interaction between the severity of aphasia, its recovery, and emotional status. In other words, scores on standard aphasia measures fail to predict communication distress in people with aphasia.

Prognostic Factors

There have been other approaches to predicting recovery based on the presence of a range of prognostic factors, for example, that significant relationships are found between certain demographic variables and outcomes. However, on many of them, there is a disagreement among research studies. Factors such as the severity of aphasia, the time postonset of stroke, aphasia type, the site and extent of brain lesion, the presence of dysarthria and bilateral damage, and the co-occurrence of other nonverbal cognitive conditions (e.g., limb apraxia or agnosia) are clearly interrelated and appear to be interdependent. There is a considerable disagreement among research studies about whether some are useful theoretical constructs at all (e.g., type of aphasia). For several variables (e.g., age, sex, and handedness), findings between studies can vary. Some studies suggest that age, for instance, is a prognostic indicator and others do not.

Such findings on recovery are not the whole story, and there is a range of small-group and single-case studies going back to the early 20th century showing that people with aphasia can make steady recovery for many years. Single-case studies of long-term aphasia show that some people continue to recover even up to 25 years. Since those early studies, more has been discovered about what aspects of aphasic symptomatology recover the earliest and the most.

The Influence of Other Cognitive Factors

There is a growing understanding of the relationships between language, the breakdown of language in aphasia, and other nonlinguistic cognitive domains. Language does not proceed in glorious isolation but is highly dependent upon other cognitive processes. These include long-term, short-term, and working memory and semantic memory; executive functions such as inhibition and initiation; as well as praxis or action processing that enables planning, programming, organizing, and coordinating speech actions. Without the involvement of these processes, language cannot proceed. The diffuse damage caused by stroke interferes with a wide range of cognitive processes, which are often significantly impaired following brain damage resulting in aphasia. In addition, a range of aphasic symptoms, such as semantic impairments, syntactic comprehension, jargon aphasia, and aphasic speech automatisms, are being investigated with the aim of determining to what extent they can be explained through damage to other cognitive processes. Investigations into impaired cognitive processes implicated in aphasic symptomology include action semantics, short-term and working memory, *anosognosia* (failure on the part of the individual to recognize that he or she has an illness or condition), and failures to inhibit unwanted behavior. These processes, directly unrelated to linguistic processes per se, are considered by many to be supportive processes for language expression and comprehension.

Mechanisms of Recovery

A wide range of mechanisms have been hypothesized to account for recovery over the years, representing a sometimes confusing mixture of neurophysiological and behavioral explanations often overlapping and conceptually indistinguishable from each other. Some neural mechanisms of recovery following damage to the brain are well established and under research in contemporary science.

In the early 1800s, Constantin Von Monokov first described one such process, *diaschisis*, which is a situation where tissue and neural networks at some distance from the lesioned brain area are negatively influenced by the radiation of a process from the damaged area that obliterates neural excitability via a neural pathway in another brain area. Von Monokov identified associative diaschisis acting in the same hemisphere as the damaged area of brain and affecting undamaged areas. Commissural diaschisis operates via the corpus callosum linking the two hemispheres. The opposite, undamaged side of the brain is affected by the damaged side. Corticospinal diaschisis operates via corticospinal neural pathways.

The effects of diaschisis are therefore seen as different from, and in addition to, the effects of the primary brain damage. The behavioral disruptions observed in the individual are therefore seen as a result of a combination of the effects of the diaschisis and the primary damage. Recovery of function is the result of the lessening effects of diaschisis with time postonset of the brain damage. Any remaining deficits are attributed to the original lesioned area. As such, diaschisis is more a sparing explanation for recovery.

The notion of neuroplasticity gets a great deal of attention and is widely used as the basis for a plethora of the so-called *brain training* programs. It is also, however, fueling much biological, neurophysiological, and behavioral research and is by no means a new idea. The notion that the brain has a certain degree of plasticity has been around at least since the late 1900s in the work of Santiago Ramón y Caya, who hypothesized that plasticity takes place at the synapse (the junction between neurons). William James first described the plasticity of the human brain in response to lifelong learning. The modern notion of neuroplasticity rests on such foundations. It can be simply defined as changes in neural circuitry in response to learning through environmental exposure, so that anything humans learn is directly explained by changes in neural circuitry and brain structure, as when learning a specific skill, such as playing a musical instrument or establishing arithmetic tables. Included in this definition are reorganizational adjustments in response to functional losses due to brain aging or brain damage, as in aphasia.

One view is that real recovery is best seen as neural sparing, where recovery is due to undamaged neural tissue. This view distinguishes the loss of function that simply cannot be recovered and behavioral deficits that are the result of attempts to shift functional control to undamaged neural systems. Behavioral deficits (e.g., the symptoms of aphasia such as agrammatism or paraphasia) are seen as compensatory responses to damaged language systems. Recovery for an individual, therefore, may occur through a combination of *restoration* (restitution) of lost cognitive functions or *compensation* (substitution) for lost functions. These basic principles of restoration and compensation, utilized in aphasia intervention, originated with Henry Charlton Bastian in the latter part of the 19th century. How much an individual's recovery may be due to restoration of a previously lost function or compensation for a lost function is not fully understood.

Differential and Symptomatic Recovery

Research since the turn of the 21st century has examined the recovery of different components of language in aphasia after stroke. Semantics and syntax appear to improve significantly for the first 6 weeks after stroke. Phonology appears to recover for the longest period over 12 months, and communication continues to recover even for decades. However, there is also a great deal of variability in the recovery of separate linguistic components between people with aphasia.

As discussed earlier, artificial *connectionist* neural networks have been developed that mimic various aspects of cognition and are then lesioned in various ways. One deep dysphasic participant's impairment in naming and repeating nonwords resulted in semantic and sound-related (formal) paraphasias and neologisms. In repetition, the individual produced mainly semantic paraphasias but also formal paraphasias and neologisms. In naming, he produced mainly formal paraphasias. The researchers explained this as resulting from a fast rate of decay. Naming a picture runs from semantic specification to lexical access to phonological specification, so semantic representations decay earlier than lexical representations, which, in turn, decay earlier than phonological ones. Anomia in severe deep dysphasia is characterized by a high rate of phonologically related words (formal paraphasias) because they are more accessible. Repetition, however, runs from acoustic analysis to phonological output and need not access semantics. The predominance of semantic paraphasias in repetition reflects rapidly decayed phonological specifications and a dependence on the semantic system.

A connectionist lesion model was developed, which mirrored the participant's recovery of naming and repetition. Improvement (decreases) in decay rate was the basis of recovering repetition and naming. For others with a similar pattern of deficits, the recovery (i.e., a decrease in decay rate) may be similarly explained.

Neuroimaging studies of the brain areas involved in recovery from aphasia are often contradictory, but meta-analyses seem to suggest that there is consistency in areas activated. Some spared left hemisphere language areas and new left hemisphere (and some right) hemisphere areas are involved. Participants with aphasia who have left inferior frontal damage recruit right inferior frontal areas more than those without damage to the inferior frontal area. In addition, areas that may hinder recovery are also recruited. Recruitment of the right hemisphere during recovery appears to depend on the location and extent of the left hemisphere lesion. Right hemisphere involvement is less where there is less extensive damage to the main left hemisphere language areas and more when the left hemisphere's language network is extensively damaged.

Chris Code

See also Anomia; Aphasia; Aphasia Intervention; Executive Function and Communication; Psychosocial Impact of Aphasia; Spontaneous Recovery

Further Readings

Cahana-Amitay, D., & Albert, M. L. (2015). *Redefining recovery from aphasia*. New York, NY: Oxford University Press.

Cappa, S. F. (2011). The neural basis of aphasia rehabilitation: Evidence from neuroimaging and neurostimulation. *Neuropsychological Rehabilitation, 21*, 742–754.

Code, C. (2001). Multifactorial processes in recovery from aphasia: Developing the foundations for a multilevelled framework. *Brain & Language, 77*, 25–44.

Denes, G. (2016). *Neural plasticity across the lifespan: How the brain can change*. Abingdon, UK: Routledge.

El Hachioui, H., van de Sandt-Koenderman, M. W. M. E., Dippel, D. W. J., Koudstaal, P. J., & Visch-Brink, E. G. (2011). A 3-year evolution of linguistic disorders in aphasia after stroke. *International Journal of Rehabilitation Research, 34*, 215–221.

Hillis, A. E. (2002). Does the right make it right? Questions about recovery of language after stroke. *Annals of Neurology, 51*, 537–538.

Jarso, S., Li, M., Faria, A., Davis, C., Leigh, R., Sebastian, R., . . . Hillis, A. E. (2014). Distinct mechanisms and timing of language recovery after stroke. *Cognitive Neuropsychology, 30*, 454–475.

Lam, J. M. C., & Wodchis, W. P. (2010). The relationship of 60 disease diagnoses and 15 conditions to preference-based health-related quality of life in Ontario hospital-based long-term care residents. *Medical Care, 48*, 380–387.

Martin, N., Saffran, E. M., & Dell, G. S. (1996). Recovery in deep dysphasia: Evidence for a relation between auditory-verbal STM capacity and lexical errors in repetition. *Brain and Language, 52*, 83–113.

Simmons-Mackie, N. N., & Damico, J. (1997). Reformulating the definition of compensatory strategies in aphasia. *Aphasiology, 11*, 761–781.

Turkeltaub, P. E., Messing, S., Norise, C., & Hamilton, R. H. (2011). Are networks for residual language function and recovery consistent across aphasic patients? *Neurology, 76*, 1726–1734.

RECURSION

Recursion is a mathematical principle that involves repeating an algorithm (a sequence of mathematical operations) any number of times. There is no limit to the number, and infinite repetition is possible. In other words, the mechanism can be used to describe infinite objects using only a finite description.

Recursion is an important principle in the theory of computation, a branch of mathematics that demonstrates whether something is computable and how. This led to the creation of computer science. Furthermore, recursion is a fundamental principle that is found in all cognitive sciences. The principle of recursion was used in linguistics by Noam Chomsky to explain how it is possible for a human being to generate an infinite number of sentences from a limited number of rules and words. Recursion is supposedly one of the basic principles that allows human brains to implement language.

There are several types of recursion in language. The most complex one is *centrally embedded recursion*. For example:

[The man filed a complaint]

[The man [the boy hit] filed a complaint]

[The man [the boy [the girl kissed] hit] filed a complaint]

In the last two sentences above, the central clause reproduces the grammatical structure of the main clause. It would be possible to add more clauses within the last sentence, but the resulting sentence would be very difficult to understand. This difficulty is explained by memory limitation because processing many embedded clauses implies having the whole sentence in mind. This limitation led Chomsky to separate the principle of competence (the theoretical knowledge of grammar) from the principle of performance (the actual production of language within the limits of the actual biological brain). For Chomsky, the principle of recursion belongs to competence and is nonlimited, which explains why language is potentially infinite.

Real examples of multiple embedded clauses in language exist although they are infrequent. Often the memory load is lighter than in the example above because the elements to be memorized are clearly different from one another. For example:

[The fact [that the teenager [who John dates] was pretty] annoyed Suzie]

Some linguists have argued against the necessity of recursion in language, explaining that recursive embedding is not the only solution used to express embedding in human languages. This seems to be the case for the Pirahã language. Although recursion is found in almost all languages in the world, it might not be a defining condition of human language.

Language Acquisition

Children demonstrate early knowledge of the structural properties of language. In the case of lexical recursive structures, as for example in "red rats eater," children make the difference between grouping "red rats" to mean "eater of red rats" (the correct interpretation) and grouping "rats eater" to mean "red rats-eater" (an incorrect and ungrammatical interpretation, although based on a much more frequent grammatical construction). However, the acquisition of complex structures and especially compound sentences is slow, and the first compound sentences acquired are based on specific grammatical structures (clefts) and not recursive structures.

Language Impairment

One of the few studies to have explicitly tested the existence of recursion in children with specific language impairment (SLI) found poorer performances on recursion measures in children with SLI when compared with age-matched normally developing children. This is not surprising, as children with SLI are known to have difficulties with complex processing. Although recursion should not be reduced to complexity, it does call for simultaneous processing; hence, processing limitations might impair recursive processing in children with SLI.

Christophe Parisse and *Christelle Maillart*

See also Clauses and Phrases; Syntax and Grammar

Further Readings

Chomsky, N. (1965). *Aspects of the theory of syntax*. Cambridge, MA: MIT Press.

Corballis, M. C. (2011). *The recursive mind: The origins of human language, thought, and civilization*. Princeton, NJ: Princeton University Press.

Karlsson, F. (2010). Syntactic recursion and iteration. In H. van der Hulst (Ed.), *Recursion and human language. Studies in generative grammar* (pp. 43–67). New York, NY: De Gruyter Mouton.

van der Hulst, H. G. (Ed.). (2010). *Recursion and human language*. Berlin, Germany: De Gruyter Mouton.

REFERENCE

Reference is a notion used in several linguistic subdisciplines. It can be conceived as a property of the meanings of words and expressions, which connects the mental concepts that speakers can entertain with specific mind-external entities that these concepts can describe. The notion of reference is tightly interwoven with the notions of sense and denotation and plays a role in the study of various communication disorders. This entry discusses technical terms related to reference, key notions, problems that can arise in patients with communication disorders, and some examples.

Key Notions

The technical term *reference* is closely connected to the terms *referent*, *act of reference*, *referential expressions*, and *refer to*. To understand how these terms are related and used, consider the place name Rome. English speakers generally use this name to refer to the capital of Italy in conversations. The referent of this expression is the real-life city, with its inhabitants and history. The act of reference is performed when speakers use this expression in a context, such as when suggesting they might go to Rome for a holiday. Reference, then, is the term used to describe this general category of linguistic concepts.

The notion of reference is tightly connected to that of *sense*, defined as the set of properties or "mental fingers" that allow speakers to use words and their meanings to refer to entities in the world. Acts of reference can thus be conceived as inherently relational, if one takes a psychological perspective. An act of reference can establish a relation between a mind-internal token instantiating the sense of a word and a referent as the mind-external object it refers to. When speakers use the place name Rome, they associate their concept of this city (i.e., its token) with the city itself (i.e., the referent). The sense of the name Rome and its use in a sentence are the linguistic elements establishing this relation.

Reference is not a notion that is restricted to names and nouns, hence the use of the term *referential expression*. For instance, indexical expressions (or *deixes*) always refer to specific aspects of the context. The spatial deixis *here* and the temporal deixis *now* always refer to the speaker's location and utterance time (deixis). Similarly, personal pronouns such as *I* always refer to the speaker of an utterance, although in often subtle manners (*semantics*). Reference can thus connect the meanings of linguistic expressions to different entities, such as cities, places, and moments in time.

Reference is generally defined at the level of phrases, one example being the definite noun phrase *the dog*. The sense of the common noun *dog* individuates a class of domestic animals. In combination with *the* and its sense, however, *the dog* is a noun phrase that can be used to refer to a specific dog in a context. For instance, one can use the sentence *the dog is barking* to refer to a specific barking dog, in this example, a dog named Sparkie. Crucially, acts of reference may be unsuccessful. If a speaker uses this sentence in a context in which there are two dogs (e.g., Sparkie and Laika), then interlocutors may not be able to figure out to which dog the speaker is referring to. The act of reference is said to fail, as the participants in this conversation cannot align themselves in the use of this referential expression.

Therefore, acts of reference allow speakers to establish *discourse referents*, the relevant entities entertained in the context of discourse or conversation. Discourse referents can be conceived as the referents that participants in a conversation focus on, if each participant can successfully establish the identity of these referents. For instance, three friends can discuss their next destination for the holidays, with one friend using the sentence, "We should go to Rome next holiday break." By using the place name Rome, the speaker introduces this city as a key discourse referent in this conversation. The other friends, once they establish that the speaker is referring to the Italian capital, can voice their opinion on this proposal. Reference is thus a dynamic notion that emerges in the context of discourse.

Experimental Evidence

Reference has played an important part in the study of language processing research. Many works have investigated how participants in conversation perform acts of reference and what communicative problems may arise when these acts are unsuccessful. For instance, the successful use of definite noun phrases in discourse usually requires speakers to offer sufficient descriptive content. In the aforementioned context with the dogs, Sparkie and Laika, one speaker can use the more informative *the female dog* to refer to Laika, to avoid reference failure. However, this use can be successful insofar as the other participants know (or can infer) that Laika is a female dog. Hence, reference acts require considerable processing resources, a fact that may lead participants to experience problems jointly establishing referents in conversation.

Given the underpinning mechanisms of reference, certain disorders can heavily affect speakers' ability to perform these acts. For instance, patients with Asperger's and autism spectrum disorders perform poorly in the use of referential expressions. These patients often have insurmountable problems in envisioning other individuals' mental processes. Therefore, they use referring expressions (e.g., definite noun phrases, indexicals) in an ambiguous manner. For instance, a patient may use a sentence such as *the dog is barking* to describe a context in which two dogs, Sparkie and Laika, are barking. As the patient cannot be aware that other speakers cannot know which of the two dogs the patient has in mind, this reference act is bound to be unsuccessful.

Equivalent problems arise in patients affected with aphasic disorders. Patients affected with Broca's aphasia are often unable to produce functional lexical items (e.g., the definite article *the* in *the dog*, thereby failing to produce full referential expressions). Wernicke's aphasia patients, given their inability to produce meaningful expressions, tend to produce expressions that fail to refer, for instance, using *the dog* when no dogs are present in a context. In these cases, patients do not face production or comprehension problems per se but rather an inability to let speakers jointly access and interpret these acts of reference in context.

Francesco-Alessio Ursini and Aijun Huang

See also Aphasia; Deixis; Semantic Disorders; Semantics; Type versus Token

Further Readings

Cohen, H., & Lefebvre, C. (Eds.). (2005). *Handbook of categorization in cognitive science*. Burlington, VT: Elsevier.

D'amico, J. S., Müller, N., & Ball, M. J. (Eds.). (2010). *The handbook of language and speech disorders*. Chichester, UK: Wiley-Blackwell.

Murphy, M. L. (2003). *Semantic relations and the lexicon*. Cambridge, UK: Cambridge University Press.

Riemer, N. (2010). *Introducing semantics*. Cambridge, UK: Cambridge University Press.

REFERRAL ISSUES

A *clinical referral* is a request for specialist attention to a suspected disease or disorder. It represents a transfer of information about an individual, as well as a transfer of clinical responsibility over that individual, and must therefore provide a rationale for that transfer. A referral initiates a process typically consisting of consultation, assessment, intervention (if necessary), and follow-up, resulting in either client discharge or further referral. Concerns over communication disorders commonly involve referrals to speech–language pathologists (SLPs), making it important to understand both how those referrals reach them and on what grounds they are made. This entry defines referrals and discusses the scope of referral to SLPs, the referral process, and what are grounds for referral.

Scope of Referral to Speech–Language Pathology

Communication disorders disrupt a communication chain that basically operates through tripartite coordination among a sender, a receiver, and a code. Sender and receiver must share the same code and use the same rules for coding and decoding a message, respectively. Communication takes place when sent and received messages match, although this ideal is difficult to judge in practice. Many factors are at play in human communication, such as sender intention (also called *illocution*) and receiver interpretation (*perlocution*), both differing from the assumed factual content of the messages (*locution*). In addition, messages may be transmitted through different physical carriers (e.g., air, telephony, or electronic means), and human communication is typically multimodal, making simultaneous and complementary use of different codes, such as gestural or body language when speaking, compounding the complexity of deciding on the causes of deficient communication.

Referrals to SLPs about communication abilities may reflect concerns about language, speech (including voice), and/or hearing, the latter involving audiology specialists. Language is a cognitive ability. It develops through social interaction via different modes that favor different senses, such as hearing for spoken languages or sight for signed and printed languages. Speech and hearing depend on the sender's and receiver's physical ability to use language through the medium of sound. Voice issues include control over, for example, loudness, pitch, or nasality, which may signal disorder where they deviate from the requisite vocal quality (also called *vocal posture*), articulatory settings, or voice settings associated with specific languages and language varieties.

Language, speech, and hearing disorders may be independent from one another or interdependent in their causal probability. A referral for speech impairment, for example, may omit mention of hearing impairment, whereas the latter often causes the former, whether language ability is intact or not. Productive language deficiencies may or may not relate to receptive disorder. Standard referrals state possible causes of disorder and purposes of the referral (e.g., reducing the client's dependency on skilled or familiar communication partners or recommending augmentative and alternative communication methods to meet clients' needs).

Process of Referral to Speech–Language Pathology

In principle, anyone can initiate a referral process, including self-referral or referral management systems that provide electronic handling of clinical paperwork. Human initiators may be laypeople (e.g., the individual's relatives) or specialists (e.g., professionals in health, education, or care services), but the referral always directs to a specialist. By following the procedures that substantiate the reasons for the referral, initiators act as gatekeepers releasing prescreening information about the client. The procedures may be informal, as in a private phone call to the family doctor, or formal, involving completion and official submission of standard documentation. Apart from obvious reasons, including traumatic accident, sudden onset of disease, or genetic disorders known to affect communication abilities (e.g., Down syndrome), attesting to the need for a referral may not be straightforward.

A referral offers a preliminary assessment about a suspected clinical condition that the initiator either lacks competence and/or authorization to handle or wishes to secure a second opinion for. Any assessment involves a comparison, typically to developmental or aging norms for children or adults, respectively, and is therefore relative, in that norms vary in time and space. Falling silent in the presence of adults, for example, may be expected or deviant child behavior depending on culture. Initiators' own expectations naturally set the standard warranting referral action.

Lay initiators commonly rely on informal assessment comparing clients to themselves, such as when a child has started stammering, or an elderly relative now fails to respond to familiar communicative exchanges, where the benchmark of normality is individual, based on the client's habitual behavior. Professional initiators rely on formal assessment methods, such as standardized language ability tests, where the benchmark of normality is statistical, based on the habitual behavior of a normed population. Both benchmarks are useful, in that the client is assumed to represent the statistically significant population that generated the assessment norms but is also an individual. Statistical criteria define deviation, but individual criteria constrain its scope, helping to avoid unnecessary referral. A child's vocabulary count, for example, may deviate from a statistical milestone at a certain age but be normal for that child, whose linguistic development is steadily progressing.

Grounds for Referral to Speech–Language Pathology

Standardized tests of language ability are relatively recent in Western clinical practice, dating from the 1950s. Standardization gives a measure of their reliability, in that they are norm referenced, but the norm itself may be unusable for several reasons.

First, the label *language ability* is misleading. Language ability is shared by all typically developing human beings, whereas language ability tests assess ability in particular languages, which is individual and depends on factors such as quantity and quality of environmental input or motivation and attitudes toward the languages in question. Poor proficiency in a language is not a reliable indicator of language disorder. If proficiency can be improved by remedying those factors (e.g., through language tuition), then there is no need for clinical intervention. In monolingual individuals, language disorder may be difficult to distinguish from deficiencies in their only language. In multilingual individuals, the decision is facilitated by the fact that language disorder affects all of their languages. This is why assessment of multilingual individuals must take into account their full linguistic repertoire, just like assessment of monolingual individuals accounts for their full linguistic repertoire, which happens to consist of a single language.

Second, language ability tests are labeled for a language (e.g., Spanish), whereas they are normed for the language variety that any population necessarily uses, including norming populations (e.g., Mexican Spanish or regional varieties of it). Linguistically, the concept of *a language* is a mere convenient abstraction. There is a norm for each variety of each language, regardless of whether it has been standardized for assessment purposes, and the vast majority of languages and language varieties lack such normed instruments.

Third, virtually all assessment instruments are normed for standard varieties of languages, which draw on social conventions rather than actual uses. Standard varieties, being prestige varieties, often associate with judgmental labels such as *good* or *correct*. These terms also appear in language assessment reports, together with their negative counterparts (e.g., *poor grasp*, *unnatural delivery*, *difficult to understand*), raising the question of *to whom*. Standards of naturalness or intelligibility are not absolute, being created by habit and familiarity.

Fourth, language ability tests commonly focus on modular components that languages are assumed to consist of. These can include grammar rules, sounds, or vocabulary items, to the detriment of rules and items defining pragmatic uses of those languages, or awareness of conventionally appropriate uses of language (e.g., toward elders or in public places, whose disruption may signal language disorder).

Finally, language ability tests are normed from and for monolingual uses of language, invalidating their use with multilingual individuals, in that multilingualism is not an addition of monolingualisms.

Referral initiators ascribe communication breakdown to the clients (the senders/receivers in the communication chain), taking the language variety that they use and the one on which they are assessed (the code) as the same. The problem may instead lie in the code, whose norming marks as atypical any uses outside the scope of the normed population. Ability tests normed for one language do not work for other languages, as little as tests normed for, say, Texan English can be used to assess Singapore English. The same holds for test translation or adaptation across languages or language varieties. Proof of healthy or disordered communication ability can only be obtained by controlling the code variable, making it constant.

Reliance on less appropriate assessment tools results in referral bias, both overreferral and underreferral. Overreferral is well-documented, for example, in the disproportionate number of referrals to SLPs or special education needs for children variously described as minority or culturally and linguistically diverse, qualifiers in common use to designate ethnic, linguistic, and/or sociocultural backgrounds that differ from the local mainstream. Referrals highlight developmental and/or academic milestones that the children fail to meet, often with no distinction or no statement of causal directionality between the two. Communicative impairment, however, may present as subpar academic performance, or vice versa, and one may be the cause or the consequence of the other. Those children's regional, social, and/or multilingual differences are interpreted as deficits. This interpretation is an artifact of assessment tools that will inevitably find deviations, in that their norms do not represent what would be normal for these children, perpetuating the myth and the associated stigmatization that, by definition, they need clinical intervention. Overreferral identifies false positives (also called *type I errors*), mistaking typical behavior for disorder and resulting in unnecessary burdening of specialist time and resources.

Underreferral misses false negatives (type II errors), mistaking disorder for typical behavior. Depending on sociocultural factors, there may be different thresholds of tolerance toward what is considered normal (e.g., degree of hearing loss among older individuals or indiscriminate use of a multilingual individual's languages). Underreferrals may also result from initiators' difficulties communicating in the language(s) of the specialists to whom referrals are directed. Underreferral fails to identify disordered behavior, including in time for early intervention, burdening families and communities with recurrent communication breakdown.

Informed referrals trigger processes that reliably pinpoint what constitutes disordered communication through shared responsibility between initiator and specialist. Initiators offer preliminary guidance, ideally gleaned from the awareness of typical communicative behavior, including where local linguistic and sociocultural backgrounds may not match their own. Referral direction that safeguards the clients' interests also lies with initiators. Two common examples of misdirected referral concern deaf children referred to hearing rather than deaf professionals and multilingual children referred to specialists with no knowledge or experience of multilingualism, jeopardizing the children's chances of developing communication skills in alternative modes or languages, respectively. The latter case relates to the lack of instruction on multilingualism in SLPs' training, not to the misconception that SLPs must be multilingual themselves or know all the languages of their clients. Dynamic assessment methods, for example, properly target language ability rather than ability in specific languages. Specialists, in turn, decide whether there is a reason for further action. This is particularly relevant where clients, or their representatives, insist on referral, claiming that only a specialist opinion will reassure them. In the absence of a gold standard (i.e., the best available agreed-upon benchmark), specialists also assess the accuracy of the referral assessment itself, which may require calibration from information about the client's normality standards.

Communicative norms that usefully serve as a benchmark for referral processes are found in the everyday exchanges to which individuals are exposed and in which they participate, as well as exploration of all their communicative resources. Children and adults may resort, for example, to prosody or gestural language to compensate for words that are not yet acquired or forgotten, respectively. Informed cooperation between health and education professionals and the client's family and broader community helps provide guidance toward streamlined referral, intervention, and rehabilitation, mitigating the serious consequences of communication disorders on individual and social well-being.

Madalena Cruz-Ferreira

See also Diagnosis of Communication Disorders; Intercultural Communication; Multilingualism; Screening for Speech and Language Disorders; Special Education; Standardized Testing

Further Readings

Cruz-Ferreira, M. (Ed.). (2010). *Multilingual norms*. Frankfurt, Germany: Peter Lang.

Harry, B., & Klingner, J. K. (2014). *Why are so many minority students in special education? Understanding race and disability in schools* (2nd ed.). New York, NY: Teachers College Press.

Hummert, M. L., & Nussbaum, J. F. (Eds.). (2001). *Aging, communication and health: Linking research and practice for successful aging*. Mahwah, NJ: Erlbaum.

MacSwan, J., & Rolstad, K. (2006). How language proficiency tests mislead us about ability: Implications for English language learner placement in special education. *Teachers College Record, 108*(11), 2304–2328.

Paul-Brown, D., & Ricker, J. H. (2003). *Evaluating and treating communication and cognitive disorders: Approaches to referral and collaboration for speech-language pathology and clinical neuropsychology* [Online]. Retrieved February 18, 2017, from http://www.asha.org/policy/TR2003-00137.htm

Regional Cerebral Blood Flow (rCBF)

Two central objectives of neurological research are the isolation and measurement of cerebral neurological activity. The collection of neural activation data is inherently challenging, as researchers are limited to relatively noninvasive procedures on live patients. Fortunately, the current research paradigm is able to estimate brain activity by isolating and measuring areas of regional cerebral blood flow (rCBF). Although it may seem counterintuitive to measure rCBF as a means to infer neural activity, the data behind this research paradigm are well founded on empirical science. This entry describes the relationship between neural activity and rCBF and details two popular methodologies that researchers use to infer neural activity from rCBF measurements.

The Relationship Between Neural Activity and rCBF

When one specific brain region has an increase in neural activity, these active nerve cells will increase their energy consumption. As neural activity increases, so will the nerve cell's glucose and oxygen consumption. Specifically, glucose consumption reflects synaptic activity by fueling the maintenance of neuronal membrane potentials and restoring neuronal ion gradients. In other words, neurons need to consume glucose as a means to continue functioning properly before, during, and after periods of activity. As such, as neural activity increases, so will glucose consumption and the demand for oxygen.

A substantial amount of research reliably links localized cerebral glucose consumption (in a specific part of the brain) with autoregulation of rCBF. *Autoregulation* refers to the body's natural ability to regulate and maintain a constant blood pressure to sustain life and to make slight changes in blood pressure to accommodate changes in cellular activity. Although the body successfully autoregulates rCBF, these mechanisms are not completely understood. Autoregulation of rCBF is believed to occur by the body constricting and dilating the diameters of cerebral blood vessels in a specific cerebral location, thereby controlling the amount of rCBF. Quite simply, a constricted vessel reduces rCBF, while a dilated vessel increases rCBF. Through autoregulation, the diameter of cerebral vessels is adjusted in response to the body's systemic blood pressure as well as changes in the blood's chemical composition. For example, autoregulation results in vessel dilation when higher levels of carbon dioxide are found in the blood and in vessel constriction when lower levels of carbon dioxide are found in the blood. As a consequence, blood flow is increased relative to the cellular activation that requires an increase in glucose and oxygen consumption. Therefore, an increase in rCBF reflects an increase in glucose and oxygen consumption, which reflects an increase in neural activity. Although this is an indirect relationship spanning over a few physiological steps, it is a valid and reliable relationship that has withstood intense empirical testing.

The Measurement of rCBF

Although there are various technologies believed to quantify rCBF as a means of inferring neural activity, some of the most common include functional magnetic resonance imaging (fMRI) and positron emission tomography (PET).

fMRI

fMRI is able to measure blood flow by using blood oxygen level–dependent contrasts. When a neuron fires and completes an action potential, it must quickly replenish energy via glucose and oxygen consumption such that the cell can re-establish itself for future activity. Through the hemodynamic response (i.e., change in blood flow) of autoregulation, the body increases blood flow to these regions of neural activity, so that oxygen and glucose can be consumed. Oxygen is transported in the blood via the red protein hemoglobin, which contains iron. As a consequence, the iron in the hemoglobin within the blood has measurable magnetic properties. In 1990, researcher Seiji Ogawa published data demonstrating that oxygenated hemoglobin has different magnetic properties from deoxygenated hemoglobin and that these differences can be detected and measured using MRI. Accordingly, fMRI measures the difference in magnetism between oxygenated and deoxygenated hemoglobin, thereby reflecting localized cellular activity of oxygen consumption. Stated differently, fMRI measures a relatively higher concentration of oxygenated hemoglobin within rCBF *upstream* from the region of neural activity, with a higher concentration of deoxygenated hemoglobin directly *downstream* from the active neurons.

PET

PET relies on some of the same assumptions regarding blood flow as fMRI to infer neural activity. For example, PET also assumes that active neurons will consume more glucose and oxygen relative to lesser active neurons. However, PET differs from fMRI in that PET measures the relative radioactivity of tissue, as opposed to fMRI measuring the magnetic properties of blood. Patients undergoing PET are injected with positron-emitting (radioactive) tracers into their bloodstream. Although there are a number of tracers used in PET, one of the most common is fludeoxyglucose, which is an analog of glucose. As neural activity increases, the cellular consumption of glucose and oxygen also increases. Thus, the more active the cell, the more it will consume fludeoxyglucose and more radioactive the cell will become. These positron-emitting cells emit gamma rays, which can be identified, recorded, and measured three-dimensionally in living patients with a PET scanner.

One of the advantages of PET over other forms of functional neural imaging is that different tracers have been developed to target different neuroreceptors. The targeted selection of specified neurotransmitters can be of great use in researching specific neurophysiatric or neurological illnesses as well as the development of new pharmaceuticals targeting specific neural functions.

Similar to fMRI, PET scans can provide a good topographic detail but at the cost of poor temporal resolution. This is to say that PET data are functionally averaged over time and cannot provide specificity relative to the timing of neural activations.

Applications and Limitations

A wealth of data correlates changes in rCBF with neural activity. In short, neural activity triggers glucose and oxygen consumption, which changes blood chemistry, stimulates autoregulation of rCBF, and dilates cerebral blood vessels, thereby increasing rCBF. As a consequence, measuring rCBF can provide a reasonable estimate of neural activity. Although fMRI and PET are the most commonly used techniques of reliable and valid indirect measures of neural activity via rCBF, it is also important to note that changes in rCBF occur after a series of physiological events. Accordingly, although indirect measures of neural activity via the measurement of rCBF have limited temporal resolution, these methods are some of the best available procedures in identifying and measuring regions of neural activity.

Gregory J. Snyder

See also Electroencephalography (EEG); Neurogenic Communication Disorders; Plasticity of Brain; Quantitative Research; Research; Technology and Communication Disorders

Further Readings

Bailey, D. L., Townsend, D. W., Valk, P. E., & Maisey, M. N. (2005). *Positron emission tomography: Basic sciences*. Secaucus, NJ: Springer-Verlag.

Jueptner, M., & Weiller, C. (1995). Review: Does measurement of regional cerebral blood flow reflect synaptic activity? Implications for PET and fMRI. *Neuroimage, 2*(2), 148–156.

Kandel, E. R., Schwartz, J. H., & Jessell, T. M. (2000). *Principles of neural science* (4th ed.). New York, NY: McGraw-Hill.

Logothetis, N. K. (2003). The underpinnings of the BOLD functional magnetic resonance imaging signal. *Journal of Neuroscience, 15*(23), 3963–3971.

Ogawa, S., Lee, T. M., Nayak, A. S., & Glynn, P. (1990). Oxygenation-sensitive contrast in magnetic resonance image of rodent brain at high magnetic fields. *Magnetic Resonance in Medicine, 14*(1), 68–78. doi:10.1002/mrm.1910140108, PMID 2161986

REHABILITATION

The word *rehabilitate* derives from the Medieval Latin word *rehabilitare*, meaning to restore or bring back to a former condition. Medical rehabilitation is a process designed to help individuals suffering from a functional difficulty to reach their highest possible level of self-sufficiency. The restorative nature of the root word implies a prior level of functioning. Thus, rehabilitation is most commonly used in reference to health-care services for individuals who have acquired difficulties. The level of independence achieved through rehabilitation depends on a variety of factors, including the disability or difficulty itself as well as the environmental and social context in which the individual participates. Thus, rehabilitation services' aims vary according to the individual's needs. Desired outcomes may include independently dressing oneself, obtaining a full-time job, gaining employment in a supported environment, and/or living independently. Common difficulties or disabilities that result in provision of rehabilitative services include, but are not limited to, amputation, spinal cord injury, stroke, traumatic brain injury, and mental illness. Rehabilitation usually involves a combination of medicine, therapy, education, and/or vocational training. This entry describes the field of physical medicine and rehabilitation (PM&R) from a historical perspective and outlines the biopsychosocial model that governs rehabilitation practices. Rehabilitation in communication sciences and disorders (CSD) is then discussed in the context of research, technology, and client care.

Habilitation and Rehabilitation

The terms *rehabilitation* and *habilitation* are sometimes used synonymously although they take on slightly different meanings in some legislative settings. Habilitation refers to services that help a person with a developmental or congenital disability to keep or improve skills, as well as to learn new skills that facilitate functioning for self-sufficient daily living (e.g., services for a child with a developmental hearing loss or cognitive difficulty). Rehabilitation includes services that focus on regaining lost skills while also maintaining and improving abilities of daily living (e.g., services for an adult with an acquired hearing loss or cognitive difficulty). Thus, the difference between habilitation and rehabilitation is primarily related to the underlying cause of the disability and client's prior functioning level, rather than the services provided. Both have a similar goal of assisting individuals to achieve independent functioning in daily living activities. The shared objectives and similar outcomes likely explain why rehabilitation is often used interchangeably with habilitation in the literature.

PM&R

The enterprise of rehabilitation medicine is known as *PM&R*, physiatry, or physical and rehabilitation medicine. This branch of medicine has the goal of enhancing and restoring functional ability and improving the quality of life for individuals with impairments. A physician having completed training in this field is referred to as a physiatrist and often serves on the interdisciplinary team of rehabilitation professionals involved in the rehabilitation process, which includes physical, occupational, and speech therapy; recreation therapy; psychology; nutrition; and social work.

Rehabilitation may occur in a variety of settings, including a hospital, an outpatient facility, or a special rehabilitation center designed for the treatment of specific disorders (e.g., psychiatric disorders or neurological disorders). Medical rehabilitation facilities often include activities of daily living facility. Activities of daily living facilities offer a simulated apartment setting for clients to learn and practice tasks they will need for everyday living.

History

The concept of rehabilitation became popular during both World Wars in the treatment of injured soldiers and laborers. During the 1940s, rehabilitation services were developed for survivors of spinal cord injuries. Sir Ludwig Guttmann, a neurologist from Britain, recognized the need for services beyond the typical nursing care of the time. He worked with others in the United States to develop extensive rehabilitation plans that would allow those with spinal injuries to achieve the highest quality of life possible and thus extended the life span of this population.

In the early 1900s, two unofficial specialties, PM&R medicine, developed separately. In practice, both specialties treated similar client populations consisting of those with disabling injuries. American physiatrist Frank Krusen was a pioneer of physical medicine. He founded the first Department of Rehabilitation at Temple Hospital in 1928 and soon thereafter coined the term *physiatry*. In 1947, the specialty of Physical Medicine was established under the authority of the American Board of Medical Specialties. However, 4 years earlier, in 1943, the Baruch Committee (a committee that awarded funds to develop physiatry programs) had defined the specialty as a combination of the two fields and laid the framework for the medical specialty of PM&R. Howard

Rusk, an internal medicine physician, was the pioneer of rehabilitation medicine, specializing in rehabilitating air force pilots during World War II. In 1949, at the insistence of Rusk and others, the specialty incorporated rehabilitation medicine and changed its name to PM&R.

In the late 1900s, disability activists and scholars' influence led to major reforms in how disability was defined and understood and shaped the outcomes of interest in research. At this time, rehabilitation technology (formerly rehabilitation engineering) developed as a component of the medical rehabilitation field. This area of medicine deals with prosthetics and orthotics.

Since the 1980s, the employment of individuals with disabilities through programs that provide them with ongoing support services for vocational rehabilitation has received increased attention. Traditionally, the most common form of supported employment in the United States was provided by sheltered workshops, facility-based vocational programs for individuals with disabilities that often received government funds and provided both services and employment to these individuals. Today, such individuals are mainstreamed into the regular workplace, with jobs modified to meet their needs. The affirmative action provisions of the U.S. Rehabilitation Act of 1973 contributed to this shift. The Rehabilitation Act is federal legislation that authorizes the grant programs of vocational rehabilitation, supported employment, independent living, and disability assistance. It also authorizes a variety of training and service discretionary grants administered by the Rehabilitation Services Administration, as well as research activities administered by the National Institute on Disability and Rehabilitation Research and the National Council on Disability. The Rehabilitation Act also includes a variety of provisions focused on rights, advocacy, reasonable accommodations, and protections for individuals with disabilities. It requires an affirmative action in employment by the federal government and government contractors. It prohibits discrimination on the basis of disability in programs conducted by federal agencies, programs receiving federal financial assistance, federal employment, and employment practices of federal contractors.

In 2006, the United Nations Convention on the Rights of Persons with Disabilities was adopted. This instigated a change in rehabilitation practices shaped by the development of disablement models, especially the International Classification of Functioning, Disability and Health (ICF), which emphasized a biopsychosocial model.

Biopsychosocial Model

Since the early 2010s, rehabilitation has assumed a central position within all health-care settings, from emergency and intensive care services to palliative and end-of-life care services. The attraction of the rehabilitation model is its attention to the individual's functional activities and social roles as a component of the medical care provided. In this way, it is expected that rehabilitation results in better client outcomes and more health-care services for the same resource commitment. This model involves a multidisciplinary team of professionals who work together to analyze the situation, identify all contributing factors, and develop a collaborative plan that can be implemented across settings as health status changes. The team serves not only to provide the individual with skills but also to deliver education and knowledge regarding how to achieve goals and self-manage their care. Thus, the client is actively involved in the planning and execution of their rehabilitation program. Culturally, health care fosters caring and risk avoidance rather than encouraging activity because activities often involve risk. Rehabilitation facilitates the introduction of such activities (e.g., physical and communicative) in supported environments so that clients can work to increase autonomy.

The process of rehabilitation largely reflects the key features of the biomedical model in that it is designed to restore health or normality. Nevertheless, the focus on functioning despite the disability and the emphasis on environmental factors means that rehabilitation is essentially a biopsychosocial model that is designed to accompany and parallel the typical biomedical model.

Rehabilitation medicine and care is based upon the conceptual framework of the World Health Organization's ICF. This model recognizes that the impairment, problem, or disease itself impacts an individual's activities and therefore the person's participation in society. The ICF framework consists of two parts: (1) functioning and disability and (2) contextual factors. Functioning and disability encompasses body functions and structures (i.e., the individual's anatomy, physiology, and psychology) as well as activity and participation (i.e., the individual's functional status, including mobility and communication). The contextual component of the model acknowledges that environmental (e.g., work, laws) and personal factors (e.g., race, gender, education) also influence this participation. Hence, although functional status may be related to a health condition, the health condition alone does not predict the individual's functional status. The World Health Organization emphasizes that health is more than the absence of disease, as it includes the physical, mental, and social functioning of a person. Thus, functioning as classified in the ICF is an essential component of health and health care.

The rehabilitation process involves the collection of information on impairments, such as motor, language, and cognitive difficulties, with the goal of understanding the cause of disability rather than diagnosing a disease. As compared to the biomedical model, rather than collecting information on symptoms and signs and merely identifying the disease and diagnosis, the biopsychosocial model has the much broader goal of understanding the situation as a whole, particularly focusing on the nature and causes of the disabilities seen. This requires an understanding of client factors, such as emotions, beliefs, goals, and expectations; information concerning context (e.g., personal, social, physical); and information about activities and roles.

Rehabilitation also involves input from a range of specialties, rather than a medical doctor or small team alone. Therefore, data collection in this biopsychosocial approach may take time, requiring a much closer and longer relationship between the client and the different professionals involved. Integration of the data collected usually requires an interdisciplinary team meeting to interpret observations and come to valid synthesis. For example, after a stroke, one might require information from nurses, a neurologist, a speech and language therapist/pathologist, a physio/physical therapist, a social worker, a nutritionist, as well as a community nurse and possibly housing services in the community. Thus, the model involves many people, from many different professions, working within several different teams and organizations, as well as parties that may not be a part of a health-related field (e.g., housing services). It is important to note that the individual's family members or caregivers are also considered an integral part of the team.

Goal setting in rehabilitation differs somewhat from the traditional biomedical model where the professional expert sets goals for the individual. The goal setting process in rehabilitation involves a team approach, which most often includes the clients themselves. Goals aim to change the individual's behavior, and the inclusion of the client in this process ensures that they are relevant to the person receiving treatment and their caregivers. Collaborative goal setting and sharing of information between all involved parties are typical of the biopsychosocial model. Many interdependent interventions may be required to target a single goal and so require planning and coordination from many professionals in the team. Thus, a successful rehabilitation model is highly collaborative.

The central process of change in this model is related to learning. The client and family members receive education on how to achieve desired goals in the presence of altered or limited skills and abilities. Practice is therefore an essential component of a successful rehabilitation model. For example, the evidence on constraint-induced therapy and the principles of neuroplasticity suggest that practice intensity is an extremely effective component of the rehabilitation and recovery process. Although practice does not always require the professional's presence, they should be involved at some level to ensure that appropriate education, feedback, and support are provided. The professional also has an integral role in facilitating the motivation of the client and family members, presenting a positive perspective, and participating in collaborative goal setting that develops achievable, challenging, measurable, and relevant goals for the individual.

In biomedical care models, the primary interventions are directed at disease control. In rehabilitation, there are usually several primary interventions aimed at various parts of the biopsychosocial model. It is not unusual for a client to need multiple services, such as exercise to improve muscle function, provision of orthotics and/or other equipment, instruction on how to use the equipment, feedback during practice of activities, help and support in adjusting expectations, training for caregivers, and organization of adaptations for transitioning to new environments as care settings change. Similarly, many clients requiring rehabilitation services may experience multiple difficulties (e.g., an individual with an acquired brain injury may experience mobility, language, cognition, emotional, and behavioral difficulties). The combination of multiple services for a single client contributes to the primary goal of providing practical functional support with a wide range of activities.

Rehabilitation aims to maximize recovery and avoid loss of fitness, skills, and confidence associated with illness and being cared for. Rehabilitation creates an environment in health-care settings that encourages practice of activities and ultimately facilitates functional independence.

Research and Technology

Some organizations are involved in rehabilitation efforts. These include the National Rehabilitation Association, the National Association of Rehabilitation Facilities, and the Office of Disability Employment Policy.

The rehabilitation field has often been critiqued for lacking supporting scholarship and theoretical grounding. In an effort to advance the research in this area, a number of rehabilitation-specific publications were developed. There are four prominent rehabilitation sciences journals: (1) *Archives of PM&R*, (2) *Clinical Rehabilitation*, (3) *Journal of Rehabilitation Medicine*, and (4) *Disability and Rehabilitation*. These are all multidisciplinary, international journals that seek to encourage an understanding of functional difficulties and promote rehabilitation science, practice, and policy. All publish peer-reviewed manuscripts on important trends and research in rehabilitation. Furthermore, there are many other fields of study and diagnosis-specific journals that publish studies in the area of rehabilitation, including many in the field of CSD. Consequently, there is a constantly growing body of research on the field of rehabilitation.

Systematic reviews support multidisciplinary rehabilitation for clients with acquired brain injury, multiple sclerosis, vestibular dysfunction, and chronic obstructive airway disease. Moreover, there is evidence that rehabilitation can benefit clients with degenerative conditions that are often considered beyond rehabilitation, such as Alzheimer's disease and motor neuron disease.

Rehabilitation is often defined in subcategories, relative to the specific focus of the services. For example, *aural rehabilitation* focuses on the rehabilitation of hearing difficulties. *Cognitive rehabilitation* involves service provision for individuals with cognitive linguistic difficulties. *Vestibular rehabilitation* includes services for individuals with balance difficulties. *Vocational rehabilitation* specifically emphasizes skills for independent employment.

Technology assumes a large role in rehabilitation. The use of both low- and high-technology supportive tools is emphasized across the different rehabilitation specialties. Aural rehabilitation may involve the use of cochlear implants and hearing aids. Rehabilitation for mobility may involve the use of wheelchairs. Rehabilitation of communication may often involve alternative augmentative communication devices. However, the technological tools used to facilitate rehabilitation are not limited to the individual, but also implemented within the environmental context (e.g., amplification tools and wheelchair accessible lifts).

Rehabilitation in CSD

It has already been noted that successful communication is an integral part of the rehabilitation process. This clear and frequent communication is necessary between professionals and the individual receiving rehabilitation services, among the team of professionals themselves, and includes the family members of the client. One of the major goals of rehabilitation is to facilitate successful navigation of the social context. It is therefore necessary that all professionals involved liaise to enable a supportive environment in which shared attitudes and expectations allow the individual to demonstrate self-sufficiency within the setting. The CSD professional is essential for this process of successful communication in rehabilitation. It is the CSD professional's role to educate the client, family, and other professionals on the optimal communication strategies for the particular individual.

In the CSD field, rehabilitation involves working to facilitate the most independent swallowing and communication skills possible. Thus, the CSD specialist will work toward the rehabilitation of individuals who experience difficulties with swallowing, motor speech (apraxia or dysarthria), language (aphasia and developmental language difficulties), voice, hearing, and cognition. Most frequently, clients seeking such rehabilitation services include those with diagnosed acquired neurological diagnoses (e.g., stroke, traumatic brain injury, degenerative diseases). Nevertheless, the population of rehabilitation clients also includes a wide variety of other acquired diagnoses (e.g., postlaryngectomy and postintubation) and often includes those with developmental disabilities (e.g., autism and Down syndrome).

As one of the integral members of the rehabilitation team, it is the CSD specialist's role to participate as a team member in assessment, goal setting, treatment, and education. *Assessment* in rehabilitation involves a comprehensive evaluation of skills, be it swallowing, voice, speech, language, hearing or cognition, and liaison with other professionals. It is important that assessment involves a holistic perspective and takes into account the accompanying challenges (e.g., general mobility and visual difficulties) and the impact such issues may have on communication. *Goal setting* is also a collaborative process that involves the client, family, and other professionals. Optimal goals will be achievable, challenging, measurable, and relevant for functional participation in everyday settings. *Treatment* involves the presentation of skills the client may practice, compensatory strategies the client may use, and environmental modifications that may facilitate the achievement of goals. The personal context is important, and from the outset, the client needs to be reminded that success requires full engagement. Hence, treatment also involves the influencing of the client's attitude and expectations. Successful rehabilitation involves educating other professionals, clients, and family members on optimal communication techniques and the environmental and contextual support that is necessary for communicative competence.

Louise C. Keegan

See also Compensatory Adaptation and Strategies; Functionalism; International Classification of Functioning, Disability and Health; Motivation; Rehabilitative Audiology; Vestibular Rehabilitation

Further Readings

Frontera, W. R. (2006). Research and the survival of physical medicine and rehabilitation. *American Journal of Physical Medicine & Rehabilitation*, 85(12), 939–944.

Gibson, B. E. (2016). *Rehabilitation: A post-critical approach*. Boca Raton, FL: CRC Press.

Lagana, R., & Esposito, S. (2012). *Rehabilitation, practices, psychology and health*. New York, NY: Nova Science.

McPherson, K., Gibson, B. E., & Leplege, A. (2015). *Rethinking rehabilitation: Theory and practice*. Boca Raton, FL: CRC Press.

Siegert, R. J., & Levack, W. M. M. (2014). *Rehabilitation goal setting: Theory, practice and evidence*. Boca Raton, FL: CRC Press.

Wade, D. (2015). Rehabilitation—A new approach. Overview and part one: The problems. *Clinical Rehabilitation*, 29, 11, 1041–1050.

Websites

National Association of Rehabilitation Facilities. Retrieved from https://www.naranet.org/

National Rehabilitation Association. Retrieved from https://www.nationalrehab.org/

Office of Disability Employment Policy. Retrieved from https://www.dol.gov/odep/

Rehabilitative Audiology

Rehabilitative audiology's overarching goal is to reduce the quality of life impacts from hearing difficulties on individuals and their communication partners. The field of audiology has its roots in rehabilitation. As a field of study and clinical practice, audiology's roots are linked to rehabilitation centers established during and immediately following World War II. Returning service members who experienced damage to their auditory systems received rehabilitative services. These services included provision of hearing aids and amplifying devices, speechreading training, auditory training, communication strategies training, and counseling. These services encompass what is termed rehabilitative audiology. This entry discusses the rehabilitative audiology.

Rehabilitative audiology has grown post–World War II, but the overarching goal remains the same. Advances in technology, understanding of the

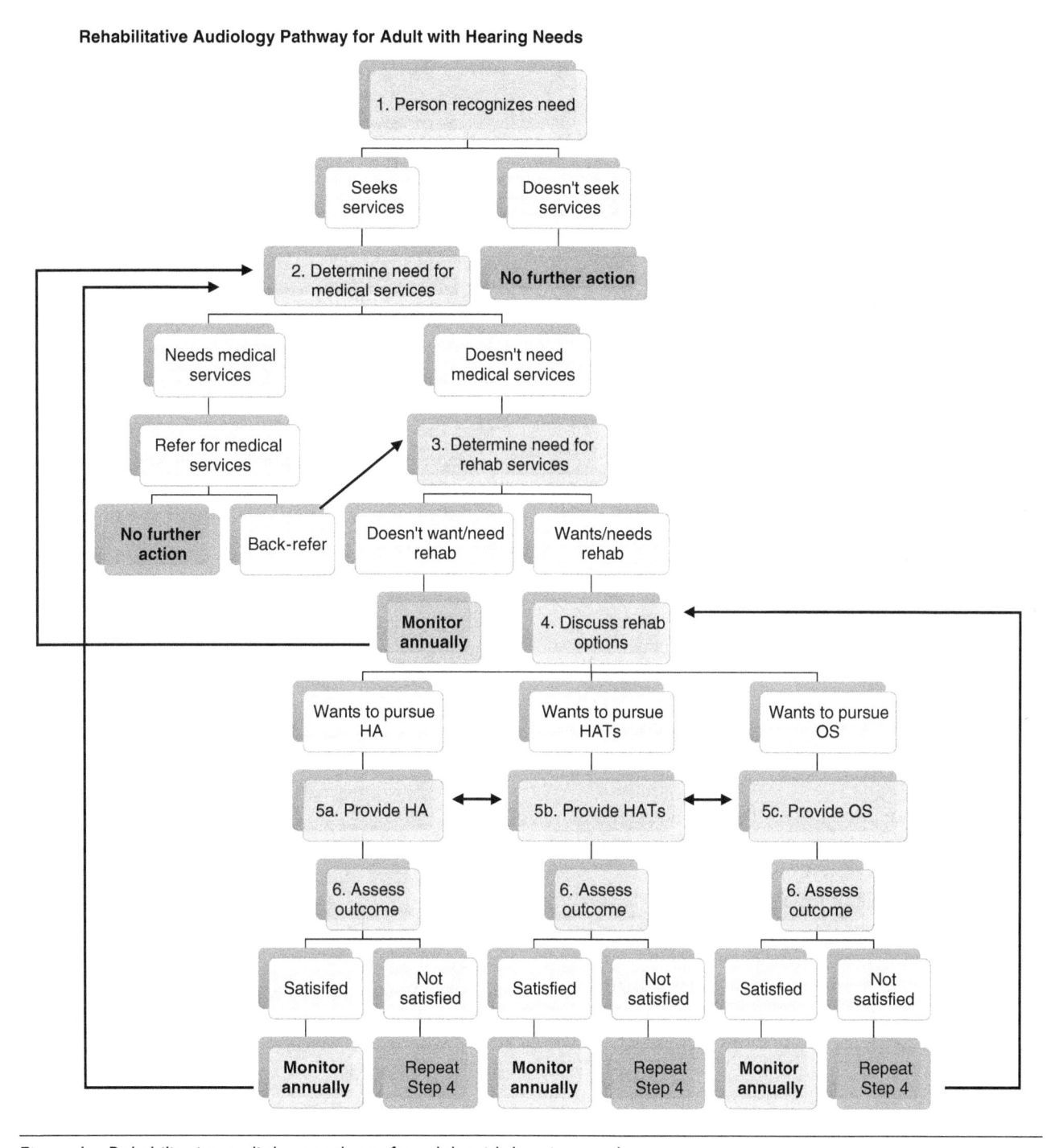

Rehabilitative Audiology Pathway for Adult with Hearing Needs

Figure 1 Rehabilitative audiology pathway for adult with hearing needs

Note: HA = hearing aids, HATs = hearing assistance technology, OS = other services.

auditory system, and the impact of hearing difficulties in daily life have expanded the scope of rehabilitative audiology. In most settings, audiologists and speech–language pathologists/therapists provide rehabilitative audiology. In other settings, these rehabilitative services may be provided by teachers of deaf and hard of hearing children, hearing therapists, and audiometrists. Rehabilitative audiology involves a holistic, person- and family-centered approach to service delivery.

A Rehabilitative Audiology Model

Figure 1 shows one rehabilitative audiology model for an adult with hearing difficulties. The pathway begins with the person recognizing hearing needs. Many adults who recognize hearing difficulties do not seek services. Those who do may elect to enter hearing health-care service from a variety of places. The decision of where to enter the hearing health-care system is based on several factors, including the nature and structure of the healthcare system. This model represents one potential pathway for a person who recognizes hearing difficulties for the first time as well as a person who has previously sought services and recognizes new hearing difficulties. The model is similar to the potential pathways for children with hearing problems. However, in many instances, the family would take the lead on decision making, rather than the child (depending on the child's age).

The next step in the pathway involves an audiologic assessment. One goal of this assessment is to determine the need for medical intervention to address the hearing difficulties. If the person's hearing difficulties arise from a medical issue, the clinician makes a referral to a medical professional. Even if medical services are required, this does not negate the possible need for rehabilitative services. Clinicians can ask for a back-referral if hearing difficulties persist beyond the provision of medical services.

If hearing difficulties persist beyond the provision of medical services or if medical services are not appropriate to address hearing difficulties, the third step in the pathway is to determine the need for rehabilitative services. If the person elects to pursue rehabilitation, the clinician can proceed with a discussion about the most appropriate option. If the person does not wish to pursue any rehabilitative option or if the clinician's assessment indicates rehabilitation is not a suitable option, the person can be monitored annually for any changes. The monitoring includes both a diagnostic assessment and a rehabilitation needs assessment (Steps 2 and 3).

If the person is a candidate for rehabilitative services and elects to pursue rehabilitation, the fourth step in the pathway involves using shared decision making to select the appropriate services for that person. These services typically fall under three categories: (1) provision of hearing aids, (2) provision of hearing assistance technology (HAT), and (3) provision of other types of rehabilitative services. It is important to note that these rehabilitative options are not mutually exclusive. For example, a person may opt to pursue hearing aids and also opt to pursue HAT and/or other services.

Shared decision making is a collaboration between the clinician, the person with hearing difficulties, and family members. In shared decision making, clinicians share their knowledge of the evidence base regarding the efficacy and effectiveness of rehabilitation options. The person with hearing difficulties and his or her family members share their values, preferences, and needs. Then, collaboratively, the team discusses how to accomplish the goal of finding the most appropriate rehabilitation option. Tools such as decision aids can help facilitate this process.

Following the shared decision-making process, the fifth step involves the provision of one or more rehabilitative services. These are discussed in detail in the next section. The final step in the pathway is to assess the outcome of rehabilitation service. This assessment process can include both objective and subjective assessment. An example of an objective assessment is performing electroacoustic measures of hearing aid performance in the person's ear. An example of a subjective assessment is administering a questionnaire to the person to determine the benefit of the rehabilitation. Significant other perception of benefit of rehabilitation can also add valuable information during this process.

If the person is satisfied with the outcome of rehabilitation, the clinician can monitor him or her annually. The monitoring includes both a diagnostic assessment and a rehabilitation needs assessment (Steps 2 and 3). If the person is not satisfied with the outcome of rehabilitation, the clinician returns to Step 4 in which shared decision making is used to select an appropriate service. For example, a person may elect to pursue hearing aids. During the outcome assessment, unmet needs may be identified. These needs may be addressed through the provision of HAT. This process continues until the person is satisfied that all needs have been met, at which time the clinician monitors the person annually.

Hearing Aids

Hearing aids have been part of rehabilitative audiology from its inception. In the early days, most rehabilitative audiology centers were located in military settings. This meant that there was a continuum of services provided in a single facility, from assessment to rehabilitation, including hearing aid provision. In the civilian sector, however, hearing aid provision was out of bounds for most audiologists. For example, it was a violation of the American Speech-Language-Hearing Association code of ethics to sell hearing aids. Over time, there was dissatisfaction with this model, and by the late 1970s, the American Speech-Language-Hearing Association code of ethics changed to allow audiologists to sell hearing aids. As of 2018, a large proportion of audiologists sell hearing aids and do so in a variety of service delivery settings.

Most hearing aids are worn externally on a person's ear and consist of a microphone, an amplifier, a signal processor, and a receiver (a speaker). There are some types of hearing aids that are surgically implanted in or near a person's ear. For example, some hearing aids are implanted in the middle ear space, and some are implanted in the bones of the skull behind the ear. Regardless of how the sound is delivered, the basic function of a hearing aid is to amplify sounds. The underlying goal of most hearing aid fittings is to improve a person's access to (audibility of) speech, while ensuring comfort and minimal distortion.

Advances in hearing aid technology allow hearing aids to process sounds in sophisticated ways. Modern hearing aids can amplify some types of sounds (e.g., speech) more than other types of sounds (e.g., noise). They can be adjusted to suit most degrees and configurations of hearing abilities. In addition, features such as directional microphones allow the hearing aids to amplify sounds coming from different directions (e.g., in front of the listener) more than sounds coming from other directions (e.g., behind the listener). This can enhance a person's ability to understand speech despite background noise.

The benefits of using hearing aids have been well documented. Direct-person benefits include improved emotional stability, improved physical and mental health, improved sense of control over life situations, improved self-image, reduction in feelings of dependence, and increased feeling of safety. Interpersonal benefits include improved communication, increased intimacy and improved sex life, and increased participation in social settings. Work-related benefits include increased income and earning potential, improved communication, and reduction in fatigue and stress. Family members of people who wear hearing aids also report benefits. These include improved relationships in the home environment, improved feelings about self, and improved social life.

Most people who wear hearing aids report being satisfied with them. The rate of overall hearing aid satisfaction has increased from around 60% in the late 1980s to over 70% in the late 2000s. It is important to note that the rate of hearing aid satisfaction varies by listening situation. People who wear hearing aids report higher satisfaction in quieter environments and smaller groups, with 80–90% of hearing aid wearers reporting satisfaction in these situations. Fewer people report satisfaction in large groups and in noisy environments, such as sporting events and classrooms, with only 60–70% of hearing aid wearers reporting satisfaction in these situations.

Some people stop wearing hearing aids after obtaining them. These are sometimes referred to as *in the drawer* hearing aids. It is difficult to quantify the rate of hearing aid disuse, partly because it is difficult to define disuse. When defining disuse as never wearing a hearing aid, it is estimated that around 12–16% of hearing aid owners stop wearing their hearing aids. This figure has remained relatively stable over the past several decades. People stop wearing hearing aids for a variety of reasons, including a lack of perceived benefit from them (particularly in noisy situations), cosmetics, perception of lack of need for wearing the hearing aids, difficulty inserting or removing the hearing aids, poor physical fit or discomfort from the hearing aids, poor sound quality of the hearing aids, and hearing aid feedback (whistling).

Not everyone who recognizes hearing difficulties will choose to own hearing aids. The rates of hearing aid ownership vary across studies and across health-care systems. It is estimated that only around 25% of adults in the United States who recognize significant hearing difficulties report owning hearing aids. However, the rate increases when there is a national funding scheme. For example, in the

United Kingdom, it is estimated that the rate of hearing aid ownership is around 42% and that around 83% of hearing aid owners received government-funded hearing aids. One factor that seems to play a role in making the decision to own hearing aids is a person's degree of hearing difficulties. As the degree of hearing difficulties increases, the rate of hearing aid ownership also increases. Another important factor is a person's age. As a general trend, as a person's age increases, so too does the rate of hearing aid ownership.

When asked about the reasons for not owning hearing aids, people report many different factors. One of the most commonly cited reasons for not owning hearing aids is the perception that the person will not benefit from hearing aids because of the type of hearing loss (e.g., level of severity). This finding is similar between countries that have a government funding scheme and those that do not. Another commonly cited reason for not owing hearing aids is the cost. In places without government-funded hearing aids, many people report that they cannot afford hearing aids. Regardless of government funding for hearing aids, many people report they do not own them because of people's attitude toward hearing aids and hearing problems.

Cochlear Implants

People with more severe hearing problems and certain types of hearing problems may not benefit from hearing aids. In these cases, cochlear implants can provide access to auditory information. A cochlear implant is not a hearing aid. It is an electronic device that delivers auditory information directly to the auditory nerve so the brain can interpret sounds. Clinicians, physicians, and the person with hearing difficulties and/or their family members use shared decision making to determine candidacy for cochlear implants. In general, to be a candidate for cochlear implants, a person must have hearing needs that are not likely to be addressed through the use of hearing aids. In most cases, the person must experience severe hearing difficulties in both ears and have difficulty understanding speech. Cochlear implants can be implanted in one or both ears. Often, this decision is based on the policies of the funding agency and the age of the person with hearing difficulties.

The evidence on the effectiveness of cochlear implants is similar to the evidence of the effectiveness of hearing aids. The vast majority (90%) of adults who receive a cochlear implant report benefits in understanding speech. Children who receive a cochlear implant show improved speech, language, and auditory development. Factors that affect the success of cochlear implantation include the length of time the person had hearing problems prior to implantation, the degree of hearing difficulties, the physical condition of the person's inner ear (cochlea), coexisting medical conditions, and support (including other rehabilitation options discussed below).

HAT

Another rehabilitation option for people with hearing difficulties is the use of HATs. HATs include different types of devices that help people with hearing difficulties in their daily lives. HATs can be described in terms of what they aim to accomplish. Some HATs aim to improve access to speech, particularly in difficult listening situations. Others' aim is alerting a person to an auditory signal.

Factors that make it difficult to understand speech in many situations can include distance between the speaker and the listener, background noise, and reverberation. HATs aimed at addressing this situation include frequency-modulated systems, infrared systems, induction loop systems, and personal sound amplification systems. These systems can be used with or without hearing aids and cochlear implants.

HATs that aim to improve access to speech do so in a variety of listening situations. HAT solutions aimed at improving access to speech over the telephone include amplified telephones, captioned telephones, relay systems, and telephone devices for the deaf. Telephone HATs can also be used with existing technology. For example, text messages, instant messaging, and e-mail can replace or support some telephonic communication.

HAT alerting devices are designed to help people with hearing difficulty gain access to various signals. One example is an alarm clock that vibrates rather than produces an auditory signal. Another example is a doorbell that flashes. Alerting devices can be an important safety consideration. For example, hearing aids and cochlear implants are not usually worn overnight or in the shower. People who are deaf or hard of hearing need to be alerted to crying babies and smoke alarms. HATs that are worn on the person, shake the bed, or flash lights can be used to alert him or her to these signals. Fire alarms can also be set to specific frequencies to enable them to be heard by people with a variety of hearing configurations. Some fire departments will provide these alarms at no charge to people with hearing difficulties.

Other Rehabilitative Services

Devices such as hearing aids, cochlear implants, and hearing assistive technology address access to sounds. Other rehabilitative services address other hearing needs. There are several types of services that can be offered to people with hearing difficulties. The goal of auditory training is to rewire the auditory pathways in the brain that have changed as a result of decreased auditory input to the brain due to hearing difficulties. There are several auditory training programs available for both adults and children. Evidence on the effectiveness of auditory training programs is somewhat mixed, however. It appears that some people benefit from it, while others do not. This is one reason why it is important for clinicians to use a shared decision-making approach to find the best option for specific individuals.

Speechreading

Speechreading refers to using auditory, visual, and any other information (such as gestures and facial expression) to understand auditory information. The underlying theory of speechreading is that people integrate auditory and visual information, which can enhance speech understanding. There is a long history of research on speechreading. This research has uncovered some factors that impact speechreading ability, including how well the talker pronounces speech; the use of facial expressions and gestures; the familiarity of the speaker; the complexity of the message; the angle, distance, lighting, and acoustics in the room; and the listener's residual hearing, emotional and physical state, and underlying language skills.

Communication Strategies

The use of communication strategies can enhance a person's ability to participate in a conversation. Communication strategies include actions taken by the person with hearing difficulty or the communication partner to improve or repair conversation. Some strategies can be used to prepare for effective communication. For example, a person may ensure that the conversation takes place in a quiet room with good lighting and few distractions. Some strategies involve telling communication partners how best to communicate (e.g., slow down, speak a little louder, remove objects from in front of the face).

Even when steps are taken to prepare for effective communication, it can still break down. In these instances, people can use communication repair strategies. These include asking the speaker to repeat, telling the speaker what was understood and asking them to repeat the rest, asking the speaker to rephrase, asking the speaker to confirm what was said, and asking the speaker to write the information. Communication strategies training can be quite simple and can take only a few sessions to accomplish.

Hearing-Related Counseling

Finally, hearing-related counseling is used to address the impacts on the quality of life due to hearing problems. This includes the impacts to the person with hearing difficulties and communication partners. Counseling can be offered in individual/family settings or group settings. Short-term benefits of group counseling have been demonstrated, both for adults who wear hearing aids and for those who do not. In addition, there is some evidence to suggest that communication partners also benefit from participating in group rehabilitation. There is ample compelling evidence to suggest that providing rehabilitation services is beneficial to people with hearing problems and their communication partners, at least in the short term. Using shared decision making, clinicians can help people with hearing difficulties and their families find a rehabilitation option that suits their needs and lifestyles.

Rebecca J. Kelly-Campbell

See also Audiovisual Integration; Auditory Training; Cochlear Implants; Hearing Aid Fitting; Hearing Aids

Further Readings

Montano, J. J., & Spitzer, J. B. (2009). *Adult audiologic rehabilitation*. San Diego, CA: Plural.

Tye-Murray, N. (2009). *Foundations of aural rehabilitation: Children, adults, and their family members*. Clifton Park, NJ: Delmar Learning.

Wong, L., & Hickson, L. (2012). *Evidence-based practice in audiology*. San Diego, CA: Plural.

REINNERVATION OF THE LARYNX

The larynx is subject to highly specialized neural control, due to its primary functions involving swallowing protection, cough, and airway maintenance. Phonation also requires specialized and rapid adjustments of motor and sensory systems. Laryngeal paralysis results from injury to the nerve supply of the larynx from peripheral or central nervous system. This can occur unilaterally or bilaterally and can affect both motor and sensory functions. *Laryngeal reinnervation* refers to the restoration of laryngeal function by the connection of different or alternate peripheral nerves to replace the injured laryngeal nerves. This entry discusses the anatomy of the larynx, history of laryngeal reinnervation, nonselective and selective reinnervation, and future directions.

The major nerve supply to the larynx involves both superior laryngeal nerve (SLN) and recurrent laryngeal nerve (RLN) on each side. These are branches of the vagus nerve, and their embryological development is as follows. The SLN divides into an internal branch SLN and external branch SLN (eSLN). The internal branch SLN goes to, and through, the thyrohyoid membrane and provides sensation to the supraglottic larynx and glottic larynx to the level of the vocal folds. The eSLN provides motor innervation to the cricothyroid muscle, with variable interconnections to the thyroarytenoid muscle through a communicating branch. The RLN supplies motor function to the other intrinsic muscles of the larynx, which have both adductor and abductor functions. It also innervates the cricopharyngeus muscle and provides sensation to the glottic and subglottic laryngeal mucosa. Neuroanatomic studies have demonstrated marked variety and variability in laryngeal nerve innervation patterns to individual muscles and interconnectedness between laryngeal nerves within the larynx. Other muscles that attach to the laryngeal cartilage are cervical strap muscles, innervated by branches of the cervical plexus called the *ansa cervicalis* and inferior pharyngeal constrictor muscles innervated by the vagus nerve. Other peripheral nerves of cranial and spinal origin also course through the neck, including spinal accessory, hypoglossal, and phrenic nerves. These nerves become options for use in laryngeal reinnervation.

Experiments with laryngeal reinnervation in animals were first reported in 1893. The first human laryngeal reinnervation was described in 1909, the repair of a transected RLN from a gunshot wound. Experiments from the 1960s through the 1990s explored different ways to reinnervate the paralyzed larynx, addressing the problems of both unilateral and bilateral vocal fold paralysis. Techniques of neurorrhaphy, direct nerve implant, and nerve–muscle pedicle have been investigated. These have addressed the issues of donor nerve morbidity, especially phrenic nerve and diaphragm paralysis. The concept of laryngeal synkinesis has been developed, describing the cross-innervation of laryngeal adductors and abductors from laryngeal nerve injury and aberrant regeneration. Reinnervation techniques have been separated into nonselective and selective approaches.

Nonselective Reinnervation

Nonselective reinnervation refers to the reinnervation of the main RLN trunk, which contains a bundle of axons going to both adductor and abductor muscles. In treating unilateral vocal fold paralysis, this has become the preferred approach through the anastomosis of a branch of the ansa cervicalis to the distal RLN. Motor fibers regenerate nonselectively to the laryngeal muscles but preferentially reinnervate adductor muscles due to a 3:1 ratio of adductor to abductor fibers. This regeneration facilitates glottic closure to provide adductor tone that restores voice and abductor tone to stabilize arytenoid position. Ansa cervicalis to RLN reinnervation was first described in 1923 and revived in the 1980s. Its efficacy in restoring voice in unilateral vocal fold paralysis has been documented since the 1980s with a series of retrospective case studies, one small randomized study, and one meta-analysis. The data support the contention that this approach is equivalent or superior to injection or medialization laryngoplasty techniques

Selective Reinnervation

Restoring vocal fold abduction and adduction to reanimate paralyzed vocal folds is a long-sought goal in laryngology. The clinical impairment in airway from bilateral vocal fold paralysis is due to the inability of the vocal folds to abduct, from the paralysis of the posterior cricoarytenoid (PCA) muscles. In selective laryngeal reinnervation, the goal is to separately reinnervate abductor and adductor laryngeal muscles. To reinnervate the PCA muscle, donor nerve from a muscle that activates with inspiration has been sought. The main candidates investigated with proximity in the neck to the larynx are the phrenic nerve, the ansa cervicalis nerve, and the eSLN nerve. With the phrenic nerve, either its main trunk or rootlets can be implanted directly into the PCA muscle via direct neurorrhaphy to the RLN abductor branch or into the PCA muscle directly. The nerve–muscle pedicle approach, now largely abandoned, used a cuff of strap muscle with attached ansa cervicalis nerve that was sewn into the PCA muscle directly. Similarly, the adductor laryngeal muscles can be selectively reinnervated by the implantation of nerve into the muscle belly through a thyroplasty window or by neurorrhaphy to the adductor RLN branch.

As of 2018, the technique of bilateral selective laryngeal reinnervation developed by Jean-Paul Marie is the most extensively studied with the largest clinical experience. In this approach, the upper C3 root of the phrenic nerve is used as a driver for the PCA muscles. They are bilaterally reinnervated through a jump graft harvested from the greater auricular nerve with branches implanted into each PCA muscle vertical belly. The adductor muscles are reinnervated from the thyrohyoid branch off the hypoglossal nerve to the RLN main trunk on each side, using a small jump graft from the greater auricular nerve. In another approach, Michael Orestes and colleagues reported two cases using the ipsilateral eSLN to drive the PCA and ansa cervicalis to adductor RLN, with sectioning of the Interarytenoid IA muscle.

Laryngeal reinnervation, as in other peripheral nerve repair procedures, depends on nerve regenerative healing capability. These have limitations from scarring, axonal degeneration, muscle atrophy, and aberrant regeneration. Time duration of nerve injury and patient's age also have been shown to affect the outcomes of laryngeal reinnervation. These reduce the functional effectiveness of nerve repair. Further advances in laryngeal reinnervation may come from bioengineering to enhance the nerve healing and regeneration process and to improve outcomes.

Marshall Smith

See also Laryngeal Disorders: Benign Vocal Fold Pathologies; Laryngectomy; Swallowing Disorders; Swallowing Intervention

Further Readings

Fancello, V., Nouraei, S. R., & Heathcote, K. J. (2017). Role of reinnervation in the management of recurrent laryngeal nerve injury: Current state and advances. *Current Opinion in Otolaryngology & Head and Neck Surgery*, 25(6), 480–485.

Gibbins, N. (2014). The evolution of laryngeal reinnervation, the current state of science and thoughts for future treatments. *Journal of Voice*, 28, 793–798.

Krishnan, G., Du, C., Fishman, J. M., Foreman, A., Lott, D. G., Farwell, G., . . . Birchall, M. A. (2017). The current status of human laryngeal transplantation in 2017: A state of the field review. *The Laryngoscope*, 127(8), 1861–1868.

Zur, K. B., & Carroll, L. M. (2018). Recurrent laryngeal nerve reinnervation for management of aspiration in a subset of children. *International Journal of Pediatric Otorhinolaryngology*, 104, 104–107.

RELATIONAL ANALYSES

A *relational analysis* is an examination of a child's speech productions in relation to the adult targets. Most typically, this process involves the comparison of a child's productions to the adult targets. It describes the difference between what the child is trying to produce and what the child actually produces. This type of analysis contrasts with an *independent analysis*, which describes a child's abilities without reference to the adult targets. An independent analysis simply lists what a child produces. For example, for a child who produces the word *cat* (/kæt/) as [dæt], a relational analysis would indicate that the child produced the word inaccurately. Specifically, the child produced the prevocalic /k/ inaccurately and instead produced [d]. An independent analysis would simply describe what the child produced (i.e., the entire production and/or its individual components). It would not consider that the child was attempting to produce prevocalic /k/ but did so inaccurately. This entry discusses how relational analyses are conducted, goals, and the most common types of relational analyses.

Relational analyses are typically conducted on children's single-word and/or connected speech samples. Single-word samples are frequently collected using standardized tests of speech sound production. As a common tool used by speech–language pathologists in the assessment of speech sound disorders (SSDs), these tests require children to label pictures of objects or actions spontaneously or sometimes in response to an examiner's model. Standardized tests serve a dual purpose in that they allow the speech–language pathologist to determine a child's eligibility for speech–language services and identify speech errors and potential targets for treatment. Connected speech samples might be collected by engaging the child in conversation about a prior event or during structured or unstructured play. These samples are then transcribed phonetically (or phonemically), either live or from recordings, before being used to form the basis of a relational analysis.

A relational analysis tends to be reserved for children who are somewhat proficient in their speech sound production abilities and for whom there is an expectation of at least a partial match between their speech and the adult targets. One goal of this type of analysis is to identify each speech sound error as a phoneme substitution, an omission, a distortion, or an addition. One also can determine the production consistency of a speech sound by looking at the number of times it is produced correctly and the number of different errors within a sample and analyze the word productions for contextual effects.

An independent analysis is typically conducted on young children with immature speech (i.e., those younger than 18 or 24 months). As these children are not expected to be highly accurate in their speech, there is less of a concern with comparing their productions to the adult targets and more interest in simply describing what they are able to produce. In these cases, an independent analysis might include a repertoire of the child's speech sounds (*phonetic inventory*), a repertoire of the syllable and word structures present in the child's speech, and a description of the speech sounds or structures that are not present in the child's speech (*constraints*).

There are several different types of relational analyses, the most common of which include a phonological process (or error pattern) analysis, a place–voice–manner analysis, and measures that reflect the severity of SSD (and to some extent intelligibility), like Lawrence Shriberg's percent consonants correct (PCC) and percent vowels correct (PVC) metrics and David Ingram's proportion of whole-word proximity. Each of these analyses compares a child's productions to the adult targets and considers the accuracy of the child's productions. A phonological process analysis identifies error patterns and categorizes them according to whether they (1) affect the syllable structure of the target word (syllable structure processes), (2) result in one phoneme being substituted for another (substitution processes), or (3) result in one phoneme becoming more like another in the target word (assimilation processes). For example, a child who produces the word *umbrella* (/ʌmbrɛlə/) as [bɛwə] would be described as using weak syllable deletion, cluster reduction (both syllable structure processes), and gliding (substitution process).

A place–voice–manner analysis is similar to a phonological process analysis in that it allows for the identification of error patterns. Unlike a phonological process analysis, a place–voice–manner analysis tallies both correct and incorrect productions of individual phonemes, grouped according to their place and manner of articulation and whether they are voiced or voiceless. For example, for a child who produces the word *dinosaur* (/daɪnəsɔr/) as [daɪnədɔə], accurate prevocalic /d/ and /n/ would be tallied. Inaccurate prevocalic /s/ and postvocalic /r/ also would be tallied, and his or her error phonemes would be noted, namely [d] and [ə], respectively.

The grouping of phonemes according to their place and manner of articulation and whether they are voiced or voiceless allows the speech–language pathologist to identify the patterns of strength and weakness according to these features.

Some relational analyses can provide a reflection of SSD severity. For instance, PCC and PVC are calculated by dividing the number of consonants or vowels produced accurately, respectively, by the total number of consonants or vowels attempted. Whole-word proximity provides an insight into how closely the child's word productions approximate the adult targets. This word-level analysis differs from PCC and PVC, both phoneme-level analyses, in that it compares words rather than phonemes. Lower PCC, PVC, and whole-word proximity scores are associated with more severe forms of SSD.

Toby Macrae and *Ruth Huntley Bahr*

See also Phonological Disorders; Phonological Processes; Phonology; Speech–Language Pathology; Speech Sound Disorders

Further Readings

Edwards, M. L., & Shriberg, L. D. (1983). *Phonology: Applications in communicative disorders.* San Diego, CA: College-Hill Press.

Elbert, M., & Gierut, J. (1986). *Handbook of clinical phonology.* San Diego, CA: College-Hill Press.

Ingram, D. (2002). The measurement of whole-word productions. *Journal of Child Language, 29,* 713–733. doi:10.1017/S0305000902005275

Kamhi, A. G., & Pollock, K. E. (2005). *Phonological disorders in children: Clinical decision making in assessment and intervention.* Baltimore, MD: Brookes.

Macrae, T. (2016). Comprehensive assessment of speech sound production in preschool children. *Perspectives of the ASHA Special Interest Groups (SIG 1), 1*(2), 39–56. doi:10.1044/persp1.SIG1.37

RELAXATION THERAPY

Systematic methodologies for eliciting a relaxed state date back to ancient times, and relaxation techniques have been incorporated into treatments for communication disorders since at least the 19th century. Relaxation therapies, which fall under the broad rubric of complementary and alternative medicine, may reduce physical tension, calm the mind to reduce mental stress, and enhance the quality of life for individuals with communication disorders and their caregivers. This entry discusses somatic and cognitive approaches in relaxation therapy, applications for cognitive and communicative disorders, efficacy, and future directions for research.

Approaches

Relaxation therapies may be subdivided into somatic (or physiological) and cognitive (or psychological) approaches. There is, however, considerable overlap among techniques. Some practitioners adopt a more holistic approach whereby relaxation therapies are viewed along a continuum from purely somatic to purely cognitive, with a wide range of approaches falling between these extremes.

Somatic approaches entail identification and objective awareness of physical tension, followed by techniques to induce a relaxed state. Somatic approaches include progressive muscle relaxation, stretching and deep breathing exercises, the Alexander technique, and biofeedback. Briefly, progressive muscle relaxation involves systematic and mindful tensing of muscles, immediately followed by purposeful relaxation. Stretching and breathing approaches are rooted in yoga. Stretching exercises focus on reducing muscular tension, whereas breathing exercises effect relaxation through deep, diaphragmatic breathing. The Alexander technique targets the postural domain (especially as related to the head, neck, and spine) to enhance efficiency of movement and to reduce tension. Finally, biofeedback methods employ instrumentation to allow an individual to monitor physiological events during relaxation training and establish volitional control.

Cognitive approaches, in contrast, focus on reducing psychological stress and anxiety, which may negatively impact health and communication. Cognitive approaches include imagery, autogenic training, and meditation. Guided imagery methods involve visualization of a pleasant place or activity, which is used to establish a relaxed state. Anxiety-evoking situations may be introduced gradually, as the client employs mental images to maintain the relaxed state. Autogenic training is derived from self-hypnosis and entails establishing a deeply relaxed state of consciousness (i.e., trance). Meditation is a contemplative practice that may lead to mental clarity and a calm relaxed state. Many forms of meditation exist, including mindfulness meditation, transcendental meditation, and object-focused meditation. Within the health sciences, the mindfulness-based stress reduction program (MBSR) has been especially influential. MBSR, developed by Jon Kabat-Zinn, is derived from Buddhist traditions and emphasizes nonjudgmental and purposeful awareness of the present moment.

Applications

Relaxation therapies have been used with a wide range of cognitive and communicative disorders. Three primary goals of relaxation therapies have been identified: (1) enhancing speech production and swallowing by reducing muscular tension, (2) reducing effects of anxiety as a barrier to cognitive–communicative functioning, and (3) enhancing quality of life by reducing the stress of living with a communicative disability, for caregivers as well as individuals with communication disorders.

Undue muscular tension can pose a barrier to speech and swallowing. Accordingly, relaxation therapies (especially somatic approaches) have been incorporated in treatments for fluency, voice, and motor speech disorders as well as dysphagia. Physical tension is often observed among individuals who stutter, and relaxation methods may enhance speech fluency by reducing tension and associated struggle behaviors. Somatic approaches, typically involving progressive muscle relaxation and surface electromyographic biofeedback, have been used in treating hyperfunctional voice disorders, spasmodic dysphonia, and spastic dysarthria. Similar methods have been used to reduce spasticity associated with dysphagia.

Many individuals with communication disorders, such as stuttering and aphasia, experience anxiety, which in turn exacerbates the effects of the disorder. Cognitive relaxation techniques may reduce anxiety and enhance communicative effectiveness. Mindfulness meditation, for example, has been used in conjunction with more traditional treatments for managing stuttering, acquired neurogenic communication disorders (e.g., aphasia, dysarthria), and cognitive disability secondary to traumatic brain injury or dementia.

Finally, relaxation therapies have been used to help individuals with communication disorders and their caregivers to deal with stress and depression. Mindfulness meditation, in particular, has been used in this manner with conditions such as stroke, autism spectrum disorder, and dementia of the Alzheimer type.

Efficacy

Although relaxation therapies have been used in the treatment of communication disorders for many years, the evidence in support of their use is largely limited to descriptive case studies and small N quasi-experimental research. Relaxation therapies have typically been evaluated as an adjunct to more traditional approaches to treatment. Findings to date suggest that relaxation may enhance outcomes and contribute to higher quality-of-life ratings.

As noted previously, there exist multiple goals and strategies for eliciting a relaxed state. Unfortunately, most relaxation methodologies are not standardized and are rarely described in detail sufficient to evaluate treatment fidelity or to enable replication. An exception to this trend is research employing MBSR, which has a standard curriculum for practitioners and materials for clients. In the medical literature, MBSR has been associated with improvements in depression and anxiety, conditions that also may negatively impact communication effectiveness. MBSR has also been associated with reduced stress and improved psychological well-being in individuals with a range of conditions, including stroke. Additional research is clearly needed to evaluate and clarify the role of relaxation therapies in the management of communication disorders.

Thomas W. Powell

See also Biofeedback; Depression; Emotional Impact of Communication Disorders; Positive Psychology and Wellness; Psychological Stress and Speech Disorders; Quality of Life and Neurogenic Communication Disorders; Quality of Life and Stuttering

Further Readings

Boyle, M. P. (2011). Mindfulness training in stuttering therapy: A tutorial for speech-language pathologists. *Journal of Fluency Disorders, 36*, 122–129.

Gilman, M., & Yaruss, J. S. (2000). Stuttering and relaxation: Applications for somatic education in stuttering treatment. *Journal of Fluency Disorders, 25*, 59–76.

Kabat-Zinn, J. (1994). *Wherever you go, there you are: Mindfulness meditation in everyday life.* New York, NY: Hyperion.

Murray, L. L., & Kim, H.-Y. (2004). A review of select alternative treatment approaches for acquired neurogenic disorders: Relaxation therapy and acupuncture. *Seminars in Speech and Language, 25*(2), 133–149.

Roy, N. (2008). Assessment and treatment of musculoskeletal tension in hyperfunctional voice disorders. *International Journal of Speech-Language Pathology, 10*, 195–209.

Relevance Theory

Relevance theory is a psychological model of pragmatic processing. In this theory, relevance is a basic psychological phenomenon involved in all aspects of cognition that arises from the fact that humans have choices about which environmental cues to attend to. The claim is that people are driven to attend to what is most relevant in each situation. In language, relevance is used as a guiding principle for understanding how people express and recognize meaning. This model explains how an individual hearing a message (the hearer) can infer the full meaning intended by the speaker of the message (the speaker) by using all the evidence available to them and by selecting the most relevant information. The available evidence includes the information from the language, context, and hearer's own knowledge and beliefs. This entry discusses the key processes described by relevance theory and explains how individuals go beyond what is said to understand what is meant.

Consider the utterance, "Did he say that?" Traditional models of language processing focus on what is said rather than what is meant and thus explains how one understands this utterance as a process of decoding. According to decoding models, communication consists of a speaker and a hearer sharing a language (or code), so that the speaker encodes the message and sends it for the hearer to decode. In relevance theory, by contrast, the hearer's understanding of this utterance requires him or her to infer what the speaker meant and to use any information available to understand what the speaker intended to convey. The information obtained by decoding the language is one example of such information, but much more information is needed to infer what the speaker meant.

In the above utterance example (Did he say that?), information from the meaning of the words (semantics) tells that a question is being asked, that an unspecified male (the referent of the word "he") might have said something (again unspecified, the referent of the word "that"), and that the hearer is being asked to verify the truth of whether that unspecified person said that unspecified thing. One clearly needs more information to fully understand what the speaker meant. Other evidence available would include the context of the utterance, including the linguistic context (what was said before this utterance) and the physical context (whether there was someone in the immediate environment who could be the referent of "he"). Still other evidence, such as knowledge about the speaker and his or her beliefs and preferences, might also be used if relevant.

Relevance theory helps to understand the cognitive processes involved in fully comprehending utterances, such as the one above, by using two central ideas or principles: (1) the cognitive principle and (2) the communicative principle. The cognitive principle states that successful interpretation of a message is a process of sifting through the evidence to find the most relevant meaning for the least cognitive effort. The communicative principle explains that each message carries with it an assumption of its own relevance. The first principle helps to make sense of the cognitive relevance of information, and it explains how a hearer decides which information to pay attention to. The second principle, however, is needed to make the system efficient and to explain the role of the speaker.

For information to be relevant to a hearer, it must connect with previous knowledge or with the context. Because the hearer assumes the speaker intended to convey a relevant message, he or she will put in as much effort as it takes to reach a plausible understanding. For the hearer to decide how much cognitive effort is enough, there is an expectation that the effort and relevance are counterbalanced. Some interpretations take more cognitive work than others, but in each case, the aim is to understand the relevance of what has been said.

In the utterance, "It is so hot in here," for example, if the hearer feels the cold more than the speaker, the speaker has a preference for saving money on heating bills by keeping the thermostat turned down, and the hearer has a habit of secretly turning the thermostat back up, all of this previous knowledge will connect with the utterance as the hearer sifts through the information to find the message's relevance. In this situation, there is likely to be some cognitive effort needed to understand this utterance is not the simple statement suggested by the form of the language that has been used. Instead, it is an accusation that the hearer has secretly turned up the heating against the speaker's preferences.

Relevance theory explains that understanding requires finding the most relevant meaning for the least cognitive effort. The model includes an input system (hearing or seeing the message) and a deductive device in which concepts from the message are manipulated and integrated in order to understand the meaning of the message. The concepts come from the words in the utterance and consist of chunks of memory linked to logical, encyclopedic, and lexical information. In other words, each concept has a mental file associated with it in which individuals file any new information they get about that concept. For example, the word "dog" supplies lexical information about the word's meaning, logical information (e.g., animal of a certain species), and encyclopedic information based on world knowledge and past experiences (e.g., barks, wags its tail when it is happy, keeps people company).

In summary, relevance theory provides a psychologically valid theoretical framework to explain how humans go beyond what is said to understand what is meant by balancing cognitive effort with the reward of finding the relevance of a message.

Lucy T. Dipper

See also Lexicon; Meaning; Pragmatics

Further Readings

Blakemore, D. (1992). *Understanding utterances: An introduction to pragmatics.* Malden, MA Wiley-Blackwell.

Sperber, D., & Wilspon, D. (1986). *Relevance: Communication and cognition* (Vol. 142). Cambridge, MA: Harvard University Press.

RELIABILITY

Reliability is a crucial component of the measurement process. It is used in the theoretical characterization of communication disorders, assessment of individuals with communication disorders, and evaluation of intervention efficacy. Measurement is a process of representing theoretical constructs through observable events scored by an observer. This entry discusses measurements' internal cohesiveness and repeatability with respect to their uses in assessing individuals and evaluating intervention efficacy.

The theoretical constructs of interest in communication disorders are often cognitive/motoric abilities developed by the person's nervous system, including understanding of spoken language, construction of language units, speech fluency, and production of speech sounds, to name a few. The largely unobservable internal neural organization of these abilities is represented in the measurement process through an operational definition in which an observable behavior represents the unobservable neural organization or ability. For example, the underlying construct of expressive language ability has been operationally defined using measures such as *mean length of utterance* (MLU; average length of a speaker's utterances in morphemes) and number of different words used.

Reliability measures degree of consistency and repeatability. *Consistency* refers to the internal cohesiveness of a measure or the degree to which components of the measurement agree with one another. *Repeatability* is the degree to which a measure will produce similar results under similar conditions for the same person.

Consistency

Measurements of underlying constructs related to oral and written communication typically involve multiple observations that are summed or averaged to form a score or set of subtest scores. A test's *internal consistency* refers to the relationships between the individual test items and the overall test score. For example, the average MLU for children between the ages of 3 years, 0 months and 3 years, 6 months is between 3.0 and 3.75 morphemes per utterance. Typical utterances of this length include talking about actions (e.g., "He walks" or "He is walking"). So an adult who asks the child questions about actions during an adult–child interaction would be providing test items like "What is he doing?" that would be consistent with the child's ability and would probably result in relatively consistent responses by the child. Test items that ask the child to identify objects in the room (e.g., "What is this?" and "Who is this doll?") would likely result in shorter utterances (e.g., "a ball" and "the mommy") with scores lower than the typical child's test average. Thus, some of the adult questions would result in child responses that are more consistent with the child's overall score than others.

Clinicians and experimenters who construct tests use measures of internal consistency to improve their test procedures. Items not consistent with the total score are, at best, an inefficient part of the measurement. At worst, a lack of relationship between a test item and overall score indicates that the item is not measuring the right underlying ability and thus is not a valid measure. Responses to the unrelated items vary randomly relative to the person's targeted ability and thus add unwanted variability to the test scores, making the scores less repeatable.

Repeatability

A measure is reliable when repeated measures of the same individual result in similar scores. The time period between these repeated measurements must be one in which the underlying construct should not have changed. The typical measure of this type of reliability is test–retest reliability in which a group of people's performance is measured twice. The degree of reliability is expressed as a correlation coefficient or a standard error of measurement (*SEM*).

A *correlation coefficient* is a descriptive statistic that measures the degree to which the individuals in a group of people obtain the same scores relative to the group on the two measures. A perfectly high correlation in which all of the people receive the same relative scores on both measures results in a correlation of 1.0. If there is no relationship between the two scores, the correlation is 0. The correlation will be high if the individuals are ordered similarly by the two tests, that is, the same people are scoring at the top of both tests, a different group of people is scoring in the mid-range of both tests, and so forth. In other words, the two test administrations assign similar scores to individuals and will rank order them approximately the same way.

Figure 1a shows a graphic representation of a group of people's test–retest performance resulting in a high correlation. Each data point

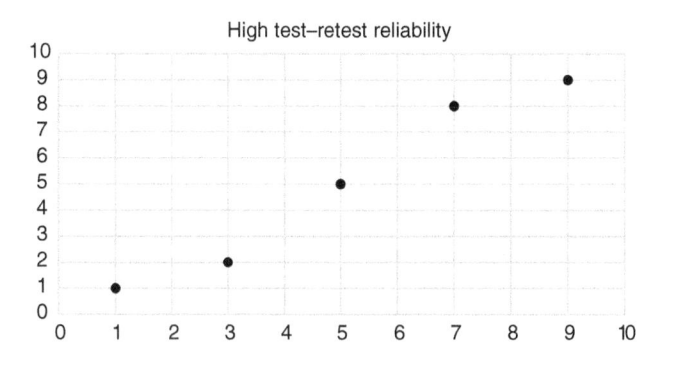

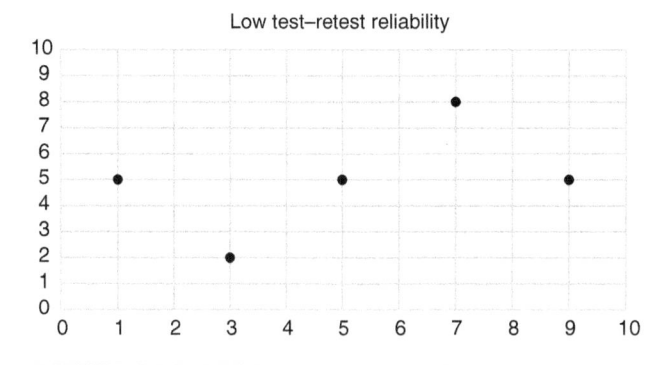

Figure 1 Scattergrams of two administrations of the same test to a group of individuals resulting in high and low test–retest reliability

represents a particular person's first score on the x-axis and the same person's second score on the y-axis. A perfect correlation would show all of the dots on a single line rising from left to right. The scores in the high test–retest correlation sample shown here resulted in a correlation coefficient of $r = .98$, compared to an $r = .45$ for the low correlation set. In the high test–retest data, the people with the lowest, middle, and highest scores in the pretest produced the same scores at posttest. The remaining two people scored either one point lower or higher in the second testing. Looking across the scores from left to right, it is shown that as the scores on the first test rise, the scores on the second test tend to rise. These characteristics would indicate that, on a group basis, this measure has good test–retest reliability.

Figure 1b shows a test with poorer test–retest reliability. The person with the lowest score on the first measurement (1) obtained a middle score (5) on the second test. The person who obtained the highest score in the pretest (9) also scored a 5 in the posttest. The end result is that there is little relationship between a person's first and second scores. If a person's first test score is unrelated to the second test score, there is little or no test reliability.

Test–retest reliability is used to calculate the SEM, which is a measure of the amount of error in a test score. It is calculated with the following formula in which SD represents the standard deviation of the second score and r represents the test–retest correlation.

$$(SEM = SD\sqrt{1-r})$$

As the test–retest correlation (r) approaches 1.0, the SEM decreases. If the test–retest correlation is perfect, then $r = 1$ and the SEM = 0. This would mean that there is no error in the measurement, and the measurement is perfectly reliable. If a child scored an MLU of 3.0, for example, this would be his or her true score. However, measurements are never perfect; there is always some error. SEM uses test–retest reliability to estimate confidence intervals for our measurements. Assuming the SD of the measurement of a 3-year-old's MLU is 1.0 (to make the calculation easier), if $r = .7$, the SEM is .55; if $r = .8$, the SEM is .44; if $r = .9$, the SEM is .32. Each improvement in test–retest reliability decreases the SEM.

The interpretation of SEM is the same as the interpretation of an SD. If a child scored a 3.0 on the MLU measure, one would be 68% confident that his or her true score is within the confidence interval from 3.0 − 1 SEM to 3.0 + 1 SEM. When the test–retest reliability is .7, the SEM is .55, and the 68% confidence interval is 2.45–3.55. If the test–retest reliability is .9, the SEM is .32, and the 68% confidence interval is 2.68–3.32.

Better confidence in a measure makes the job of evaluating intervention efficacy more reliable. If an individual's preintervention MLU is 3.0 and the SEM for this measure is .5, his or her real pretest score is likely to be in confidence interval of 2.5–3.5. So if a period of intervention raises the individual's pretest score from 3.0 to 3.25, it is unclear if the intervention was effective because his or her posttest score is within the confidence interval of the pretest. On the other hand, if the postintervention score is 4.0, one can be more confident that there has been a change in the individual's underlying ability.

Reliability is a characteristic of measurement that expresses the degree to which a measure is internally consistent and repeatable. Internal consistency is measured by correlating test items with the overall measurement scores. It is used to improve tests so that all parts of a measurement are tapping the same underlying ability. Test–retest reliability is used to measure measurement consistency. As a measure becomes more reliable, the confidence interval of scores that includes the underlying true score shrinks, and the user becomes more confident in the measurement. The confidence interval of a preintervention score provides a guide to how much improvement should be made to conclude that an intervention caused a change in the underlying ability.

Paul R. Hoffman

See also Diagnosis of Communication Disorders; Statistics: Descriptive; Statistics: Inferential; Test–Retest Approach; Validity

Further Readings

Anastasi, A., & Urbina, S. (1997). *Psychological testing* (7th ed.). Upper Saddle, NJ: Prentice Hall.

Groth-Marnat, G. (2009). *Handbook of psychological assessment*. Hoboken, NJ: John Wiley.

Shipley, K. G., & McAfee, J. G. (2018). *Assessment in speech-language pathology: A resource manual* (4th ed.). New York, NY: Delmar Cengage.

RESEARCH

Research in communication sciences and disorders is a broad topic that encompasses many different methods and procedures. Research in disciplines such as audiology, speech–language pathology, and speech and hearing science refers to approaches to inquiry that are preplanned and systematic in nature. The term *scientific research* is used to set this kind of research apart from everyday forms of information gathering and research that members of the public conduct. This entry offers a comprehensive discussion of the nature of scientific research, presenting its various types and methods (e.g., empirical vs. nonempirical, basic vs. applied, and translational) and explaining in detail the differences between the forms that research designs can take and the ways in which variables are defined and used by the researchers. The entry then continues with a discussion of ethics in research and concludes with an outline of how study findings are disseminated throughout the research community.

Scientific research employs well-documented, specifically defined research methods in the information gathering process. The term is plural because researchers have many different approaches for investigating a research question. Even with these differences, all scientific research shares the characteristics of being preplanned and systematic in nature. This feature is important because using well-defined methods to conduct a study allows other researchers to easily conduct similar studies and replicate the findings.

Another commonality among the various research approaches is a clearly stated aim. The aim might take the form of a statement of purpose, a research question, or a formal research hypothesis. A well-designed study always has at least one clearly stated purpose or question, but often, researchers design studies that provide information related to more than one purpose. Investigations in communication sciences and disorders have addressed issues that were the most interesting and relevant. In developing these questions, researchers identified a lack of evidence or the need to confirm the findings of prior studies and also considered questions that could be studied in an ethical manner.

Investigators sometimes develop a research hypothesis instead of a research question. A research *hypothesis* is a formal statement of the expected outcome of a study based on the researcher's prior knowledge of the subject, possible theoretical explanations, and prior, related research. This hypothesis might be a statement about the relationship between two measures (a positive or negative association) or a statement about the causal relationship between a factor that the researcher manipulates and an outcome measure. In communication sciences and disorders, the outcomes often are measures of participants' auditory perception, language, speech, voice, or swallowing. The factors that researchers manipulate in studies usually are therapeutic in nature. When researchers generate formal hypotheses to capture the intent of a study, the tradition is to state such hypotheses in the negative as a *null hypothesis*. The null hypothesis is a statement that two measures have no association, two groups are not different, or the factor manipulated in the research had no effect on the outcome measure. The null hypothesis is the basis for statistical analysis of the results, and the researcher's goal is to reject the null hypothesis. That is, the aim of research is to identify significant relationships and differences and thus demonstrate that the null hypothesis was not viable. The term *hypothesis testing* refers to an approach to research that includes stating a formal null hypothesis and conducting appropriate statistical tests to determine the viability of that hypothesis.

Types of Research

As previously stated, research in the field of communication sciences and disorders falls into multiple categories. One classification is the distinction between empirical and nonempirical research. Research that is *empirical* involves the collection of new information such as responses and samples from the participants in a study. In communication sciences and disorders, the participants most often are human beings; although, the term *participant* broadly includes other entities including anatomical specimens, animals, or organizations. Research that is *nonempirical* utilizes existing information from previous, usually published, research on a topic.

When conducted according to well-documented, predefined methods, nonempirical studies fall under the category of scientific research. A high-quality, nonempirical study has all or most of the following characteristics. First, the study has a clearly stated focus or research question. Second, the researcher should conduct a thorough search for existing information on the topic and document that search in the write-up of the study. Additionally, the researcher usually has a predefined set of criteria for determining what prior research fits the study (criteria for inclusion and exclusion of prior research), completes a critical appraisal of the included research to document the quality of the various studies, draws conclusions about the similarities and differences among the various research findings, and finally clearly states how the findings address the research question. These typically are the procedures followed in systematic reviews and meta-analyses, which are examples of high-quality, nonempirical research. In a systematic review, the authors organize their findings in tables and report conclusions in a verbal manner. A meta-analysis has those features plus an additional statistical analysis of the combined results across multiple, comparable studies.

One of the key concepts associated with *empirical research* is the collection of original *data*. The term *data* refers to the measurements or observations the researcher makes over the course of a study. The term is the plural form, and *datum* is the singular form referring to a single measurement. In common usage, often, the term *data* is used in a singular context. The types of data collected in the field of communication sciences and disorders are highly varied. Measurements and observations of auditory perception, speech, language, voice, and swallowing range from physiological and electrophysiological measurements (e.g., airflow measurements of respiration during speech or evoked potentials reflecting activity in the brain) to acoustic measures of speech and voice, to scores from standardized tests, and to analyses of orthographic and phonetic transcriptions of speech and language samples. The data obtained during a study are the basis for answering the research questions and testing hypotheses.

Within the category of empirical research, professionals often make a distinction between basic research and applied research. The aim of *basic research* is to better understand a particular phenomenon, such as how one learns language or produces and perceives speech. Basic research in communication sciences and disorders has contributed to a better understanding of the normative aspects of speech and language acquisition, the way listeners process a speech signal, the production of speech from thought to oral-motor movements, among many other topics. Basic research involves studies that occur in a laboratory under carefully controlled conditions. Speech and hearing scientists conduct much of the basic research that provides the foundation for audiology and speech–language pathology, but these professions also draw on research from related disciplines such as linguistics, neuroscience, and psychology. Basic research is essential for establishing the foundation for applied disciplines including speech–language pathology or audiology but does not lead directly to approaches for assessing and treating speech, language, and hearing disorders.

The focus of *applied research* is on identifying solutions to practical issues and problems. In communication sciences and disorders, applied research usually addresses prevention, assessment, and treatment of communication and swallowing disorders. Applied research also encompasses studies aimed at developing new products and technologies to improve people's lives. Applied research in communication sciences and disorders has addressed issues such as the reliability and validity of objective measures of speech and voice; the most effective treatment approaches for speech and language disorders; the effectiveness of different service delivery models such as parent and clinician delivered, telepractice, and online delivery; and the most beneficial technologies to aid hearing and speech. Although applied research might be conducted in academic and laboratory settings, applied studies also take place in the community and in school clinical and medical settings. Applied research has a relationship to the scope of practice for audiologists and speech–language pathologists and provides direct evidence to guide clinical services.

Translational research is another category of research that has some similarities to applied research. When conducting a translational study, researchers use the knowledge gained through basic research to design and investigate prevention, assessment, and treatment approaches that will benefit individuals and the population at large. Translational research often occurs in several phases. The first phase is to use knowledge and information gained through basic research to generate new clinical procedures and to test those new procedures under relatively controlled conditions. If the findings from the initial studies are promising, the next phase is a broader study of the new procedures in typical service delivery settings such as clinics, hospitals, and schools. The ultimate aim of translational research in communication sciences and disorders is to improve the population's overall health and well-being in areas such as speech and language, hearing, and swallowing.

Research Design

The starting point for most empirical research is a *research design*, which is a plan for conducting the study. The design includes information such as the procedures for gathering data, the identity and number of participants, the time frame for the investigation, the measurements and observations, and the strategies for data analysis. As described in the following sections, empirical studies in communication sciences and disorders employ many different research designs.

Longitudinal Research

The plan for observing participants over time is a primary design feature. In *longitudinal research*, the investigators gather data from participants at multiple occasions over the course of the study. The specific length is variable depending on the research question. Longitudinal research designs have been employed in the field of communication sciences and disorders to study the typical development of speech and language from infancy through the preschool years, to study the effects of aging on speech, language and hearing, and to study recovery from a stroke. Although longitudinal research often is observational in nature, researchers sometimes add a longitudinal component to treatment studies to evaluate the long-term effects.

In longitudinal investigations of typical speech and language development, the researchers have recruited a group of participants who are all approximately of the same age. These participants often were relatively young, such as 1-year-olds, when they began the studies. Typical observation schedules for these studies were every 4 months or every 6 months, and the studies continued until the children reached a specific age. In longitudinal investigations of the effects of normal aging, the participants usually started the study at an older age such as between the ages of 50 and 65. These studies might continue for a decade or more, and in some instances, older adults took part until a very advanced age. All of the participants in observational, longitudinal research are similar at the start of the study based on criteria such as age, education, health status, geographic location, cultural and linguistic background, and so forth.

In treatment research with a long-term component, the researchers usually aim to compare different groups of participants—one that received a particular treatment and one that did not. In such studies, the participants typically complete a test prior to the study (a pretest) and a test immediately at the conclusion of the study (a posttest). Scheduling an additional test several months or even a year after the conclusion of the study provides information about the lasting effects of the treatment.

An alternative to a longitudinal research design is cross-sectional research. In *cross-sectional research*, all observations and testing occur within a relatively short period of time. To make comparisons across age groups, the investigators recruit different groups of individuals to represent each age group. A cross-sectional approach to studying typical speech and language development would involve recruiting groups of children who represented each age of interest (e.g., a group of 1-year-olds, a group of 2-year-olds, a group of 3-year-olds). For studies of the effects of aging, the participants might include separate groups of adults who are 50, 60, 70, and 80 years old. An advantage of cross-sectional research is that the study can be completed in a relatively short time. A longitudinal study of changes in communication and swallowing from age 50 to 80 would take 30 years to complete. Using a cross-sectional approach, the researchers could complete data collection within a few months. However, cross-sectional designs do not allow researchers to study changes in the same individuals as they mature and age naturally. Many factors related to speech, language, and hearing could be different for 80-year-olds who were born in the 1930s compared to 50-year-olds who were born in the 1960s. These possible differences in experiences create challenges for interpreting the findings of cross-sectional research.

Although age is often a variable in cross-sectional research, other comparisons are possible. In communication sciences and disorders, examining differences between individuals with speech, language, and hearing impairments and those without such impairments is a common research design. Examples of this type of research include studies of children with and without language impairments, subgroups of children with language impairments, adults with normal and impaired hearing, and children with different degrees of hearing impairment. These investigations allow researchers to document differences between groups on a multiplicity of variables, but such studies cannot establish causal relationships between these variables and the presence of communication disorders.

Qualitative and Quantitative Research

Another difference among research designs is the distinction between qualitative and quantitative research. *Qualitative research* designs are a group of methodologies that employ naturalistic observation, focus on in-depth understanding of the experiences of a particular individual or group, and utilize inductive reasoning. An inductive approach involves gathering specific observations and identifying commonalities, patterns, or themes that emerge from the data. Some qualitative investigations extend beyond identification of themes to the development of a theory, proposed as a probable explanation for the observed phenomena. Examples of the observations obtained in qualitative studies are detailed descriptions, transcripts of conversations and interviews, and work samples (e.g., drawing, writing samples). Many methodologies fall under the umbrella of qualitative research: Case study, conversation analysis, ethnography, grounded theory, phenomenology, and thematic analysis are among the approaches employed in communication sciences and disorders.

Although researchers in communication sciences and disorders have used qualitative methodologies, quantitative research designs are far more common in the field. Quantitative research studies most often take place in controlled or even laboratory situations, utilize measures that are numerical in nature, and employ statistical analysis to identify differences and relationships. Conducting research in controlled situations provides for a degree of experimental control over extraneous factors that might confound the results of a study. Quantitative research encompasses the traditional methods of science including generating theories and testing hypotheses that arise from those theories.

The *scientific method* is a deductive, step-by-step approach that begins with a problem or question that motivates the research. The next step is to thoroughly study background information related to the question. This leads to a more refined research question or formal research hypothesis. Subsequently, the researcher designs and conducts a study to obtain relevant evidence or data. The next step is the data analysis usually with some type of statistical procedure. The analysis yields the information needed to draw conclusions about the research question or hypothesis. The scientific method is an iterative process, and each study leads to new questions and further investigation. The scientific method reflects a process of deductive reasoning from general models and theories to specific predictions of possible outcomes that the research findings either confirm or refute.

Quantitative approaches have been used to study many aspects of auditory perception and hearing, speech and language, and swallowing. In these studies, the researchers utilized numerical measures to quantify some phenomenon associated with communication, including measures of accuracy, duration, frequency of occurrence, or magnitude.

Most studies in communication sciences and disorders could be classified as purely qualitative or quantitative in nature. However, *mixed methods* research that combines qualitative and quantitative approaches are possible. In mixed methods approaches, the researchers might collect the quantitative and qualitative data concurrently or sequentially. A common mixed methods approach is to obtain quantitative data from a questionnaire and qualitative data from interviews. In a concurrent approach, administration of the questionnaire and completion of the interviews occur in the same time frame and often with the same group of participants. In a sequential approach, the researchers complete one form of data collection first, for example, administering questionnaires to a large group of participants and completing a quantitative analysis of the questionnaire responses. Subsequently, the researchers might interview another, smaller group of participants and complete in-depth, qualitative analyses of those responses. Studies employing mixed methods designs are less common in communication sciences and disorder publications than studies with purely quantitative design. Nevertheless, researchers have employed mixed methods designs to study a variety of topics including aphasia, assistive technology and augmentative communication, child language disorders, clinical service delivery models, hearing impairment and deafness, and stuttering.

Experimental and Nonexperimental Research

An additional distinguishing characteristic among studies is whether the research was experimental or nonexperimental. The category of *nonexperimental research* encompasses studies that investigate existing, naturally occurring phenomena. A variety of descriptive or observational investigations fall into this category, including case studies and observational group studies such as correlation, case–control or comparative, cohort, cross-sectional, prevalence, and survey research.

A case study could be qualitative, quantitative, or both. As the term implies, a case study is an in-depth investigation of an individual, often a person with a rare diagnosis or other unique characteristics. In correlational studies, the researchers administer two or more tests to a group of individuals to determine the relationship between the measures. Correlation studies yield information about the direction and strength of the relationship. The direction might be direct (positive) or inverse (negative), and the strength ranges from negligible (a correlation of 0 or close to ±0) to perfect or nearly perfect (close to ±1.0).

A case–control or comparative study has two or more groups of participants who differ on some characteristic. The research literature in communication sciences and disorders includes many studies that compare persons with a particular communication disorder (the cases) and persons with typical communication (the controls). The cases and controls are similar on other variables such as age, education, ethnicity, and linguistic background. The aim of case–control studies is to compare persons with communication disorders, such as hearing impairments, language impairments, stuttering, and voice disorders, and their matched controls on measures of interest to the researchers.

A cohort study often is longitudinal in nature. The cohort consists of a group of participants recruited because they share a characteristic of interest to the researchers. The investigators follow the cohort over time to determine what differences emerge. Investigators typically conduct prevalence and survey research with a sample of participants thought to represent a larger population. In communication sciences and disorders, prevalence studies provided evidence regarding the percentage of individuals in the sample and, by inference in the larger population, affected by a speech, language, or hearing disorders. Survey research is common in many fields of study. Surveys generate evidence in the form of self-reported characteristics and opinions. The types of questions used in surveys range from yes/no, to multiple choice, to rating scales, and to open-ended responses. The persons recruited to participate in survey studies depend on the aims of the study. In communication sciences and disorders survey, participants have included service providers such as audiologists and speech–language pathologists, parents or family members, or persons with communication disorders.

In *experimental research*, the investigators actively manipulate one or more variables to create different conditions for the participants in the study. A true experimental study has the added component of random assignment of participants to groups. Following random assignment, the groups take part in the study under different conditions. One common experimental approach is a pretest–posttest, randomized control group design. These investigations might have just two groups of participants, one serving as the experimental group and the other serving as the control group. Both groups complete a pretest prior to the study and a posttest at the end of the study. If the purpose of the study is to investigate the effectiveness of a treatment, the experimental group receives the treatment between the pretest and posttest, whereas the control group only completes the pretest and posttest. If the treatment and control groups performed in a similar manner on the pretest and differently on the posttest, the difference most likely occurred due to the treatment. A randomized pretest–posttest design is also known as a *randomized control trial*. This type of research design has a special role in education and healthcare fields such as audiology and speech–language pathology because randomized control trials are essential for documenting the effectiveness of education and treatment procedures. Variations on the basic randomized pretest–posttest design include replacing the control group with an alternate treatment group, including a third group (e.g., experimental treatment, comparison treatment, no treatment control), or adding a long-term posttest.

In many pretest–posttest, randomized designs, the researchers manipulate just one variable, most often a treatment variable. In more complex designs, called *factorial research designs*, the investigators manipulate more than one variable. For example, investigators might study different treatment procedures along with different levels of treatment intensity. Such designs allow researchers to study combinations of variables, such as different treatments delivered with low intensity compared with high intensity.

In some situations, randomly assigning participants to a treatment or control group is not practical. In such instances, the researchers still could conduct the investigation, but the study would be *quasi-experimental*. Quasi-experimental research is research with intact groups such as classrooms, communities, or patients served by different medical centers. These studies are experimental in nature with manipulation of at least one variable. The findings from quasi-experimental investigations are less conclusive because intact groups could differ on experiences or traits that are outside the researchers' control.

Group and Single-Subject Research

One final division to consider, within the topic of research design, is the distinction between group research designs and single-subject research designs. The term *single-subject research design* implies the notion of a study conducted with only one participant, but that is not necessarily the case. The number of participants is not the defining difference between single-subject and group research. Rather, the way subjects (i.e., participants) take part in the experimental and control conditions of the investigation and the way researchers report the findings delimit the two research approaches. In *group research*, the investigators select a group of individuals who represent a larger population to take part in the study. Under the best sampling conditions, the researchers should obtain an unbiased sample that embodies the characteristics of the population as a whole. In many instances, the investigators specifically define the population characteristics, such as persons between the ages of 60 and 70 who suffered a left-hemisphere, ischemic stroke, children from ages 1 to 3 with bilateral, sensorineural hearing loss, or children from ages 5 to 7 with specific language impairment. As noted above, the key to obtaining an unbiased sample is random sampling. The size of the sample or group depends on the nature of the phenomenon and the size of the population under study. Experimental group studies have the additional step of random assignment of participants to treatment and control groups. The goal of group research is to generalize the findings of the investigation to the larger population rather than just understand the behaviors of the actual participants in the study.

In analyzing the findings of a group study, the investigators aggregate the observations obtained from individual participants and generate measures that reflect group performance. These measures include common descriptive statistics such as the mean and median to represent central tendency and the standard deviation to represent variability. Other statistical procedures, such as correlation and regression analyses, yield information about the relationships between measure, whereas another set of statistical procedures, including *t*-tests and analysis of variance, yield information about group differences.

In *single-subject research*, the investigators recruit participants with characteristics that are a good fit for the predefined aims of the study. Researchers most often utilize single-subject designs to study low-prevalence populations or in the early phases of treatment efficacy research. Although single-subject studies could have just one participant, many such studies have multiple participants to provide replication of the findings. Readers should draw an important distinction between descriptive case studies and single-subject research designs. Single-subject research designs are experimental approaches with comparisons of control and treatment conditions. In single-subject research, the control condition is referred to as the *baseline phase*, and the treatment condition is the *treatment phase*. The subjects take part in both the baseline and treatment phases of the study; thus, subjects serve as their own controls. This is a key distinction between a true, experimental study and single-subject studies. In true experiments, random assignment places some subjects in the treatment group and the other subjects in the control group. The subjects only participate in one of the conditions.

The basic single-subject design consists of a single baseline and treatment sequence. Variations on this basic design include repeating the baseline and treatment phases, replication across participants or a multiple baseline across-subjects designs, and replication across behaviors or a multiple baseline across-behaviors designs.

A second crucial distinction between single-subject and group designs is apparent in reporting the results. Authors report the findings from single-subject research individually for each participant. If a study had four participants, the authors would present the baseline and treatment findings for each participant separately, most often in a series of graphs. Analysis of the findings from single-subject research begins with visual inspection of the graphs. If the study demonstrated a treatment effect, this would be apparent in definitive differences between measures from the baseline phase compared with measures from the treatment phase. The investigators might supplement the visual displays with statistical analyses, but the statistics are less central to understanding the findings than the statistics associated with group research.

Variables

The concept of a variable is important to understanding research in any field of study, including communication sciences and disorders. A variable is something that can change or be different in some manner. In communication sciences and disorders, the variables are most often behavioral and experiential. Any useful variable must be measurable and observable. Investigators often designate variables as either independent variables or dependent variables. Independent variables are the ones the researchers manipulate over the course of the study. The manipulations could be short-term experiments in which the investigators modify the conditions for completing a task or long-term manipulations such as the ones that occur in treatment research. Dependent variables are the outcome measures employed in a study. Researchers in communication sciences and disorders have techniques to evaluate or measure a variety of human communication behaviors. Some examples include acoustic analyses of speech and voice, behavioral measures of auditory perception and language processing, electromyograms of muscle activity, and notation systems such as phonetic transcription. In experimental research, the aim is to determine how the independent variable or experimental manipulation affects the dependent variable or outcome measure. In some nonexperimental research, the purpose is to determine how well the independent variable predicts the dependent variable. In conducting the study, the researchers also might control or hold constant other potential variables that otherwise might influence the outcome of the study. Maintaining this control over confounding influences is one way to assure that research findings are reliable and valid.

Ethics

As previously stated, the aim of empirical research in communication sciences and disorders is to investigate and potentially answer questions of wide-ranging interest. A pivotal factor in selecting research topics is the ability to study the topic in an ethical manner. Three general principles form the foundation for ethical conduct of research—respect for persons, beneficence, and justice. All three focus on the protection of the individuals who participate in research. The principle of *respect for persons* encompasses the concepts of informed consent and voluntary participation. Respect for persons also means that individuals have the right to discontinue their involvement in a study at any point. Protecting the well-being of participants is the focus of the principle of *beneficence*. Researchers should design studies in a way that minimizes any potential risks to participants and should discontinue the investigation if any unforeseen problems emerge. Researchers also need to safeguard the identity of participants by maintaining the confidentiality and security of their research records. Finally, the principle of *justice* means that members of society should share equally in the benefits and risks associated with participating in research. Researchers should not discriminate against any particular class of individuals in identifying research volunteers, nor should they take advantage of vulnerable groups within society. The principles for ethical conduct of research are embodied in federal law as well as in the code of ethics of professional organizations such as the American Speech-Language-Hearing Association and the American Academy of Audiology.

Dissemination

Although scientific curiosity is a strong motivation for conducting research, investigators often have the goal of presenting and/or publishing their findings as well. Through their presentations at state, national, and international conferences and publications in professional journals, researchers contribute to the evidence base for the professions of audiology, speech–language pathology, and speech and hearing science. The research base for communication sciences and disorders is extensive; the best way to identify information on a particular topic is to utilize online databases and search engines. Although some search engines are available by subscription only, the tools that are available for free provide comprehensive coverage of publications in communication sciences and disorders and a useful set of strategies for conducting the search. Three to consider are Google Scholar (https://scholar.google.com/) for general searches, PubMed (https://www.ncbi.nlm.nih.gov/pubmed/) for searches with a health science or medical focus, and ERIC (https://eric.ed.gov/) for searches with an educational focus.

Scientific research is essential for establishing a strong evidence base for the field of communication sciences and disorders. Research is a topic that is relevant across all professional settings, including educational and health care as well as academic and laboratory settings. Attending professional conferences and reading articles in scholarly publications are ways for audiologists and speech–language pathologists to maintain their professional competence. Additionally, clinicians contribute directly to the research base of the professions by conducting practice-based or applied research.

Lauren K. Nelson

See also Databases in Communication Disorders; Efficacy and Effectiveness of Treatment Studies; Ethics in Communication Disorders Research; Evidence-Based Practice; Experimental Research; Qualitative Research; Quantitative Research; Treatment Research

Further Readings

American Speech-Language-Hearing Association. (2004). *Evidence-based practice in communication disorders: An introduction* [Technical report]. Retrieved from www.asha.org/policy

Byiers, B. J., Reichle, J., & Symons, F. J. (2012). Single-subject experimental design for evidence-based practice. *American Journal of Speech-Language Pathology, 21*, 397–414. doi:10.1044/1058–0360(2012/11–0036)

Damico, J. S., & Simmons-Mackie, N. N. (2003). Qualitative research and speech-language pathology: A tutorial for the clinical realm. *American Journal of Speech-Language Pathology, 12*, 131–143.

Dollaghan, C. A. (2004). Evidence-based practice in communication disorders: What do we know and when do we know it? *Journal of Communication Disorders, 37*, 391–400. doi:10.1016/j.jcomdis.2004.04.002

Horner, J., & Minifie, F. (2011). Research ethics I: Responsible conduct of research (RCR)—Historical and contemporary issues pertaining to human and animal experimentation. *Journal of Speech-Language-Hearing Research, 54,* S303–S329. doi:10.1044/10924388(2010/09–0265)

Horner, R. H., Carr, E. G., Halle, J., McGee, G., Odom, S., & Wolery, M. (2005). The use of single-subject research to identify evidence-based practice in special education. *Exceptional Children, 71,* 165–179.

Irwin, D. L., Pannbacker, M., Norman, J., & Lass, N. J. (2013). *Clinical research methods in speech-language pathology and audiology* (2nd ed.). San Diego, CA: Plural.

Jones, S. M., & Mock, B. E. (2007). Responsible conduct of research in audiology. *Seminars in Hearing, 28*(3), 206–215. doi:10.1055/s-2007-982902

Meline, T. (2010). *Research primer in communication sciences and disorders.* Boston, MA: Pearson.

Nelson, L. K. (2017). *Research in communication sciences and disorders: Methods for systematic inquiry* (3rd ed.). San Diego, CA: Plural.

Orlikoff, R. G., Schiavetti, N. E., & Metz, D. E. (2015). *Evaluating research in communication disorders* (7th ed.). Boston, MA: Pearson.

Patten, M. L. (2014). *Understanding research methods: An overview of the essentials* (9th ed.). Glendale, CA: Pyrczak.

Ratner, N. B. (2006). Evidence-based practice: An examination of its ramifications for the practice of speech-language pathology. *Language, Speech, and Hearing Services in Schools, 37,* 257–267.

Salkind, N. J. (2010). *Encyclopedia of research design: Volume 1.* Thousand Oaks, CA: Sage.

Trochim, W. M. K., Donnelly, J. P., & Arora, K. (2016). *Research methods: The essential knowledge base* (2nd ed.). Boston, MA: Cengage Learning.

Residual Speech Sound Errors

Residual speech sound errors are misarticulations that persist past the normative age of sound mastery and are typically observed in children 9 years or above. Many, but not all, children with residual speech sound errors have received long-term intervention for speech disorder. It is commonly believed that most residual speech sound errors are normalized by adulthood. Although prevalence data are limited, it is estimated that less than 2% of adults present with residual speech sound errors.

Speech sound disorder classification systems typically identify a subtype characterized by phonetically based residual speech sound errors. Some researchers make a further distinction between residual and persistent speech sound errors. According to this view, residual speech sound errors may be remnants of a more widespread speech sound disorder that probably involved omission or substitution error patterns. Although children with residual speech sound errors are likely to have made progress in speech production, they continue to have difficulty articulating the target sound beyond the age when most children have mastered its production. For other children, speech sound errors appear not to have been related to a broader system-wide problem. Instead, distortion of a small number of sounds—often just one (e.g., /ɹ/)—persists beyond the typical age of mastery. It has been proposed that the term *persistent speech sound error* may be more appropriate than *residual* for such children.

Characteristics

Among English speakers, residual and persistent speech sound errors typically impact one or more sounds with late ages of mastery, often described as the *late eight* sounds (i.e., /ɹ, l, s, z, θ, ð, ʃ,* and tʃ/). Of these, the sounds most often cited as residual errors are /ɹ/, /s/, /z/, and /l/. Often, residual speech sound errors involve distorted productions, as opposed to omission or substitution errors, which are more common among younger children with nonresidual speech sound disorders. For example, speakers with residual speech sound errors may derhoticize production of /ɹ/ (e.g., [ʊ] for /ɹ/) or produce lateralized sibilants (such as [ɬ] for /s/). Residual speech sound errors are likely to impact production of various allophones of the target phoneme (e.g., vocalic and consonantal allophones of /ɹ/ in English dialects that are rhotic). Further, the distortion is likely to affect production of the sound both as a singleton and in consonant clusters.

Children with residual speech sound errors may present with concomitant disorders impacting perceptual (auditory discrimination), metaphonological (phonological awareness and memory), and cognitive skills (e.g., cognitive flexibility, short- and long-term memory, and self-monitoring). Children with residual errors may experience teasing or bullying, and they may have associated self-esteem issues. Such problems seem to be more common as speakers get older, at least during the school-age years.

Assessment

Children with residual speech sound errors typically have intelligible speech and present with a small number of sounds in error. Naturalistic speech samples and standardized single-word elicitation tests may be used with younger children to document the breadth and severity of the disorder. If the speaker is able to read, then phonetically balanced reading passages may be administered. Assessment of coarticulatory effects is desirable to evaluate consistency of the error across allophones and in a variety of phonetic contexts (abutting various vowels and consonants). Such assessment may uncover facilitative phonetic environments that can be capitalized on during the treatment process. Dynamic assessment methods can be used to determine the effects of imitation and linguistic level upon sound production (stimulability). Evaluation of articulatory control and prosodic features may include rate modification tasks, production of polysyllabic words, and emphatic stress tasks. Instrumental assessment (e.g., acoustic analysis, ultrasonography) may provide important details regarding the nature of the disorder. Because children with residual speech sound errors are at risk of disorders of perceptual, metaphonological, and cognitive skills, evaluation of these areas should be considered. Procedures for assessing residual speech sound errors of bilingual speakers have also been described in the literature.

Treatment

Some individuals with residual or persistent speech sound errors benefit from traditional motor-based treatments involving phonetic placement cues, facilitative phonetic environments, shaping (i.e., reinforcement of successive approximations), and self-monitoring. Alternative treatment approaches are necessary, however, for many speakers. Instrumental biofeedback approaches, such as electropalatography and ultrasound, have been used to successfully treat residual speech sound errors. Electropalatography has been used successfully to modify sibilant errors, including lateralization. Less often, electropalatography has been used in the remediation of /ɹ/. Ultrasound-based treatments, too, have been found effective for establishing production of /ɹ/ as well as other targets. Multimodal treatments that include visual biofeedback and principles of motor learning have also been described. Few efficiency studies have been published that directly compare treatment options for residual speech sound errors. Findings document considerable differences among individual outcomes, suggesting an interaction between participant characteristics and treatment conditions that require additional research.

Thomas W. Powell

See also Articulation Therapy (Phonetic Intervention); Electropalatography (EPG); Speech Sound Disorders; Ultrasonography

Further Readings

McAllister Byun, T., & Preston, J. L. (Eds.). (2015). Residual speech errors: Causes, implications, treatment. *Seminars in Speech and Language*, 36(4), 215–216.

McAuliffe, M. J., & Cornwell, P. L. (2008). Intervention for lateral /s/ using electropalatography (EPG) biofeedback and an intensive motor learning approach: A case report. *International Journal of Language and Communication Disorders*, 43, 219–229.

Preston, J. L., & Edwards, M. L. (2007). Phonological processing skills of adolescents with residual speech sound errors. *Language, Speech, and Hearing Services in Schools*, 38, 297–308.

Preston, J. L., Leece, M. C., & Maas, E. (2017). Motor-based treatment with and without ultrasound feedback for residual speech-sound errors. *International Journal of Language and Communication Disorders*, 52, 80–94.

Preston, J. L., McCabe, P., Rivera-Campos, A., Whittle, J. L., Landry, E., & Maas, E. (2014). Ultrasound visual feedback treatment and practice variability for residual speech sound errors. *Journal of Speech, Language, and Hearing Research*, 57, 2102–2115.

Resilience

Resilience is the ability to construct and experience positive outcomes amid serious threats to adaptation or development. Resilience commonly refers to an individual's capacity to adapt or return to a state of functional equilibrium following destabilizing threats. Often, resilience includes the transformation of the system to a new, yet stable, status of functionality. When an individual experiences challenges, such as a communication disorder, and develops patterns of functioning that allow him or her to adapt or rehabilitate, these changes are viewed as resiliency. This entry discusses how resilience is assessed and measured and traces the three waves of resilience research.

Resilience is assessed and measured through a number of data collection and analysis methods. Descriptive and directed interviews have been used to assess resilience as well as participant observations and detailed personal and familial case histories aimed at describing the protective and stress-related risk factors present in the client's life. However, researchers have most routinely relied upon checklists and scales of resilience, with preference for standardized questionnaires rating self-control, affective responsiveness, cognitive functioning, attachment, and initiative. Resilient individuals hold the belief that they can influence life events and have the capacity to translate that belief into action. In essence, resilient individuals hold some control over significant aspects of their lives even if the control extends only to how they choose to perceive life's experiences. Resilient individuals are observed to respond to change and adversity as an opportunity to grow as opposed to stressors that incapacitate.

Historically, resilience research has benefited from three major evolving waves. Within the first wave of resilience, some of the earliest attempts at defining and measuring resilience and understanding what makes a difference in one's capacity to experience positive outcomes are found. Leading expert in resilience research Ann S. Masten recognizes that all humans experience adversity and stress and routinely overcome these challenges. Her work positions resilience as an ordinary phenomenon most individuals frequently display as they experience stressors throughout a lifetime. Challenges and threats to development and positive life outcomes are common, but some experiences (e.g., catastrophe, trauma, illness, persistent and pervasive limitations) may overwhelm the individual's capacity to absorb or spring back. Adversity in life and developmental vulnerability are conceptualized as risk factors. Risk factors represent an elevated probability of undesirable life outcomes. Risk factors vary depending upon when they are assessed, the individual makeup, and individual response to factors associated with the context. Poverty, natural disasters, maltreatment, parental divorce or neglect, ineffective schools or health-care systems, and high community crime rates are among the external risk factors consistently found to negatively impact resilience in individuals. Internal risk factors include impaired cognition, presence of an illness or disorder, unresponsive temperament, emotional regulation challenges, or issues with explanatory style.

The first wave of resilience research also developed an understanding of the protective factors, attributes, and assets displayed by individuals capable of overcoming adversity. In most instances, protective factors included the polar opposite of the risk factors. Protective factors are conceptualized in terms of prosocial variables associated with the individual, family, and community of interest. Thus, external protective factors include effective schools and accessible health-care systems, stable and safe families, homes and communities, and established supportive interpersonal networks. Internal protective factors include effective problem solving, adequate cognition for contextual demands, and physical and emotional development that meet societal expectations. A positive self-perception, a sense of meaning and purpose in life, the ability to self-regulate emotions, and an overall sense that one's social group values one's talents further protectively contribute to resilience. Understanding of these factors informed the second wave of resilience research.

The second wave reflected an advanced conceptualization of resilience beyond a set of characteristics, to the dynamic process individuals engage in to recover or cope with adversity. The focus in second wave research centers on how resilience functions and how the protective and risk factors influence individual outcomes. Resilience can be promoted by protective factors. It is believed that variables modify the individual's response to negative or adverse events, thereby avoiding negative outcomes. Second wave understandings have valued the interplay of protective and risk factors. For example, the presence of risk factors may inhibit resilience but does not always result in undesirable outcomes. Ineffective schools have been identified as a risk factor for children, for example, however, protective factors of familial supports and effective cognitive functioning may overwhelm and counter the risks constructing positive outcomes within the specific child. Protective and risk factors are dynamic and consequently impact individuals in uniquely personal ways. The second wave of resilience more effectively explains the interrelatedness and compounding effect of risk variables. For example, an individual with a healthy biological background, living in poverty might have limited access health care, effective schools, or strong prosocial parental relationships due to the parents' need to work long hours at multiple jobs in attempts to make ends meet. The presence of multiple risk factors then presents a cumulative or cascading effect that contributes to negative life outcomes. Conversely, second wave resilience has described protective factors as potential buffers against risks with potential for therapeutic positive cascading impacts focused on in the third wave of resilience research.

Better understanding of the dynamic nature of resilience-related factors informed the third wave of resilience research. The third wave suggests resilience can be taught and learned through purposeful activities that yield measurable results reflective of prosocial capacities. Because many risk factors are beyond the influence of clinicians, resilience-enhancing interventions primarily develop strengths and assets as resources. Resilience-building strategies are tailored to the individual's abilities and contexts. Clinicians mediate the development of resilience through therapeutic experiences that allow successful authentic social interactions. Central to therapeutic success in building resilience is the client's awareness of individual control responses to communicative challenges. Work support networks and external influences foster connection of close relationships with caring individuals. For children, this may include incorporating family members into the intervention. For adults, external resilience building may facilitate a spouse's ability to advocate for the client or the welcoming and ongoing encouragement of support group members.

Resilience is content- and context-specific. An individual facing one type of risk in a certain setting may be overwhelmed, while a different risk in the same setting may not negatively impact resilience. The uniqueness of context and individual attributes contribute to the challenge of studying resilience and in research efforts to identify universal protective factors and outcomes. Professionals desiring to make comparisons across groups and populations are challenged by individuals' uniqueness.

Ryan Nelson

See also Adaptation Theory; Compensatory Adaptation and Strategies; Positive Psychology and Wellness; Socialization

Further Readings

Lyons, R., & Roulstone, S. (2018). Well-being and resilience in children with speech and language disorders. *Journal of Speech, Language and Hearing Research, 61*, 324–344.

Masten, A. S. (2014). *Ordinary magic: Resilience development*. New York, NY: The Guilford Press.

Ungar, M. (2014). Practitioner review: Diagnosing childhood resilience a systemic approach to the diagnosis of adaptation in adverse social and physical ecologies. *Journal of Child Psychology and Psychiatry, 56*, 4–17.

Zolkoski, S. M., & Bullock, L. M. (2012). Resilience in children and youth: A review. *Children and Youth Services Review, 34*, 2295–2303.

Resonance Disorders

Like articulation and phonation, resonance is a fundamental feature of speech production. Resonance is an acoustic phenomenon affected by the physical characteristics of the pharyngeal, oral, and nasal cavities. The oral, pharyngeal, and nasal cavities are tubelike structures that have specific resonance characteristics. During normal speech, the acoustic signal generated by the larynx (voiced sound) is filtered, as the articulators (lips, tongue, mandible, soft palate, and pharyngeal walls) move continuously to change the shape of the oral and pharyngeal cavities. As these cavities change shape, their resonance characteristics will also change, affecting the acoustic signal that is emitted from the oral cavity. Thus, various vocal tract shapes are associated with specific voiced speech sounds such as vowels.

If the vocal tract does not allow voiced sound to propagate through the pharyngeal and oral cavities as it should, either the oral or nasal resonance characteristics of speech can be altered, and a resonance disorder can result. This entry is an overview of resonance disorders that can occur, the various causes, assessment for diagnosis, and various treatment approaches to correcting resonance disorders.

Types of Abnormal Resonance

Resonance is a speech characteristic that is present in all speakers. Most individuals exhibit a resonance that is within the range of *normal*, meaning that it does not cause a listener to hear them as sounding *different*. This section reviews the resonance characteristics that are considered *abnormal*.

Hypernasality

During normal speech, the nasal cavity is separated from the oral cavity for the majority of speech sounds. This is made possible by the movements of the soft palate and pharyngeal walls, which can close the port that couples the nasal cavity to the oral cavity (referred to as the *velopharyngeal port*). In doing so, the voiced sound transmitted up from the pharyngeal cavity can be directed through the oral cavity. During the production of the phonemes /m/, /n/, and /ng/ (referred to as *nasal consonants*), the velopharyngeal port is left open, thus allowing some of the voiced sound to resonate within the nasal cavity. For all other speech sounds, the velopharyngeal port should be closed (or nearly closed). When the nasal cavity is coupled to the oral cavity to an excessive extent during the production of vowels and voiced consonants (not including nasal consonants), the speech is characterized as being *hypernasal*. Hypernasality is a perceptual phenomenon that can only occur during the production of voiced speech sounds.

The degree of hypernasality perceived by a listener is influenced greatly by the size of the velopharyngeal port opening during speech. In general, the larger the velopharyngeal port (or the greater the extent to which the nasal cavity is coupled to the oral cavity), the greater the degree of hypernasality. It should be noted, however, that the degree of perceived hypernasality is dependent upon the acoustic impedance relationship between the nasal and oral cavities. Acoustic impedance within the oral cavity is determined by the shape of the oral cavity, which is influenced largely by the position of the tongue. If the tongue is positioned high and posteriorly in the oral cavity, oral acoustic impedance will be high, and it may be more likely that voiced sound will propagate (and resonate) within the nasal cavity. Therefore, for any given velopharyngeal port opening, the position of the tongue will influence the degree of nasal resonance that a listener perceives.

Hyponasality

During normal speech, a slight degree of nasal resonance occurs, primarily due to sound being transmitted across the mucosal tissues of the soft palate and pharynx. Whereas hypernasality is characterized by the presence of too much nasal resonance, *hyponasality* occurs when too little nasal resonance occurs. Hyponasality is most commonly perceived when the nasal cavity is obstructed, such as when an individual has nasal congestion due to an upper respiratory infection. In cases like these, voiced sound cannot resonate or propagate through the nasal cavity because the nasal mucosa are swollen and filled with mucous. Once the swelling resolves and the mucous clears, normal resonance returns.

Cul-de-sac Resonance

Unlike hypernasality and hyponasality, *cul-de-sac resonance* does not involve excessive coupling or decoupling of the nasal cavity. Rather, it is characterized by the abnormal way the voiced sound resonates within the oral and pharyngeal cavities. A cul-de-sac resonance occurs when the voiced sound resonates within the oropharyngeal space but does not propagate through the oral cavity in a normal manner due to an abnormal constriction at the entrance to the oral cavity. Like the name implies, the voiced sound reaches a *dead end* in the oropharynx, and speech is perceived as rather muffled.

Causes

Resonance disorders can have various etiologies, but the underlying cause is either an abnormal structural, neurological, or functional alteration of the oral or pharyngeal cavity, or the abnormal coupling or decoupling of the nasal cavity relative to the oral cavity. These abnormal alterations will result in distinctive acoustic–perceptual features. The following sections summarize the most common causes of resonance disorders.

Structural Causes

If the oral, nasal, or pharyngeal cavities are altered structurally, or if the hard/soft palate, tongue, or pharyngeal walls are anatomically different from normal, this can lead to the production of abnormal resonance. This section reviews the most common structural causes of resonance disorders.

Cleft Palate

According to the Centers for Disease Control, cleft palate is one of the most common birth defects. In this condition, the soft and hard palates do not develop in utero, so that at birth, there is no separation of the oral and nasal cavities. Even if the palate is surgically repaired during infancy, it is not uncommon for the soft palate and pharyngeal structures to be deficient in separating the oral and nasal cavities during speech. This condition, known as *velopharyngeal insufficiency*, results in excessive nasal resonance (hypernasality). The severity of hypernasality can vary across individuals, but it should be noted that the majority of children and adults with repaired cleft palates achieve normal resonance. Typically, the greater the extent of nasal cavity coupling, the greater the degree of perceived hypernasality.

Lingual–Palatal–Pharyngeal Cancer

Individuals who have malignant masses or lesions within the lingual–palatal–pharyngeal structures may ultimately exhibit some type of resonance disorder. The type and extent of the resonance problem will depend on several factors. First, surgical removal of cancerous masses can result in structural alteration of the oral and/or pharyngeal cavities. Second, radiation therapy of the affected structures can hinder a speaker's ability to move the lingual–pharyngeal–palatal structures in a normal fashion; this too can alter the shape of the oral and pharyngeal cavities and affect the resonance characteristics of the oral–pharyngeal cavities. In addition to these types of structural alteration, damage to the nerves and muscles responsible for movement of the tongue and pharyngeal structures can also impair a speaker's ability to control oral–pharyngeal spaces for normal resonance.

Surgical excision of a cancerous lesion within the hard and/or soft palate can result in a sizable oral–nasal fistula causing excessive coupling of the nasal cavity to the oral cavity. Perceptually, the result is excessive nasal resonance that sounds similar to an individual with velopharyngeal insufficiency. In general, the extent of the excessive nasal resonance is influenced by the size of the palatal defect. These defects may be surgically closed or covered with a dental appliance that resembles a modified retainer.

Trauma

Individuals who are subjected to some type of physical trauma to the facial skeleton or neck may suffer structural damage to the oral, palatal, and/or pharyngeal structures. As mentioned above, surgical excision of diseased tissue can cause damage to the oral and pharyngeal cavities. Damage caused by trauma can be more extensive, and surgical repair may not be as optimal because there may be a paucity of healthy tissue for reconstruction. Thus, the alteration of the oral–pharyngeal cavities may be more significant, and the resonance disorder will become more severe.

Hypertrophic Tonsils and Adenoids

It is not uncommon for children or young adults who are otherwise healthy to develop enlarged tonsils and/or enlarged adenoids. In many instances, hypertrophic tonsils and adenoids may not alter the speaker's oral, pharyngeal, or nasal resonance. However, if these tissues become excessively large, a resonance disorder can occur.

The tonsils can become so enlarged that they fill the oropharynx, touching at midline. When this condition occurs, the voiced sound cannot propagate into the oral cavity, and the sound tends to resonate in the upper pharynx, resulting in a cul-de-sac resonance. If it is deemed necessary to remove the tonsils surgically, normal resonance is typically restored postoperatively.

The adenoids are located along the superior aspect of the posterior pharyngeal wall, typically just above the velopharyngeal port. Typically, adenoids are evident during childhood, but the size of the tissue does not prevent the propagation of voice sound into the nasal cavity. However, it is possible for the adenoids to become hypertrophic. In extreme cases, the tissue can obstruct the velopharyngeal port and even fill part of the posterior nasal cavity. When adenoids become hypertrophic, voiced sound cannot resonate within the nasal cavity, and hyponasality is perceived. If it is deemed necessary to remove the adenoids surgically, and the individual exhibits normal velopharyngeal anatomy, normal resonance is typically restored postoperatively.

Neurological Causes

Whereas structural disorders result in an alteration to the physical dimensions of the oral or pharyngeal cavities or result in a permanent coupling of the oral and nasal cavities, neurological disorders tend to impair a speaker's ability to move the articulators. Consequently, vocal tract shape cannot be changed in a dynamic fashion, and the nasal cavity cannot be functionally separated from the oral cavity.

Stroke/Traumatic Brain Injury

Individuals who suffer a stroke or a traumatic brain injury will have damage to either the cortex, subcortical area, or brain stem. In many instances, damage to these areas will impair motor function for speech. The articulators may (a) move more slowly than normal, (b) move with less range of motion, or (c) a combination of both. These impairments can result in the speaker's ability to affect precise vocal tract shapes to maintain adequate oral–pharyngeal resonance. In addition, the inability of the velopharyngeal structures to move effectively can result in excessive nasal cavity coupling.

Neurodegenerative Disease

Individuals who are affected by neurodegenerative diseases typically exhibit mild neurological symptoms during the early stages of the disease. This is true for conditions such as Parkinson's disease and amyotrophic lateral sclerosis. During this time, hypernasality may be one of those early symptoms, as the velopharyngeal structures may begin to move more slowly or with decreased range of motion. As the disease progresses, the hypernasality may become more severe.

Functional Resonance Disorders

Functional speech disorders occur in individuals who have normal speech anatomy and physiology but who exhibit maladaptive speech behaviors. In essence, individuals with functional resonance disorders have adopted articulation patterns that result in abnormal resonance. Functional resonance disorders can be characterized by hypernasality, hyponasality, or cul-de-sac resonance, depending on how the speaker is manipulating the articulators. In most cases, the individual may be positioning the soft palate or the tongue incorrectly. If the tongue carriage is too posterior, oral acoustic impedance can be increased, and voice sound may be more likely to be transmitted into the nasal cavity. If the tongue is positioned too posteriorly and too high in the posterior aspect of the oral cavity, voiced sound may be trapped in the oropharynx, and a cul-de-sac resonance is perceived. Lastly, although it is an uncommon occurrence, it is possible to exhibit functional hyponasality if the speaker maintains relatively tight velopharyngeal closure during the production of all speech sounds, even for nasal consonants.

Measurement of Disordered Resonance

Clinicians and researchers who study resonance disorders characterize the presence/absence and severity of the disorder using two approaches. One approach involves perceptual assessment and the other involves using instrumentation to measure the physical presence of the resonance abnormality. It is important to note that perceptual assessment continues to be the most critical aspect of evaluating resonance. Instrumental assessment can complement perceptual assessment, but it does not replace perceptual judgment.

Although this entry has covered several types of resonance disorder, the only one of these resonance phenomena that has received considerable attention is hypernasality. This section focuses on measurement of hypernasality.

Perceptual Assessment of Nasality

Perceptual assessment of nasality is a subjective exercise. The task seems rather simple. It involves listening to a speech sample (e.g., conversational speech), then determining the extent to which the sample is different from *normal*. Certainly, rating the presence or absence and severity of nasality requires training, and it is assumed that clinicians with more experience listening to nasality are more reliable as raters. It is problematic that there is no standardized approach to rating nasality. Thus, in the clinical environment, speech pathologists have used various approaches to documenting the presence and severity of it. Some have reported descriptive judgments of severity, such as *mild, moderate,* or *severe*. Equal-appearing interval scales have been used extensively in the clinical setting. These scales are numerical; some are five-point scales, and some are seven-point scales. In each case, one represents *normal*, and the highest number on the scale is *most severe hypernasality*. Although the assumption is that the broader the scale (e.g., seven points vs five points), the greater the resolution to the assigned rating, there is no evidence to suggest that one scaling approach is superior. Further, there is evidence to show that equal-appearing interval scales do not capture the perception of nasality as completely as another approach, referred to as *direct magnitude estimation*. The direct magnitude estimation procedure is somewhat cumbersome and is difficult to employ in the clinical setting, but it has been recommended for use in research involving perceived nasality by, for example, Tara Whitehill and colleagues.

Instrumental Measurement of Nasality

Although the acoustic correlates of nasalization are well known, there are few clinical instruments available that provide a physical measurement of resonance that quantifies perceived nasality. The most commonly used instrument is the Nasometer by KayPENTAX, which uses two microphones to measure nasal acoustic activity and oral acoustic activity, then calculates a ratio signal—nasal acoustic intensity/(nasal + oral acoustic intensity) × 100—which is referred to as the *nasalance signal*. Increases in nasalance have been highly correlated with increases in perceived hypernasality.

Treatment

An individual who exhibits a resonance disorder may be a candidate for treatment, depending on the etiology and severity of the problem. The treatment approaches may involve physical alteration of the nasopharyngeal space (surgical or prosthodontic management) or behavioral management (speech therapy).

Speech Therapy

Individuals who may benefit from speech therapy for a resonance disorder may fit one of the following profiles:

- The individual has normal oral–pharyngeal anatomy, and it appears that the resonance disorder is due to maladaptive articulatory behaviors.
- The individual exhibits a mild resonance disorder that may be due to an anatomic abnormality, but the individual has the potential to learn articulatory patterns to compensate for the anatomic deficiency.

In cases where the individual may have either hypernasality or a cul-de-sac resonance due to maladaptive articulation, the goal of speech therapy will be to entrain tongue movements/positions that are lower and more anterior within the oral cavity, which increases the likelihood of oral transmission of voiced sound. In some instances, increasing mouth opening may bring a similar result, although there are limitations to this approach.

If an individual exhibits a mild degree of hypernasality, and it is determined that the etiology is a small velopharyngeal opening, a trial period of speech therapy may be warranted. For these individuals, speech therapy may focus on increasing articulatory effort to facilitate improved velopharyngeal closure, or it may focus on manipulating tongue position or mouth opening. In these cases, speech therapy should be implemented on a short-term basis. If no improvement is observed, speech therapy should be terminated.

Surgical Management

In cases where hypernasality is due to structural insufficiency (such as a short soft palate), surgical alteration of the velopharyngeal structures is common. The approach to surgery entails using existing tissue from either the soft palate or the posterior or lateral walls of the pharynx to create a velopharyngeal port that is smaller at rest and therefore more readily closed during speech. It is not advisable to use the tissues to *overclose* the port, as this will result in nasopharyngeal obstruction and hyponasal speech. Thus, if surgical management of the velopharynx is to be successful, it is essential that the individual demonstrates some degree of velopharyngeal movement to complete closure of the smaller velopharyngeal port during speech.

Prosthodontic Management

There are instances when surgical management of the velopharyngeal structures is not advisable. Some individuals are not candidates for surgery if they are medically fragile. Others may exhibit normal anatomy but may have a significant neurological deficiency. Individuals for whom surgery is not warranted may be candidates for prosthodontic management. There are two general approaches to prosthodontic management: an obturator or a palatal lift. These are appliances fabricated by a dental specialist with input from the speech pathologist.

An obturator is warranted in cases where hypernasality is caused by a significant structural deficiency. The *obturator* is an acrylic bulb that is attached to the back of a dental retainer. The bulb is positioned within the velopharyngeal space, so that during speech, the velopharyngeal structures move and close against the bulb. The size of the bulb depends on the extent of velopharyngeal movements exhibited by the individual (the more movement, the smaller the bulb needs to be). The appliance is removable for cleaning, and it does not need to be worn during sleep.

A palatal lift is warranted in cases where the individual has normal anatomic structures, but the soft palate is relatively immobile due to a neurological deficiency. In these cases, the lack of mobility decreases the likelihood that surgical management would be successful. The *palatal lift* is similar to an obturator in that it relies on a dental retainer. The difference is that, instead of a bulb that fits in the velopharyngeal space, the palatal lift is composed of a paddlelike extension from the retainer that pushes the soft palate into the velopharyngeal space to allow for velopharyngeal closure. Like the obturator, the palatal lift is removable for cleaning and need not to be worn during sleep.

David L. Jones

See also Anatomy of the Human Articulators; Cleft Lip and Palate: Speech Effects; Craniofacial Anomalies; Dysarthria; Nasalance and Nasometry; Nasality; Neurogenic Communication Disorders

Further Readings

Kummer, A. W. (2008). *Cleft palate and craniofacial anomalies* (2nd ed.). Clifton Park, NY: Thomson Delmar Learning.

Peterson-Falzone, S. J., Hardin-Jones, M. A., & Karnell, M. P. (2010). *Cleft palate speech* (4th ed.). St. Louis, MO: Mosby-Elsevier.

Whitehill, T. L., Lee, A. S. Y., & Chun, J. C. (2002). Direct magnitude estimation and interval scaling of hypernasality. *Journal of Speech, Language, and Hearing Research, 45*, 80–88.

Zajac, D. J., & Vallino, L. D. (2016). *Evaluation and management of cleft lip and palate: A developmental perspective*. San Diego, CA: Plural.

Response to Intervention (RtI)

Response to intervention (RtI), also referred to as *Multi-Tiered System of Supports*, is a framework intended both to support learners facing academic challenges and to select from among these students those who will be diagnosed as having a specific learning disability (SLD). This entry describes the origins of this model and the typical organizational structure and instructional protocols it employs. It also provides an overview of key research on the subject and a listing of challenges faced by this policy moving forward.

Historical Foundations

In the United States, the Individuals with Disabilities Education Act (IDEA), passed in 1975, was that country's first concerted, systematic effort to designate children as having SLDs. The process involved two steps: (1) a child was given a test designed to measure the intellectual ability and (2) he or she was given norm-referenced achievement tests. If assessments showed a significant discrepancy between results of the intelligence and the achievement tests (i.e., the student's estimated ability was shown to be substantially higher than his or her level of achievement), he or she would be designated as having a learning disability. If there were not a significant discrepancy, the student would be labeled what Keith Stanovich termed a *garden-variety* poor reader, the assumption being that the child was working up to capacity and would not benefit from special education services.

However, research ultimately offered two key findings. First, those students who failed to qualify as SLD were very similar to those so designated, and second, when provided with the same assistance, they made the same progress. This research called into question the use of the discrepancy formula to determine SLD status. In response, the 2004 reauthorization of IDEA (called the *Individuals with Disabilities Education Improvement Act*) recommended, although did not require, a different approach called *RtI*. Rather than employing assessments as key determinants of SLD, it was assumed that struggling students were not benefiting sufficiently from instruction. Under RtI, students received interventions of ever-increasing intensity until they achieved at an adequate rate. If these interventions failed to bring about this change, the student received a learning disability designation. In this way, it was the intent of RtI to both avoid a learning disability diagnosis and to provide a mechanism for such a determination, if ultimately needed. To facilitate the implementation of these prediagnosis interventions, school districts in the United States were allowed to use as much as 15% of their special education funding to serve non–special education students.

Structure of Interventions

Although the Individuals with Disabilities Education Improvement Act did not address the number or type of interventions expected, RtI is often described in terms of three or four tiers. One framework consists of the following tiers and assessments.

Tier 1 is strong, research-based core instruction in the regular classroom, including differentiated teaching within that setting as needed. It is expected that about 80% of students will succeed with Tier 1 instruction alone. A screening measure is given to all, or nearly all, students early in the school year to suggest which students might need Tier 2 support.

Tier 2 is small group instruction provided by the classroom teacher (above and beyond Tier 1) and/or by a specialist. An additional 15% of students should make sufficient progress given this Tier 2 support. Progress-monitoring assessments focused on specific curricular elements used in Tier 2 classes determine which students are doing well enough to leave Tier 2, which need to continue, and which would benefit from Tier 3 instruction.

Tier 3 occurs at a teacher/student ratio of about 1:1 or 1:2. The curriculum for this intervention is designed to reflect the very specific and individual needs of qualifying students and should raise to about 99%, the number of students who function successfully. The remaining 1% or so would then receive a SLD designation.

It should be noted that, even within school districts adopting much of the RtI model, there is a tendency to skip the intensive tutoring step. This practice is likely due to the cost of serving students with such a high teacher-to-student ratio. In this case, students are referred for special education assessment after they have received Tier 2 intervention; a discrepancy formula is once again used to determine SLD status, with special education resource room placement serving as Tier 3. A return to use of the discrepancy formula model undermines RtI principles and may result in students receiving services in an environment with a lower teacher-to-student ratio than they had received in Tier 2. This step backward is unfortunate because studies of U.S. students placed in resource room settings have shown that, on average, they make only minimally better progress than similar students who remain in the regular classroom. On the other hand, research is beginning to demonstrate that, when implemented with integrity, RtI programs typically lower the number of students enrolled in special education.

Instructional Protocols

There are two commonly used protocols for Tiers 2 and 3 instruction within the RtI framework. The first is the *standard treatment protocol*. In this model, curriculum is commonly scripted and administered with fidelity for a specified period of time. All children in need of assistance at a given grade level often receive the same intervention, whether or not the intervention is well suited to their individual needs (despite research findings showing that learners who struggle do so for different reasons and require different instruction). Commonly, standard treatment protocol interventions that address reading are oriented toward word recognition and decoding. Alternatively, they attempt to cover the full gamut of reading elements from phonemic awareness through comprehension, with minimal time spent on each. Due to the clear and straightforward character of standard treatment protocol interventions, they are often provided by noncertified staff.

The second is the *problem-solving protocol*. In this approach, students receive an individualized plan based on results from the screening assessment and in collaboration with school staff familiar with the child's learning profile. They are assigned to interventions that meet their particular needs. In reality, instruction in this model may also be highly standardized, although there is more differentiation from student to student. Despite the inherently individualized nature of Tier 3 expectations, standardized approaches are often found at this level as well.

RtI Research

As of 2017, there exists a relative dearth of research examining Tier 1 instruction. Key findings demonstrate, however, that employing a research-based curriculum is important, although not necessarily one of the scripted programs that are often selected. Setting aside uninterrupted blocks of time and increasing the amount of instruction provided in differentiated small groups is also beneficial, as is peer tutoring. Similarly, there is little research looking at Tier 3 interventions, and the available research generates more questions than answers. It is unclear just how different the content of Tier 3 instruction should be from that provided in Tier 2, and only one description of Tier 3 protocols is found in RtI research. It is also uncertain whether it is possible to predict early on whether some students are likely to need Tier 3 support and can fruitfully skip over less intensive interventions.

Most RtI research is concerned with instruction at Tier 2. This research shows that students can progress within programs based on differing theoretical frameworks. Needier students benefit more than those who are less far behind, and younger children are more likely to catch up with peers than are older students. The question of intensity remains unresolved. Some studies suggest that student make greater progress if they receive more lessons in a shorter period of time. Some studies, however, seem to demonstrate that double the amount of instruction in the same time period is no more beneficial than less intense interventions. Even when Tier 2 teaching emphasizes print-based skills, it is crucial to maintain a focus on meaning making so that the purpose of reading remains front and center.

Challenges for RtI Moving Forward

Although RtI is a promising approach to providing support for students who struggle, the framework faces a number of challenges moving forward.

One challenge is how educators address the fact that there remains a predominantly deficit-oriented view of the learner associated with this model. It is the intent of RtI to place responsibility for inadequate academic progress squarely in the court of instructional design, rather than blaming students for their failure. Nevertheless, it appears that students exhibit the same degree of shame and hopelessness within this model as has been the case with other intervention efforts.

Second is what adjustments should be made when supporting culturally and linguistically diverse students. It is crucial that schools communicate effectively with families and communities, viewing them as resources rather than roadblocks. Parents and other community members serve as links to what Norma Gonzalez and Luis Moll have termed *funds of knowledge*, information and practices children bring to school that can be drawn upon to support these learners.

A third challenge is determining what assessments are most useful in selecting students for levels of intervention, planning for instruction, and monitoring progress. Commonly, standardized assessments that measure only low-level skills are employed. However, informal measures, such as miscue analysis, provide rich data to inform instruction.

Fourth is how educators can adjust interventions that prove effective at younger ages to intervene with older children, and what an effective secondary-level program looks like. There are few studies examining middle and high school interventions. Those available demonstrate that students who have received this instruction, even at high rates of intensity and over long periods of time, rarely achieve at the level of their peers.

A fifth challenge is, given the personnel demands of a productive RtI approach, how school districts can best use limited resources. Classroom teachers provide Tier 1 instruction and can offer a Tier 2 program for some students. However, support staff, and certificated teachers whenever possible, are also needed. This is particularly true for Tier 3 tutoring, which requires a deeply sensitive and responsive teacher for the neediest students.

Finally, another challenge is how the RtI framework must adapt to the advent of more sophisticated standards, such as the Common Core State Standards adopted by most of the United States. Books and articles addressing Common Core State Standards say little about the needs of students who are already struggling, and the focus of Tier 2 and Tier 3 interventions has typically been on low-level skills. Integration of both policies is necessary to ensure student success.

In sum, RtI offers a better theorized and generally effective model for supporting students who struggle academically and, when necessary, for determining which students qualify for an SLD diagnosis. Interventions of ever-increasing intensity are provided for students who need assistance. This is accomplished using either a standard treatment protocol with clearly delineated instructional practices or a problem-solving protocol that appears to be more responsive to the needs of individual students. Additional research is required to demonstrate with clarity what the content and approach of curriculum should be. Districts face other challenges when implementing this design, including responding to linguistic and cultural differences, selecting appropriate assessments, effectively serving children across the age spectrum, addressing high-level standards, and using district resources effectively and efficiently.

Elizabeth L. Jaeger

See also Learning Disabilities; Reading and Reading Disorders; Special Education; Standardized Testing; Writing and Writing Disorders

Further Readings

Artiles, A. J. (2015). Beyond responsiveness to identity badges: Future research on culture in disability and implications for response to intervention. *Educational Review*, 67(1), 1–22.

Brozo, W. G. (2009/2010). Response to intervention or responsive instruction? Challenges and possibilities of response to intervention for adolescent literacy. *Journal of Adolescent and Adult Literacy*, 53(4), 277–281.

Fuchs, D., Fuchs, L. S., & Compton, D. L. (2012). Smart RTI: A next-generation approach to multi-level prevention. *Exceptional Children*, 78(3), 263–279.

Jaeger, E. L. (2017a). Learning through responsive and collaborative mediation in a tutoring context. *Australian Journal of Language and Literacy*, 40(3), 210–224.

Jaeger, E. L. (2017b). Implementation of Common Core-based curriculum in a fourth-grade literacy classroom: An exploratory study. *Reading Horizons*, 56(1), 45–68.

Jaeger, E. L. (in press). Bella here and there: Forming and re-forming identities across school contexts. *Reading and Writing Quarterly*

Jaeger, E. L. (2018). Bella here and there: Forming and re-forming identities across school contexts. *Reading and Writing Quarterly*, 34, 306–321.

Johnston, P. H. (2011). Response to intervention in literacy: Problems and possibilities. *Elementary School Journal*, 111(4), 511–534.

Orosco, M. J. (2010). A sociocultural examination of response to intervention with Latino English language learners. *Theory into Practice, 49*(4), 265–272.

Stephens, D., Cox, R., Downs, A., Goforth, J., Jaeger, L., Matheny, A., . . . Wilcox, C. (2012). I know there ain't no pigs with wigs: Challenges of Tier 2 intervention. *The Reading Teacher, 66*(2), 93–103.

van Kraayenoord, C. E. (2010). Response to intervention: New ways and wariness. *Reading Research Quarterly, 43*(3), 363–376.

Wixson, K. K., & Lipson, M. Y. (2012). Relations between the CCSS and RTI in literacy and language. *The Reading Teacher, 65*(6), 387–391.

RETROCOCHLEAR HEARING LOSS

Retrocochlear hearing loss, sometimes called *neural hearing loss*, is a type of sensorineural hearing loss characterized by normal inner ear structures but impaired propagation of neural signals from the inner ear to the central nervous system (CNS). Most commonly, retrocochlear hearing loss results from disorders of the cochlear nerve. Although distinct from cochlear hearing loss (also known as *sensory hearing loss*), both conditions may exist simultaneously. Audiological testing patterns may sometimes, but not always, distinguish between sensory (cochlear) hearing loss and neural (retrocochlear) hearing loss. The most common etiology of a retrocochlear hearing loss is a tumor involving the vestibulocochlear nerve. This entry discusses the diagnosis of retrocochlear hearing loss and the most common etiologies encountered.

Conductive and Sensorineural Hearing Losses

The human ear is a finely tuned organ that senses ambient pressure waves, termed *sound waves*. Sound is sensed when sound waves pass through the pinna of the ear and external auditory canal, vibrate the tympanic membrane, vibrate the middle ear ossicles, and propagate as fluid waves within the fluid of the inner ear. These fluid waves cause mechanical deflections in the hair cells of the cochlea of the inner ear, which transduce the mechanical signal into electrical signals that are relayed to the CNS along the auditory nerve.

Any derangement of the sound transmission pathway results in a hearing loss. When the transmission is interrupted at the outer or middle ear, the loss is termed a *conductive hearing loss*. If the inner ear is unable to sense the fluid waves or transduce them into electrical signals, a sensory, or cochlear, hearing loss results. If the neural impulses are unable to propagate to the CNS, or if the CNS is unable to process the impulses, the loss is termed a *neural*, or *retrocochlear*, *hearing loss*. Together, sensory (cochlear) and neural (retrocochlear) hearing losses are grouped into the broader entity of *sensorineural hearing losses*.

Hearing losses are diagnosed with audiometric testing. A full audiometric battery consists of pure-tone thresholds, speech reception thresholds, speech recognition testing, tympanometry, acoustic reflex testing, and otoacoustic emissions (a detailed description of the full audiometric battery is out of the scope of this entry). In the context of this entry, pure-tone threshold testing ascertains the sensitivity of the test ear to sinusoidal pressure waves. Pure-tone testing is performed both for *air conduction* (AC), which tests the entire auditory pathway, and for *bone conduction* (BC), which bypasses the tympanic membrane and ossicles and tests the inner ear and distal portion of the auditory pathway. Sensorineural hearing losses present with no or minimal difference between AC and BC thresholds.

Diagnosing Cochlear and Retrocochlear Hearing Losses

Once a sensorineural hearing loss has been diagnosed, distinguishing between a cochlear and retrocochlear hearing loss requires further testing. Otoacoustic emissions are sounds generated by the outer hair cells of the cochlea either spontaneously or in response to an auditory stimulus, and the absence of otoacoustic emission indicates a cochlear hearing loss. If a patient presents with a unilateral or an asymmetric sensorineural hearing loss, one must have a high level of suspicion for retrocochlear pathology. Additional testing is almost always mandated in such cases.

Auditory brainstem response testing is abnormal in patients with a retrocochlear hearing loss. When an auditory brainstem response is performed, auditory stimuli are presented to the ears, and scalp surface electrodes record the various neural responses to these stimuli. An increased latency of neural responses to the auditory stimulus signifies a retrocochlear hearing loss. Acoustic reflex testing, which quantifies the physiologic contraction of the stapedius muscle in response to loud auditory stimuli, is nonspecific and may be affected in cochlear, retrocochlear, and conductive hearing losses.

If a retrocochlear hearing loss is diagnosed, imaging is mandatory to rule out the presence of a tumor along the course of the auditory nerve. The most commonly utilized imaging study is magnetic resonance imaging with intravenous contrast, which will reveal a tumor, such as a vestibular schwannoma.

Vestibular Schwannomas

The most commonly diagnosed retrocochlear pathology is a *vestibular schwannoma* (also called an *acoustic neuroma*), a benign tumor arising from the Schwann cells of the superior or the inferior vestibular nerve. The superior and inferior vestibular nerves are two of the three components of the eighth cranial nerve, the vestibulocochlear nerve, the third part of which is the cochlear, or auditory, nerve.

The vestibulocochlear nerve arises from the brainstem and travels through a bony canal, the internal auditory canal (IAC), before reaching the cochlea and vestibule. It is accompanied within the IAC by the seventh cranial nerve, the facial nerve. A large portion of the vestibulocochlear nerve fibers is myelinated, owing to the presence of Schwann cells along the nerve, thus enhancing conduction of nerve impulses. A schwannoma is a benign tumor resulting from an abnormal proliferation of Schwann cells, and when schwannomas are found within the IAC, they arise almost exclusively from either the superior or inferior vestibular nerves, not the cochlear (auditory) or facial nerves.

Vestibular schwannomas occur unilaterally in the vast majority of cases, and their incidence has been estimated around one per 100,000 individuals per year. In patients with neurofibromatosis type 2 (NF2), however, bilateral vestibular schwannomas are present. NF2 results from mutations in the NF2 gene, which encodes for the protein merlin. In addition to bilateral vestibular schwannomas, patients affected by NF2 often present with additional neural tumors, such as meningiomas and spinal ependymomas.

As a vestibular schwannoma grows, it exerts pressure on the surrounding structures, including the cochlear nerve. Increasingly severe compression leads to inhibition of normal nerve conduction along the cochlear nerve, thus resulting in a progressive hearing loss. The facial nerve, which is a motor nerve that provides innervation to the muscles of the face, is more robust, and a similar degree of compression of the facial nerve usually does not result in facial weakness or paralysis.

Over time, an untreated vestibular schwannoma generally enlarges and fills the IAC. It then begins to grow outside of the IAC, into the cerebellopontine angle. If growth remains unchecked, a vestibular schwannoma can cause compression of the brainstem and ventricles, hydrocephalus, and death. Treatment is aimed at removal of the tumor via surgical resection or at arresting the growth of the tumor, as with stereotactic radiation therapy.

Other Causes of Retrocochlear Hearing Loss

Although tumors account for the majority of retrocochlear hearing losses, other conditions may present similarly. In pediatric patients, auditory neuropathy often presents as a congenital hearing loss. Although the etiology of auditory neuropathy is unclear, affected patients demonstrate a mild to profound hearing loss in the affected ear(s), and auditory brainstem response testing is abnormal.

In individuals with multiple sclerosis, demyelination in the CNS may cause derangements of neural conduction along the auditory pathway. Pathologic plaques are frequently seen on magnetic resonance imaging. A cerebrovascular accident, also called a *stroke*, may similarly cause impaired neural conduction and result in a hearing loss. Finally, impingement of the cochleovestibular nerve by a vascular structure, such as a cerebellar artery, a vertebral artery, or the basilar artery, may cause hearing loss in certain cases. Treatment is directed at addressing the underlying pathology.

Kevin A. Peng and Eric P. Wilkinson

See also Anatomy of the Hearing Mechanism and Central Audiology Nervous System; Auditory Neuropathy Spectrum Disorder; Cochlear Hearing Loss; Hearing Disability and Disorders; Hearing Tests; Noise-Induced Hearing Loss and Its Prevention; Physiological Basis for Hearing

Further Readings

Brackmann, D., Shelton, C., & Arriaga, M. A. (2015). *Otologic surgery*. Elsevier Health Sciences. Amsterdam, Netherlands.

Cueva, R. A. (2004). Auditory brainstem response versus magnetic resonance imaging for the evaluation of asymmetric sensorineural hearing loss. *The Laryngoscope, 114*(10), 1686–1692.

Hirsch, B. E., Durrant, J. D., Yetiser, S., Kamerer, D. B., & Martin, W. H. (1996). Localizing retrocochlear hearing loss. *Otology & Neurotology, 17*(4), 537–546.

House, J. W., & Brackmann, D. E. (1979). Brainstem audiometry in neurotologic diagnosis. *Archives of Otolaryngology, 105*(6), 305–309.

Ruckenstein, M. J., Cueva, R. A., Morrison, D. H., & Press, G. (1996). A prospective study of ABR and MRI in the screening for vestibular schwannomas. *Otology & Neurotology, 17*(2), 317–320.

REVALUING READING

Revaluing involves renegotiating and repositioning readers' literacy perceptions and beliefs, ultimately reconstructing readers' literacy identities. Ken Goodman conceived the term *revaluing* to counter deficit-based notions of *fixing* problems or remediating readers. Revaluing is identifying and recognizing language strengths in reading and valuing personal abilities to learn. Revaluing supports readers in shifting toward a view of reading that emphasizes understanding and the construction of meaning. This entry emphasizes the need to shift from traditional notions of medical remediation and deficiencies of the reader to focusing on the value a reader attributes to both the reading process and their ability as a reader.

Common-sense beliefs about reading focus on word recognition and phonics and may overemphasize fluency and error proofreading. Young readers are caught in an internal conflict as they attempt to construct meaning during reading, while also preoccupied with word accuracy. Readers can become overly concerned with trying to achieve word accuracy. They can become victims of an unbalanced and decontextualized skills approach to reading. Dynamic Indicator of Basic Early Literacy Skills and timed reading assessments that focus on word accuracy and speed undermine literacy and may penalize readers for taking necessary time to construct meaning while they read. Students can become frustrated and depressed and may resent both reading and school. A reader identified as vulnerable may work hard with limited strategies, such as sounding out, as a result of overemphasis on decoding. As readers gain new insights into reading as meaning making, they develop awareness of various meaning-making strategies and language cueing systems. Readers navigating texts confidently decide for themselves which strategies they need to construct meaning.

Opportunities to Revalue

Semiotics is the study of meaning making and the way meaning is conceptualized. According to Charles Peirce, shifting conceptualizations or beliefs require an element of doubt, or else unchallenged perceptions remain indefinitely. Once doubt enters the mind, an individual imagines and contemplates the thought and seeks to work out its relevance as new opportunities and experiences occur that either validate or contradict new thinking. In this way, an individual is prepared to test new ideas and thinking. Beliefs (or habits, as Peirce prefers) position individuals toward action and vice versa. Actions further mediate thinking in a process of infinite semiosis. Klaus Jensen defines belief from the perspective of a semiotician as readiness to engage and to act. Similarly, the work of Yetta Goodman, Dorothy Watson, and Carolyn Burke further discusses ways in which literacy beliefs position readers toward literacy.

By means of experiences that cause readers to doubt the value of word accuracy during reading, individuals begin to revalue reading as meaning making. It isn't enough to simply teach that reading is comprehending. Readers must determine it for themselves.

Ken Goodman and Yetta Goodman's work and research in miscue analysis and retrospective miscue analysis (RMA) support revaluing traditional word-focused views. A *miscue* occurs when what is read is different than the expected reading. As individuals construct meaning during reading, they use cues to make predictions, which are reflected in their miscues. Through RMA, readers examine their own miscues and talk about them. Readers engaging in RMA examine their own meaning-making processes at work and take ownership of the reading process as they self-monitor and self-correct in efforts to make sense. Readers view themselves as resourceful and competent meaning makers and, hence, good readers.

This comprehensive model of reading explains how readers begin observing miscues everywhere in the world. As they reflect, challenge, and doubt conceptions that reading is about word accuracy, they shift toward a meaning-making model of reading.

Revaluing Leads to Shifts in Reading Behavior

Confidence during reading is required for revaluing. As a result of understanding and valuing how personal experiences and background knowledge support reading, identifying personal strengths as a reader, and seeing the good things individuals do during reading, readers come to see that miscues are a natural part of the reading process. They shed deficit views of themselves as readers and develop confidence in their reading. The more comfortable people are during reading, the more willing and successful they will be promoting and extending their own reading abilities. Figure 1 illustrates this cycle of revaluing and the importance of reader confidence.

A Case Study of Revaluing: "Well, It's Usually Easy for Other Kids But It's Not Easy for Me"

Wyatt was a vulnerable 8-year-old, third-grade reader. He was labeled with a specific learning disability in reading by the school and falling far below school standards. During out-of-school tutoring at the start of third grade with Kelly Murphy, Wyatt was given a Burke Reading Interview used to identify readers' perceptions and attitudes. The following dialogue occurred during this interview:

Kelly: When you are reading and you come to something you don't know, what do you do?

Wyatt: I try to . . . skip the word and start reading it again . . . I go read it again . . . until I can figure out the word.

Kelly: How did you learn to read?

Wyatt: I still don't know how to read.

Kelly: Do you think you are a good reader?

Wyatt: No . . . because everybody in my whole class says I'm not . . . especially on the reading tests.

Kelly: Tell me about the reading tests.

Wyatt: Well, it's usually easy for other kids but it's not easy for me.

Wyatt's responses indicated a word-focused view of reading and poor perception of himself as a reader and of his reading. Wyatt was regularly timed during reading, and according to his school, he read 34 words per minute (wpm) at the start of third grade. The goal for readers was arbitrarily set at 100 wpm by end of third grade. Wyatt knew exactly how many words he read per minute and was unhappy with his score. His mother was concerned about his reading and about his diminishing self-concepts as a learner.

Initially in tutoring outside of school, Wyatt resisted reading. When he did read, it was for speed, appearing less concerned with making sense, which was possibly a product of the pressure he felt to increase his wpm score. Though

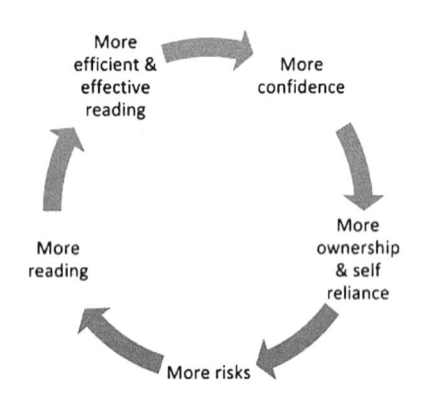

Figure 1 Revaluing cycle

Source: Adapted from Goodman and Marek (1996, p. 206).

reluctant and hesitant to read at the beginning of the school year, language experience provided Wyatt with a safe place to explore his own process of literacy as he orally self-authored stories about his dog. Wyatt's own stories served as a segue to other texts and tutoring activities, including RMA.

Wyatt was excited and willing to tell stories, read them, and study and reflect on his miscues. Through RMA conversations, Wyatt moved away from preexisting word-focused views of reading and found ways to construct meaning. Wyatt evaluated his own miscues in terms of their quality and came to see miscues as part of the reading process.

Throughout the school year, Wyatt revalued reading: the ways he conceptualized reading and his own reading ability. Wyatt began to appreciate himself as a meaning maker and, hence, a reader. As he became more efficient in constructing meaning, his fluency improved. Wyatt's wpm score doubled over the course of the school year, from 34 to 75.

During another Burke Reading Interview during tutoring toward the end of third grade, the following exchange took place:

Kelly: How did you learn to read?

Wyatt: My mind helped me learn how to read.

Kelly: Do you think you are a good reader?

Wyatt: Yes, I do think I am a good reader.

Kelly: Do you know you are a good reader?

Wyatt: Yes!

The interview was filled with tangents about a book Wyatt read about the Underground Railroad and a young child hiding in a cornfield, a *Minecraft* book Wyatt borrowed from a friend at school, and a new story he wanted to tell as part of language experience during tutoring. Wyatt was excited to talk about books; excited to author more language experience stories; and willing to engage in reading experiences where he felt safe, comfortable, and successful. Tutoring experiences avoided deficit-based approaches to reading instruction and honed in on positive meaning-making strategies that Wyatt could connect with. As Wyatt took risks and opened himself up to the study of his own reading and those positive things he already did while reading, his new insights into the reading process supported him in challenging and renegotiating his negative self-perceptions as a reader. Wyatt was revaluing his reading and himself as a reader.

Revaluing is not instructing readers to read differently. Revaluing is about empowering readers to become aware of what readers do when they read. Revaluing is about helping people take ownership of their own reading by relying on their own meaning maker—their brain—to comprehend. In the process of revaluing the reading process, individuals revalue themselves as readers.

Kelly Allen Murphy and Ken S. Goodman

See also Metacognition; Metalinguistics; Miscue Analysis; Reading and Reading Disorders; Reading Fluency; Response to Intervention (RtI); Scientific Realism; Skills Versus Strategies

Further Readings

Goodman, K. (1967). Reading: A psycholinguistic guessing game. *Journal of the Reading Specialist, 6*(4), 126–135.

Goodman, K. (2014). Revaluing readers and reading. In K. Goodman & Y. Goodman (Eds.), *Making sense of learners making sense of written language: The selected works of Kenneth S. Goodman and Yetta M. Goodman* (pp. 189–196). New York, NY: Routledge.

Goodman, K., & Goodman, Y. (2011). Learning to read: A comprehensive model. In R. Meyer & K. Whitmore (Eds.), *Reclaiming reading: Teachers, students and researchers regaining spaces for thinking and action* (pp. 19–41). New York, NY: Taylor & Francis.

Goodman, Y. (1999). Retrospective miscue analysis: Illuminating the voice of the reader. In A. Marek & C. Edelsky (Eds.), *Reflections and connections: Essays in honor of Kenneth S. Goodman's influence on language education* (pp. 311–331). Cresskill, NH: Hampton Press.

Goodman, Y., Flurkey, A., & Martens, P. (2014). *Retrospective miscue analysis: A window into readers' thinking*. Katonah, NY: Richard C. Owen.

Goodman, Y., & Goodman, K. (2014). To err is human: Learning about language processes by analyzing miscues. In K. Goodman & Y. Goodman (Eds.), *Making sense of learners making sense of written language: The selected works of Kenneth S. Goodman and Yetta M. Goodman* (pp. 115–134). New York, NY: Routledge.

Goodman, Y., & Marek, A. (1996). Revaluing readers and reading. In Y. Goodman & A. Marek (Eds.), *Retrospective miscue analysis: Revaluing readers and reading* (pp. 203–207). Katonah, NY: Richard C. Owen Publishers.

Goodman, Y., Watson, D., & Burke, C. (2005). *Reading miscue inventory: From evaluation to instruction.* Katonah, NY: Richard C. Owen.

Pearson, D. (2006). Foreword. In K. Goodman (Ed.), *The truth about DIBELS: What it is, what it does* (pp. 40–49). Portsmouth, NH: Heinemann.

Savan, D. (1988). *An introduction to C.S. Peirce's full system of semeiotic.* Toronto, Canada: Toronto Semiotic Circle.

Right Hemisphere Cognitive–Communication Disorders

The right side of the brain, although traditionally considered nondominant for language, plays an important role in communication. Damage to the right cerebral hemisphere in adulthood can result in a variety of communication and other cognitive deficits, although there is substantial heterogeneity in the presentation of deficits across individuals. Cognitive deficits typically impact attention and executive functions. Communication disorders can impact speech, language, and/or pragmatics, which is the social use of language for communication.

There is no single commonly accepted label for the deficits associated with right hemisphere damage (RHD). In this entry, the term *cognitive–communication deficits* will be used. Approximately, 50% of all individuals with damage to the right cerebral hemisphere will exhibit some deficits. Of those patients who are admitted to an inpatient rehabilitation unit, the prevalence is greater than 80%. There are few predictable patterns of co-occurrence of the various deficits, resulting in substantial heterogeneity across patients.

RHD can be caused by stroke, tumors, or traumatic brain injury. Strokes affecting the right cerebral hemisphere occur at nearly the same frequency as those in the left hemisphere; however, compared to those with left hemisphere strokes, individuals with RHD are less likely to arrive at a hospital in time to receive state-of-the-art medical treatments, more likely to have larger lesions, and less likely to receive rehabilitation for subsequent cognitive–communication deficits.

History

Descriptions of cognitive and communication deficits associated with RHD appeared in the 1940s, beginning with visuoperception and visuoconstruction impairments. This was followed by descriptions of difficulties with the expression and comprehension of emotions and emotional language. Research from the 1970s and 1980s supported the idea that deficits lie in complex language processes, such as understanding the gist or theme of a story; interpreting nonliteral language, humor, or abstract meanings; and understanding intended meaning. Production was characterized as tangential, overpersonalized, and poorly organized. The descriptive studies paved the way for the development of theories of underlying deficits in the 1990s. Empirical studies of treatments for the RHD deficits began to appear in the late 2000s. To date, there remains a critical need for more treatment research to provide evidence of the efficacy of proposed treatments.

Cognitive Disorders

Cognitive disorders include disorders of attention, memory, and executive function (e.g., planning, reasoning, problem solving, and awareness).

Attention and Neglect

Attentional deficits can affect focused, sustained, alternating, or divided attention. In addition to these general attentional deficits is unilateral neglect. Neglect is a deficit of directed attention in which sensory stimuli on the opposite side of the brain injury are not fully processed. While either side can be affected, left neglect due to RHD is more common and more likely to persist into the chronic stages than right neglect after left hemisphere brain damage.

Neglect can affect visual, auditory, and tactile modalities. Individuals with neglect will act as if they cannot see (visual), hear (auditory), or feel (tactile) stimuli on the side opposite of the brain damage. Importantly, the deficit is not in the sensory pathways or initial cortical processing but in attending to and consciously processing those sensory signals. Motor neglect also can occur, in which a patient does not use one side of the body to the extent possible. For example, someone with left motor neglect may try to screw a cap onto a tube of toothpaste using only the right hand instead of both the hands.

The most common and most well understood form of neglect is visuospatial neglect. It affects approximately 25% of individuals with RHD but often spontaneously recovers within the first days or weeks poststroke. While the visual pathways to the cortex are intact and visual images are processed in the occipital lobe, the cerebral damage reduces attention to the left side of space. There are multiple forms of neglect defined by what region of space is affected. Personal neglect refers to neglect of one's own body, in which the left side of the body is not dressed or groomed. Peri-personal neglect affects the region of space within an arm's reach and is generally assessed through paper/pencil tasks. Extrapersonal neglect involves the space beyond an arm's reach. Individuals with extrapersonal neglect may have difficulty with navigation (e.g., bumping into doorframes on the left). These three forms of neglect are dissociable and may co-occur in any combination. Two additional forms of neglect are viewer-centered (egocentric) and object- or stimulus-centered (allocentric). Viewer-centered neglect affects the region of space defined by the visual field, such that the left side is defined as the region to the left of the patient's midline. In stimulus-centered neglect, the left side of individual items is neglected, regardless of where they lie within the visual field. The most commonly diagnosed type of neglect is viewer-centered peri-personal neglect; however, this is also the form most often assessed, likely resulting in an overrepresentation of this type compared to the others.

Memory and Executive Functions

Memory and executive function deficits associated with RHD are less well studied and understood. Memory deficits generally impair working memory or the ability to simultaneously store and process information. Executive function deficits can occur in planning, organizing, reasoning, and problem solving. One of the most striking cognitive disorders is anosognosia or reduced awareness of deficits. Individuals may not be completely aware of their motor, sensory, communication, or cognitive deficits. Anosognosia for neglect is common. Some individuals may be able to acknowledge deficits but may not fully understand the implications of them. For example, even if a patient can report that he/she has left hemiparesis, he/she may not understand that the hemiparesis will affect her ability to drive.

Communication Disorders

Communication disorders can affect speech, language, and pragmatics. As with all of the disorders described thus far, not everyone with RHD will exhibit the same deficits, and the patterns of co-occurrence are unpredictable.

Speech Disorders

Aprosodia is a deficit in the production (expressive aprosodia) and/or comprehension (receptive aprosodia) of prosodic contours. Prosody refers to the melody of speech and the use of intonation to express intent and emotion. Linguistic prosody is used to mark phrase boundaries, to emphasize important words or phrases, and to differentiate types of utterances, such as statements versus questions. Emotional prosody conveys a person's mood or emotional state. Expressive aprosodia is characterized by limited intonation, resulting in *flat* or monotone-sounding speech. Individuals with receptive aprosodia will have difficulty interpreting emotion or intent expressed through intonation or tone of voice.

Language Disorders

Expressive language disorders may take the form of extremes of quantity (verbosity or paucity of speech), disorganization, overpersonalization, and tangentiality. Comprehension deficits affect the ability to integrate and synthesize multiple sentences. Problems also can occur in understanding the intent of a statement when there is more than one possible interpretation, such as understanding the contextually appropriate meaning of idioms, metaphors, jokes, or sarcasm.

Pragmatic Disorders

Deficits in pragmatics are considered by some to be the defining characteristic of RHD. Communicative interactions may be awkward, inefficient, or somewhat inappropriate. Some of the problems may be linked to difficulty interpreting nonverbal communication such as facial expressions or body language. Others can be associated with language and cognitive deficits. For example, comprehension deficits can cause misinterpretations of a speaker's intent or the gist of a story or conversation. Memory and problem-solving deficits can make it difficult to follow conversations with multiple people contributing or figure out how to fix a communication breakdown. Expressive deficits affecting quantity, organization, and content influence the effectiveness and efficiency of communication.

Theories of Communication Disorders

There are several theories of underlying language-processing deficits that impact general comprehension. Connie Tompkins's *suppression deficit* hypothesis posits that RHD can cause inefficiency in suppression of competing meanings of ambiguous words or phrases and that the degree of inefficiency is associated with the degree of discourse comprehension problems. When confronted with an ambiguous word (e.g., *organ*), normal language processes activate multiple meanings of that word (musical instrument and body part) and quickly suppress the meaning that is not supported by the context. For example, in the sentence "He transplanted the organ," initially both meanings of *organ* would be activated, but the musical instrument meaning would quickly be suppressed based on the contextual bias. This suppression process is slow or inefficient in some adults with RHD, and the inefficiency is related to general comprehension ability.

A second explanation is Mark Beeman's *coarse coding* hypothesis. According to the model, the intact left hemisphere quickly activates and selects the most common or relevant meanings and features of words. The right hemisphere, in contrast, more *coarsely* codes the language stimuli and weakly activates many meanings and features, including some that are only distantly related to the core meaning. For example, in the left hemisphere, the word *apple* would activate meanings such as *fruit, red, crunchy,* and *tree*. In the right hemisphere, additional features such as *green, healthy,* and *rotten* might be activated. The right hemisphere processing is presumed to be critical for generation of inferences and interpretation of less-common or nonliteral meanings. The hypothesis suggests that RHD impairs the coarse coding function of the right hemisphere, resulting in overly literal language comprehension and deficits in inference generation. This explanation has been widely used to explain both normal right hemisphere language processes and RHD comprehension deficits, although not all studies report strong relationships between coarse coding function and discourse comprehension.

A third theory, suggested by Francesca Happe and colleagues, is that RHD impairs *theory of mind* or the ability to understand that other people have knowledge, beliefs, and points of view that differ from one's own. Deficits in theory of mind result in problems understanding others' beliefs and actions. Theory of mind is a complex ability, and complex tasks are required to assess it. Thus, it is not clear whether RHD specifically impairs theory of mind, or if poor performance on the tasks is related to complexity of the tasks themselves.

A final explanation of the communication disorders is that there is a problem in using contextual cues. This explanation appeared in much of the work in the 1980s and was first described as a source of broader communication disorders by Penny Myers in her *inference failure* hypothesis. More research is needed to systematically test the idea, but converging evidence suggests that adults with RHD benefit from multiple strong contextual cues that consistently support a single interpretation. Difficulties arise, however, when multiple disparate cues must be integrated to generate a single interpretation.

These various hypotheses are not necessarily exclusive, and some evidence suggests that they can co-occur and possibly interact. For example, coarse coding and suppression deficits have been found to co-occur. Additionally, difficulties integrating multiple contextual cues may be related to inefficient suppression processes.

Assessment and Treatment

Assessment of cognitive–communication disorders typically involves a mixture of standardized and informal tasks and observations. The majority of treatments for the communication disorders are symptom based, such as working on interpretation of idioms and metaphors instead of focusing on the underlying impairments, such as suppression and coarse coding. Much work is needed to develop valid, sensitive measures for assessment and treatments that improve underlying deficits, which will result in broad improvements in communication.

Margaret Lehman Blake

See also Aphasia; Cognition; Executive Function and Communication; Pragmatics; Prosodic Disorders

Further Readings

Blake, M. L. (2016). Cognitive communication disorders associated with right hemisphere brain damage. In M. L. Kimbarow (Ed.), *Cognitive communication disorders* (2nd ed.). Plural.

Blake, M. L., Duffy, J. R., Myers, P. S., & Tompkins, C. A. (2002). Prevalence and patterns of right hemisphere cognitive/communicative deficits: Retrospective data from an inpatient rehabilitation unit. *Aphasiology, 16,* 537–548.

Blake, M. L., Frymark, T., & Venedikov, R. (2013). An evidence-based systematic review on communication treatments for individuals with right hemisphere brain damage. San Diego, CA. *American Journal of Speech-Language Pathology, 22,* 146–160. doi:10.1044/1058-0360 (2012/12–0021)

Tompkins, C. A., Klepousniotou, E., & Gibbs Scott, A. (2012). Nature and assessment of right hemisphere disorders. In I. Papathanasiou, P. Coppens, & C. Potagas (Eds.), *Aphasia and related neurogenic communication disorders* (pp. 297–343). Sudbury, MA: Jones & Bartlett.

Room Acoustics

Room acoustics is concerned with the behavior of sound generated within an enclosure. The basic influence on sound due to the enclosure is to generate many *sound reflections*: A large, plane, hard surface will produce a mirrorlike reflection of sound. The number of reflections we might be dealing with is considerable: An audience member in a large theater space receives about 40,000 reflections in the first second after the first sound arrives at the listener's ears. After this first second, sound rays in the theater have experienced about 45 reflections. Another significant complication is that not all surfaces are flat; a bumpy surface will produce an impure reflection that is somewhat scattered. Comparison with behavior for light is instructive: Pure reflection occurs with a mirror; a scattered reflection comes from a matte white surface. The difference, compared with sound, is related to the roughness of the surface at the scale of wavelength for light.

A surface that reflects sound is generally *hard*; reflective materials include stone, brick, plaster, thick timber, and glass. As for light, many surfaces are of course not white and reflective; a black surface, for example, will absorb most of the light falling on it. Analogous to a black surface, sound-absorbing surfaces are porous and thick, which is effective at most frequencies. Sound-absorbing surfaces include upholstery, curtains, and carpets, while the most efficient absorbing materials are mineral wool, fiberglass, and acoustic open-cell foam. Many proprietary materials for acoustic absorption are available. Often, most surfaces in rooms are hard and reflect sound; people, however, absorb sound because of their clothing, which is why an occupied room will sound different than an empty one. To continue the visual analogy, light reflections usually involve color, and in acoustic terms, some frequencies are absorbed more than others. For example, porous absorbers are usually efficient at high frequencies and become progressively less so at lower frequencies. Thicker porous absorbers (e.g., 50 mm or more) are more effective at low frequencies than thinner absorbers; 25 mm is normally considered the minimum worthwhile thickness. As outlined in the following sections, introduction of sound absorbers on room boundaries is the most common acoustic intervention in practice, though not in large single-use auditoria.

To understand the behavior of sound in rooms, it is also important to take account of the ways in which our ears interpret what they hear. There is clear evidence that our ears have adapted to sound in enclosures, in particular our ability to determine the location of a single source of sound, what is known as *localization*, in spite of all the reflections we receive coming from all directions.

What Our Ears Hear in a Room

Figure 1 shows a simplified representation, known as an *impulse response*, of what a listener receives in time for a brief sound emitted from a single source. The first element is the direct sound, which travels directly from the source to the listener and drops off in amplitude with distance. In a room intended for communicating speech or music, one aims to have good sight lines, which will also guarantee good propagation of the direct sound. The direct sound is followed by first reflections, which come from the floor, walls, or ceiling; they arrive later because they have had to travel greater distances than the direct sound. These reflections have been found to be important since they enhance speech intelligibility or clarity with music. Subsequently, the number of reflections increases, though their individual strength decreases because they have had to travel farther and have been influenced by absorption at some surfaces included in their paths.

It turns out that the most important component of what is received by the listener concerns the later section. When reflection energies are averaged, the decay of sound pressure in the later section follows an exponential curve; however, when converted into decibels (dB), this decay *becomes* linear. The slope of the decibel decay is the crucial parameter, expressed in terms of the duration for a 60-dB reduction, which is known as the *reverberation time* (RT), measured in seconds. The choice of 60 dB is based on the approximate time during which a decay can be heard; this allows estimation of the RT in a cathedral-type space, for instance, where the RT can be 4–12 s. Shorter RTs, as say in a classroom, cannot be heard explicitly but the effects of reverberation can still be appreciated. For good speech transmission, an RT of 1 s or less is appropriate. For a large concert hall, the goal is normally around 2 s.

In 1900, a lecturer at Harvard University, W. C. Sabine, investigated reverberation and proposed an equation now named after him: the Sabine equation. This states that the RT is proportional to the ratio between the volume (V) of the space and the total amount of acoustic absorption. Absorption of a material is quantified by a coefficient, taking values between 0 and 1, the latter referring to 100% absorption. The total acoustic absorption is calculated by considering all room surfaces and summing the product of the area (S) and absorption coefficient (α) for each surface. Thus,

$$RT = \frac{0.16 V}{\Sigma S \alpha} s.$$

The constant here assumes volumes and areas are in meters. Sabine's equation is still used regularly today. However, one requirement for accuracy with the equation is that sound during the decay is traveling with equal probability in all directions, in what is known as a *diffuse space*. A sports hall is an example, where this may not be the case (see section Small Halls).

The RT of a room varies with frequency but is generally quoted as the value at midfrequencies (the mean value at 500 and 1000 Hz). In many cases, the RT at low frequencies (such as 125 Hz) should also be considered. Frequently in practice, the ceiling height is important for the actual RT, for reasons linked to the Sabine equation.

A second concern in many rooms is the loudness or amplitude of sound. The direct sound is not of course influenced by the enclosure and decreases 6 dB per doubling of distance.

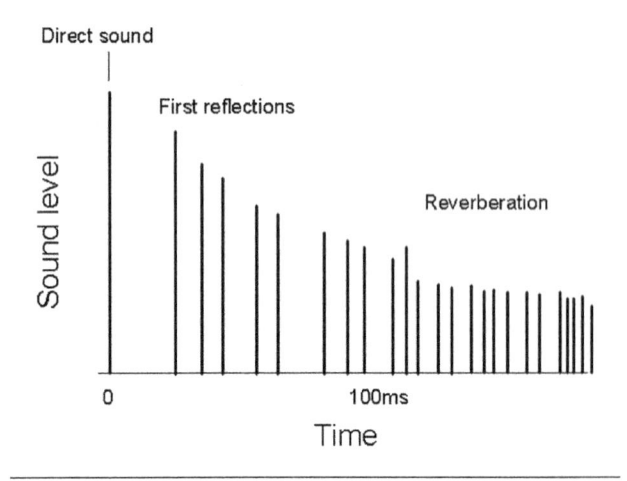

Figure 1 The time sequence of sound received by a listener in a room with a source emitting a brief sound, known as the *impulse response*

Source: Author.

The presence of the enclosure means that the loudness does not decrease so much with distance, which can be valuable to allow "people to hear at the back." There are thus two components contributing to the overall loudness: the direct sound and the reflected, room sound. The magnitude of the room sound is influenced by the total amount of absorption in the room. The more absorption it contains, the quieter the room sound will be; larger rooms often have more absorption in them and are hence quieter. In reality, certain spaces may be perceived as too quiet and certain spaces too loud.

Different rooms have different acoustic priorities. In the past, the RT value for each room type has been the dominant concern; in several room types, however, a more sophisticated approach is appropriate. The optimum acoustic criteria for a space are either based on providing a pleasant acoustic environment or controlling communication of speech or music. A suitable background noise level (e.g., due to assisted ventilation) is an additional requirement and is outside the scope of this entry.

Circulation Spaces

Circulation spaces containing significant amounts of acoustic absorption have a more relaxing character, whether they be atria, corridors, or spaces in between. Recommendations for school circulation spaces may include sound absorption to create a more calming environment.

Classrooms

The acoustic treatment of classrooms is required to create a calm atmosphere and allow easy communication between teachers and students. This can be achieved by introduction of large areas of sound-absorbing material.

Many countries have regulations concerning school acoustics. To conform to requirements, classroom ceilings are generally made fully sound absorbing, though some additional absorption on the walls is often required. Carpets on floors are also desirable. Regulations often specify midfrequency RTs, such as in Britain a maximum RT of 0.8 s for secondary classrooms and 0.6 s for primary schools. For hearing-impaired students, an even shorter maximum value of 0.4 s is stipulated.

Acoustically absorbent pinboard is an option for walls without losing usable area. Acoustic requirements for open-plan classrooms tend to be more demanding compared with the conventional seated arrangement.

Lecture Rooms

Lecture rooms have the acoustic benefit that the lecturer is mostly facing the audience, which allows for much higher numbers of audience and lesser requirements for acoustic absorption. The room should not have ceilings higher than what makes sense from a visual perspective. Contrary to classrooms, in lecture rooms of moderate to large size, the front portion of the ceiling should be made reflective (with a hard surface) to preserve an early sound reflection, which will enhance speech intelligibility. A midfrequency RT of less than 0.8 s is recommended; for larger lecture rooms, a limit of 1 s can be applied. Some low-frequency absorption is also suggested to avoid *boomy* conditions that can be detrimental to speech.

For lecture halls holding more than 50 people, a raked (i.e., angled) floor is preferred both for visual and acoustic reasons. In more formal spaces, placing speakers on a platform will assist speech propagation. Sound-absorbing treatment is often placed on the rear wall opposite the speaker.

Small Halls

School assembly spaces and similar public halls are often multipurpose, and the acoustic requirements would ideally vary depending on usage. Optimum conditions are different for speech and music, a space with a longer RT being favored for music. In either case, modestly absorbing (that is upholstered) seating is recommended to limit the change of RT with occupancy.

If the hall is also used as a gymnasium or for indoor sports, the seating will be cleared away yet some control of reverberation is still necessary. It is common to have hard (nonabsorbing) surfaces at person level, but this creates a nondiffuse space (sound bounces principally between low vertical surfaces), which will result in a long effective RT. Sound-absorbing treatment able to withstand physical impacts is available and should be used for low-level walls to control this.

To return to the conflicting requirements for speech and music, the former normally takes precedence, leading to recommended RTs at midfrequencies in the range 0.8–1.2 s. Again, a significant rise in low-frequency RT is to be avoided by using low-frequency absorption. It is important not to have curved concave room surfaces, which can cause undesirable focusing.

Large Halls—Auditoria

At the large scale, acoustic requirements become more demanding. For speech, the principal issue is good speech intelligibility, with drama theaters a main example. For music, there are several more criteria beyond RT, relating for instance to the need for musical clarity and the sense of being involved with the performance, what is often called *acoustical intimacy*. With large audience numbers, it is important to maintain sufficient loudness for the speech or music, which means that, beyond the inevitable absorption provided by the audience and performers or their seating, there should be little added absorbing treatment. Since RT remains important (slightly below 1 s for speech and approaching 2 s for music), the Sabine equation indicates the need to carefully consider the overall volume and probably the ceiling height. A rise in low-frequency RT is advantageous for music but not for speech.

Design in plan should begin with the stage, sized to accommodate the required number of performers. For drama, several stage–audience relationships exist, from proscenium theaters to the opposite extreme of theater-in-the-round. An important concern for drama is that the human speaker radiates sound directionally; more sound is emitted forward than backward. An early acoustic reflection, generally from the ceiling, often helps intelligibility. Theater-in-the-round is particularly demanding acoustically, allowing for smaller maximum audience numbers for this configuration of around 700 maximum. Shorter RTs also help in this case (0.8 rather than 1 s).

Raked seating is much to be preferred for all auditoria. Concert halls are generally either end-on, with the stage at one end, or surround halls, with some audience to the side and behind the stage. Balconies for all auditoria should not have too many rows of seating below them.

Audiology Spaces

Spaces to test individual hearing require a particularly low amount of room sound plus very quiet conditions with inaudible background noise. Special construction may be needed to control noise from neighboring spaces within the same building. Maximum RTs of 0.25 s are specified, which should be achievable with highly sound-absorbing walls and ceiling. Where tests involve loudspeakers, a minimum floor area of 8–9 m^2 is appropriate. More detailed information is available from relevant authoritative sources.

Concluding Remarks

It is a common observation that in small domestic spaces, the acoustics often looks after itself. This comes about because the acoustics of small spaces tend to be less critical, and there is inevitable absorbing material included: carpets, seating, sofas, books, and so on. In public spaces, this convenience will often not exist, requiring acoustic intervention. In larger spaces, there is often a good case for engaging a competent acoustic consultant; experience of a similar building type is usually valuable.

Mike Barron

See also Acoustics; Audiology; Decibel; Intelligibility

Further Readings

(2015, November). *Acoustics of schools: A design guide*. St. Albans, UK: Institute of Acoustics/Croydon, UK: Association of noise consultants [Online]. Retrieved August 2017 from http://www.association-of-noise-consultants.co.uk/wp-content/uploads/2015/11/Acoustics-of-Schools-a-design-guide-November-2015.pdf

Barron, M. (2010). *Auditorium acoustics and architectural design* (2nd ed.). London, UK: Spon Press.

BB93: acoustic design of schools—Performance standards. UK: Department of Education [Online]. Retrieved August 2017, from https://www.gov.uk/government/publications/bb93-acoustic-design-of-schools-performance-standards

RULE-GOVERNED ALTERNATIONS

The term *rule-governed alternations* is used to describe variations in language based on predictable patterns. This entry describes alternations that occur in adult forms of English and in the speech of children acquiring English. In phonology and morphology, many alternations in pronunciation are associated with particular phonetic conditions. For example, to create a plural noun in English, *s* is added to the singular form, as in cats (from cat), dogs (from dog), and bees (from bee). This description works for written forms but does not reflect variations in pronunciation. There are, in fact, three pronunciations of the plural: [s], [z], and [əz], determined by the phonetic features of the segment preceding the plural marker:

(1) When the singular form ends in an affricate /tʃ dʒ/ or a palatal or alveolar fricative /s z ʃ ʒ/, the plural ending is /əz/.

(2) When the singular form ends in a voiceless consonant, other than those listed in (1), the plural ending is /s/.

(3) When the singular form ends in a vowel or a voiced consonant other than those listed in (1), the plural ending is /z/.

Rule-governed alternations also occur in child speech whereby a segment varies from correct (i.e., adultlike) to incorrect as children acquire the phonology of their language. Examples of phonetically conditioned changes in child speech related to word position, neighboring segments, and/or stress placement are provided subsequently.

In terms of word position, there are two common alternations, both based on voicing. *Voiceless aspirated stops* in word-initial position are produced without aspiration, or with very little aspiration, and are perceived as their voiced cognate. Thus, the word *two*, with the voiceless stop /t/, sounds like *do*, and *pat* sounds like *bat*. In *word-final position*, the opposite occurs: *word-final voiced obstruents* (stops, fricatives, and affricates) are produced as their voiceless cognates. For example, the final /b/ of *bib* is heard as [p] and final /g/ of *dog* is heard as [k].

There are two types of rule-governed alternations associated with the sequence of phonemes in a word, one affecting contiguous segments and the other affecting noncontiguous segments. In the early stages of word learning, most children produce both labial stops (/p/ and /b/) and alveolar stops (/t/ and /d/) in accordance with place of articulation of the target consonant. For some children, however, there is a pattern of alternations conditioned by the vowel of a consonant–vowel sequence: for words in which a labial consonant is followed by a front vowel, the labial target is produced as an alveolar. For these children, the words *ball* and *bird* are produced with an initial labial [b], but the words *pee*, *beep-beep*, and *baby* are with an alveolar [d]. This pattern seems to disappear relatively early in the developing system. A similar alternation has been documented for target velars (/k/ and /g/); in the early stages of development, some children produce all target velars as alveolars, a phonological process referred to as *velar fronting*. As velar consonants begin to emerge, their appearance is conditioned by phonetic features of the neighboring vowel: In words with a consonant–vowel sequence of a velar followed by a central or back vowel, place of articulation of the velar is accurate. Thus, words such as *good*, *go*, *come*, and *call* are produced with a velar stop, whereas the words *key*, *cap*, and *give* are produced with an alveolar stop. This pattern of rule-governed *fronting* before front vowels is often maintained until a child is 3–4 years old.

Alternations affecting noncontiguous segments in a word are usually characterized as some type of assimilation, wherein two segments in a word become more similar (i.e., assimilate). Common examples of assimilation in child speech involve alternations in the place or manner of consonants. *Velar assimilation*, a pattern (or process) in which a nonvelar consonant is produced as a velar, is well-documented; examples from one child include the targets *walk*, *sock*, *talk*, and *duck* all produced as [gak]. In these cases, the place of articulation of the initial consonant takes on to the place of articulation of the final velar consonant. Assimilations of this sort can be categorized as either progressive or regressive. *Progressive assimilation* occurs when a consonant earlier in the target word affects a consonant later in the word, as in the word *coffee* /kafi/ produced as [kaki]. *Regressive assimilation* occurs when a consonant later in the target word affects a consonant earlier in the word, as in the targets *walk, sock, talk,* and *duck* produced as [gak]. Although most alternations involve place of articulation, rule-governed noncontiguous alternations can also affect manner of articulation. In children, one can witness productions with nasal assimilation, such as [mʌni] for *money* and [mænts] for *pants*, and lateral assimilation, as in [l ɛ l o] for *yellow.*

The third type of rule-governed alternations is related to variations in production linked to the position of a segment within the syllable and/or to the stress pattern of a word. Again, the clearest examples are with the production of velar consonants. Although some children produce all velars as alveolars (the process of *velar fronting*), for many children, the place of articulation varies according to the position of the target within the syllable. Syllable-final velars are produced correctly, but syllable-initial velars are produced as alveolars. Thus, word-final /k/ in the word *talk* is produced as a velar, but word-initial /k/ in *caught* is produced as [t]. For some children, syllable stress is also a factor. Syllable-initial velars in stressed position are fronted to alveolars, while those in unstressed position are produced as velars. Thus, the word *cookie*, with two syllable-initial /k/ targets, may be pronounced [tʊki], with target /k/ in the stressed syllable produced as [t] but as [k] in the unstressed syllable. This stress-related phenomenon is also evident in the pronunciations of *my key* and *Mikey*. In the two-word phrase, target /k/ of the stressed word *key* is produced as [ti], while target /k/ of the unstressed syllable of *Mikey* is produced accurately, as [k].

Carol Stoel-Gammon

See also Phonological Development; Phonological Processes

Further Readings

Bernhardt, B., & Stemberger, J. (1998). *Handbook of phonological development.* San Diego, CA: Academic Press.

Stoel-Gammon, C. (1996). On the acquisition of velars in English. In B. H. Bernhardt, J. Gilbert, & D. Ingram (Eds.), *Proceedings of the UBC International Conference on Phonological Acquisition* (pp. 201–214). Somerville, MA: Cascadilla Press.

CPSIA information can be obtained
at www.ICGtesting.com
Printed in the USA
LVHW100139130220
646810LV00002B/6